CLINICAL
MANUAL OF
EMERGENCY
PEDIATRICS

Notice

CLINICAL MANUAL OF EMERGENCY PEDIATRICS

FOURTH EDITION

Ellen F. Crain, M.D., Ph.D.
Professor of Pediatrics and Emergency Medicine
Albert Einstein College of Medicine
Director, Pediatric Emergency Services
Jacobi Medical Center
Bronx, New York

Jeffrey C. Gershel, M.D.
Associate Professor of Clinical Pediatrics
Albert Einstein College of Medicine
Chief of Pediatrics
Jacobi Medical Center
Bronx, New York

Assistant Editors:
Jeremy Halberstadt, M.D.
Rachel J. Katz-Sidlow, M.D.

McGRAW-HILL
Medical Publishing Division

New York   Chicago   San Francisco   Lisbon   London   Madrid   Mexico City
Milan   New Delhi   San Juan   Seoul   Singapore   Sydney   Toronto

CLINICAL MANUAL OF EMERGENCY PEDIATRICS, 4/e

4 5 6 7 8 9 0   DOC/DOC   0 9 8 7 6

ISBN 0-07-137750-6

This book was set in Times Roman by V&M Graphics, Inc.
The editors were Andrea Seils, Susan R. Noujaim, and Muza Navrozov;
the production supervisor was Richard Ruzycka;
the cover designer was Marsha Cohen.
Alexandra Nickerson created the index.
RR Donnelley was printer and binder.

This book is printed on acid-free paper.

Library of Congress Cataloging-in-Publication Data

Clinical manual of emergency pediatrics / [edited by] Ellen F. Crain, Jeffrey C.
  Gershel.—4th ed.
    p. ; cm.
    Includes bibliographical references and index.
    ISBN 0-07-137750-6
    1. Pediatric emergencies—Handbooks, manuals, etc.   I. Crain, Ellen F.
  II. Gershel, Jeffrey C.
    [DNLM: 1. Emergencies—Child—Handbooks.   2. Emergencies—Infant
  Handbooks   3. Emergency Medicine—methods—Child—Handbooks.
  4. Emergency Medicine—methods—Infant—Handbooks.   5. Pediatrics—
  methods—Handbooks.   WS 39 C641 2003]
  RJ370.C55 2003
  618.92′0025—dc21

                                                                    2002016693

INTERNATIONAL EDITION ISBN 0-07-121251-5
Copyright © 2003. Exclusive rights by the McGraw-Hill Companies, Inc., for man-
ufacture and export. This book cannot be re-exported from the country to which it
is consigned by McGraw-Hill. The International Edition is not available in North
America.

Contents

Contents

Contents

Assistant Editors

Jeremy Halberstadt, M.D.
Instructor in Pediatrics
Albert Einstein College of Medicine
Jacobi Medical Center
Bronx, New York

Rachel J. Katz-Sidlow, M.D.
Assistant Clinical Professor of Pediatrics
Albert Einstein College of Medicine
Jacobi Medical Center
Bronx, New York

Chapter Editors

David E. Bank, M.D.
Associate in Clinical Dermatology
College of Physicians and Surgeons
Columbia University
New York, New York

Alison Brent, M.D.
Assistant Clinical Professor of Pediatrics
University of South Florida College of Medicine
Tampa, Florida

Bonnie Bunch, M.D., Ph.D.
Assistant Professor of Child Neurology
University of South Dakota School of Medicine
Sioux Falls, South Dakota

Anthony J. Ciorciari, M.D.
Assistant Professor of Emergency Medicine
Albert Einstein College of Medicine
Jacobi Medical Center
Bronx, New York

Sandra J. Cunningham, M.D.
Associate Professor of Clinical Pediatrics and Clinical Emergency Medicine
Albert Einstein College of Medicine
Jacobi Medical Center
Bronx, New York

Chester M. Edelmann, Jr., M.D.
Professor of Pediatrics
Senior Associate Dean Emeritus
Albert Einstein College of Medicine
Bronx, New York

Joel Fein, M.D.
Associate Professor of Pediatrics and Emergency Medicine
The University of Pennsylvania School of Medicine
Children's Hospital of Philadelphia
Philadelphia, Pennsylvania

Michael H. Gewitz, M.D.
Professor of Pediatrics
New York Medical College
Westchester County Medical Center
Valhalla, New York

Waseem Hafeez, M.D.
Associate Professor of Clinical Pediatrics
Albert Einstein College of Medicine
Children's Hospital at Montefiore
Bronx, New York

Richard Hamilton, M.D.
Associate Professor of Emergency Medicine
Medical College of Pennsylvania
Hahnemann University
Philadelphia, Pennsylvania

Robert Hendrickson, M.D.
Instructor in Emergency Medicine
Medical College of Pennsylvania
Hahnemann University
Philadelphia, Pennsylvania

David M. Jaffe, M.D.
Professor of Pediatrics
Washington University School of Medicine
St. Louis Children's Hospital
St. Louis, Missouri

Jeffrey Keller, M.D.
Assistant Professor of Otolaryngology, Head & Neck Surgery
College of Physicians and Surgeons
Columbia University
New York, New York

Carolyn M. Kercsmar, M.D.
Professor of Pediatrics
Case Western Reserve University
Rainbow Babies & Children's Hospital
Cleveland, Ohio

Alfred Kohan, M.D.
Attending Urologist
Winthrop University Hospital
Mineola, New York

Steven Krauss, D.D.S.
Assistant Clinical Professor of Dentistry
Albert Einstein College of Medicine
Rose F. Kennedy Center
Bronx, New York

Caroline Lederman, M.D.
Clinical Instructor in Ophthalmology
College of Physicians and Surgeons
Columbia University
New York, New York

Martin Lederman, M.D.
Assistant Professor of Ophthalmology
New York Medical College
Valhalla, New York

Frederick Leickly, M.D.
Clinical Professor of Pediatrics
Indiana University School of Medicine
James Whitcomb Riley Hospital for Children
Indianapolis, Indiana

Jeremiah J. Levine, M.D.
Professor of Pediatrics
Albert Einstein College of Medicine
Long Island Jewish Medical Center
New Hyde Park, New York

Stephen Ludwig, M.D.
Professor of Pediatrics
University of Pennsylvania School of Medicine
Children's Hospital of Philadelphia
Philadelphia, Pennsylvania

Ronald L. Mann, M.D.
Clinical Instructor in Orthopedics
New York Medical College
Valhalla, New York

Robert W. Marion, M.D.
Professor of Pediatrics
Albert Einstein College of Medicine
Children's Hospital at Montefiore
Bronx, New York

B. J. Mistry, D.D.S., M.D.S.
Assistant Clinical Professor of Dentistry
Albert Einstein College of Medicine
Bronx, New York

Gregg Rusczyk, M.D.
Fellow in Pediatric Emergency Medicine
Washington University School of Medicine
St. Louis Children's Hospital
St. Louis, Missouri

Holly Schachner, M.D.
Assistant Professor of Clinical Pediatrics
College of Physicians and Surgeons
Columbia University
New York, New York

James Seidel, M.D., Ph.D.
Professor of Pediatrics
UCLA School of Medicine
Harbor-UCLA Medical Center
Torrance, California

Miriam Silfen, M.D.
Assistant Professor of Pediatrics
Albert Einstein College of Medicine
Jacobi Medical Center
Bronx, New York

Jodi J. Sutton, M.D.
Attending Physician
Northern Westchester Hospital Center
Mt. Kisco, New York

Michael Touger, M.D.
Associate Professor of
    Clinical Emergency Medicine
    and Clinical Family Medicine
Albert Einstein College of Medicine
Jacobi Medical Center
Bronx, New York

Mark Weinblatt, M.D.
Associate Professor of Clinical Pediatrics
New York University of Medicine
Winthrop Hospital
Mineola, New York

Toba A. Weinstein, M.D.
Assistant Professor of Pediatrics
Albert Einstein College of Medicine
Long Island Jewish Medical Center
New Hyde Park, New York

Alfred Winkler, M.D.
Assistant Professor of Urology
Albert Einstein College of Medicine
Jacobi Medical Center
Bronx, New York

Paul K. Woolf, M.D.
Assistant Professor of Pediatrics
New York Medical College
Westchester County Medical Center
Valhalla, New York

Chapter Contributors

Dan Barlev, M.D.
Assisstant Professor of Radiology and Pediatrics
Albert Einstein College of Medicine
Jacobi Medical Center
Bronx, New York

Katherine J. Chou, M.D.
Assistant Professor of Pediatrics and Emergency Medicine
Albert Einstein College of Medicine
Jacobi Medical Center
Bronx, New York

Alfred DeSimone, R.Ph.
Senior Associate Pharmacist IV
Jacobi Medical Center
Bronx, New York

Madeline Garcia-Bigelow, J.D.
Co-director, Sanctuary for Families
Bronx, New York

Jeremy Halberstadt, M.D.
Instructor in Pediatrics
Albert Einstein College of Medicine
Jacobi Medical Center
Bronx, New York

Fred Henretig, M.D.
Professor of Pediatrics and Emergency Medicine
University of Pennsylvania School of Medicine
Children's Hospital of Philadelphia
Philadelphia, Pennsylvania

Olga Jimenez, M.D.
Assistant Professor of Pediatrics
Albert Einstein College of Medicine
Jacobi Medical Center
Bronx, New York

Ashutosh Kacker, M.D.
Assistant Professor
Department of Otorhinolaryngology
New York Presbyterian Hospital
New York, New York

Steven R. Levine, M.D.
Clinical Instructor of Pediatrics
Albert Einstein College of Medicine
Jacobi Medical Center
Bronx, New York

Frank Maffei, M.D.
Assistant Professor of Pediatrics and Emergency Medicine
University of Rochester School of Medicine and Dentistry
Strong Children's Hospital
Rochester, New York

Diane Rhee, M.D.
Fellow in Pediatric Cardiology
College of Physicians and Surgeons
Columbia University
New York, New York

Kirsten Roberts, M.D.
Assistant Professor of Pediatrics
Albert Einstein College of Medicine
Jacobi Medical Center
Bronx, New York

Michael Rosenberg, M.D., Ph.D.
Assistant Professor of Pediatrics
Albert Einstein College of Medicine
Jacobi Medical Center
Bronx, New York

Deborah Saltzberg, M.D.
Assistant Clinical Professor of Pediatrics,
    Community Medicine, and Emergency Medicine
Mt. Sinai School of Medicine
New York, New York

Melissa Sheinker, M.D.
Pediatrician
Boca Raton Pediatrics
Boca Raton, Florida

Eric Small, M.D.
Assistant Clinical Professor of Pediatrics,
    Orthopedics, and Rehabilitation Medicine
Mount Sinai School of Medicine
New York, New York

Arthur Smerling, M.D.
Associate Professor of Clinical Pediatrics
    and Anesthesiology
College of Physicians and Surgeons
Columbia University
New York, New York

Linda Volpe, M.D.
Assistant Professor of Pediatrics
Albert Einstein College of Medicine
Jacobi Medical Center
Bronx, New York

Loren Yellin, M.D.
Assistant Professor of Pediatrics
Albert Einstein College of Medicine
Jacobi Medical Center
Bronx, New York

Preface

In the fourth edition of the *Clinical Manual of Emergency Pediatrics*, we have endeavored to remain true to our original intention: to provide a concise, portable handbook summarizing the majority of conditions that are seen in a pediatric emergency department. For each topic, we have included essential points and priorities for diagnosis, management, and follow-up care, as well as indications for hospitalization and a bibliography to guide further reading.

Hospital emergency department practitioners encounter patients with a variety of acute complaints, from the life-threatening to the mundane. Meanwhile, primary care providers are now expected to manage acute illnesses in ambulatory settings. Ill children are hospitalized less often, and are discharged back to their primary care providers sooner than ever before. Increasing numbers of chronically ill and medically fragile children are receiving care in ambulatory sites. As a result of these shifting practices, providers working in settings such as private offices and clinics may be faced with potential, or real, pediatric emergencies. These caregivers, as well as emergency physicians, may benefit from a practical handbook.

In the fourth edition, we have maintained the book's unique features while making many changes that should increase the manual's utility. Because the scope of childhood illnesses and injuries seen in acute care settings is constantly increasing, we have revised and updated every chapter. We have added new sections on back pain, emergency radiology, failure to thrive, implantable devices, ingestions (ADHD medications, antidepressants, antipsychotics, cold medications, inhalants, rat poison), interpersonal violence, rehabilitation of orthopedic injuries, the abnormal CBC, the critically ill infant, and the cross-cultural encounter. In response to the changing times, we have also added a section on biological and chemical terrorism.

A word of caution is in order. Although a manual for emergency care can be very useful, it may tempt physicians, particularly those still in training, to look for automatic solutions. It is not our intent that this text be used as a protocol book. Students and housestaff in training should not use this manual to substitute for their own critical thinking and sensitivity when caring for children and their families.

Our thanks go to the contributors to the third edition: J. R. Avner, D. E. Bank, R. M. Barkin, P. Belamarich, L. Bernstein, A. Brent, B. L. Bunch, A. A. Caldamone, K. J. Chou, A. Ciorciari, A. Cooper, S. J. Cunningham, J. DeBellis, M. H. Gewitz, D. M. Jaffe, J. Joseph,

D. Hodge III, C. M. Kercsmar, M. E. Lederman, S. R. Levine, L. Levy, W. J. Lewander, K. Lillis, S. Ludwig, F. Maffei, R. L. Mann, R. W. Marion, S. Z. Miller, B. J. Mistry, J. Rosenfeld, D. Saltzberg, D. Saunders, S. Schwartz, J. Seidel, J. Shliozberg, A. Smerling. S. Smith, R. E. K. Stein, J. J. Sutton, M. Tenenbein, H. Trachtman, A. Walker, M. Weinblatt, P. K. Woolf, and R. H. K. Wu. Without their efforts in the third edition, there would be no fourth edition. In addition, we owe special thanks to Jeremy Halberstadt and Rachel J. Katz-Sidlow whose tireless efforts ensured the successful completion of this edition. Although the quality of this fourth edition reflects the hard work of all the contributors and section editors, the final manuscript reflects our approach to any given illness or problem. We are responsible for the book's content.

We are grateful to our families and colleagues who tolerated our preoccupation with this book. By what they have taught us and by their example we are especially grateful to the pediatric emergency department nurses, attendings, nurse practitioners, physicians' assistants and nurses at the Jacobi Medical Center. We have become better teachers and caregivers by observing them and their interactions with patients and families. We are indebted to the pediatric and emergency medicine housestaffs and the pediatric emergency medicine fellows at the Jacobi Medical Center, and the medical students of the Albert Einstein College of Medicine whom we have had the privilege of teaching and learning from over the years. Their thoughtful questions provided the impetus for this manual.

This book is dedicated to the memory of Dr. Lewis M. Fraad, our beloved mentor, whose name has been memorialized in the name of our department, the Lewis M. Fraad Department of Pediatrics at Jacobi Medical Center. Day in and day out he set an example for all of us by combining intellectual rigor with a deep respect for children and their families. He will always be with us when we are at our best.

Ellen F. Crain
Jeffrey C. Gershel
August 2002

CHAPTER 1

Resuscitation

James Seidel—Editor
- **Arthur Smerling and Deborah Saltzberg—Contributors**

AIRWAY MANAGEMENT

Airway support is critical in treating respiratory compromise and vital in the management of other pediatric emergencies. Immediate goals in the emergency department (ED) include reversing hypoxemia, supporting ventilation, maintaining airway patency, and protecting the airway from secretions and vomitus.

Equipment for Airway Support

Nasal Cannula The actual O_2 concentration delivered is unpredictable, so this method is appropriate only for patients who require minimal O_2 supplementation. An O_2 flow rate <3 L/min is usually well tolerated by older children. Small children will accept the nasal cannula if the prongs are trimmed so that the plastic does not tickle the patient's nares.

Oxygen Hood A high flow rate (>7 L/min) will keep the delivered O_2 concentration close to the administered concentration and ensure that the exhaled gas is flushed out of the system. This method is well tolerated by infants and permits excellent access to the chest, abdomen, and extremities.

Simple O_2 Mask The actual O_2 concentration that the patient receives is dependent on the O_2 flow rate and the patient's ventilatory pattern, as room air enters through the ventilation holes in the sides of the mask. Oxygen flow rates > 6 L/min will deliver 30–60% O_2 and prevent the rebreathing of exhaled gas.

O_2 Mask with Reservoir This system consists of a simple mask attached to a reservoir bag that is connected to an O_2 source. Some models contain one-way valves at the ventilatory holes to prevent the entrainment of room air and/or valves at the reservoir bag to prevent the entry of exhaled gas into the reservoir bag. Ensure that the oxygen flow rate is greater than the patient's minute volume (7 mL $\times$ weight in kg $\times$ breaths per minute in a younger child; 6–10 L/min in an older child). The reservoir bag must

1

be larger than the patient's tidal volume (5–7 mL/kg); it should remain inflated during inspiration. Oxygen concentrations up to 60% in valveless systems and greater than 90% in systems with valves can be achieved if the oxygen flow rate is adequate and there is a good seal around the face mask. These masks are available in various sizes in order to fit snugly over the patient's face.

Nasopharyngeal Airway   This device is particularly helpful in patients with upper airway obstruction from tongue or palatal problems; obtunded patients tolerate it well. Insert the airway gently along the floor of the nostril to avoid lacerating the nasal mucosa or adenoids. A nasopharyngeal airway is contraindicated in a trauma patient pending evaluation for head injury. Also, do not use it in a patient with a coagulopathy or a possible basilar skull fracture. The appropriately sized airway extends to the base of the tongue without compressing the epiglottis. This is the distance from the tip of the nose to the tragus of the ear.

Oropharyngeal Airway   The oropharyngeal airway is often helpful when ventilating a comatose patient. It is used to keep the base of the tongue off the posterior pharyngeal wall and maintain a patent airway. The first part of the airway is very firm and is designed to be placed between the teeth to prevent biting (the endotracheal tube or your finger). However, it can precipitate vomiting and laryngospasm in the awake or obtunded patient. It may be helpful to depress and extend the tongue when inserting the airway. When placed next to the patient's face, an appropriately sized airway extends from the central incisors to the angle of the jaw. Oropharyngeal airways that are too small have been aspirated, and airways that are too large can push the tongue back and obstruct the air passage. The best airways have a central air channel and closed sides (Guedel-type); open-sided airways may lacerate the tonsillar tissue.

Suction Catheters   These must be available in sizes small enough to pass through the smallest available endotracheal tube (ETT). A 5 Fr catheter will pass through a 2.5-mm ETT. Large rigid plastic suction catheters (Yankauer-type) are very useful for clearing blood and secretions from the mouth.

Bag and Mask   The most common system used to ventilate a nonbreathing patient consists of an O_2 reservoir (corrugated tubing), self-inflating bag (Ambu Bag), valve, and mask. These bags do not need a constant flow of O_2 to refill; they entrain room air. Transparent masks are available in multiple sizes (premature; infant; toddler; child; small, medium, and large adult) to ensure a snug fit over the bridge of the nose and mouth; the eyes must not be covered. If the bag has a pop-off valve set at 35 cm H_2O, there must be a way to override it. One can quickly check to make sure that the O_2 is connected by listening to the flow in the reservoir.

Laryngoscope and ETTs   These must be available in various sizes along with spare handles, bulbs, and batteries. The most popular blades are

Table 1-1 **Appropriate Laryngoscope Blades, Endotracheal Tubes**
(ETTs), and Suction Catheters

LARYNGOSCOPE BLADES

Premature–newborn	Miller 0
1 month–toddler	Miller 1
18 months–8 years	Miller 2, Macintosh 2
>8 years	Macintosh 3

ETTs AND SUCTION CATHETERS

AGE	*ETT*	*SUCTION CATHETER*
Premature	2.5-mm ID*	5 Fr
Newborn	3.0- to 3.5-mm ID	8 Fr
One month	3.5-mm ID	10 Fr
One year	4.0-mm ID	10 Fr
Older	4 + [(age in years)/4]	

*Internal diameter.

listed in Table 1-1. Often straight blades (Miller) are easier to use than
curved blades (Macintosh) in young children.

Always have available ETTs 0.5 mm larger and smaller than the calculated size. Cuffed ETTs are used in children over 8 years of age [>5.5 mm
inner diameter (ID)].

Laryngeal Mask Airway (LMA).   This device consists of a Silastic tube
that is diagonally attached to an inflatable cuff (Figs. 1-1 and 1-2). When

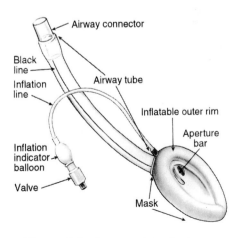

Figure 1-1   Laryngeal mask airway.

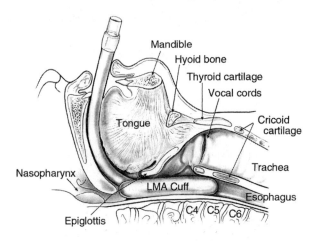

Figure 1-2   Laryngeal mask airway in place.

the cuff is inserted into the mouth, it sits above the vocal cords. It is used in patients with decreased airway reflexes (i.e., locally anesthetized, obtunded, or comatose). When properly placed, the LMA directs air into the trachea and avoids gastric distention. Unlike an ETT, it will not stop gastric contents from being aspirated into the trachea. It is particularly helpful in patients who are difficult to ventilate with a bag and mask because of a large tongue, small mouth, or retrognathic jaw. It can also be used as an aid to fiberoptic bronchoscopy and "blind" intubation, because anything inserted through a properly placed LMA will be directed into the trachea. Details describing the proper insertion technique for the device come with the package. It is reusable and must be sterilized between uses. It is available in sizes that will fit newborns to adults (Table 1-2).

Ventilation and Intubation

Ventilation   Ventilate the apneic patient with a bag-mask apparatus until it is certain that the appropriate equipment and personnel for intubation are assembled. Place an older child in the "sniffing" position with the head elevated on a small pad or folded towel. For an infant, keep the head

Table 1-2   Sizes of Laryngeal Mask Airways

Size 1	< 5 kg
Size 1.5	5–10 kg
Size 2	10–20 kg
Size 2.5	20–30 kg
Size 3	30–50 kg
Size 4	50–70 kg
Size 5	> 70 kg

midline and slightly extended (no pillow). Flexing or overextending the neck may interfere with adequate ventilation. Place the fifth finger of your left hand behind the angle of the patient's jaw and lift the jaw so that the lower teeth are in front of the upper teeth. The left thumb and index finger can hold the mask snugly to the face, with the bottom of the mask between the chin and the lip. Using the E-C clamp technique, apply upward pressure on the angle of the jaw and downward pressure on the bottom of the mask to keep the mouth open, but avoid compressing the neck with the middle, ring and small fingers.

Adequate ventilation causes symmetric movement of the chest wall and good breath sounds by auscultation. If the patient is making any respiratory effort at all, it is best to time the breaths with his or her efforts. If positive pressure ventilation is distending the stomach, gentle pressure on the cricoid cartilage (Sellick maneuver) will occlude the esophagus and prevent air from entering the stomach. Aggressive cricoid pressure may kink the trachea and prevent air from entering the lungs.

Intubation   To intubate the patient, place the thumb and index finger of your gloved right hand into the rightmost part of the patient's mouth. Place the index finger on the patient's upper teeth and the thumb on the patient's lower teeth. Open the mouth as wide as possible. Imagine that the patient's face is a clock with the chin at 12 o'clock and the nose at 6 o'clock. Place the blade of the laryngoscope into the mouth as far to the right as you can, with the handle pointing to 3 o'clock. Once the blade is advanced as far as necessary, rotate the handle to 12 o'clock. This rotation will sweep the tongue out of your line of vision. Pull the handle of the laryngoscope up and away from you at a 45° angle to the floor. Be careful not to touch the upper teeth with the handle or the blade. If the blade is in too deep, slowly withdraw it until the glottis pops into view. Place a curved blade in the patient's vallecula and use it to pull the epiglottis upward. Straight blades may be placed below the epiglottis and used to elevate it.

Once the epiglottis is exposed, take care to introduce the ETT from the rightmost side of the mouth so that you do not obscure the view of the cords. Advance the ETT until the cuff just passes beyond the cords (Table 1-3). Uncuffed tubes often have a mark at the distal end of the tube, which—when placed at the level of the cords—will position the distal tip of the ETT in the midtrachea. This mark is useful only if the ETT is the appropriate size and the patient has a normal-size trachea. Hold the tube securely against the upper teeth (or gums). Carefully withdraw the laryngoscope.

The cricoid ring is the narrowest part of a child's airway. An ETT may easily pass the cords, but if it meets resistance in the subglottic area, replace it with a smaller tube.

Table 1-3   Appropriate ETT Depth (at gum line)

1-kg infant	7 cm
2-kg infant	8 cm
3-kg infant	9 cm
> 1 year	[(age in years)/2] + 12

Confirming Position   After successful intubation, confirm that both sides of the chest rise symmetrically and that breath sounds can be heard equally in both axillae. Confirm the presence of exhaled CO_2 from the ETT with either a colorimetric CO_2 detector or a CO_2 analyzer. If breath sounds are louder in the stomach than in the chest, remove the ETT and ventilate by mask. If you are unsure whether the ETT is in the trachea, check the position with a laryngoscope. Extending or rotating the head brings the ETT higher. Flexing the neck pushes the ETT deeper. On chest radiograph, confirm that the tip of the ETT is opposite T2 (one finger-breadth above the carina).

Medications for Sedating and Paralyzing

Individual patients may be difficult to ventilate by mask and/or to intubate under direct visualization. Do not use sedation or muscle relaxation if there is any concern that bag-mask ventilation will be inadequate—for example, when the airway is partially obstructed by facial trauma or epiglottitis. Anticipate a difficult intubation and request help if the patient has restricted neck extension or an obvious neck mass or if the tip of the uvula is not visible when the mouth is opened. Summon an experienced laryngoscopist to perform an awake laryngoscopy in a patient with a difficult airway or to paralyze a patient before intubation.

**NEVER SEDATE OR PARALYZE A PATIENT WHOM
YOU MAY NOT BE ABLE TO VENTILATE!**

When rapid control of the airway is required and regurgitation is a concern, perform a rapid sequence intubation. Begin by having the patient breathe 100% oxygen for at least 3 min; use a bag-mask if the patient is apneic. This will replace the nitrogen in the patient's functional residual capacity with oxygen. Small children and anxious adolescents can have increased vagal tone. Give atropine (0.02 mg/kg IV) prophylactically to prevent the profound bradycardia that occasionally occurs during laryngoscopy. Once the equipment is assembled (Table 1-4), give the patient a short-acting sedative (e.g., thiopental, etomidate, ketamine, or propofol), followed immediately by a short-acting muscle relaxant (e.g., succinylcholine or rocuronium). After the patient loses consciousness, have an assistant apply pressure to the cricoid cartilage, thereby occluding the esophagus against the vertebral bodies and preventing passive regurgitation. Do not ventilate by mask or release the cricoid pressure until placement of the ETT has been confirmed. Intubate the trachea once the patient is paralyzed (<60 s). If the intubation cannot be performed in < 20 s, ventilate the patient with bag and mask while another person maintains cricoid pressure and call for help. Change the laryngoscope blade, ETT size, patient's position, or laryngoscopist before attempting another intubation. Repeated intubation attempts will cause edema and bleeding and make mask ventilation more difficult. If you cannot intubate or ventilate by mask, insert a LMA or call for a surgeon to perform a cricothyrotomy.

Table 1-4   Equipment for Intubation

Suction (large-bore)
O_2 source
Bag and mask
Oral airway
Laryngoscope with assorted blades
ETT (one-half size larger and one-half
    size smaller than expected)
Stylette
Laryngeal mask airway
Medications
An assistant

Drugs for Intubation

Atropine (0.01–0.02 mg/kg IV)   Atropine, an anticholinergic, will dry secretions and prevent vagally induced bradycardia.

Lidocaine (1 mg/kg IV)   Lidocaine prevents a rise in ICP associated with laryngoscopy.

Thiopental (4–6 mg/kg IV)   This barbiturate induces rapid loss of consciousness and also apnea. It causes dose-dependent vasodilatation and hypotension, which can be profound in a patient with dehydration or traumatic blood loss or one who is taking antihypertensive drugs. Since thiopental is rapidly redistributed from the brain, the effects are short-lived in this dose range.

Succinylcholine (2 mg/kg IV)   This short-acting muscle relaxant blocks the neuromuscular junction. Muscle fasciculations may occur soon after IV administration, followed by relaxation lasting less than 10 min. Premedicate 1–3 minutes before giving the succinylcholine with vecuronium (0.01 mg/kg IV) or rocuronium (0.06 mg/kg IV) to prevent fasciculations. Patients may develop tachyarrhythmias (usually well tolerated) or serious bradyarrhythmias that are responsive to atropine. Succinylcholine may cause an acute rise in intracranial and intraocular pressure. Patients with abnormal muscle membrane receptors may develop hyperkalemia (Table 1-5).

Table 1-5   Succinylcholine-Related Hyperkalemia

Burns >24 h old
Massive trauma >24 h old
Progressive upper motor neuron disease
Stable (nonprogressive) upper motor
    neuron disease <12 months of age
Diffuse muscle wasting
Serious abdominal infection

Midazolam (0.1 mg/kg IV)   This short-acting benzodiazepine produces sedation and amnesia.

Vecuronium (0.1 mg/kg IV)   Vecuronium is a muscle relaxant with minimal hemodynamic effects, even with large doses. A dose of 0.1 mg/kg IV wears off in under a half hour.

Rocuronium (0.6 to 1 mg/kg IV)   Rocuronium is a muscle relaxant with minimal hemodynamic side effects and a shorter duration of action than vecuronium.

Ketamine (1 to 2 mg/kg IV)   Ketamine provides analgesia and amnesia. Pretreat the patient with atropine to decrease secretions. Ketamine is useful for asthmatic patients requiring intubation since it provides bronchodilation in addition to sedation. It can cause tachycardia and vasoconstriction, but these side effects are usually well tolerated.

Etomidate (0.3 mg/kg IV)   Etomidate is a short-acting (3–5 min) anesthetic that has minimal hemodynamic effects. It may cause a short, self-limited episode of myoclonus and will depress cortisol levels.

Transporting an Intubated Patient

The principles of transport are the same regardless of the distance: The patient must be as stable as possible, and there must be adequate equipment (Table 1-6), personnel, and monitoring available for resuscitation during transport.

The most common oxygen tanks taken on transport are sizes D (396 L) and E (659 L). The oxygen flow rate determines the length of time a tank will last. For example, at 10 L/min, a D tank will last only 40 min and an E tank 1 hour. Take spare tanks for long transports.

Portable suction devices are notoriously unreliable. A useful device can be constructed from a 60-mL catheter-tip syringe connected to a length of suction tubing attached to a suction catheter. A colleague drawing back on the syringe can generate adequate suction to clear small amounts of material.

Table 1-6   Equipment for Transport

Oxygen tank
Bag and mask
Suction apparatus and catheters
ETT (appropriate size and one-half size smaller)
Stylette, oral airway, tape, and laryngoscope
Portable monitor with ECG, oximetry, end-tidal
   CO_2, and noninvasive blood pressure
Oximeter
Drugs for resuscitation, sedation, and paralysis
   (as appropriate)

Electronic monitors are now available with portable power supplies. However, a stethoscope, finger on the pulse, and observation of the patient's color remain important, reliable, and low-maintenance monitors. Vigilance is required to diagnose potentially catastrophic ventilation problems en route. The ETT can easily slip into the patient's esophagus without any movement of the tube at the mouth, causing decreased chest excursion and decreased breath sounds bilaterally. Frequent auscultation and laryngoscopy, if necessary, will identify problems. Plugging of the ETT causes high inspiratory pressure in addition to decreased chest excursion and faint breath sounds bilaterally. This can usually be corrected with suctioning, but occasionally requires reintubation. Endobronchial intubation (right more common than left) causes high inspiratory pressure and unilateral decreased breath sounds, although a pneumothorax is another cause of unilateral decreased breath sounds.

BIBLIOGRAPHY

Levy RJ, Helfaer MA: Pediatric airway issues. *Crit Care Clin* 2000;16:489–504.
McAllister JD, Gnauck KA: Rapid sequence intubation of the pediatric patient. *Pediatr Clin North Am* 1999;46:1249–1284.
Motoyama EK: Endotracheal intubation, in Motoyama EK, Davis PJ (eds): *Smith's Anesthesia for Infants and Children,* 5th ed. St. Louis: Mosby, 1990, pp 217–256.
Sullivan KJ, Kissoon N: Securing the child's airway in the emergency department. *Pediatr Emerg Care* 2002;18:108–121.

CARDIOPULMONARY RESUSCITATION

Cardiopulmonary arrest in infants and children is rarely a sudden event. Rather, it occurs after deterioration from a preexisting condition, which has resulted in respiratory or circulatory failure. Many underlying disorders may lead to cardiopulmonary arrest, including trauma, sepsis, respiratory illness, foreign-body aspiration, poisoning, or metabolic disease. Primary cardiac arrest is relatively rare in the pediatric age group and is usually secondary to congenital heart disease, direct trauma to the thorax, or electrocution. However, ventricular tachycardia and ventricular fibrillation may be more common in pediatric patients than had previously been suspected.

The outcome of unwitnessed cardiopulmonary arrest in infants and children is poor. Only 8.4% of pediatric patients who have out-of-hospital cardiac arrest survive to discharge, and most are neurologically impaired. If there is only a respiratory arrest without loss of pulse, 88% of patients will have a good outcome. The best reported outcomes have been in children who receive bystander cardiopulmonary resuscitation (CPR) and have a rapid Emergency Medical Service (EMS) response and in those who present with a ventricular rhythm disturbance that responds to early defibrillation.

ED Priorities

To optimize outcome, impending respiratory distress, respiratory failure, and circulatory failure must be recognized early in the evolution of the disease process, prior to the development of full cardiopulmonary arrest.

All equipment, supplies, and drugs must be available and organized for easy access, and it is imperative for the staff to be trained in pediatric resuscitation and to practice these techniques routinely.

Organize the physician and nursing staff into a resuscitation team, with each member knowing his or her role. Identify a team leader whose only responsibility is to oversee the resuscitation and give orders. With adequate personnel, a complete team consists of members with the following roles: leader, vascular access, airway, chest compressions, history, medications, recording nurse, and runner. Ideally, a respiratory therapist will assist the team. A clock must be nearby to facilitate record keeping.

Airway

Airway management is always the first priority. Place the head in a neutral position to open the airway, using the head tilt–chin lift and jaw-thrust maneuvers. If there has been trauma or the etiology of the arrest is unclear, use only the jaw thrust and protect the cervical spine until it has been cleared by clinical and radiographic examination. Suction any secretions from the mouth and hypopharynx.

Breathing, Oxygenation, and Ventilation

Provide ventilation using a bag-mask device with an appropriate-size mask. The minimum volume for the bag is 450 mL, and it must be equipped with a reservoir to ensure that 100% oxygen is delivered. The rate of assisted ventilation can be facilitated if the rescuer squeezes the bag, watches for the chest rise, and says, "squeeze, release." Use a rate of 20 breaths per minute for a child and at least 20 breaths per minute for an infant (Table 1-7); give enough time for inspiration of the oxygen (1–1.5 s). Bagging too rapidly or at too high a pressure causes inflation of the stomach and barotrauma. Observe the chest rise and listen for breath sounds. If ventilation is difficult or breath sounds are unequal, reposition and suction the airway and consider foreign-body aspiration. An oral or nasopharyngeal airway may be of help in maintaining a patent airway during bag-mask resuscitation. If the patient is ventilated with a bag-mask device for more than a few minutes, place a nasogastric tube to remove air from the stomach.

Endotracheal intubation (see "Airway Management," pp 5–6) is the best way to manage the airway during cardiopulmonary arrest. The indications for endotracheal intubation include the following:

- Need for assisted ventilation to maintain effective alveolar gas exchange
- Inadequate central nervous system control of ventilation, resulting in apnea or inadequate respiratory effort
- Excessive work of breathing, leading to fatigue
- Lack of airway protective reflexes (gag)
- Airway obstruction
- Need to control the airway during procedures or diagnostic studies

Table 1-7   Summary of BLS Maneuvers in Infants and Children

MANEUVER	INFANT (<1 YEAR)	CHILD (1 TO 8 YEARS)
Airway	Head tilt–chin lift (use jaw thrust for trauma victim)	Head tilt–chin lift (use jaw thrust for trauma victim)
Breathing		
Initial	Two breaths at 1–1½ s/breath	Two breaths at 1–1½ s/breath
Subsequent	20 breaths/min	20 breaths/min (approximate)
Circulation		
Pulse check	Brachial/femoral	Carotid
Compression area	Lower half of sternum	Lower half of sternum
Compression width	Two thumbs	Heel of one hand
Depth	Approximately ⅓–½ depth of the chest	Approximately ⅓–½ depth of the chest
Rate	At least 100/min	100/min
Compression/ ventilation ratio	5:1 (pause for ventilation)	5:1 (pause for ventilation)
Foreign-body obstruction	Back blows/chest thrusts	Heimlich maneuver

Adapted from Hazinski MF (ed): *PALS Provider Manual.* Dallas: American Heart Association, 2002, pp 43–80, with permission.

Estimate the ETT size by matching the diameter of the ETT to the width of the nail of the patient's fifth finger or the diameter of the nares. Alternatively, use a formula: [4+ (age in years/4)]. A tape which correlates weight with length and gives fairly precise sizes of supplies, including ETT sizes, as well as appropriate drug doses is commercially available (Broselow tape, Vital Signs Corporation, Totowa, NJ; Fig. 1-3). Always have immediately available one tube a size larger and another a size smaller than the one estimated. A straight Miller laryngoscope blade is generally used for pediatric intubation. Cricoid pressure (the Sellick maneuver) during intubation may help visualize the airway and prevent regurgitation of stomach contents. Always have a tonsil-tipped suction device (Yankauer) and an appropriate-sized suction catheter readily available during intubation. If trauma to the cervical spine is a concern, have an assistant maintain in-line stabilization during the intubation; avoid traction or movement of the neck. Verify tube placement by clinical examination: listen for equal breath sounds in the axillae and observe a good chest rise with ventilation. A chest radiograph or direct visualization through a laryngoscope will confirm proper ETT placement. Use end-tidal CO_2 monitoring with capnography or a disposable colorimetric device for

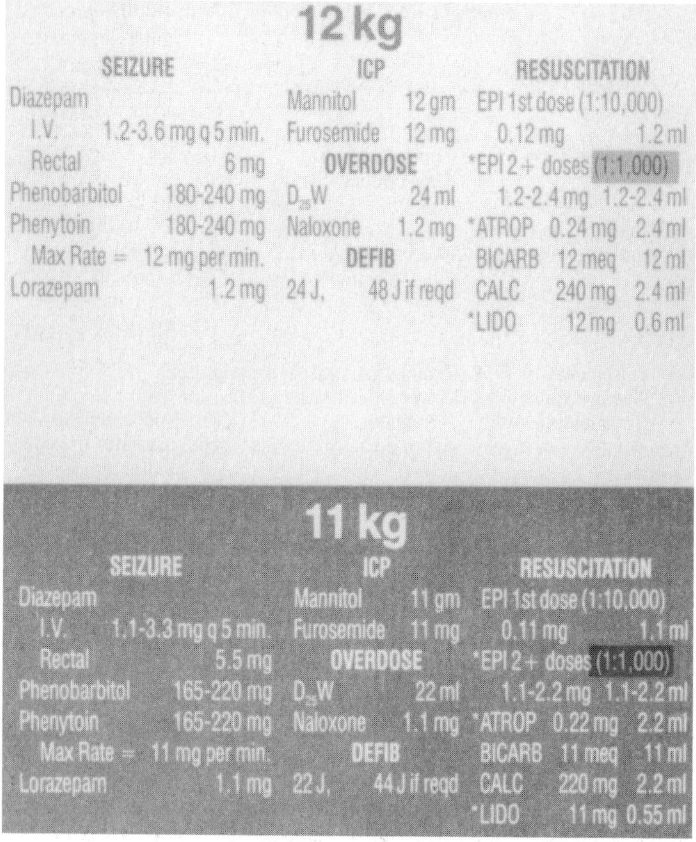

12 kg

SEIZURE		ICP		RESUSCITATION		
Diazepam		Mannitol	12 gm	EPI 1st dose (1:10,000)		
I.V.	1.2-3.6 mg q 5 min.	Furosemide	12 mg	0.12 mg		1.2 ml
Rectal	6 mg	**OVERDOSE**		*EPI 2+ doses (1:1,000)		
Phenobarbitol	180-240 mg	D₂₅W	24 ml	1.2-2.4 mg	1.2-2.4 ml	
Phenytoin	180-240 mg	Naloxone	1.2 mg	*ATROP	0.24 mg	2.4 ml
Max Rate =	12 mg per min.	**DEFIB**		BICARB	12 meq	12 ml
Lorazepam	1.2 mg	24 J,	48 J if reqd	CALC	240 mg	2.4 ml
				*LIDO	12 mg	0.6 ml

11 kg

SEIZURE		ICP		RESUSCITATION		
Diazepam		Mannitol	11 gm	EPI 1st dose (1:10,000)		
I.V.	1.1-3.3 mg q 5 min.	Furosemide	11 mg	0.11 mg		1.1 ml
Rectal	5.5 mg	**OVERDOSE**		*EPI 2+ doses (1:1,000)		
Phenobarbitol	165-220 mg	D₂₅W	22 ml	1.1-2.2 mg	1.1-2.2 ml	
Phenytoin	165-220 mg	Naloxone	1.1 mg	*ATROP	0.22 mg	2.2 ml
Max Rate =	11 mg per min.	**DEFIB**		BICARB	11 meq	11 ml
Lorazepam	1.1 mg	22 J,	44 J if reqd	CALC	220 mg	2.2 ml
				*LIDO	11 mg	0.55 ml

Figure 1-3   Broselow tape.

confirmation of ETT placement. A positive test during CPR confirms proper tube placement; however, a negative test may indicate a misplaced tube or poor perfusion.

Remember the mnemonic DOPE if the patient deteriorates after endotracheal intubation. This development may be due to Displacement of the tube, Obstruction of the tube, Pneumothorax, or Equipment failure.

Circulation

A combination of the "heart pump" and the "thoracic pump" theories probably accounts for blood circulation during chest compressions. There is some evidence that chest compressions in pediatric patients facilitate circulation by direct compression of the heart (heart pump), while changes in intrathoracic pressure generated by compressions cause the flow of blood through the heart to the systemic circulation (thoracic pump).

Infant   The two-thumb hand-encircling technique is now the preferred method for chest compressions in an infant. Place two thumbs in the midline just below the nipple line and encircle the chest with the hands. Be sure not to compress the lateral walls of the chest with the hands. Deliver chest compressions on the sternum with the two thumbs. If the infant is too large for this technique, use the two-finger method. Place two or three fingers one fingerbreadth below the intermammary line. Compress the sternum to a relative depth of approximately one-third to one-half the anterior/posterior diameter of the chest at a rate of at least 100/min. Adequate compressions usually generate a pulse.

Child   Place the heel of the hand one fingerbreadth above the intersection of the ribs and sternum. Compress the sternum to a relative depth of approximately one-third to one-half the anterior/posterior diameter of the chest at a rate of 100/min.

For all patients, ensure that each compression and relaxation phase is of equal length and that the fingers or hands are not removed from the chest during the relaxation phase of chest compressions. Coordinate compressions and ventilation in a 5:1 ratio. Simultaneous compression and ventilation may transiently increase blood flow, but this effect may not be important in pediatrics.

Obstructed Airway

If airway obstruction from a foreign body is suspected and the patient is awake and can speak, make no attempts to remove the object. Call an otolaryngologist or surgeon. If the patient deteriorates, use the following procedures:

Infants Younger Than 1 Year   With the rescuer sitting, place the infant prone, straddling the rescuer's legs, with the head supported in a dependent position. Give five sharp back blows between the baby's scapulae. If this fails to dislodge the object, turn the infant over and give five chest thrusts using two fingers on the midsternum. Repeat these maneuvers until the object is expelled or the infant becomes unconscious.

Unconscious Infant   First open the airway, using a tongue–jaw lift maneuver, and look for a foreign body. If an object is seen, remove it. If there is no improvement, attempt rescue breathing. If the rescuer is unable to deliver breaths, reposition the head and try again. Proceed with advanced airway maneuvers until respirations have been restored.

Children Older Than 1 Year   Use the Heimlich maneuver. Place the child face up and kneel at his or her feet. Position the heel of the hand in the midline of the epigastrium and, with the second hand on top of the first, give a series of upward thrusts. Each thrust should be a separate and distinct movement. If the patient loses consciousness, position the head and attempt rescue breathing as above.

Foreign bodies may also be removed under direct visualization with a laryngoscope and Magill forceps. On rare occasions, if there is total obstruction of the proximal upper airway, cricothyrotomy may be needed. Tracheal or laryngeal foreign bodies that are located more distally may require removal through a flexible bronchoscope. Blind sweeps of the oropharynx are never indicated. After attempting to clear the airway, resume bag-mask ventilation and reassess. Repeat the maneuvers if the airway still seems obstructed after two or three attempts at bag-mask ventilation.

Vascular Access

Spend no more than 1 to 2 min attempting to obtain peripheral vascular access. If skilled personnel are present, attempt central venous access through the femoral route. However, the intraosseous (IO) approach allows for rapid access to the circulation and should be attempted immediately while other vascular sites are secured. Intraosseous needle placement is no longer restricted to children under 6 years of age.

The site for IO infusion is the proximal medial tibia about two fingerbreadths below the tibial tuberosity. Direct a 14- or 16-gauge IO needle away from the growth plate almost perpendicular to the bone (Fig. 1-4). Use steady pressure and a screwing motion until a "give" is felt. Once the needle has gone into the marrow cavity, it will be stable and will not need taping. It is not necessary to draw back on the syringe and aspirate marrow, but one should be able to push fluid easily without extravasation. If the fluid extravasates (the calf expands or feels cold), remove the needle and make an attempt on the other side. Never attempt intraosseous access through an infected wound or fracture site. Any drugs or fluid, including blood products, can be given via the intraosseous route, although high flow rates are not possible without applying pressure to the IV bag or pushing the fluid directly through a large syringe. Dilute hyperosmolar solutions—such as 50% dextrose and 7.5% sodium bicarbonate—before infusion into the marrow cavity.

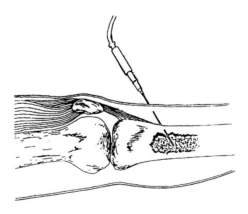

Figure 1-4   Placement of an intraosseous needle.

Fluid Administration

Shock and circulatory collapse may be the primary causes of cardiopulmonary arrest. Give an initial volume expansion of 20 mL/kg of isotonic crystalloid to patients in shock. The type of fluid used, lactated Ringer's or normal saline, depends on institutional preference.

Drugs

Tracheal Drug Administration   The ETT provides a rapid route for the delivery of drug therapy via absorption from the tracheobronchial tree. Medications that may be given via the ETT include lidocaine (2%), atropine, naloxone, and epinephrine. Dilute all drugs with 5 mL of normal saline prior to direct instillation into the ETT. Alternatively, instill the medications through a catheter that extends beyond the tip of the ETT and follow with a 5-mL normal saline flush. Follow ETT administration with five manual ventilations. Although the time to peak concentration of some drugs is similar to that for IV administration, higher doses may be required to achieve an appropriate therapeutic level. For epinephrine, the exact ET dose is not known, but higher than standard doses are recommended (0.1 mL/kg of 1:1000 solution).

Epinephrine   Epinephrine is the most important drug used in resuscitation. The alpha effects are important for increasing blood flow, particularly to the myocardium and central nervous system. Epinephrine increases the heart rate, myocardial contractility, systemic vascular resistance, and cardiac automaticity. The suggested standard dose is 0.01 mg/kg (0.1 mL/kg) of the 1:10,000 concentration IV or IO. In cardiopulmonary arrest, high-dose epinephrine (0.1–0.2 mg/kg of the 1:1,000 concentration) has been suggested when the standard dose fails to produce a perfusing rhythm. This is still controversial, and although there may be return to spontaneous circulation, few data suggest that this therapy improves final outcome.

Atropine   Atropine is a parasympatholytic drug that accelerates the atrial pacemakers and atrioventricular conduction. It is indicated for symptomatic bradycardia with evidence of poor perfusion or hypotension. Hypoxia may be the underlying cause of bradycardia, particularly in small infants. Thus, oxygenation and efforts to improve perfusion must precede the administration of atropine. The dose is 0.02 mg/kg (1.0 mg per dose maximum) every 5 min, up to 2 mg maximum total dose; use at least 0.1 mg to prevent a paradoxical bradycardia. Always reassess the airway and the equipment if the patient becomes bradycardic after a normal sinus rhythm has been reestablished.

Calcium Chloride   There are only four indications for calcium therapy in cardiopulmonary arrest: documented hypocalcemia, hyperkalemia, hypermagnesemia, and calcium channel blocker overdose. The dose is 5 to 7 mg/kg of elemental calcium (0.2–0.25 mL/kg of 10% calcium chloride). This may be repeated once in 10 min, but subsequent doses are dictated by the measured calcium.

Sodium Bicarbonate   The use of sodium bicarbonate during cardiopulmonary resuscitation is controversial. Although severe disturbances of acid-base balance virtually always accompany cardiopulmonary failure, they are better corrected by adequate ventilation and restoration of circulation than by administration of base. Adequate ventilation removes carbon dioxide, and restoration of volume allows for removal of organic acids by the kidney. Bicarbonate may further depress cardiac contractility; therefore its use is contraindicated in cardiac arrest until adequate ventilation and circulation have been established. For a persistently low pH (<7.20) or a prolonged cardiopulmonary arrest, give 1 mEq/kg. Use arterial blood gases (ABGs) to determine base deficits and the need for continued base therapy.

Lidocaine   Rhythm disturbances are rare in children. Lidocaine may help depress ectopic foci after attempts to convert ventricular fibrillation or pulseless ventricular tachycardia by defibrillation. The initial dose is 1 mg/kg. If subsequent doses are required, use a continuous infusion. Place 120 mg of lidocaine in 100 mL of D_5W and run at 1 to 2.5 mL/kg/h (20–50 µg/kg/min).

Amiodarone   This lipid-soluble antiarrhythmic drug is recommended for a wide range of atrial and ventricular rhythm disturbances. It is a noncompetitive inhibitor of both alpha- and beta-adrenergic receptors. It prolongs the QT interval, and this is thought to be the major action in converting abnormal rhythms. For both supraventricular and ventricular rhythm disturbances, give a loading dose of 5 mg/kg over 1 min to 1 h to a maximum of 15 mg/kg/day. Do not give with procainamide.

Adenosine   This is an endogenous nucleoside that slows conduction through the atrioventricular (AV) node of the heart. It is the drug of choice for treatment of stable or unstable supraventricular tachycardia (SVT, pp 32–38). It has a half-life of about 10 s, and the side effects are minimal. It may be safely used in patients with Wolff-Parkinson-White (WPW) syndrome. The dose is 0.1 mg/kg (12 mg maximum) as a rapid push into a proximal IV site.

Procainamide   A sodium channel–blocking antiarrhythmic agent, procainamide prolongs the refractory period of the atria and ventricles and depresses the conduction velocity within the heart. It is effective in the treatment of atrial fibrillation, flutter, and SVT and may be used in postoperative junctional ectopic tachycardia. Infuse a loading dose of 15 mg/kg over 30 to 60 min with continuous monitoring of the electrocardiogram (ECG) and blood pressure. If the QRS complex widens by more than 50%, stop the infusion.

Glucose   If there is documented hypoglycemia, give a 0.5 g/kg bolus of glucose as soon as possible. Because of the risk of intraventricular hemorrhage, use a 10% solution (5 mL/kg) in neonates (premix syringe without preservative or dilute D_{50} 1:4 with sterile water). In older infants, use 2 mL/kg of a 25% solution.

Table 1-8   Calculating Infusions: The Rule of 6's

DRUG	CALCULATION
Epinephrine Norepinephrine	$0.6 \times$ body weight (in kg) = mg of drug to add to 100 mL D$_5$W
	Then, an IV rate of 1 mL/h delivers 0.1 μg/kg/min of drug
Dopamine Dobutamine Nitroprusside	$6 \times$ body weight (in kg) = mg of drug to add to 100 mL D$_5$W
	Then an IV rate of 1 mL/h delivers 1 μg/kg/min of drug

Infusions

Epinephrine   An epinephrine infusion is helpful in patients who are still hypotensive after cardiopulmonary resuscitation. The dose is 0.1 to 1.0 μg/kg/min (Table 1-8).

Dopamine   This is an endogenous catecholamine with complex effects on the heart and circulation. It has relatively few chronotropic effects with low doses. It may be particularly helpful for patients in cardiogenic shock but may not be as efficacious as epinephrine or dobutamine in patients with poor myocardial function. The advantage of dopamine is its effect on renal and splanchnic perfusion. Its actions are dose-dependent (titrate to desired effect), with some overlap:

2 to 4 μg/kg/min	Dopaminergic action: dilates renal and mesenteric vessels
4 to 10 μg/kg/min	Mixed alpha and beta effects: increases contractility with modest effects on heart rate and blood pressure
10 to 20 μg/kg/min	Alpha effect predominates: increases blood pressure due to vasoconstriction

Dobutamine   Owing to its selective action on beta-adrenergic receptors, dobutamine is an effective inotrope for patients with poor perfusion despite normal blood pressure or those with hypoperfusion and high systemic vascular resistance. The dose is 5 to 20 μg/kg/min.

Cardioversion and Defibrillation

Cardioversion is synchronized electrical conversion of a rhythm disturbance using relatively low energy doses. It is indicated for unstable SVT when the patient shows clinical signs of shock or is deteriorating. The initial dose is 0.5 to 1 J/kg to a maximum of 100 J.

Treat unstable or pulseless ventricular tachycardia (pp 40–41) or ventricular fibrillation (pp 41–42) with immediate defibrillation with an initial charge of 2 J/kg (200 J maximum). If the rhythm does not convert to normal, double the dose to 4 J/kg (360 J maximum) and repeat the defibrillation attempt. Although the sequence for treating ventricular fibrillation in children has not been studied, follow the adult decision tree in the

American Heart Association's guidelines (see Bibliography, below) if further efforts are needed.

Synchronized precordial leads must be attached to the patient, and the *synchronize button on the defibrillator must be activated* to avoid potentially lethal torsades arrhythmia. This will be evident by a light on the machine and a mark over the R wave on the ECG. Double the energy dose if subsequent cardioversion is needed.

Asystole

Treat asystole and nonperfusing rhythms with assisted ventilation and chest compressions.

Bradycardia

Bradycardia in the pediatric patient is defined as a heart rate less than 60 beats per minute. To a greater degree than older children, small infants are dependent on heart rate to maintain cardiac output, so they are more often symptomatic from bradycardia. Always treat clinically significant bradycardia by providing adequate oxygenation and ventilation. Epinephrine is the most useful drug for treating bradycardia that does not respond to oxygen. The only exceptions are symptomatic bradycardia caused by AV heart block or increased vagal tone; in those cases, give atropine. In the rare instance when bradycardia is due to complete heart block, immediately consult a cardiologist to arrange for pacing. However, pacing has not been shown to be effective in postarrest hypoxic/ischemic myocardial insult or in the treatment of asystole in children.

BIBLIOGRAPHY

Eisenberg MS, Mengert TJ: Cardiac resuscitation. *N Engl J Med* 2001;344: 1304–1313.
Fiser DH: Intraosseous infusions. *N Engl J Med* 1990;322:1579–1581.
Hazinski MF (ed): *PALS Provider Manual.* Dallas: American Heart Association 2002;81–153.
Young K, Seidel JS: Pediatric cardiopulmonary resuscitation: a collective review. *Ann Emerg Med* 1999;33:195–205.

SHOCK

The cardiovascular system delivers a constant supply of oxygen and nutrients to body tissues in order to maintain cellular function, and it removes the products of cellular metabolism, including carbon dioxide. Shock occurs when perfusion is inadequate to meet the metabolic demands of the tissues. If shock persists, there may be deterioration of organ function leading to multiple end-organ failure and death.

The many causes of shock in childhood may be classified by the mechanisms producing the poor perfusion: hypovolemic, cardiogenic, distributive, and obstructive shock (Table 1-9).

Effective perfusion requires sufficient substrate of oxygen and glucose, adequate myocardial function (including the capability to sustain an appropriate heart rate and stroke volume), and the ability to regulate systemic vascular resistance. Cardiac output is the product of stroke volume

Table 1-9   Classification and Etiologies of Shock

TYPE OF SHOCK	ETIOLOGY
Hypovolemic: Pump is empty	Trauma (hemorrhage) Dehydration (vomiting, diarrhea, poor intake) Metabolic disease (diabetes) Excessive sweating (infant)
Cardiogenic: Weak/sick pump	Rhythm disturbances Congestive heart failure Cardiomyopathy Postresuscitation
Distributive: Fluid distribution	Sepsis Anaphylaxis Spinal cord injury Third spacing of fluids
Obstructive: Obstruction of outflow	Tension pneumothorax Cardiac tamponade Pulmonary embolism

and heart rate; in children, the cardiac output is primarily maintained by changes in heart rate. Children may compensate for hypovolemia or decreased systemic vascular resistance with a dramatic increase in the heart rate. A heart rate between 160 and 200 beats per minute may signal impending circulatory failure; when the cardiac output falls by 25%, rapid decompensation may ensue. Bradycardia and hypotension are seen in uncompensated shock, which can rapidly progress to irreversible shock. Therefore do not be reassured by a normal blood pressure if there are other signs of circulatory compromise.

Hypovolemic Shock   Hypovolemia, the most common etiology of shock in infants and children, is caused by a drop in blood volume secondary to fluid loss. A child's normal blood volume is 80 mL/kg; thus, what may seem like a minor hemorrhage can represent a significant percentage of blood volume. The fluid loss stimulates adrenergic receptors, leading to an increase in systemic vascular resistance and a redistribution of intravascular perfusion to the heart, brain, and kidneys. The shunting of blood flow away from the skin causes the changes in skin color, temperature, and moisture seen in compensated shock. However, compensatory mechanisms cannot be maintained indefinitely, so the increase in systemic vascular resistance and afterload leads to increased myocardial oxygen consumption. The lack of sufficient oxygen can cause bradycardia and subsequent cardiopulmonary arrest.

Cardiogenic Shock   Cardiogenic shock occurs when there is compromised cardiac output secondary to myocardial dysfunction. This is most often seen with congenital heart disease and myocarditis and in the post-operative period after cardiac surgery. Cardiogenic shock is a terminal complication of virtually all types of shock because of the heart's requirement for a high oxygen concentration.

Distributive Shock   Distributive shock occurs when there is a redistribution of fluid within the vascular space. The most common causes are sepsis and neurologic injury. Septic shock may be seen in the first few hours of an illness (particularly in young infants) or as a result of a protracted illness in a patient with a compromised immune system. The early phases of septic shock may not be clinically apparent because of the absence of abnormal skin signs. The pulses, however, will be rapid, full, and bounding.

Obstructive Shock   Obstructive shock occurs when the pumping action of the heart is inhibited by constriction. It can be secondary to pericardial tamponade, tension pneumothorax, or pulmonary embolism. These conditions must be corrected with appropriate therapy such as pericardiocentesis or a chest tube to reverse the condition.

Clinical Presentation

The clinical presentation depends on the cardiac output relative to end-organ demand. If the compensatory mechanisms are adequate to maintain perfusion of vital organs, the patient is in "compensated shock." The blood pressure is normal, although there may be tachycardia and irritability. Once 20 to 30% of the effective circulating blood volume is lost, the patient will decompensate and become hypotensive ("decompensated shock"). As the process continues untreated, there is multiple end-organ failure and death from "irreversible shock." The signs of shock are summarized in Table 1-10.

Diagnosis

The initial assessment includes the general appearance; airway, breathing, and circulation (the ABCs); mental status; a brief history of the present illness and pertinent past history; a complete set of vital signs; and evaluation of skin signs (color, warmth, and capillary refill). However, during the

Table 1-10   Signs of Shock

EARLY	LATE
Narrowed pulse pressure	Decreased systolic pressure
Orthostatic changes (older patients)	Decreased diastolic pressure
Delayed capillary filling	Cold, pale skin
Tachycardia	Altered mental status
Hyperventilation	Confusion and lethargy
	Diaphoresis
	Decreased urine output

assessment, do not delay providing critical interventions, including positioning, supplemental oxygen, and vascular or intraosseous access. Maintain a high index of suspicion, since the signs of early shock are subtle.

Assessment   While rapidly performing the assessment, proceed with the concurrent institution of critical interventions. Strict attention to the ABCs will help improve the outcome.

General Appearance   Note the patient's general appearance and reaction to the caretaker and the surrounding environment. In infants and young children, this may be accomplished with the patient on the caretaker's lap. Note the child's level of activity; type of cry; whether the patient is consolable, playful, attentive, or irritable; and his or her reaction to painful stimuli.

In older patients who do not appear seriously ill, assess changes in the pulse and blood pressure in the supine and erect positions. Check the pulse with the patient supine; repeat after the patient has been sitting upright for 2 min. A pulse increase of 20 or more beats per minute is an indication of orthostatic hypotension. Orthostatic changes are difficult to detect in younger patients; do not waste time with these maneuvers.

ABCs   Immediately evaluate airway, breathing (ventilation and oxygenation), and circulation. The assessment of vital signs is extremely important. Evaluate the rate, rhythm, and depth of respirations and work of breathing. Feel for central and peripheral pulses, noting their rate and quality. One of the early signs of shock is tachycardia. Bounding pulses may occur in the early stages of septic shock, while thready pulses with a narrowed pulse pressure occur in hypovolemic shock. Obtain an accurate blood pressure using an appropriately sized cuff. It may be necessary to use the Doppler method. If hypotension is present, the patient is, by definition, in the decompensated phase and needs critical intervention to prevent permanent morbidity and death.

Skin Signs   Observe for central and/or peripheral cyanosis and feel for skin temperature and moisture. Cool, clammy extremities are important signs of shock. Check for capillary refill. Although capillary refill may be delayed in normal individuals, an increase is a clinical indicator of shock. With the patient's fingers at the level of the heart, apply pressure to one of the palmar fingertips until it blanches, then release, timing the interval until the fingertip "pinks up." A delay greater than 2 s is associated with poor perfusion.

ED Management

The most common error in treating shock is underestimating the severity of the condition. If there are signs of compensated shock, treat early and aggressively to prevent a bad outcome. All patients require an IV, oxygen therapy, and cardiopulmonary monitoring.

1. *Position*: Allow a conscious patient to assume a position of comfort.

2. *Oxygen*: Give 100% supplemental oxygen.

3. *Assisted ventilation:* If there is evidence of airway compromise, assist ventilation with either a bag-mask device or endotracheal intubation.

4. *Intravenous access*: Start two large-bore IV lines via peripheral veins or a central approach. If venous access is not possible or delayed, use the intraosseous approach. In critically ill or injured patients, do not spend more than 1 to 2 min attempting to establish peripheral vascular access. The effort may be resumed after the intraosseous line is secured.

5. *Fluid*: Infuse a fluid challenge of 20 mL/kg of isotonic crystalloid (lactated Ringer's or normal saline) as rapidly as possible. Several boluses may be required. The trauma patient will require blood to replace ongoing losses; use O negative or type-specific blood if available. Pneumatic anti-shock trousers have not been shown to improve patient outcome and are no longer recommended in the treatment of shock. Trauma patients who remain hypotensive after fluid resuscitation may require immediate operative intervention.

6. *Reassess:* After each intervention, look for improvement in vital signs, skin signs, and level of consciousness. Insert a Foley catheter and monitor urine output; the goal is 1 to 2 mL/kg/h.

7. *Inotropes*: With the exception of hypovolemic shock, inotropic agents may be helpful in stabilizing blood pressure if the patient remains hypotensive after fluid resuscitation. Details of using inotropic drips are given in the discussion of cardiopulmonary resuscitation, above (p 17).

a. *Epinephrine* is the infusion of choice for hypotensive patients; the rate is 0.1 to 1.0 µg/kg/min. Monitor the patient carefully and switch to a less potent agent once the blood pressure has improved.

b. *Dobutamine* is the infusion of choice for patients in cardiogenic shock who are not severely hypotensive; the rate is 5 to 20 µg/kg/min.

c. *Dopamine* may be helpful for the patient with distributive shock after successful fluid resuscitation. The rate is 5 to 20 µg/kg/min—although, to achieve the desired alpha-constriction effect, more than 10 to 15 µg/kg/min may be needed.

8. *Cardiogenic shock*: These patients may get worse after a fluid challenge; this can be treated with diuretics. Treat supraventricular tachycardia with adenosine or synchronized cardioversion (p 35) and ventricular fibrillation with defibrillation (p 42).

BIBLIOGRAPHY

Butt W: Septic shock. *Pediatr Clin North Am* 2001;48:601–625.

Hazinski MF (ed): *PALS Provider Manual.* Dallas: American Heart Association, 2002;23–42.

Hazinksi MF, Barkin RM: Shock, in Barkin RM (ed): *Pediatric Emergency Medicine: Concepts and Clinical Practice.* St. Louis: Mosby–Year Book, 1992.

Tobias JD: Shock in children: the first 60 minutes. *Pediatr Ann* 1996;24:330–338.

CHAPTER 2

Allergic Emergencies

Frederick Leickly

ANAPHYLAXIS

Anaphylaxis is the most serious manifestation of allergy. It is a severe, abrupt, untoward immunologic event that results from the generation and massive release of potent mediators from mast cells and basophils. These mediators cause increased vascular permeability, vasodilation, myocardial depression, and smooth muscle contraction. Anaphylaxis may be triggered by a classic type I, IgE-mediated response or by release of mediators through a variety of other mechanisms.

IgE-mediated anaphylaxis has been implicated in reactions caused by drugs (most often antibiotics), foreign proteins, foods, latex, and insect stings. Although any food can cause anaphylaxis, the most common are peanuts, tree nuts, shellfish, egg, milk, soy, wheat, and fish. Stinging insects of the hymenoptera family (yellow jacket, hornet, wasp, honeybee, fire ant) are associated with anaphylactic reactions. Latex, ubiquitous in many medical settings, has proven to be a potent allergen as well. Patients who have had multiple surgical procedures are at particular risk for latex reactions (e.g., children with spina bifida or urinary tract abnormalities).

When IgE is not involved, the reaction is called anaphylactoid; such reactions occur most commonly with blood or blood product infusions. Other causative agents include hyperosmolar radiocontrast materials and nonsteroidal anti-inflammatory drugs (NSAIDs). Nevertheless, anaphylactic and anaphylactoid reactions are clinically indistinguishable and are managed in the same way.

Clinical Presentation

A reaction can occur as rapidly as seconds after exposure, or it may be delayed for hours. In some individuals the reaction is biphasic, with both an immediate reaction and a more serious one 6 to 8 h later.

Anaphylaxis usually involves at least two organ systems. The skin is most frequently involved, with urticaria or angioedema occurring in nearly 90% of episodes. The next most commonly involved organ systems include the respiratory tract, the cardiovascular system, and/or the

23

Table 2-1   Clinical Findings in Anaphylaxis

ORGAN SYSTEM	CLINICAL FINDINGS
Skin	Angioedema, flushing, urticaria, pruritus
Cardiovascular	Arrhythmias, palpitations, tachycardia, syncope, hypotension
Gastrointestinal	Distention, nausea, vomiting, diarrhea, cramps
Respiratory	Rhinorrhea, dyspnea, choking, hoarseness, stridor, wheezing
Other	Sense of impending doom, diaphoresis, fecal and/or urinary incontinence, ocular irritation, sneezing, metallic taste

gastrointestinal tract. Respiratory symptoms are seen in about 70% of cases of anaphylaxis.

The signs and symptoms of anaphylaxis are summarized in Table 2-1.

Diagnosis

The diagnosis of anaphylaxis is based on the clinical manifestations and the association of exposure. Criteria include the following:

- Presence of an allergic sign or symptom: urticaria, angioedema, sneezing, pruritus
- Involvement of at least two organ systems
- Exposure to an agent(s) or activity known to be capable of inducing anaphylaxis or evidence of an IgE-mediated response to an agent
- Absence of any condition that can mimic anaphylaxis

Making the diagnosis of anaphylaxis is generally not difficult, although *syncopal* or *vasovagal episodes* can involve hypotension and gastrointestinal complaints. In contrast to anaphylaxis, there is an absence of bronchospasm, urticaria, and pruritus. A patient with a vasovagal response is usually markedly pallid, and bradycardia is much more common than with anaphylaxis.

Hyperventilation may cause breathlessness and dizziness but is not typically associated with other systemic symptoms except for peripheral and perioral tingling. Laryngeal edema, especially when recurrent, raises the possibility of *hereditary angioedema*. This is usually seen in adolescents and is associated with abnormal levels or abnormal functioning of an inhibitor of the first component of complement (C-1 esterase inhibitor).

Urticaria (pp 26–28) is frequently seen with anaphylaxis but often occurs without other signs of anaphylaxis; always investigate for other organ system involvement in such a patient. The bronchopulmonary manifestations of anaphylaxis are likewise indistinguishable from *asthma*. *Serum sickness* can present with urticaria and/or angioedema, but it is not usually an acute event; it is also associated with fever, lymphadenopathy, arthralgias, and arthritis.

The differential diagnosis of anaphylaxis is summarized in Table 2-2.

Table 2-2   **Differential Diagnosis of Anaphylaxis**

Embolism	Vasovagal reaction
Arrhythmia	Globus hystericus
Cardiac tamponade	Hereditary angioedema
Cardiac infarction	Serum sickness
Sepsis	Mastocytosis
Seizure	Scombroid poisoning
Insulin reaction	

ED Management

Anaphylaxis is a *medical emergency* requiring *immediate attention.* Institute the ABCs (attention to airway, breathing, and circulation) of emergency care and limit any continued exposure. Discontinue any intravenous agents immediately. Avoid using latex products when caring for a latex-allergic patient. If the affected patient is taking beta-blocking medication, be prepared for a very difficult recovery; sometimes extraordinary efforts are required to overcome beta blockade associated with concurrent anaphylaxis.

The first priority is to maintain airway patency. Allow the patient to assume a position of comfort. If adequate ventilation and oxygenation are documented by pulse oximetry, do not change the patient's position but administer 100% oxygen as tolerated. If stridor is present, and initial therapy with epinephrine is not effective, prepare to perform intubation or cricothyrotomy. Monitor the electrocardiogram (ECG) and oxygen saturation continuously and establish IV access. Make a rapid assessment of the rate of progression and the extent of the reaction.

The mainstay in the treatment of anaphylaxis is aqueous epinephrine. If the patient is not hypotensive, give 0.01 mL/kg (0.5 mL maximum) of 1:1000 epinephrine *intramuscularly.* This will achieve a faster peak level than subcutaneous administration. Repeat the dose every 15 min as needed. Immediately *after* the epinephrine, give diphenhydramine. This is not a substitute for epinephrine but can help reduce symptoms rapidly and may shorten the time course of the reaction. If the oral route is used, liquids or chewable tablets allow for quicker absorption. The dose is 5 mg/kg/day divided q 6 h (50 mg/dose maximum) IM, IV, or PO. The H_2 class of antihistamines may be helpful in reducing histamine-induced cardiac arrhythmias in selected cases. Give famotidine 1 to 2 mg/kg (50 mg maximum) slowly IV.

Glucocorticosteroids are not helpful for treating the acute reaction but can abrogate a late-phase response. Give IV hydrocortisone (5 mg/kg q 6 h, 100 mg maximum) or methylprednisolone (1–2 mg/kg q 6 h, 60 mg maximum), or oral prednisolone (2 mg/kg, 60 mg maximum).

Treat hypotension and cardiovascular shock aggressively. Give 1:10,000 epinephrine IV (0.1 mL/kg, 10 mL maximum). If venous access is not available, administer epinephrine (0.1 mL/kg of 1:1000) via the endotracheal tube. If the initial response is inadequate, use an intravenous drip, starting with 0.1 μg/kg/min (1.5 μg/kg/min maximum). Also give an initial fluid bolus of 20 mL/kg of isotonic crystalloid (see "Shock," pp 18–22). Repeat the boluses as necessary. On occasion, a patient taking a beta blocker may have hypotension that does not respond to epinephrine. In such a case, give IV glucagon, 1-mg bolus, followed by a continuous infusion of 1 to 5 mg/h, titrating the dose to the response.

Treat bronchospasm with nebulized albuterol, 0.03 mL/kg (1.0 mL maximum) diluted in 2.0 mL of saline, either q 1 h or continuously. See "Asthma" (pp 571–574) for the treatment of bronchospasm not responsive to albuterol.

Discharge Considerations

- Observe for 6 h. Late-phase reactions occur within this time period.
- Give prednisone 2 mg/kg qd (60 mg maximum) for 5 days.
- Give diphenhydramine (5 mg/kg/d divided q 6 h, maximum 50 mg/dose) for 5 days to treat urticaria.
- Prescribe injectable epinephrine (Epi Pen Jr. <15 kg, Epi Pen >15 kg) and instruct the patient and family on when and how to use it.
- Educate the family regarding avoidance of the trigger(s).
- Inform family about MedicAlert bracelets (1-888-633-4298 or www.medicalert.org).

Refer all patients with an episode of anaphylaxis to an allergist.

Follow-up

- Primary care follow-up within 2 to 3 days

Indications for Admission

- Persistent bronchospasm
- Hypotension requiring vasopressors
- Significant hypoxia
- Patient resides some distance from medical facilities

BIBLIOGRAPHY

Dibs SD, Baker MD: Anaphylaxis in children. A 5 year experience. *Pediatrics* 1997;99(1). http://www.pediatrics.org/egi/content/full/99/1/e7.

Kagy L, Blass MS: Anaphylaxis in children. *Pediatr Ann* 1998;27:727–734.

Simons FER, Roberts JR, Gu A, et al: Epinephrine absorption in children with a history of anaphylaxis. *J Allergy Clin Immunol* 1998;101:33–37.

URTICARIA

Urticaria, or hives, is a common cutaneous reaction caused by release of chemical mediators, especially histamine, from mast cells or basophils. Angioedema is a similar process occurring in the deep dermis or subcutaneous tissues.

Acute urticaria lasts less than 6 to 8 weeks, while chronic urticaria is defined as hives persisting beyond this time frame. In 80% of these cases, the etiology is unknown, although chronic urticaria can be associated with systemic illnesses such as juvenile rheumatoid arthritis (JRA), systemic lupus erythematosus (SLE), viral hepatitis, lymphomas, and thyroid disease. The most common causes are listed in Table 2-3.

Table 2-3   Common Etiologies of Urticaria

Allergic reactions—IgE-mediated	"Other" allergic reactions
Pollen	Serum sickness
Animal dander	Transfusions
Foods	Autoimmune reactions
Eggs	
Milk	**Nonallergic reactions**
Wheat	Radiographic contrast media
Soy	Nonsteroidal anti-inflammatory
Peanuts	drugs
Tree nuts	
Shellfish	**Physical causes**
Drugs: antibiotics	Cold
Insect bites	Heat
Latex	Pressure
Idiopathic	Sunlight
Infection	Water
	Vibration

Clinical Presentation

A hive is a well-circumscribed, raised, evanescent area of skin edema on an erythematous base. Acute urticaria usually develops within minutes of exposure to the causative agent. The size of individual hives may vary from a few millimeters to centimeters (giant urticaria), and the lesions are virtually always pruritic. Simple hives tend to come and go in crops, with individual lesions usually lasting for less than a day. On rare occasions a hive will persist for up to 48 h. Angioedema may be associated more with pain than with itching and may take days to resolve completely.

Diagnosis

The key feature in making the diagnosis of hives is the duration of the lesions. Lesions that remain fixed in place for longer than 24 to 48 h are not typical hives. A violet hue within the lesion or the absence of pruritus also suggests alternative etiologies.

Obtain a complete history, seeking a possible offending agent. Determine the time of onset, site, duration, and frequency of the lesions. Inquire about recent medication use, injections, insect bites, illness, and other triggers or provoking factors. For patients with chronic urticaria, ascertain if there are any associated symptoms, such as fever, joint pain, abdominal pain, weight loss, or poor circulation in the hands or feet.

A priority is to assess for signs of associated respiratory, cardiovascular, or gastrointestinal involvement, which would imply that the urticaria is a manifestation of an anaphylactic episode. Similarly, look for the presence of associated angioedema on physical examination.

In general, no laboratory testing is required, and it is not necessary to identify the trigger for a patient with acute urticaria who is otherwise well and in whom the history and physical examination do not suggest a cause. However, if the patient presents with chronic urticaria and the history and physical examination do not suggest an etiology, obtain a complete blood count (CBC) with differential, erythrocyte sedimentation rate (ESR), liver function tests, and a urinalysis.

ED Management

The priority for all patients with urticaria or angioedema is to rule out anaphylaxis (see "Anaphylaxis," pp 23–26).

The best treatment for urticaria is removing or avoiding the offending agent if it can be identified. For both acute and chronic urticaria, the drugs of choice are oral first-generation H_1 antihistamines, such as hydroxyzine (2 mg/kg/day, divided tid, 50 mg maximum) or diphenhydramine (5 mg/kg/day, divided qid, 50 mg maximum). If sedation is a concern, use a second-generation oral antihistamine, such as loratadine (>3 years: 5 mg qd if <30 kg or 10 mg qd if >30 kg), cetirizine (2–5 years: 2.5 mg qd; >6 years: 5–10 mg qd), or fexofenadine (>12 years: 60 mg bid). The antiserotoninergic agent cyproheptadine is particularly useful for treating physical forms of urticaria (give 0.25 to 0.5 mg/kg/day divided q 8–12 h, 12 mg/day maximum if 2–6 years old, 16 mg/day maximum if 7–14 years old, and 32 mg/day maximum if >14 years old). If the patient has particularly severe pruritus or angioedema, give subcutaneous 1:1000 epinephrine (0.01 mL/kg up to 0.3 mL). This will afford prompt but brief relief until the antihistamines take effect.

Follow-up

- Acute urticaria: if no improvement; primary care in 3 to 5 days
- Allergy referral in 1 to 2 weeks: peanut- or latex-induced urticaria, urticarial vasculitis, urticaria with systemic manifestations, urticaria with angioedema, urticaria that responds poorly to therapy, and if the results of the ED evaluation do not suggest an etiology for chronic urticaria

BIBLIOGRAPHY

Charlesworth E: Urticaria and angioedema: a clinical spectrum. *Ann Allergy Asthma Immunol* 1996;76:484–495.

Leickly FE: When the road gets bumpy: managing chronic urticaria. *Contemp Pediatr* 2000;17:58–71.

Mortureux P, Leaute-Labreze C, Legrain-Liferman V, et al: Acute urticaria in infancy and early childhood. *Arch Dermatol* 1998;134:319–323.

CHAPTER 3

Cardiac Emergencies

Michael H. Gewitz and Paul K. Woolf

ARRHYTHMIAS

Pediatric arrhythmias are increasing in prevalence secondary to improved survival following cardiac surgery and more extensive use of electrocardiographic (ECG) monitoring. Proper management includes accurate ECG diagnosis, careful clinical evaluation, and initiation of appropriate therapy. With all rhythm disturbances, the approach to the patient begins with a 12-lead ECG; but if there is hemodynamic instability, a single-lead ECG will suffice.

Cardiac arrhythmias requiring emergency therapy can be classified simply into tachycardias and bradycardias. The tachycardias can be further divided into narrow– and wide–QRS complex groups. Rhythms in the narrow-complex group include atrial fibrillation, atrial flutter, and supraventricular tachycardia. The most common narrow-complex tachycardia is sinus tachycardia.

Atrial Fibrillation

Atrial fibrillation is usually associated with dilatation of the right or left atrium. It most commonly occurs in patients with mitral valve disease, chronic atrioventricular (AV) valve insufficiency, Wolff-Parkinson-White syndrome, or following the Fontan procedure in patients with only one functional ventricle. Other associations include hyperthyroidism, Ebstein's anomaly, atrial septal defect, or atrial tumor. Atrial fibrillation suggests significant disease of the atrial conduction system and is usually a chronic problem. "Lone" atrial fibrillation, in the absence of other cardiac abnormalities, is rare in children.

Clinical Presentation and Diagnosis

Suspect atrial fibrillation when the pulse is "irregularly irregular." Heart sounds may vary in intensity, a pulse deficit may be present, and the cardiac impulse shows marked variability. The ECG shows chaotic

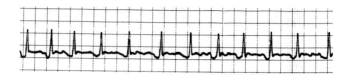

Figure 3-1   Atrial fibrillation.

fibrillatory waves of varying amplitude, morphology, and duration, causing variation of the baseline. The RR interval is irregularly irregular. The ventricular rate varies between 100 and 200 bpm (Fig. 3-1).

The atrial rate is generally >350 bpm, while in *supraventricular tachycardia* (SVT) the rate is slower (150–300 bpm) and the RR interval is constant.

ED Management

Treatment can usually be delayed until the patient is admitted to an intensive care setting, where therapy is aimed at control of ventricular rate, conversion to sinus rhythm, and prevention of stroke. However, in the ED, use synchronized cardioversion (1 J/kg) to treat acute atrial fibrillation associated with a rapid ventricular rate and signs of hemodynamic compromise.

If the patient is hemodynamically stable, consult a pediatric cardiologist before initiating pharmacologic cardioversion, which can most frequently be accomplished with ibutilide or amiodarone. Rate control is best accomplished with diltiazem or digitalis. Digitalis is contraindicated if the patient is known to have Wolff-Parkinson-White syndrome, since it may facilitate conduction through an accessory AV connection, leading to ventricular fibrillation.

Although atrial thrombus is uncommon in children with atrial fibrillation, anticoagulation is recommended if there is chronic (>48 h) atrial fibrillation. Obtain an echocardiogram in order to document the presence of a thrombus.

Indications for Admission

- Acute onset of atrial fibrillation
- Chronic atrial fibrillation with an increase in ventricular rate requiring treatment with a new antiarrhythmic medication

BIBLIOGRAPHY

Applegate TE: Atrial arrhythmias. *Prim Care* 2000;27:677–708.

Fish F, Benson DW: Disorders of cardiac rhythm and conduction, in Emmanouildes GC, Riemenschneider TA, Allen HD, Gutgesell HP (eds): *Moss and Adams Heart Disease in Infants, Children, and Adolescents,* 5th ed. Baltimore: Williams & Wilkins, 1995, pp 1580–1583.

Gold MR, Josephson ME: Cardiac arrhythmias: current therapy. *Hosp Pract* 1999; 34:27–38.

Atrial Flutter

Atrial flutter can occur spontaneously in the newborn, or it may be a manifestation of pre- or postoperative structural cardiac disease, cardiomyopathy, or primary electrical disease. Atrial flutter is relatively rare in childhood, although the incidence is increasing because more patients are surviving complex atrial surgery, such as the Fontan procedure or the Mustard repair for transposition of the great vessels.

Clinical Presentation and Diagnosis

Atrial flutter is characterized by an atrial tachycardia with a rate between 300 and 480 bpm. The atrial rhythm is extremely regular, and flutter waves are usually present. These form a continuous sawtooth undulation of the baseline P waves (Fig. 3-2). The ventricular rate is dependent on AV conduction, which is most commonly 2:1. When 1:1 conduction is present, the flutter waves may not be apparent.

When the diagnosis is in doubt, use vagal maneuvers or adenosine (pp 34–35) to increase the degree of AV block and slow the ventricular rate. This may make the flutter waves more apparent.

In *SVT* the atrial rate is 180 to 240 bpm, with 1:1 AV conduction and a fixed RR interval. Vagal maneuvers may terminate SVT, while in atrial flutter the degree of AV block may increase, slowing the ventricular rate, but the rhythm does not convert to sinus.

ED Management

Hemodynamically Unstable Patient   If the patient is hemodynamically unstable, presenting with hypotension or congestive heart failure, cardiovert using 0.5 to 1.0 J/kg, in the synchronized mode, as the initial dose. If the patient is taking digoxin, give IV lidocaine, 1 mg/kg, prior to cardioversion to prevent ventricular arrhythmias. If initial cardioversion is unsuccessful, increase the dose to 2 J/kg.

Hemodynamically Stable Patient   If the patient is hemodynamically stable, first attempt pharmacologic treatment. Use IV digoxin [total digitalizing dose (TDD) = 30 µg/kg; give one-half of the TDD initially, followed by one-quarter of the TDD q 6–8 h × 2], IV amiodarone (5 mg/kg over 10–15 min), or IV ibutilide (0.01 mg/kg over 10 min) in order to slow the ventricular rate or convert to sinus rhythm. If these measures

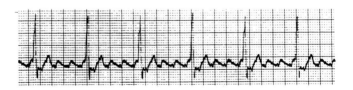

Figure 3-2   Atrial flutter.

are unsuccessful, elective electrical cardioversion may be required. Begin with 0.5 to 1.0 J/kg; double the dose if there is no response.

Indications for Admission

- New-onset atrial flutter
- Difficult-to-control atrial flutter for observation or for electrical or drug therapy

BIBLIOGRAPHY

Applegate TE: Atrial arrhythmias. *Prim Care* 2000;27:677–708.

Fish F, Benson DW: Disorders of cardiac rhythm and conduction, in Emmanouildes GC, Riemenschneider TA, Allen HD, Gutgesell HP (eds): *Moss and Adams Heart Disease in Infants, Children, and Adolescents,* 5th ed. Baltimore: Williams & Wilkins, 1995, pp 1580–1583.

Gow RM: Atrial fibrillation and flutter in children and in young adults with congenital heart disease. *Can J Cardiol* 1996;12(suppl A):45A–48A.

Sinus Tachycardia

Sinus tachycardia (ST) is an increased heart rate for age originating from the sinus node. The most common causes of ST are anxiety, fever, anemia, hypovolemia, congestive heart failure, exercise, hyperthyroidism, emotional upset, and medications (bronchodilators, decongestants).

Clinical Presentation and Diagnosis

Since normal hemodynamics are generally maintained, ST is usually an incidental finding in a patient with some other presentation. The rate is generally between 100 and 180 bpm, although in infants it may reach 240 bpm.

Sinus tachycardia must be differentiated from *SVT,* in which the rate can be as rapid as 340 bpm and the QRS complexes may not be preceded by recognizable P waves. In some cases of SVT, the QRS complexes may be preceded by abnormally directed P waves that are negative in leads I and aVF. Also, the rate may vary in ST, while in SVT the RR interval is consistent. Increasing the ECG paper speed to 50 mm/s may help to identify normal P waves.

ED Management

Most often, ST is encountered in the settings mentioned above, so therapy is directed toward identifying and treating these conditions.

BIBLIOGRAPHY

Applegate TE: Atrial arrhythmias. *Prim Care* 2000;27:677–708.

Supraventricular Tachycardia

SVT is the most common significant pediatric cardiac arrhythmia. The mechanism of SVT is usually reentry, secondary to microreentrant circuits, as in sinus or AV node reentry, or macroreentrant circuits involving an AV bypass tract, as in Wolff-Parkinson-White (WPW) syndrome. In

Table 3-1   Factors Predisposing to Supraventricular Tachycardia

Primary electrical disease	Sepsis
Atrioventricular bypass tract	Hyperthyroidism
(WPW)	Fever
Dual AV nodal pathways	Drugs
Myocarditis	Epinephrine
Cardiomyopathy	Decongestants
Ebstein's anomaly	Ephedrine
Mitral valve prolapse	Methylphenidate
Previous cardiac surgery	
(Mustard or Senning procedure for	
TPGV; Fontan; TAPVR repair)	

WPW, Wolff-Parkinson-White syndrome; TPGV, transposition of the great vessels; TAPVR, total anomalous pulmonary venous return.

20% of patients there is a trigger, such as infection or the use of cold remedies containing sympathomimetics (Table 3-1). Congenital heart disease, such as Ebstein's anomaly or corrected transposition, occurs in approximately 20% of patients.

Clinical Presentation

The presentation depends on the age of the patient, duration of the tachycardia, and whether there is preexisting heart disease. Common clinical findings include palpitations, shortness of breath, chest pain, respiratory distress, dizziness, syncope, irritability, pallor, and poor feeding in infants. The heart rate is usually between 150 and 300 bpm. Heart failure is uncommon in patients over 1 year of age and is usually associated with congenital heart disease, SVT for longer than 24 h, and heart rates greater than 200 bpm.

Diagnosis

The ECG in SVT is diagnostic and typically reveals a narrow-complex tachycardia at a rate of 150 to 300 bpm. The P wave may not be seen, may be inverted just after the QRS complex, or may precede the QRS but have an abnormal axis (negative in leads I or aVF). The ventricular complexes are usually normal in contour, although aberrant conduction can cause slight widening. The RR interval is fixed (Fig. 3-3).

SVT must be differentiated from *sinus tachycardia*. In the latter, the rate is usually less than 180 bpm (240 bpm in infants), a P wave with

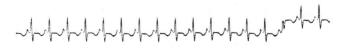

Figure 3-3   Supraventricular tachycardia.

normal axis precedes the QRS complex, and some variation in the RR interval may be present.

SVT with aberrant conduction and wide QRS complexes may be difficult to differentiate from *VT*, which is suggested by the presence of atrioventricular dissociation, a sicker patient, slower rate of the tachycardia, and isolated premature ventricular contractions elsewhere on the ECG. *Assume that all wide-complex tachycardias in children are ventricular tachycardia unless the diagnosis of SVT is absolutely certain.*

ED Management

Perform a history and physical examination, carefully evaluate the patient's hemodynamic status, and continuously monitor the ECG and blood pressure. Congestive heart failure or hemodynamic compromise are indications for rapid termination of the arrhythmia. After successful conversion to a sinus rhythm, obtain a complete ECG, looking for WPW, and refer the patient to a pediatric cardiologist.

Vagal Maneuvers
Vagal nerve stimulation causes a slowing of the spontaneous rate of the sinus pacemaker and potential atrial and junctional pacemakers and increases the effective refractory period of the AV node. Continuously monitor the ECG when vagal maneuvers are attempted. If they are successful, the tachycardia breaks abruptly and is replaced by a normal sinus rhythm (Fig. 3-4). Transient slowing of the ventricular rate suggests that either sinus tachycardia or atrial flutter was misdiagnosed as SVT. Eyeball pressure is not recommended, as retinal detachment can occur. Gagging and inducing vomiting may be effective but may lead to aspiration in infants or agitated patients. Commonly employed vagal techniques include the following:

Eliciting the Diving Reflex   Submerge the face of an older child in ice-cold water or place an ice bag with equal volumes of ice and water over the face for 10 to 20 s. This may cause an intense vagal stimulation; use only if facilities are available to perform full CPR.

Unilateral Carotid Massage   Perform the massage at the junction of the carotid artery and the mandible. This is much more likely to be successful in the older child or adolescent.

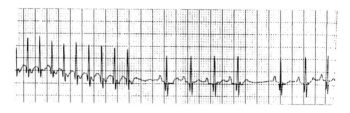

Figure 3-4   SVT response to ice bag.

Valsalva Maneuver   Ask the patient to "bear down" or "strain" as if attempting to move his or her bowels. If this is unsuccessful, have the patient stand on his or her head for 15 to 30 s.

Pharmacotherapy

Adenosine   Adenosine, an endogenous purine metabolite, is the drug of choice for the treatment of SVT. It terminates SVT by blocking conduction in the AV node and thus breaks the reentry circuit. It has been shown to be safe and effective, even in the presence of severe hemodynamic compromise. Give an initial dose of 0.1 mg/kg (6 mg maximum) as a rapid IV bolus, preferably at a proximal IV site. If ineffective in 2 to 3 min, double the dose (12 mg maximum). The onset of action is 10 to 15 s and the half-life is about 15 s. Bradycardia or transient asystole may occur after termination of the arrhythmia; flushing, wheezing, and cough are transient side effects.

Verapamil   Verapamil is a calcium slow-channel blocker that is extremely effective in treating SVT. The dose is 0.075 to 0.15 mg/kg, given slowly IV. This can be repeated twice at 15-min intervals. Verapamil is contraindicated under 1 year of age because of possible cardiovascular collapse; other contraindications include congestive heart failure and beta-blocker (propranolol) use. Side effects may include bradycardia and hypotension; treat with atropine (0.02 mg/kg), isoproterenol (0.1 µg/kg/min infusion), and calcium chloride (5–7 mg/kg of elemental calcium = 0.2–0.25 mL/kg of calcium chloride).

Digoxin   Digoxin terminates SVT through its vagal effect. While digoxin remains the mainstay of treatment for chronic SVT, it has been replaced by adenosine for acute SVT. The major drawback of digoxin is the delayed onset of action; SVT may not be terminated for 6 to 24 h after beginning therapy. The IV total digitalizing dose (TDD) is 30 µg/kg. Give one-half of the TDD initially, then one-quarter of the TDD at 6- to 8-h intervals. Digoxin is contraindicated in patients with WPW syndrome, as it shortens the refractory period of a bypass tract in up to one-third of these patients.

Cardioversion

Synchronous cardioversion is indicated when there is hemodynamic compromise (heart failure, shock, acidosis) or if other treatment modalities have failed. The dose is 0.5 to 1 J/kg, which can be repeated, doubling the dose to a maximum of 2 J/kg. Sedate older patients with midazolam (0.1 mg/kg IV) prior to cardioversion. To prevent ventricular dysrhythmias, give lidocaine (1 mg/kg IV) to digitalized patients prior to attempting cardioversion. Prior to cardioversion, *be certain of synchronized mode setting* to avoid potentially lethal ventricular arrhythmias.

Consult a pediatric cardiologist if the patient is refractory to vagal maneuvers, adenosine, verapamil and cardioversion. The Pediatric Advanced Life Support algorithms for tachycardia with adequate and poor perfusion are summarized in Figs. 3-5 and 3-6.

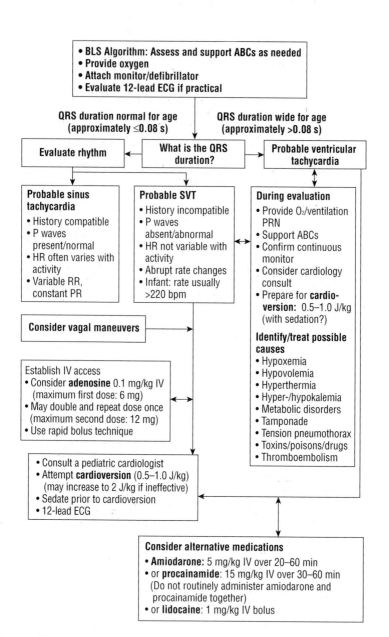

Figure 3-5 PALS algorithm for tachycardia with adequate perfusion.

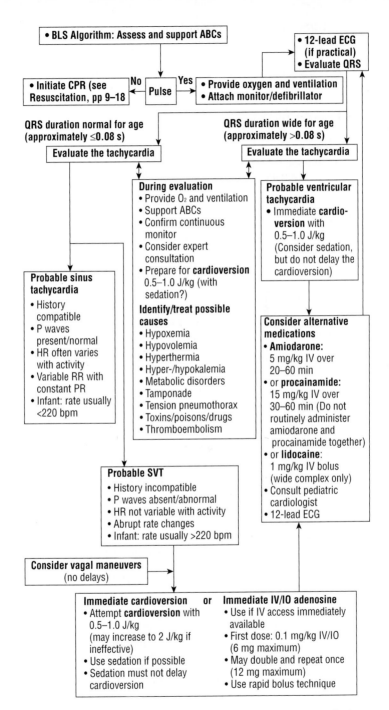

Figure 3-6 PALS algorithm for tachycardia with poor perfusion.

Follow-up

- SVT, without hemodynamic compromise, terminated in ED: 2 to 3 days

Indications for Admission

- First episode of SVT with parental anxiety or need for parental education
- SVT causing hemodynamic compromise
- Patient receiving a medication with proarrhythmic potential (flecainide, sotalol, amiodarone)

BIBLIOGRAPHY

Etheridge SP, Judd VE: Supraventricular tachycardia in infancy. *Arch Pediatr Adolesc Med* 1999;153:267–271.

Fish F, Benson DW: Disorders of cardiac rhythm and conduction, in Emmanouildes GC, Riemenschneider TA, Allen HD, Gutgesell HP (eds): *Moss and Adams Heart Disease in Infants, Children, and Adolescents,* 5th ed. Baltimore: Williams & Wilkins, 1995, pp 1572–1579.

Kugler JD, Danford DA: Management of infants, children, and adolescents with paroxysmal supraventricular tachycardia. *J Pediatr* 1996;129:324–338.

Losek JD, Endom E, Dietrich A, et al: Adenosine and pediatric supraventricular tachycardia in the emergency department: multicenter study and review. *Ann Emerg Med* 1999;33:185–191.

Ventricular Premature Contractions

Ventricular premature contractions (VPCs) most commonly occur in asymptomatic adolescents without structural heart disease. Other etiologies include ingestions (tobacco, sympathomimetic agents, tricyclic antidepressants, digoxin, caffeine), electrolyte imbalances (hypokalemia, hypocalcemia), anesthesia, and underlying heart disease (mitral valve prolapse, myocarditis, cardiomyopathy, coronary artery disease).

Clinical Presentation

Most cases are discovered during the routine examination of an asymptomatic patient, when an irregular heartbeat is noted. However, some patients complain of chest discomfort, palpitations, chest pain, or syncope.

Diagnosis

VPCs are characterized by bizarre, widened QRS complexes that are not preceded by a P wave (Fig. 3-7). They may occur in a fixed ratio with normal beats (bigeminy 1:1; trigeminy 2:1) (Fig. 3-8). They can be designated as uniform (identical ECG appearance with consistent interval from the preceding QRS) or multiform (dissimilar ECG appearances with varying coupling intervals with the preceding QRS). It is possible for the VPC to fall on the T wave of the preceding normal complex (R-on-T phenomenon) and initiate ventricular tachycardia.

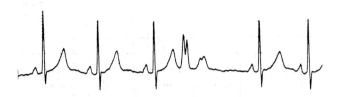

Figure 3-7   Ventricular premature contraction.

VPCs can also be divided into benign and ominous categories. *Benign VPCs* are asymptomatic, uniform, single, and infrequent with a normal resting ECG, including the QTc interval (<0.45); they are not associated with an R-on-T phenomenon or structural heart disease. Benign VPCs can be suppressed by exercise, such as 20 s of "jumping jacks."

Ominous VPCs may be symptomatic, multiform, paired, and associated with a prolonged QTc interval, an R-on-T phenomenon, or structural heart disease. Exercise either has no effect or increases the VPC frequency. Ominous VPCs indicate an increased risk of ventricular tachycardia (three or more consecutive VPCs).

ED Management

Benign VPCs   No treatment is necessary. However, for reassurance, elective referral to a pediatric cardiologist may be indicated.

Ominous VPCs   Consult with a pediatric cardiologist, who may recommend admission and/or treatment.

Follow-up
- Benign VPCs: primary care follow-up in 1 to 2 weeks.

Indication for Admission
- Ominous VPCs

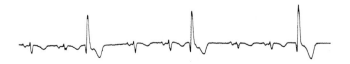

Figure 3-8   VPC in trigeminal pattern.

BIBLIOGRAPHY

Alexander ME, Berul CI: Ventricular arrhythmias: when to worry. *Pediatr Cardiol* 2000;21:532–541.

Carboni MP, Garson A Jr: Ventricular arrhythmias, in Garson A Jr, Bricker TJ, Fisher DJ, Neish SR (eds): *The Science and Practice of Pediatric Cardiology,* 2nd ed. Baltimore: Williams & Wilkins, 1998, pp 2121–2168.

Fish F, Benson DW: Disorders of cardiac rhythm and conduction, in Emmanouildes GC, Riemenschneider TA, Allen HD, Gutgesell HP (eds): *Moss and Adams Heart Disease in Infants, Children, and Adolescents,* 5th ed. Baltimore: Williams & Wilkins, 1995, pp 1587–1596.

Ventricular Tachycardia

Wide-complex tachycardias are uncommon in children, but they are often difficult to diagnose and potentially more dangerous than narrow-complex tachycardias. Wide-complex tachycardias may be ventricular or supraventricular (with aberrancy secondary to a bundle branch block or WPW syndrome) in origin. However, in the ED, *assume that a wide-complex tachycardia is VT* and treat accordingly. Erroneous treatment of VT as SVT can be devastating.

Nonetheless, it is important to remember that the upper limit of normal QRS duration varies with age. For example, a tachycardia with a QRS duration of 0.10 s is wide-complex in a newborn but narrow-complex in a 10-year-old.

VT is defined as a series of three or more consecutive ectopic beats. Etiologies include primary electrical disease (long-QTc syndrome), hypoxemia, arrhythmogenic right ventricular dysplasia, electrolyte imbalance (hyperkalemia), and ingestions (tricyclics, digoxin). Ventricular tachycardia can degenerate into ventricular fibrillation, either as a terminal event or in the setting of a prolonged QT interval.

Clinical Presentation

The symptomatology depends on the rate and duration of the tachycardia and the presence or absence of underlying structural heart disease. Occasional patients are asymptomatic, although chest pain, syncope, and palpitations are common, and lethargy, disorientation, hypotension, and hemodynamic collapse can occur.

Diagnosis

VT is a wide-QRS-complex tachycardia. The rate of ventricular tachycardia (Fig. 3-9) is 120 to 200 bpm, which is slower than *SVT* with aberrant conduction. VT is suggested by AV dissociation or if the QRS morphology resembles that of a single VPC appearing during sinus rhythm elsewhere on the ECG.

ED Management

Regardless of the patient's status, consult a pediatric cardiologist.

Hemodynamically Stable   Give a bolus of IV lidocaine (1 mg/kg), followed by a continuous infusion (20–50 µg/kg/min). If the lidocaine is not

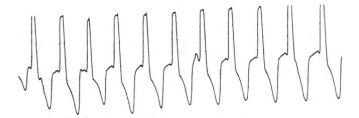

Figure 3-9 Ventricular tachycardia.

successful at restoring normal sinus rhythm, use IV amiodarone (5 mg/kg over 10–15 min). Consult a pediatric cardiologist for further management in an intensive care setting. Bretylium is contraindicated in VT, as its use may precipitate ventricular fibrillation.

Hemodynamically Compromised with Palpable Pulses   The treatment of choice is synchronized cardioversion at an initial dose of 0.5 J/kg; double the dose and repeat if not successful. If the rhythm does not convert, give an IV lidocaine bolus (1 mg/kg) followed by a third attempt at cardioversion. Ventricular pacing by a cardiologist may be required. The treatment is summarized in Fig. 3-5.

Hemodynamically Compromised without Pulses   Defibrillate with 2 J/kg, double to 4 J/kg for a maximum of three consecutive defibrillations or until conversion to sinus rhythm. The treatment is summarized in Fig. 3-6.

Indications for Admission
• Newly diagnosed or difficult-to-control VT.

BIBLIOGRAPHY

Bardella IJ. Pediatric advanced life support: a review of the AHA recommendations. *Am Fam Physician* 1999;60:1743–1750.

Fish F, Benson DW: Disorders of cardiac rhythm and conduction, in Emmanouildes GC, Riemenschneider TA, Allen HD, Gutgesell HP (eds): *Moss and Adams Heart Disease in Infants, Children, and Adolescents,* 5th ed. Baltimore: Williams & Wilkins, 1995, pp 1587–1596.

Flinders DC, Roberts SD: Ventricular arrhythmias. *Prim Care* 2000;27:709–724.

Ventricular Fibrillation

VT can degenerate into ventricular fibrillation, either as a terminal event or when there is a prolonged QT interval or R-on-T phenomenon.

Clinical Presentation

Patients with ventricular fibrillation are generally unresponsive and pulseless.

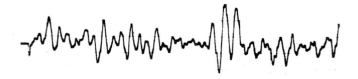

Figure 3-10   Ventricular fibrillation.

Diagnosis

In ventricular fibrillation (Fig. 3-10) there is a wavy, sinusoidal line without any true QRS complexes.

ED Management

If the VT degenerates into ventricular fibrillation, immediately defibrillate using 2 J/kg. If unsuccessful, double to 4 J/kg for three consecutive defibrillations. If unsuccessful, also give IV lidocaine (1 mg/kg) alternating with epinephrine IV or IO (0.01 mg/kg of 1:10,000) or ET (0.1 mg/kg of 1:1000). If fibrillation recurs, start a continuous infusion of lidocaine (20–50 µg/kg/min).

Indication for Admission

- Any patient who survives after treatment for ventricular fibrillation.

BIBLIOGRAPHY

Bardella IJ: Pediatric advanced life support: a review of the AHA recommendations. *Am Fam Physician* 1999;60:1743–1750.

Fish F, Benson DW: Disorders of cardiac rhythm and conduction, in Emmanouildes GC, Riemenschneider TA, Allen HD, Gutgesell HP (eds): *Moss and Adams Heart Disease in Infants, Children, and Adolescents,* 5th ed. Baltimore: Williams & Wilkins, 1995, pp 1587–1596.

Flinders DC, Roberts SD: Ventricular arrhythmias. *Prim Care* 2000;27:709–724.

Heart Block

Heart block is secondary to abnormal atrioventricular conduction. It can be primary, as in patients with congenital complete heart block, or secondary, as with Lyme disease.

Clinical Presentation and Diagnosis

First-Degree Block   First-degree block is a rate-related prolongation of the PR interval (Fig. 3-11). Patients are asymptomatic. It may be seen with increased vagal tone, digoxin administration, myocarditis, acute rheumatic fever, or diphtheria, or it may be a primary electrical phenomenon.

Second-Degree Block   Second-degree block may be secondary to acute or chronic heart disease, or it may occasionally occur in otherwise normal

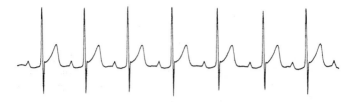

Figure 3-11   First-degree heart block.

children. With *Mobitz type I* (Wenckebach), there is progressive lengthening of the PR interval until the impulse is not conducted and a ventricular beat is dropped (Fig. 3-12). Mobitz type I is thought to occur at the AV node, is more likely to be benign, and can occur in normal patients. In *Mobitz type II,* ventricular beats are dropped without prior prolongation of the PR interval (Fig. 3-13). In Mobitz type II, the site of block is in the more distal AV conduction system; therefore there is a greater chance of progression to complete (third-degree) heart block.

Third-Degree Block   Third-degree heart block represents absolute failure of conduction of the atrial impulses to the ventricles. There is AV dissociation; the atria and ventricles beat completely independently (Fig. 3-14). Generally, the lower the location of the pacemaker within the ventricular conduction system, the slower the rate and the wider the QRS complexes. The etiology may be congenital (isolated or associated with congenital heart disease) or acquired (postoperative, acute rheumatic fever, Lyme disease, streptococcal infection, digoxin toxicity, or hyper- and hypocalcemia).

Many patients with congenital third-degree heart block are asymptomatic. However, a patient may exhibit decreased exercise tolerance, congestive heart failure, dizziness, or syncope. Acquired complete heart block is usually symptomatic, with syncope, congestive heart failure, shock, or sudden death. Symptoms are more likely with an awake pulse <50 bpm, VPCs, structural heart disease, and cardiomegaly.

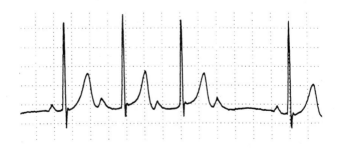

Figure 3-12   Mobitz I second-degree heart block.

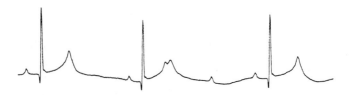

Figure 3-13   Mobitz II second-degree heart block.

ED Management

First-Degree Block   No treatment is required other than determining the etiology of the disturbance.

Second-Degree Block   In addition to determining the etiology, an ambulatory 24-h Holter ECG is indicated. Admit symptomatic patients (dizzy spells or syncope) and consult a pediatric cardiologist to evaluate for possible pacemaker implantation.

Third-Degree Block   Congenital complete heart block sometimes requires pacemaker insertion. Infants with congestive heart failure, hydrops, rates <50 bpm, or VPCs and patients with acquired third-degree blocks require temporary or permanent pacing. The ventricular rate may occasionally be increased by beta-adrenergic agents (isoproterenol) or vagolytics (atropine) in patients awaiting pacemaker placement. Consult a pediatric cardiologist prior to instituting pharmacotherapy.

Follow-up

- Cardiology follow-up within 1 week.

Indications for Admission

- First degree: Serious underlying disease
- Second degree: Newly diagnosed, postoperative, or symptomatic
- Third degree: Congestive failure, newly diagnosed, or syncope

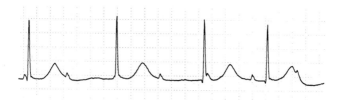

Figure 3-14   Third-degree heart block.

BIBLIOGRAPHY

Eronen M, Sirèn MK, Ekblad H, et al: Short- and long-term outcome of children with congenital complete heart block diagnosed in utero or as a newborn. *Pediatrics* 2000;106:86–91.

Fish F, Benson DW: Disorders of cardiac rhythm and conduction, in Emmanouildes GC, Riemenschneider TA, Allen HD, Gutgesell HP (eds): *Moss and Adams Heart Disease in Infants, Children, and Adolescents*, 5th ed. Baltimore: Williams & Wilkins, 1995, pp 1566–1570.

Ross BA, Trippel DL: Atrioventricular block, in Garson A Jr., Bricker TJ, Fisher DJ, Neish SR (eds): *The Science and Practice of Pediatric Cardiology*, 2nd ed. Baltimore: Williams & Wilkins, 1998, pp 2047–2057.

CHEST PAIN

Chest pain is a common complaint in late childhood and adolescence. It is often a manifestation of underlying cardiac disease in the adult population. In children, however, chest pain is commonly associated with asthma, while cardiac disease is an infrequent etiology. However, it is important to rule out a cardiac etiology.

Clinical Presentation and Diagnosis

Note the characteristics of the pain, including the subjective quality (e.g., sharp, dull, aching), the position in which it is greatest, radiation, duration, and alleviating or exacerbating factors. Cardiac pain is typically associated with exercise and improves with rest. Associated symptoms may be especially useful in determining the etiology of the pain. Also ask about a family history of sudden death (particularly during exercise), cardiomyopathy, or "heart attacks" at early ages.

Noncardiac Etiologies

Musculoskeletal Problems   Musculoskeletal problems are common causes of chest pain in the pediatric population. Tietze's syndrome (costochondritis) is characterized by anterior chest pain and tenderness to palpation over the sternocostal or costochondral junctions. Reproduction of the patient's pain on palpation is the most helpful sign. Intercostal muscle cramping (precordial catch syndrome) in the left substernal area may mimic this condition.

Psychogenic Causes   Although psychogenic causes are the second most frequent, always consider them to be diagnoses of exclusion. An adolescent with hyperventilation or anxiety can present with chest pain. The history may reveal repeated episodes of hysterical behavior, recent personal or family stresses, or a relative with heart disease. Typical complaints include shortness of breath, palpitations, or tingling of the extremities. The pain often mimics one or more organic conditions, but usually it suggests several conditions in the differential diagnosis.

Pulmonary Chest Pain   Chest pain can be pleuritic in nature, exacerbated by deep inspiration, swallowing, and coughing. It is caused by inflammation or irritation of the pleura and is seen most commonly in pneumonia, pleurodynia (coxsackievirus), or pneumothorax, although pulmonary embolism or infarction can present similarly. Bronchospasm may be the most common pulmonary cause of chest pain. A careful history of associated symptoms (fever, cough, preceding upper respiratory infection), oral contraceptive use, and underlying chronic disease (sickle cell anemia, cystic fibrosis, asthma, lupus) is useful for differentiating among these etiologies.

Gastroesophageal Disease   Gastrointestinal reflux, esophagitis, gastritis, and gastrointestinal spasm can all cause precordial pain. While upper esophageal pain is usually well localized, mid- and lower esophageal pain may be noted from the epigastrium to the suprasternal notch and may radiate to the back or arms. The heart and esophagus have similar segmental innervation, so the substernal "burning" pain may mimic angina pectoris, which is distinctly uncommon in the pediatric age group. The discomfort may be associated with eating (postprandially or in the early morning before breakfast), accentuated in the recumbent position and with straining, and relieved with antacids or cold milk.

Cardiac Etiologies
Pericarditis   Pericarditis can present with pleuritic-type chest pain that is relieved by sitting up. Patients are often unable to assume the supine position, and the pain is frequently referred to the neck, shoulders, and abdomen. On physical examination, a pericardial friction rub may be noted in the midprecordial area with the patient supine or in the left lateral decubitus position. The ECG typically shows ST-segment elevation, and a chest x-ray may reveal cardiomegaly if there is a moderately large pericardial effusion. An echocardiogram is useful in excluding a significant pericardial effusion.

Arrhythmias   Inadequate coronary blood flow secondary to an arrhythmia can cause chest pain.

Prolapse of the Mitral Valve   Vague anterior chest pain has been described in patients found to have prolapse of the mitral valve, although this occurs much less frequently than previously thought. Rarely, it may be part of a constellation of symptoms in this condition (dyspnea, palpitations, near syncope, and fatigue). The diagnosis is suggested by auscultation (midsystolic click or clicks and late systolic murmur) and confirmed by two-dimensional echocardiography.

Aortic Dissection   Although aortic dissection is extremely rare in childhood, consider it in a patient with a connective tissue disorder (Marfan's syndrome or Ehlers-Danlos syndrome). The severe pain is typically sudden in onset and "tearing" in quality. Radiation is from the anterior chest to the neck and back.

Coronary Artery Disease Coronary artery disease (myocardial ischemia, angina pectoris, myocardial infarction) is extremely rare in the pediatric population. Patients with arteritis and cocaine use may present with the pain of myocardial ischemia or infarction. Severe, persistent irritability has been noted in infants with aberrant origin of the left coronary artery from the pulmonary artery; rarely, older children present with recurrent episodes of chest pain after exercise. Patients with a history of Kawasaki disease, who are at risk for coronary artery thrombosis and aneurysm, may present with pallor, diaphoresis, or irritability. Coronary artery spasm leading to myocardial ischemia can also be seen.

ED Management

Most cases of chest pain are either musculoskeletal, gastroesophageal, pulmonary, or psychogenic in origin. Therefore a careful history, palpation of the chest wall, and pulmonary and cardiac auscultation usually suffice to determine the etiology and initiate appropriate therapy. Ask an adolescent about the possibility of recent cocaine use. Treat costochondritis with ibuprofen 10 mg/kg q 6 h.

If a cardiac etiology is suspected (irregular pulse, auscultation of an organic murmur, a systolic click, or a friction rub), obtain an ECG and check for ST- or T-wave abnormalities, chamber enlargement or hypertrophy, conduction abnormality, or arrhythmia. Many patients with noncardiac chest pain are concerned about the possibility of heart disease and are reassured by a normal ECG.

Further evaluation is dictated by the history and physical findings. A chest x-ray is indicated for patients with pleuritic chest pain, dyspnea, tachycardia, or cyanosis. Obtain a complete blood count (CBC), erythrocyte sedimentation rate (ESR), and ECG if acute pericarditis or myocarditis is suspected and cardiac enzymes if myocardial infarction is a possibility. If mitral valve prolapse or intermittent arrhythmia is suspected, refer the patient to a cardiologist for a nonemergent evaluation.

Follow-up

- Stable patient with noncardiac chest pain: primary care follow-up in 1 to 2 weeks

Indications for Admission

- Suspected coronary artery disease, pleural effusion, myocarditis, pericarditis, or aortic dissection
- Severe chest pain of unknown etiology

BIBLIOGRAPHY

Kocis KC: Chest pain in pediatrics. *Pediatr Clin North Am* 1999;46:189–203.
Selbst SM: Chest pain in children. *Pediatr Rev* 1997;18:169–173.
Talnor NS, Carboni MP: Chest pain in the adolescent and young adult. *Cardiol Rev* 2000;8:49–56.

CONGESTIVE HEART FAILURE

By definition, congestive heart failure (CHF) occurs when the heart cannot maintain adequate tissue perfusion to meet the body's basal metabolic requirements, which in children includes growth.

Four principal factors determine cardiac function: preload (ventricular end-diastolic volume), contractility (force of ventricular contraction), afterload (force opposing ventricular ejection or intramyocardial tension during ejection), and heart rate. Changes in heart rate or stroke volume directly affect cardiac output, which, in turn, is a major determinant of blood pressure.

In general, physiologic problems include excessive pressure loads, excessive volume loads, inotropic depression from impaired muscle, and rhythm disturbances. Either congenital structural heart defects or acquired diseases affecting the strength of the heart muscle or both can lead to CHF (Table 3-2).

Clinical Presentation

The clinical manifestations of CHF reflect these physiologic adjustments to reduced cardiac function. They include mechanical (hypertrophy and dilatation), biochemical (cardiac cellular energetic changes), neurohumoral (adrenergic nervous system), hematologic (oxygen transport effects), and pulmonary responses (tachypnea).

On examination, the patient is usually tachycardic and tachypneic. Pulmonary congestion causes rales, rhonchi, and wheezing, which may be confused with primary pulmonary disease. In infants, rales may be absent despite considerable tachypnea, while in older children dyspnea on exertion or orthopnea may be present. A chronic cough may be associated with the pulmonary congestion.

Table 3-2   Etiologies of Congestive Heart Failure

Congenital heart disease	**Extracardiac diseases**
Structural problems	Metabolic-endocrine diseases
Left ventricular outflow obstruction	Hypoglycemia
Coarctation of the aorta	Hypocalcemia
Critical aortic stenosis	Electrolyte disorders
Large shunt lesions	Hypothyroidism and thyroid
Severe valvular regurgitation	storm
Rhythm disorders	Sepsis
Postoperative cardiac problems	Lipid disorders
Ischemic cardiomyopathy	
AV valve regurgitation	**Toxins**
	Primary cardiac medicines
Acquired heart disease	Cancer chemotherapy (Adriamycin)
Inflammatory conditions	Digoxin
Myocarditis	Antiarrhythmics
Kawasaki disease	Cocaine
Rheumatic fever	Cardiac depressants
Cardiomyopathy	Phenytoin
Endocarditis	Lidocaine

On cardiac auscultation, there may be a third heart sound (S_3), the ventricular gallop, which is a sign of poor ventricular compliance and increased resistance to filling. A fourth heart sound (S_4), the atrial gallop, can also be heard, particularly in older children, although sometimes both of these can be present with otherwise normal cardiac findings. Not infrequently, a holosystolic, blowing murmur associated with mitral regurgitation can be heard, associated with left ventricular dilatation.

There may also be central and peripheral edema, although this is unusual in infants. Liver enlargement, jugular venous distention, and other signs of tissue fluid accumulation may be seen. The extremities may be pale and cool secondary to compensatory vasoconstriction. Pulsus alternans (beat-to-beat variability in pulse strength) also may be a palpable sign of poor myocardial strength. With chronic CHF, growth failure, especially in young infants, reflects increased caloric expenditure as well as undernutrition associated with feeding difficulties. CHF can also be associated with tachypnea and diaphoresis, particularly during feeding.

Cardiac enlargement results from ventricular dilatation and is usually readily apparent on the chest x-ray, along with pulmonary congestion. Often, cardiomegaly can also be detected by palpation of a laterally displaced cardiac impulse. Cardiac hypertrophy is usually easily noted on an ECG (left or combined ventricular hypertrophy).

Diagnosis

Obtain a thorough history, as the presence of preexisting cardiac disease or of conditions related to myocardial dysfunction can be important indicators of the possibility of CHF. Ask about a history of thalassemia or other chronic anemia, systemic infections such as HIV, systemic illnesses such as collagen vascular disease, or other acquired diseases such as rheumatic fever or Kawasaki disease.

Often, an older child with overt CHF presents with a combination of wheezing, respiratory distress, bibasilar rales, and hepatomegaly. In general, however, wheezing is most often secondary to *asthma*. There may be a history of asthma and allergies or a family history of allergies, or the patient may have eczema. *Bronchiolitis* also causes similar findings during seasonal epidemics. The patient may have fever, rhonchi, and rales in addition to wheezing.

Other causes of tachypnea, respiratory distress, and cough are *pneumonia* (fever, localized fine end-inspiratory rales, no hepatomegaly), *croup* (fever, inspiratory stridor), and *foreign-body aspiration* (sudden onset of inspiratory stridor). Most etiologies of hepatomegaly (pp 233–234) are not associated with tachypnea or respiratory distress. When the diagnosis is in doubt, obtain a chest x-ray to look for cardiomegaly and pulmonary vascular congestion.

ED Management

Although the etiology dictates the specific therapy, begin with general treatment. Give supplemental humidified oxygen and elevate the head and shoulders. Start an IV and obtain blood for arterial blood gases (ABGs), electrolytes, and a CBC. Obtain an ECG early in the course, as therapy for an underlying arrhythmia may be necessary. Inquire about the chronic use of cardiac medications. Consult with a cardiologist to help confirm the diagnosis and develop a specific treatment strategy. The patient may be discharged once the CHF is compensated and the vital signs are stable.

Give IV diuretics (furosemide 1–2 mg/kg) unless pericardial tamponade (p 20) is suspected. Give morphine sulfate (0.05–0.1 mg/kg subcutaneously) if there is pulmonary edema and consequent air hunger and restlessness. A slow transfusion of packed RBCs (10 mL/kg) is indicated for severe anemia (hematocrit <28%). Give sodium bicarbonate (1–2 mEq/kg) only for severe acidosis (pH <7.1); the airway must be secure, since respiratory decompensation may elevate Pco_2 and cerebral edema can develop.

Occasionally, respiratory support including intubation and mechanical ventilation may be required; inotropic support is then usually also needed. In the acute setting, dobutamine or dopamine (3–5 µg/kg/min to start) is preferred. Digoxin may also be given, but its onset of action is longer and specific control over dosage is less precise. In severe cases, addition of afterload-reducing agents (nitroprusside or enalapril) may be required once indwelling pressure monitoring has been secured and a cardiologist is present.

Two-dimensional echocardiography may help identify the cause of the CHF and document the magnitude of the decrease in ventricular function (ejection fraction) as well as the extent of cardiac chamber enlargement and valvar regurgitation. Long-term management usually includes an angiotensin converting enzyme (ACE) inhibitor or beta blocker.

Follow-up

- CHF successfully treated in the ED: 1 to 2 days

Indications for Admission

- Newly diagnosed or worsening CHF
- New arrhythmia or a newly acquired complication, such as endocarditis, which requires urgent attention.

BIBLIOGRAPHY

Balagurur D, Artman M, Auslender M: Management of heart failure in children. *Curr Probl Pediatr* 2000;30:1–35.

O'Laughlin MP: Congestive heart failure in children. *Pediatr Clin North Am* 1999; 46:263–273.

Shaddy RE, Tanc LY, Gidding SS, et al: Beta blocker treatment of dilated cardiomyopathy with congestive heart failure in children: a multi-institutional experience. *J Heart Lung Transplant* 1999;18:269–274.

CYANOSIS

Cyanosis specifically refers to a bluish tone visible in the mucous membranes and skin when desaturated or abnormal hemoglobin is present in the peripheral circulation. At least 5 g/dL of reduced hemoglobin is required for cyanosis to be visible. Thus, systemic desaturation may be substantial but inapparent to the eye if there is an associated anemia. Conversely, abnormal hemoglobins may be fully saturated with oxygen yet unable to release it to the tissues, so cyanosis will also be visible. Methemoglobinemia is the classic example of this situation.

Central cyanosis occurs when poorly oxygenated blood enters the systemic circulation. This usually occurs through a cardiac defect allowing systemic venous blood to bypass the pulmonary capillary bed. This is termed a *right-to-left shunt* and may occur within the heart or in the pulmonary circulation itself or when there is primary parenchymal lung disease or neurologic disease causing alveolar hypoventilation.

Typical cyanotic lesions are the "five Ts" of congenital heart disease (tetralogy of Fallot, transposition of the great vessels, total anomalous pulmonary venous return, tricuspid atresia, and truncus arteriosus), but others may also be present. Pulmonary diseases causing cyanosis can occur anywhere along the airway, from upper airway obstructive problems (croup, epiglottitis) to lower airway diseases (asthma, cystic fibrosis, pneumonia with lobar consolidation).

Peripheral cyanosis, on the other hand, usually does not reflect reduced systemic arterial oxygenation but is typically found in otherwise healthy patients who are exposed to cold or who have a vasoconstrictor response to fever. Peripheral cyanosis, visible particularly in the nail beds but absent from the perioral mucous membranes or conjunctivae, can occur as a result of circulatory insufficiency or chronic neuromuscular disease with changes in peripheral vasomotor tone.

Clinical Presentation and Diagnosis

Observation for the presence of cyanosis requires proper ambient conditions. Neon lighting, for example, may cause a false bluish tint, while cyanosis may be difficult to discern in a dark-skinned patient unless there is a strong light source.

Respiratory findings are of vital importance and may help to differentiate among the possible causes of cyanosis. Tachypnea may be present with most pulmonary diseases or with cardiac conditions associated with excess pulmonary blood flow. Shallow respirations, not necessarily associated with an increase in rate, may indicate a neurologic problem. Hyperpnea, or deep breathing with only a mild increase in rate, is more characteristic of a primary cardiac disorder where alveolar ventilation is maximized but pulmonary blood flow is reduced. Hyperpnea can also reflect metabolic acidosis or elevated intracranial pressure.

Differentiating cardiac from pulmonary etiologies is critical. In many, though not all, cases of cardiac disease, the breath sounds will be normal and the pattern of chest excursions symmetric, while wheezes, rhonchi, and chest wall abnormalities usually accompany a pulmonary process. In either case there is reduced oxygen saturation, but the patient with cyanotic cardiac disease has little response to increased ambient oxygen; whereas with pulmonary disease, the increase in saturation may be dramatic (hyperoxia test). An ABG may also be useful, since an elevated P_{CO_2} indicating impaired ventilatory status is usually not seen with cyanotic congenital heart disease unless there is associated pulmonary congestion. The chest x-ray may reveal cardiomegaly, an abnormal pulmonary circulatory pattern, or overt pulmonary parenchymal abnormalities such as atelectasis or pneumothorax.

The absence of a heart murmur does not rule out cyanotic cardiac disease; in most conditions with right-to-left shunting, there is no murmur. Also, in some conditions, such as tetralogy of Fallot, the murmur may lessen as the cyanosis becomes more intense secondary to decreased pulmonary blood flow.

ED Management

See p 53 for the treatment of an acute hypoxemic attack ("spell"). For chronic cyanotic congenital heart conditions, supportive treatment is all that can be offered until a surgical or catheter-directed intervention can be accomplished. Give supplemental oxygen, even though dramatic changes in saturation will not occur with oxygen alone. Secure IV access and give fluid to maintain an adequate circulating volume. Treat systemic acidosis once adequate ventilation is assured. Most of all, immediately consult with a cardiovascular specialist to arrange for more definitive treatment and to prevent unnecessary interventions.

Indication for Admission

- Central cyanosis.

BIBLIOGRAPHY

Gewitz MH: Introduction to the clinical examination, in Gewitz MH (ed): *Primary Pediatric Cardiology.* Mt. Kisco, NY: Futura, 1995, pp 25–57.
Grifka RG: Cyanotic congenital heart disease with increased pulmonary blood flow. *Pediatr Clin North Am* 1999;46:405–425.
Tingelstadt J: Consultation with the specialist: nonrespiratory cyanosis. *Pediatr Rev* 1999;20:350–352.

CYANOTIC ("TET") SPELLS

Acute hypoxemic attacks represent a true emergency, and initial treatment is crucial to long-term outcome. Usually, the underlying diagnosis is tetralogy of Fallot or a variant, hence the pseudonym for these attacks is *tet spells.*

In a tet spell, an acute increase in obstruction to pulmonary blood flow has occurred, either at the level of the right ventricular outflow tract within the heart or at the level of the pulmonary circulation, with a consequent increase in right-to-left shunting through an intracardiac septal defect. Alternatively, if systemic perfusion is reduced, as with hypovolemia or the development of a tachyarrhythmia, right-to-left shunting will also increase and a cyanotic spell develop.

Clinical Presentation and Diagnosis

Spells are particularly common in the early morning, shortly after the patient awakens, when there is a rapid shift in circulatory dynamics from the recumbent sleeping state. Prolonged agitation and crying are also cited as precipitants, but it is sometimes unclear whether the developing hypoxemia itself has caused the agitated state, which is then first noticed by the parent. Also, noxious stimuli, such as blood drawing or a bee sting, or any circumstance that leads to enhanced catecholamine output, can precipitate a spell in a susceptible child.

When caring for an acutely hypoxemic infant or child, inquire about a history of congenital heart disease, which raises the possibility that a spell has occurred. Rapid diagnosis of the presence of any form of tetralogy of Fallot is a priority. Obtain a chest x-ray, which may reveal poor pulmonary blood flow and the typical *coeur en sabot* (boot-shaped heart), while the pulmonary parenchyma will be normal. An ECG is useful to show right ventricular hypertrophy and a rightward axis and to rule out an underlying tachyarrhythmia. In such cases, the absence of a heart murmur is a worrisome indicator that pulmonary blood flow is severely compromised.

ED Management

Management is directed at manipulating the relative resistances of the systemic and pulmonary vascular beds as well as maintenance of appropriate circulating volume and heart rate. Flex the child's knees to the chest to help raise systemic tone. Some older patients will instinctively squat to achieve the same result. Give 100% oxygen, which also increases systemic resistance and may help enhance oxygen delivery. Treat any underlying arrhythmia and correct hypovolemia.

If oxygen and position changes do not break the spell, establish IV access and give morphine sulfate (0.1 mg/kg IV or subcutaneously). Although the precise mechanism of action is unclear, morphine may cause pulmonary vasodilation and also provide a beneficial sedative effect, with consequent reduction of catecholamine secretion.

If the patient fails to demonstrate improved oxygen saturation promptly or is obtunded, give an IV fluid bolus of 20 mL/kg normal saline and obtain an ABG. Treat metabolic acidosis with sodium bicarbonate, 1 to 2 mEq/kg by *slow* IV, only if ventilation is adequate (low or normal Pco_2). If cyanosis persists, give phenylephrine (10 µg/kg by slow IV push) to pharmacologically increase the systemic vascular resistance. Intubation and mechanical ventilation may also be necessary in severe, protracted spells.

Follow-up

- Tet spell responding to positional maneuvers: 3 to 5 days

Indication for Admission

- Any hypoxemic attack requiring medical attention (not responding to simple positional maneuvers)

BIBLIOGRAPHY

Driscoll DJ: Evaluation of the cyanotic newborn. *Pediatr Clin North Am* 1990; 37:1–27.

Gewitz MH: Introduction to the clinical examination, in Gewitz MH (ed): *Primary Pediatric Cardiology*. Mt. Kisco, NY: Futura, 1995, pp 25–57.

Walsman JD, Wernly JA: Cyanotic congenital heart disease with decreased pulmonary blood flow in children. *Pediatr Clin North Am* 1999;46:385–404.

HEART MURMURS

Although congenital heart disease is present in only about 0.8% of the general population, the prevalence of heart murmurs in children approaches 50 to 60%. Most murmurs, therefore, are "innocent" or "functional" and not pathologic.

Clinical Presentation and Diagnosis

Innocent Murmur
An innocent murmur is systolic, is short in duration, stops well before the second heart sound, and is midfrequency or "vibratory" in quality. The intensity is less than or equal to grade III/VI and decreases when the patient is in the upright position or during a Valsalva maneuver. It is usually best heard in the second or third left intercostal space and is not associated with other findings suggestive of cardiovascular disease (wide, fixed, or paradoxical splitting of S_2; ejection click). Types of innocent murmurs include the following:

Still's Murmur   Still's murmur occurs in over 50% of children between 4 and 10 years of age. It is vibratory, musical, or squeaking, heard best in the midprecordium between the lower left sternal border and the apex; it is generally grade II to III/VI in intensity. There is a normal S_2, no ejection click, and no thrill.

Pulmonic Ejection Murmur   A pulmonic ejection murmur is noted most often in older children and young adolescents. It is early- to midsystolic, diamond-shaped, grade I to III/VI in intensity, and blowing rather than vibratory in quality. It is best detected in the second left intercostal space. There is a normal S_2 and no thrill, click, or diastolic murmur.

Venous Hum   A venous hum can be appreciated in over 60% of children 3 to 6 years of age. It is heard best in the supraclavicular area, especially on the right. It is systolic-diastolic in nature with diastolic accentuation and generally grade I to III/VI in intensity. However, the loudness may change with rotation of the head and generally diminishes with compression of the jugular vein; release of pressure causes accentuation of the murmur for a few seconds. There is no thrill, systolic accentuation, or increased peripheral pulsation.

Functional Murmurs

Like innocent murmurs, functional murmurs occur in association with normal cardiac anatomy but are generally associated with conditions in which stroke volume is increased (fever, anemia, hyperthyroidism).

Organic Murmurs

In contrast to the conditions described above, organic murmurs are the result of turbulent blood flow through abnormal cardiac structures or communications. Murmurs that are diastolic (other than a venous hum); right-sided; holosystolic; harsh in quality; associated with a thrill, ejection click, or fixed S_2 splitting; or accompanied by physical findings consistent with heart disease (cyanosis, clubbing, absent lower extremity pulses, signs of congestive heart failure) suggest that a murmur is organic.

ED Management

With the exception of possible bacterial endocarditis, a murmur itself does not require acute management. Rather, intervention may be necessary for the underlying disease causing the murmur. Refer all patients with murmurs that do not meet the strict criteria of an innocent or functional murmur to a pediatric cardiologist.

Most patients with organic murmurs require subacute bacterial endocarditis (SBE) prophylaxis prior to undergoing dental or genitourinary manipulation. Patients with murmurs secondary to rheumatic heart disease require rheumatic fever prophylaxis. The fact that a child is receiving rheumatic fever prophylaxis does not obviate the need for SBE prophylaxis.

Indications for Admission

- Signs of congestive heart failure or acute rheumatic fever
- Suspected or proven infective endocarditis

BIBLIOGRAPHY

Danford DA: Effective use of the consultant, laboratory testing, and echocardiography for the pediatric patient with heart murmur. *Pediatr Ann* 2000;29:482–488.
Gessner IH: What makes a heart murmur innocent? *Pediatr Ann* 1997;26:82–91.
Pelech AN: Evaluation of the pediatric patient with a cardiac murmur. *Pediatr Clin North Am* 1999;46:167–188.

INFECTIVE ENDOCARDITIS

Infective endocarditis (IE) is an infection of the endothelium of the heart valves or great vessels. It most commonly develops in a patient with pre-existing congenital heart disease, particularly valvular anomalies (aortic stenosis, prosthetic valve) and conditions associated with increased turbulence of blood flow (ventricular septal defect, aortic regurgitation). In this regard, conditions such as isolated secundum atrial septal defect are not likely to be related to IE.

A substantial percentage of IE cases occur in patients with no preexisting cardiac anomaly. These children have developed acute bacterial endocarditis and may suddenly become extremely ill.

For IE to occur, the endocardium must be exposed to potentially pathogenic bacteria. Dental treatments can result in bacteremia even without periodontal disease. Similarly, certain surgical procedures (tonsillectomy, urologic surgery) or the presence of a chronic indwelling parenteral catheter also place the patient at risk.

Clinical Presentation and Diagnosis

Diligence is required to suspect and treat IE and to refrain from other incorrect therapy. Inquire about any factors establishing a milieu for IE, particularly recent dental and surgical procedures, the presence of a venous catheter, and IV drug use.

Although fever in any patient with congenital heart disease raises the possibility of IE, certain situations are particularly worrisome. These are a protracted febrile illness, particularly without any obvious focus, even if thought to be of "viral" etiology; a documented change in the clinical picture, such as the development of a new heart murmur or congestive heart failure; the onset of hematuria; signs of either cutaneous emboli or embolic events to other organs; a new neurologic finding; or a focal infection such as pneumonia or meningitis.

Frequently, early signs and symptoms may be subtle. Classic findings such as change in a murmur, evidence of emboli, and splenomegaly may not be easily discernible. Nonetheless, carefully examine the conjunctivae, nail beds, palms, soles of the feet, and other skin surfaces to search for evidence of emboli, including tender nodules in the finger or toe pads (Osler nodes), small hemorrhages on the palms or soles (Janeway lesions), and linear subungual lesions (splinter hemorrhages). Perform a careful fundoscopic exam and serial auscultations, as murmurs may be transient and change may be rapid. Conversely, in fulminant acute IE, only the signs of severely compromised circulatory status may be present, without any heart murmur.

Obtain blood for a CBC, ESR, blood culture, and urinalysis. The diagnosis is ultimately confirmed by obtaining positive blood cultures. There may be a leukocytosis with a leftward shift, anemia, and an elevated ESR. The urinalysis may reveal pyuria, hematuria, and proteinuria. Infective endocarditis is a cause of immune complex nephritis. Scrape any cutaneous emboli and examine after Gram's staining. If IE is being considered, consult a cardiologist to arrange for a two-dimensional echocardiogram. If a vegetation is identified, the study can confirm the diagnosis before the blood results have become available.

ED Management

While it may sometimes be crucial to initiate treatment rapidly, it is always imperative that an alternative diagnosis not be obscured. The treatment of IE involves protracted use of appropriate antibiotics, depending on culture and sensitivity results. Attempt to obtain at least two sets of blood cultures from any febrile child at risk for IE (congenital heart disease, normal heart but chronic indwelling catheter) *before antibiotics are administered*. Once the cultures have been obtained, give broad-spectrum IV antibiotics such as penicillin (200,000 U/kg/day divided q 4 h, 18 million U/day maximum) or ceftriaxone (100 mg/kg/day, 4 g/day maximum) combined with gentamicin (3 mg/kg/day divided q 8 h, 240 mg/day maximum). If there is particular suspicion for a gram-negative organism, as in an immunocompromised patient, use ampicillin (300 mg/kg/day divided q 6 h, 12 g/day maximum) or ceftriaxone combined with gentamicin.

Indication for Admission

- Suspected or proven infective endocarditis

BIBLIOGRAPHY

Bayer AS, Bolger AF, Taubert KA, et al: Diagnosis and management of infective endocarditis and its complications. *Circulation* 1998;48:2936–2948.

Brook MM: Pediatric bacterial endocarditis: treatment and prophylaxis. *Pediatr Clin North Am* 1999;46:275–287.

Martin JM, Neches WH, Wald ER: Infective endocarditis: 35 years of experience at a children's hospital. *Clin Infect Dis* 1997;24:669–675.

PERICARDIAL DISEASE

Three distinct disease processes can involve the pericardium: pericarditis, pericardial effusion, and pericardial tamponade. Infections are the most common etiology of pericardial diseases, but there are a variety of other causes in childhood (Table 3-3).

Pericarditis   Pericarditis is inflammation of the pericardium (infectious or noninfectious).

Pericardial Effusion   A pericardial effusion is the accumulation of fluid in the pericardial space.

Pericardial Tamponade   Pericardial tamponade is impaired cardiac output secondary to reduced ventricular filling. This is caused either by fluid accumulation in the pericardial space or by constriction of the heart from an abnormally thickened pericardium. The rapid accumulation of a small amount of fluid can produce tamponade, while chronic slow accumulation is more readily tolerated.

Clinical Presentation and Diagnosis

Pericarditis   Chest pain is the initial symptom in acute pericarditis. It is a constant, sharp sensation across the anterior precordium and is frequently associated with shoulder discomfort. The pain varies with position, being worse when the patient is supine and relieved when he

Table 3-3   Etiologies of Pericarditis

Infectious	Traumatic
Bacterial	Postpericardiotomy syndrome
H. influenzae	Chest wall injury
Staphylococcus	
Streptococcus	**Oncologic**
Pneumococcus	Leukemia
Viral	Lymphoma
Other	
(Tuberculosis, fungal)	**Other**
	Drug-induced (minoxidil)
Inflammatory	Blood dyscrasias
Rheumatic	
Collagen	

or she is upright. Respiratory symptoms, particularly tachypnea, typically accompany the pain. There is often a history of a preceding upper respiratory tract infection. Fever is usually present, and the patient may also complain of abdominal pain. There may be a history of open heart surgery in the past 10 to 14 days (postpericardiotomy syndrome).

Pericardial Effusion   When a substantial pericardial effusion is present, the symptoms may mimic CHF. There may be tachypnea with chest retractions and nasal flaring. With impaired cardiac output, tachycardia and vasoconstriction occur, with pallor, low blood pressure, and cool extremities. Other findings secondary to systemic congestion are hepatosplenomegaly and neck vein distention.

Pericardial Tamponade   Cardiac tamponade is a true medical emergency. Classic findings include hypotension, distended neck veins, muffled heart sounds, and the presence of pulsus paradoxus, a greater than 10 mmHg fall in systolic blood pressure associated with inspiration. A fall in the blood pressure of more than 20 mmHg is serious. Pulsus paradoxus may also be found in respiratory disorders such as *asthma* and in *congestive heart failure.*

On auscultation, findings depend on the amount of fluid accumulated. When inflammation is present without fluid, as in acute pericarditis, there is often a loud friction rub. This is a scratchy, harsh sound heard throughout the cardiac cycle. The pericardial rub diminishes in proportion to the volume of the fluid collection. The heart sounds in general decrease in intensity in direct proportion to pericardial fluid volume. Particularly ominous is the agitated child with signs of reduced cardiac output and a "quiet" auscultatory examination.

Obtain an ECG and chest x-ray. With pericarditis, the ECG reveals elevated ST segments and often generalized T-wave inversions. Diminished precordial voltage usually indicates pericardial fluid accumulation. On x-ray, the heart size is increased with pericardial effusion but may be small with pericardial constriction without fluid (constrictive pericarditis). Other laboratory tests are nonspecific. With purulent pericarditis, there is leukocytosis and an elevated ESR. However, viral diseases will often be associated with normal values of both parameters, and the highest acute-phase reactants can be seen with rheumatologic pericarditis.

ED Management

The approach to the child with pericardial disease varies depending on whether there is an effusion.

Pericarditis   For pericarditis without fluid accumulation, invasive treatment is not warranted. Admit the patient, give analgesics (aspirin, ibuprofen, or indomethacin), and observe for the development of complications (effusion, tamponade, myocarditis). Steroids are usually not indicated for initial management.

Pericardial Effusion   Closely follow the vital signs and degree of pulsus paradoxus, as pericardial fluid accumulation is usually a dynamic process. Rapidly changing circumstances may precipitate an acute crisis. Consult a cardiologist and admit the patient. Diagnostic pericardiocentesis may be required, especially if purulent pericarditis is suspected.

If purulent pericarditis is suspected, provide supplemental oxygen, establish IV access, and arrange for pericardiocentesis. Obtain blood and pericardial fluid specimens and begin broad-spectrum antibiotics with *Staphylococcus aureus* and *Haemophilus influenzae* type B coverage (nafcillin 150 mg/kg/day divided q 6 h and cefotaxime 150–200 mg/kg/day divided q 6 h). The incidence of pericarditis caused by *H. influenzae* type B has decreased dramatically since the advent of immunization against it.

Pericardial Tamponade   When a substantial volume of pericardial fluid has accumulated, tamponade can develop rapidly. Arrange for immediate therapeutic drainage.

Indications for Admission

- Pericardial effusion (unless chronic)
- Pericarditis
- Pericardial tamponade

BIBLIOGRAPHY

Rheuban K: Pericardial disease, in Allen HD, Gutgesall HP, Clark EB, Driscoll D (eds): *Moss and Adams' Heart Disease in Infants, Children and Adolescents*, 6th ed. New York: Lippincott Williams & Wilkins, 2001, pp 1287–1296.
Roodpeyma S, Sadeghian N: Acute pericarditis in childhood: a 10-year experience. *Pediatr Cardiol* 2000;21:363–367.
Towbin JA: Myocarditis and pericarditis in adolescents. *Adolesc Med* 2001;12:47–67.

SYNCOPE

Syncope is a transient loss of consciousness accompanied by loss of postural tone resulting from decreased cerebral perfusion.

Clinical Presentation

The unconscious period may be preceded by a history of an inciting factor, such as a noxious stimulus, an excessively warm environment, emotional upset, or exercise. The patient may report a prodrome of dizziness, diaphoresis, headache, chest pain, palpitations, visual or auditory phenomena, or respiratory distress. There may be a history of recurrent episodes. Findings on physical examination may include diaphoresis, hypotension (sometimes postural), tachycardia or bradycardia, lethargy, or dilated pupils. Mechanisms of syncope can be classified into three groups: neurocardiovascular, cardiac, or nonneurocardiovascular.

Neurocardiovascular

Vasovagal
Vasodilatation, with pooling of blood in capacitance vessels, causes decreased blood pressure with a resultant decrease in cerebral perfusion. Usually, an associated increase in vagal tone results in bradycardia and diaphoresis. Vasodepressor syncope is often precipitated by noxious stimuli, strong emotions, or fatigue and is common in adolescents.

Orthostatic Hypotensive Syncope   This occurs on assuming an erect posture. It is rare in young children but not uncommon in normal adolescents. It may also occur if the patient is dehydrated, chronically fatigued or malnourished, has suffered an acute blood loss, or is taking vasodilator drugs. These patients can have tachycardia associated with the syncope, the so-called postural orthostatic tachycardia syndrome.

Cardioinhibitory   Parasympathetic impulses cause a severe bradycardic response.

Cardiac

Although uncommon, cardiac causes of syncope can be life-threatening. The mechanism may involve hypoxemia due to cyanotic heart disease or decreased cardiac output secondary to myocardial dysfunction, arrhythmias, or obstructive lesions.

Structural Lesions
Syncope can occur in patients with obstructive lesions (severe valvar or subvalvar aortic stenosis, pulmonary hypertension) secondary to low cardiac output, cyanotic heart disease (tetralogy of Fallot) secondary to hypoxia, or mitral valve prolapse. Most of these episodes occur during physical exertion; this history suggests a cardiac etiology. Generally, there are auscultatory abnormalities, such as a murmur or abnormality of the second heart sound or evidence of ventricular hypertrophy on the ECG.

Arrhythmias
Arrhythmias such as atrioventricular block (second- or third-degree) may cause syncope. Sick sinus syndrome is usually seen in the setting of repaired congenital heart disease. These patients may develop syncope secondary to severe bradycardia or sinus arrest. Syncope can also be associated with paroxysmal supraventricular tachycardia, atrial flutter, and atrial fibrillation, especially in patients with WPW syndrome. Ventricular tachycardia or ventricular fibrillation may present with syncope in patients with repaired congenital heart disease, arrhythmogenic right ventricular dysplasia, or primary electrical disease.

Syncope is also associated with long-QT syndrome (LQTS), either congenital (the Romano-Ward syndrome, deafness-associated Jervell-Lange-Neilsen syndrome) or acquired [many drugs, including antibiotics (clarithromycin, erythromycin), antiarrhythmics (sotalol, ibutilide, flecainide, quinidine), tricyclic antidepressants, antipsychotics, electrolyte imbalance, or starvation diets]. LQTS can lead to a specific dysrhythmia, a polymorphic ventricular tachycardia called torsades de pointes. Consider LQTS in children with a history of syncope and a corrected QT interval greater than 0.45 s.

Nonneurocardiovascular Syncope

Cerebral Hypoxemia
Hypoxia and anemia (rare) can cause syncope secondary to decreased cerebral oxygen delivery despite normal cardiac output. Respiratory causes include breath-holding spells in infants and toddlers (pp 449–450) and hyperventilation in adolescents. The infant or child with a breath-holding spell becomes pallid or cyanotic before losing consciousness, while hyperventilating adolescents may have paresthesias or carpopedal spasm. In both, there is usually a history of emotional upset.

Hysterical Fainting
Hysterical fainting occurs primarily in patients with a histrionic (theatrical) personality style. These episodes can last for up to 1 h and usually occur in front of others. The pulse and blood pressure are normal, and there is never any associated injury.

Fasting Hypoglycemia
Fasting hypoglycemia is the most common metabolic cause of syncope. Inquire about a history of diabetes or insulin use. Weakness, diaphoresis, confusion, and palpitations may occur prior to the actual syncopal episode, which is gradual in onset. Also, aspirin and ethanol ingestions can be associated with hypoglycemia.

Consider *seizures* in the differential diagnosis, although true syncope lacks convulsive movements, an aura, or a postictal state. Frequent episodes of loss of consciousness suggest epilepsy. *Migraine headaches* involving the vertebrobasilar system can cause syncope preceded by an aura and followed by the headache.

Diagnosis

A careful history usually suggests the diagnosis. Especially important is a description of the events leading up to the episode, particularly whether the syncope was abrupt and without warning or was preceded by light-headedness, dizziness, sweating, palpitations, chest pain, or respiratory distress. *Cardiac syncope* can be sudden, without any warning. Inquire about the frequency of the attacks, any sequelae after the episode, possible drug ingestion, and family history of arrhythmia, syncope, sudden death, or deafness (which may be associated with the LQTS).

On physical examination check for orthostatic vital sign changes, odors on the breath (ethanol, ketones), and murmurs. Most cardiac etiologies can be ruled out by auscultation and a 12-lead ECG with a long rhythm strip. Causative arrhythmias such as SVT, ventricular tachycardia, sick sinus syndrome, or heart block are usually not present on admission, but underlying predisposing conditions such as WPW syndrome and prolonged LQTS may be identified. If these are not found and the history does not suggest another etiology for the syncope, 24-h ambulatory monitoring is indicated.

ED Management

Unless it is clear that the patient has suffered a vasovagal episode, obtain an ECG with rhythm strip and blood for hematocrit, Dextrostix, and serum glucose. The diagnosis and management of hypoglycemia (pp 165–168) and anemia (pp 299–302) are discussed elsewhere.

Instruct patients with *orthostatic syncope* to get up slowly after lying or sitting and discontinue any implicated medications. Suggest increased fluid intake, and if the blood pressure is normal, recommend additional salt intake. The autonomic dysfunction can be documented by tilt-table testing. Reassurance and primary care follow-up are all that are usually needed for *hyperventilation* or *breath-holding.* Consult with a pediatric cardiologist for *LQTS* or other causes of cardiac syncope.

Follow-up

- Vasovagal, hyperventilation, or breath-holding episode: primary care follow-up in 1 week.

Indications for Admission

- Recurrent syncope
- Cardiac syncope likely
- Significant injury caused by the syncopal episode

BIBLIOGRAPHY

Lewis DA, Dhala A: Syncope in the pediatric patient. *Pediatr Clin North Am* 1999;
    46:205–219.
Stewart J, Gewitz M, Munoz JL, et al: Orthostatic intolerance in adolescent chronic
    fatigue syndrome. *Pediatrics* 1999;103:116–121.
Tanel RE, Walsh EP: Syncope in the pediatric patient. *Cardiol Clin* 1997;15:
    277–294.

CHAPTER 4

Dental Emergencies

B. J. Mistry and Steven Krauss

NORMAL DENTITION AND ASSOCIATED COMPLAINTS

Children may present to the emergency department (ED) with a primary dental or oral soft tissue complaint. Alternatively, a dental problem may be secondary or incidental to another problem. Dental anatomy is shown in Fig. 4-1.

Natal Teeth   Natal teeth are primary lower central incisors that are either present at birth or erupt shortly thereafter. If they are painful to a nursing mother, refer the patient to a pediatric dentist or oral surgeon for extraction

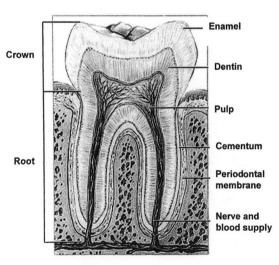

Figure 4-1   Tooth anatomy.

Table 4-1   Chronology of Tooth Eruption

Tooth	PRIMARY TEETH (MONTHS)		PERMANENT TEETH (YEARS)	
	Maxillary	*Mandibular*	*Maxillary*	*Mandibular*
Central incisor	7½	6	7–8	6–7
Lateral incisor	9	7	8–9	7–8
Cuspid	18	16	11–12	9–10
First bicuspid	—	—	10–11	10–12
Second bicuspid	—	—	10–12	11–12
First molar	14	12	6–7	6–7
Second molar	24	20	12–13	11–13
Third molar	—	—	17–21	17–21

at the parent's convenience. Loose natal teeth are an aspiration hazard. Refer the patient for immediate extraction. Otherwise, these teeth can remain until the normal exfoliation at about age 6.

Delayed Eruption   As shown in Table 4-1, typically the lower (mandibular) central incisors are the first teeth to erupt at about 6 months of age, followed by the upper (maxillary) central incisors. However, the pattern can vary, so defer concerns of eruption timing or sequence to an elective pediatric dental referral. There is even more variability in the eruption of the permanent dentition.

Minor Teething Pain   This is best treated with a teething toy that can be frozen. The cold and biting pressure often alleviate the discomfort. Acetaminophen (15 mg/kg q 4 h), ibuprofen (10 mg/kg q 6 h), or teething remedies containing 10 to 20% benzocaine. While it is controversial whether teething causes symptoms such as low-grade fever, excessive drooling, crankiness, decreased feeding, and loose stools, many infants and children remain asymptomatic.

Eruption Cyst   An eruption cyst is a fluctuant, fluid-filled sac overlying an erupting primary or permanent tooth. It will resolve spontaneously upon eruption of the tooth.

Eruption Hematoma   An eruption hematoma is a bluish or reddish blood-filled sac overlying an erupting primary or permanent tooth. It will resolve spontaneously upon eruption of the tooth.

Eruption Gingivitis This is a localized inflammation of gum tissue overlying a partially erupted tooth. In adolescents with erupting or impacted wisdom teeth, entrapped debris and microorganisms may lead to infection (pericoronitis), with localized swelling and tenderness or, in severe cases, fever, facial swelling, trismus, and dysphagia.

Follow-up

- Loose natal tooth: dentist or oral surgeon immediately.

BIBLIOGRAPHY

Cunha RF, Boer FA, Torriani DD, et al: Natal and neonatal teeth: review of the literature. *Pediatr Dent* 2001;23:158–162.

Frank J, Drezner J: Is teething in infants associated with fever or other symptoms? *J Fam Pract* 2001;50:257.

Wake M, Hesketh K, Lucas J: Teething and tooth eruption in infants: a cohort study. *Pediatrics* 2000;106:1374–1379.

CARIES AND DENTAL INFECTIONS

The most common cause of dental pain is *caries*. Dental caries (cavities) result from the interaction of normal oral flora (*Streptococcus mutans*) and easily fermentable carbohydrates, particularly sucrose. Dental infections during childhood are caused by pulp necrosis secondary to caries or tooth trauma. Infection then spreads through the root canal into the periapical (periodontal) tissue, causing an acute dentoalveolar abscess. The most common organisms are anaerobes and *Streptococcus viridans*.

Clinical Presentation

Cavity Caries most commonly occur on occlusal surfaces (pits and fissures), proximal surfaces of back molars, and the gingival parts of free smooth surfaces. They initially appear as dull, opaque, white discolorations that cavitate and then acquire yellow to brown discoloration. Cavities remain asymptomatic until the infection spreads through the enamel and dentin into the viable pulp tissue; therefore they are often visible before symptoms occur. Initially, pain may present only upon ingestion of sweet or cold foods. As the infection spreads, symptoms include local or diffuse pain, gingival swelling, and percussion sensitivity without excessive mobility.

Nursing-Bottle Caries Nursing-bottle caries occur in children between 1 and 4 years of age. The condition is caused by prolonged contact with cariogenic liquids (milk, fruit juices, soda), usually secondary to sleeping with a bottle at night or prolonged breast feeding. Although different liquids differ in their cariogenicity, any liquid other than water can cause decay if the teeth are bathed in it all night. A similar clinical picture can be caused by sucrose-sweetened medicine, pacifiers dipped in sugar, and, rarely, excessive breast feeding. Typically, the labial and palatal surfaces of the primary maxillary incisors and primary first molars are affected, while the mandibular incisors are usually spared. Extensive tooth discoloration and gross destruction of the crowns can occur.

Dental Abscess   A dental abscess can be caused by periapical infection of a necrotic tooth, often secondary to previous carious lesions or trauma to an intact tooth. An abscess presents with gingival erythema, mild to severe pain, percussion tenderness, soft tissue swelling, and lymphadenopathy. The tooth may be mobile and extruded from the socket. Sometimes a fistulous tract develops and opens onto the buccal or lingual gingival mucosa, forming a parulis (gum boil). The pain is alleviated by drainage, which may occur spontaneously or upon palpation of the tooth or gingiva. On occasion, the abscess extends into the skin, causing a facial cellulitis.

Facial Cellulitis   Infection from a severely decayed tooth can spread through soft tissues, causing a cellulitis, most often in the buccal area. Cellulitis may present with fever, pain, tenderness, trismus, swelling of the face or neck, and regional lymphadenopathy. Always examine the gingiva and teeth of a patient with facial cellulitis, as it may be secondary to a spreading dental infection.

Fat necrosis of the cheeks may be caused by cold exposure, usually from sucking on ice pops ("popsicle panniculitis"). The patient is afebrile and nontoxic, and the lesions are indurated and only minimally tender.

Deep Fascial Space Infections   Oral infections may spread to the deep fascial spaces of the head and neck. Depending on the tooth and drainage area involved, varying degrees of pain, swelling, and trismus occur. In severe cases, involvement of the sublingual, pharyngeal, retropharyngeal, parapharyngeal, or pretracheal areas can occur, leading to respiratory compromise, dysphagia, and dyspnea. In Ludwig's angina, a dental abscess beginning behind the first permanent molar can expand rapidly. The mass can then cross the midline and impinge upon and compromise the airway.

Diagnosis

Inquire about a history of recent or past dental trauma or dental work. In young children with carious lesions of the primary teeth, ask about feeding practices, particularly whether the child is put to bed with a bottle containing milk or juice. Inspect the oral cavity for obvious caries, gingival swelling and erythema, or a gum boil. Palpate the gums and molar occlusal surfaces for swelling and tenderness, tap each tooth with a tongue blade to identify percussion sensitivity, and check for tooth mobility.

ED Management

Caries   Refer all patients with caries to a dentist within a few days. Children with nursing-bottle caries require comprehensive dental care. Inform the parents of the serious nature of this condition and educate them to discontinue permitting the child to sleep with the bottle (unless it contains only water) or on the mother's breast. Refer the child to a pediatric dentist as soon as possible.

Dental Abscess   Treat a dental abscess with penicillin (50 mg/kg/day divided qid) or clindamycin (20 mg/kg/day divided qid). If the child is relatively comfortable, delay dental referral until the next day. Give ibuprofen (10 mg/kg q 6 h) or, if the patient reports pain despite ibuprofen, acetaminophen with codeine (0.5 mg/kg of codeine q 6 h). If the infection has spread beyond the teeth and gums or the patient has high fever, appears toxic, is immunocompromised, or is unable to drink, admit, treat with IV penicillin (100,000 U/kg/day divided q 6 h) or clindamycin (40 mg/kg/day divided q 6 h) and obtain a dental consultation.

Facial Cellulitis   Admit the patient and treat facial cellulitis secondary to a dental infection with IV penicillin (100,000 U/kg/day divided q 6 h) or clindamycin (40 mg/kg/day divided q 6 h), warm oral rinses, and parenteral hydration if necessary. Admit patients with deep fascial space infections and immediately consult an oral surgeon and otolaryngologist. Any suggestion of airway compromise is an indication for prophylactic intubation.

Follow-up

- Caries: dentist in 1 to 2 weeks
- Dental abscess: dentist within 24 h

Indications for Admission

- Dental abscess associated with fever >39.4°C (103°F), toxicity, or inability to take fluids orally
- Facial cellulitis secondary to a dental infection
- Evidence of deep space infection (neck swelling, severe dysphagia, dyspnea)

BIBLIOGRAPHY

Barakate MS, Jensen MJ, Hemli JM: Ludwig's angina: report of a case and review of management issues. *Ann Otol Rhinol Laryngol* 2001;110:453–456.

Martof A: Consultation with the specialist: dental care. *Pediatr Rev* 2001;22:13–15.

Sheller B, Williams BJ, Lombardi SM: Diagnosis and treatment of dental caries–related emergencies in a children's hospital. *Pediatr Dent* 1997;19:470–475.

ORAL TRAUMA

Oral trauma can result from inflicted or accidental injury. Common causes include falls, seizures, sports injuries, motor vehicle accidents, and punch injuries. Injuries to the teeth are often associated with lacerations, contusions, and abrasions of the gingiva or the oral mucosa. There may also be fractures to the supporting bone, alveolar socket, alveolar process, or maxilla. While dental injury may be overlooked secondary to distracting injuries in a victim of multiple trauma, dental trauma requires immediate attention, since injured teeth can suffer permanent damage if not treated expeditiously.

Clinical Presentation

Injuries to the Hard Dental Tissues and the Pulp
Enamel Infraction   These injuries are associated with an incomplete fracture (crack) of the enamel only, without loss of tooth substance (see Fig. 4-2).

Uncomplicated Crown Fracture   The fracture may be confined to the enamel (enamel fracture) only, so the tooth appears normal in color, with a piece of the edge missing. A more serious fracture may extend into the yellow dentin (enamel-dentin fracture).

Uncomplicated Crown-Root Fracture   The fracture involves the enamel, dentin, and cementum.

Complicated Crown and Crown-Root Fractures   Crown and crown-root fractures are classified as complicated if there is exposure of pulp. Pulp exposure is nearly always painful and is suggested by a pink or red color.

Root Fracture   A root fracture involves the dentin, cementum, and pulp. There may be associated crown fractures and excessive mobility of adjacent teeth.

Injuries to the Periodontal Tissues
Concussion   A concussion is a minor injury to the tooth's supporting structures without loosening or displacement. The tooth is sensitive when percussed but does not move when pressure is applied.

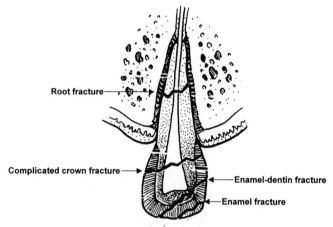

Root fracture

Complicated crown fracture

Enamel-dentin fracture

Enamel fracture

Figure 4-2   Dental fractures.

Subluxation   A subluxation is a more serious injury to the tooth's supporting structures causing abnormal loosening of the tooth without displacement. There is excessive horizontal mobility along with percussion sensitivity.

Luxation   A luxation is displacement of a tooth from its usual position. The luxation may be extrusive (partial displacement out of the socket), intrusive (displacement into the alveolar bone), or lateral (displacement other than axially). An exarticulation or avulsion is the complete displacement of the tooth out of its socket.

Lacerations   Lacerations of the lips, tongue, and oral mucosa are very common, particularly in children just beginning to walk. Lip lacerations that cross the vermilion border may present a cosmetic problem, since precise opposition of the wound margins is necessary for proper repair. Often, a child will present with lacerations of both the inner and outer surface of the lip. It is essential to identify whether these are two separate and shallow lesions or are, in fact, a communicating through-and-through laceration (uncommon). Isolated tears of the frenulum are very common.

Punctures   Falling while running with an object in the mouth can cause a puncture wound to the palate. This may appear minor but may represent a significant injury, especially if the soft palate is involved. Of particular concern are deep or dirty wounds, foreign-body contamination, and ongoing bleeding.

Mandibular Fractures   Mandibular fractures are uncommon but may occur in the area of the condyles (below the temporomandibular joints) or along the rami where the teeth are developing. With unilateral fractures, the mandible deviates toward the ipsilateral side when the mouth is opened; with bilateral fractures, the mouth may remain slightly open at all times. There is malocclusion along with the usual signs of a fracture (local swelling, ecchymoses, pain, tenderness).

Alveolar Bone Fractures   Alveolar bone fractures involve the bony processes into which the teeth are embedded and typically affect the maxillary incisors. There is displacement and mobility of the involved tooth and alveolar process, mobility of adjacent teeth, and bleeding from the adjacent gingiva.

Diagnosis

A systematic approach is necessary so that subtle injuries are not missed. Obtain a medical and dental history, including tetanus status, current medications, history of cardiac disease [subacute bacterial endocarditis (SBE) prophylaxis required], bleeding disorder, or seizure disorder. Inquire about the details of the traumatic incident, including when, where, and how the injury occurred and the time elapsed since the injury.

Extraoral Examination

First, note any extraoral wounds and bruises. Palpate the facial skeleton for tenderness or discontinuities that may represent a fracture. Assess the integrity of the facial skeleton by rocking the maxillary arch back and forth. Use the LeFort classification if abnormal mobility is found (LeFort I: hard palate and upper teeth move; LeFort II: the nose moves; LeFort III: the entire face moves). Examine the mandible and temporomandibular joints for swelling, clicking, or crepitus and check mandibular movement in all directions. Ask the patient to bite down in normal occlusion and note any deviation or pain. Then, have the patient bite down on a tongue depressor. With a mandibular fracture, the patient is unable to prevent the examiner from pulling the blade out of the mouth. If posterior neck pain is noted, delay further examination until an evaluation for cervical spine injury is completed (pp 641–644).

Intraoral Examination

Examine all soft tissues inside the mouth for swelling, bleeding, lacerations, contusions, and abrasions. Check lacerations for any foreign matter such as tooth fragments or soil. Probe any lip laceration to assess whether it is through-and-through.

Examine each tooth for crown fracture, pulp exposure, and dislocation. In some crown fractures, only a very thin layer of dentin remains over the pulp, so that the outline of the pulp can be seen as a pink tinge on the dentin.

Note any tooth displacement as well as horizontal and vertical tooth mobility. Suspect an alveolar process fracture if several adjacent teeth move when one tooth is being checked. However, excessive mobility may be difficult to evaluate clinically in a primary tooth, as it increases with normal root resorption prior to exfoliation. Tap each tooth with a fingernail or tongue blade. Percussion sensitivity in the absence of mobility is a concussion and not a serious injury.

ED Management

Elective dental referral is all that is necessary for *concussions, enamel infractions*, and *fractures of the enamel*. Immediate pediatric dental consultation is required for *subluxations, intrusions, extrusions*, and *fractures of the dentin* or *root*, or when the *pulp is exposed*. Immediately consult an oral surgeon for *mandibular, alveolar bone,* and *LeFort fractures*. If a dentist is not immediately available and a primary tooth is so loose as to be an aspiration hazard, extract it. Grab the tooth firmly with gauze and twist it out.

Reimplant *avulsed permanent teeth* if less than 1 h has elapsed since the injury. If it is not clear whether the tooth is primary or permanent, reimplant it pending consultation with a dentist or oral surgeon. Gently rinse, but do not scrub, the tooth in water or saline, reimplant it using a gentle rotating motion, then maintain firm finger pressure for 5 min. Once the tooth has been reimplanted, have the patient bite down firmly on a piece of folded gauze and immediately consult a pediatric dentist or an oral surgeon so the tooth can be stabilized. If the tooth cannot be reimplanted immediately and the child can cooperate without risk of aspiration, store it under the patient's tongue or in the buccal fold. Alternatives are the parent's mouth, a cup of milk, saliva, or a clean, moistened towel, but do not soak an avulsed tooth in water. Immediately refer the patient to a pediatric dentist or an oral surgeon. Do not reimplant an *avulsed primary tooth*. Refer the patient to the pediatric dentist the same day for evaluation of the socket and the remaining teeth.

Tongue and lip lacerations that are small and have well-approximated margins (during normal function) do not require suturing. Suture tongue and lip lacerations that are deep or gaping and continue to bleed, lip lacerations that cross the vermilion border, and through-and-through lip lacerations. Suture deep wounds with gaping edges using absorbable suture material (3-0 gut) after irrigation and careful inspection to rule out the presence of foreign bodies. For local anesthesia use bilateral inferior alveolar blocks rather than infiltration. If necessary, place a silk suture through the tip of the tongue to pull the tongue out for access. Alternatively, refer tongue and lip lacerations that require suturing to a plastic or oral surgeon for cosmetic repair. Give prophylactic antibiotics for through-and-through lip lacerations [10 mg/kg (450 mg max) of clindamycin tid]. Provide tetanus prophylaxis if needed (pp 682–683).

Puncture wounds to the palate may be complicated by vascular injury, foreign bodies, or pharyngeal abscesses. Consult an oral surgeon or otolaryngologist.

Isolated tears of the frenulum require no treatment.

Follow-up

- Concussion, enamel infraction or fracture: dentist in 2 to 4 weeks
- Avulsed tooth: dental follow-up immediately

Indication for Admission

- Mandibular or alveolar bone fracture

BIBLIOGRAPHY

Garcia-Godoy F, Pulver F: Treatment of trauma to the primary and young permanent dentitions. *Dent Clin North Am* 2000;44:597–632.

McTigue DJ: Diagnosis and management of dental injuries in children. *Pediatr Clin North Am* 2000;47:1067–1084.

Nelson LP, Shusterman S: Emergency management of oral trauma in children. *Curr Opin Pediatr* 1997;9:242–245.

DISCOLORED TEETH

Patients with poor oral hygiene may have discolored teeth from extrinsic substances that have adhered to the outer surfaces of the teeth; alternatively, intrinsic pigments may be incorporated into the tooth during development. In addition, an early carious lesion can present as (intrinsic) tooth discoloration.

Clinical Presentation and Diagnosis

Extrinsic Discoloration　Extrinsic discoloration may be brown to black (iron, smoking, coffee, tea), green (chromogenic bacteria or fungi), or orange to red (changes in oral flora due to antibiotic intake). These extrinsic stains can be readily removed from the surface by a dentist with tooth polishing.

Intrinsic Discoloration　The most common cause of intrinsic discoloration (dark gray) of isolated teeth is pulp necrosis secondary to trauma. Intrinsic discoloration may also be caused by tetracycline, given to the mother prenatally or to the child on more than one occasion before the age of 8 (the time most permanent teeth erupt). This causes yellow to brown staining of the permanent dentition. Chronic fluoride overdose can cause whitish mottling or brown spots. Children may ingest excessive fluoride from swallowing toothpastes or mouthwashes containing fluoride. Some systemic diseases can cause tooth discoloration, such as hepatic failure (brown to gray), erythroblastosis fetalis (green to blue to orange discoloration of the primary but not the permanent teeth), and porphyria (reddish to brown).

Caries　The early stage of nursing-bottle caries can appear as snow-white spots (decalcification of enamel) or brown spots on the labial or palatal surfaces of the primary maxillary incisors.

ED Management

Tooth discoloration does not constitute an urgent problem, and no acute management is indicated or available. A careful history often suggests the diagnosis. For extrinsic causes, stop the offending agent and recommend regular daily brushing. If fluorosis is diagnosed, have the family discontinue any possible fluoride sources, including supplements, vitamins, and fluoridated toothpaste and rinses. Refer patients to a pediatric dentist whenever intrinsic tooth discoloration or an early carious lesion is suspected. Refer patients suspected of having a systemic cause to the appropriate specialist.

BIBLIOGRAPHY

Warren JJ, Levy SM, Kanellis MJ: Prevalence of dental fluorosis in the primary dentition. *J Public Health Dent* 2001;61:87–91.

DISEASES OF THE GUMS, TONGUE, AND ORAL MUCOSA

In most cases, infections, inflammation, and changes of the gums, tongue, and oral mucosa are not serious disorders, although they are frustrating management problems. There are a number of distinct disease entities, but no specific therapy exists for most.

Clinical Presentation and Diagnosis

Infections
Herpes Simplex　Primary herpetic gingivostomatitis (HSV I) is a common cause of gingivostomatitis in 1- to 3-year-olds. After a 1- to 2-day prodrome

of fever, malaise, and vomiting, small vesicles appear anywhere on the oral mucosa, lips, tongue, perioral skin, or cheeks. These rapidly rupture, forming 2- to 10-mm lesions covered by a yellowish membrane. The membrane then sloughs, leaving a shallow ulcer on an erythematous base. Fever up to 40.5°C (105°F), excessive salivation, diminished oral intake leading to dehydration, and marked local lymphadenopathy can also occur. Healing begins within 4 to 5 days and is usually completed within 1 to 2 weeks.

Recurrent Herpes   Recurrent herpes ("cold sores," herpes labialis) is thought to be secondary to stress (fever, menses, sunlight exposure). It presents with small vesicles limited to the outer aspects of the lips and adjacent skin. These rupture, coalesce, and become crusted. Healing takes 1 to 2 weeks.

Herpangina   Herpangina is a summertime infection caused by a number of type A coxsackieviruses. The lesions are found only in the posterior oral cavity, which distinguishes them from *herpes* or *aphthous ulcers*. The soft palate, uvula, tonsils, and anterior tonsillar pillars are the sites of multiple, superficial, painful ulcers. Infants may be markedly irritable with fever and drooling, and severe dysphagia can lead to dehydration. The lesions heal spontaneously after 3 to 5 days.

Hand-Foot-Mouth Disease   Hand-foot-mouth disease is caused primarily by type A16 coxsackievirus. Vesicles and ulcers occurring anywhere in the oral cavity are accompanied by fever, malaise, and abdominal pain. Many patients also have a characteristic exanthem consisting of vesicles on an erythematous base located in one or more of the following sites: the palms and soles, dorsum of the hands and feet, and dorsal aspects of the fingers and toes. The lesions usually resolve within 2 weeks.

Acute Necrotizing Ulcerative Gingivostomatitis   Acute necrotizing ulcerative gingivostomatitis (ANUG, Vincent's angina, trench mouth) is an uncommon infectious disease of adolescents and young adults, probably caused by *Fusobacterium* and spirochetes. It is more common during times of stress, although in rare cases there is underlying malnutrition or immune deficiency. Characteristic findings are painful gingiva that bleed easily, ulcerated interdental papillae covered by a grayish membrane, and foul-smelling breath in addition to lymphadenopathy, malaise, and fever. ANUG is differentiated from acute primary herpes by the punched-out appearance of the interdental papillae, the lack of vesicles, and the older age of patients with ANUG.

Candidal Thrush   Thrush is common in the first year of life. The complaint is diminished oral intake or white spots in the oral cavity. On inspection, the oral mucosa is beefy red with a curd-like white exudate on the tongue, gingiva, hard palate, or buccal mucosa. This can resemble milk, but it is not easily removed by scraping with a tongue depressor. On occasion, cracking or fissuring at the angle of the mouth, or cheilitis, is seen. Many infants simultaneously have a typical candidal diaper rash.

Thrush beyond the first year of life occurs in patients who have received broad-spectrum antibiotics and those with autoimmune diseases and nutritional deficiencies. Persistent or recurrent thrush suggests possible HIV infection.

Noninfectious Ulcers

Aphthous Ulcers   Aphthous ulcers, or canker sores, are solitary or multiple (five or fewer) painful lesions anywhere on the oral mucosa. They begin as erythematous papules that become well-circumscribed ulcers with a gray fibrinous exudate on an erythematous base. The etiology is unknown, although their appearance is thought to be related to stress (allergies, infections, drugs, trauma, emotional upset). Fever is less common than with herpes. The ulcers usually last 10 to 14 days, and recurrent episodes are the rule.

Traumatic Ulcer   Ulcers of various sizes, shapes, and locations may occur. Inquire as to recent ingestion of hot foods (pizza often causes burns to the anterior palate), recent dental treatment (children often bite the lip or tongue while it is numb, or the dental drill may have scratched the tongue or cheek), and oral habits (fingernail scratches of the gingiva, chewing on inside of cheek). In the absence of repeated trauma, the lesion usually heals uneventfully within 2 weeks.

Inflammation of the Gums and Tongue

Geographic Tongue   Geographic tongue, or benign migratory glossitis, is a self-limited condition of unknown etiology. It presents as pink to red, round or irregularly shaped areas of dekeratinized and desquamated papillae, with white or yellow elevated margins on the dorsal and lateral surfaces of the tongue and a changing pattern (hence the name). It is usually asymptomatic but may be painful when inflamed.

Drug-Induced Gingival Overgrowth   Phenytoin, cyclosporine, and nifedipine can induce gingival hyperplasia. This presents as generalized overgrowth of the gingiva, with subsequent secondary infection and inhibition of tooth eruption. The overgrowth can be exacerbated by plaque-induced inflammation in patients who do not practice adequate oral hygiene. Pain and difficulty with mastication can occur if the gingiva overgrow the occlusal surfaces of the teeth. In contrast, *gingivitis* presents with edematous and hemorrhagic gums.

Juvenile Periodontitis   Juvenile periodontitis presents with generalized, rapid periodontal bone loss associated with impaired neutrophil function. It occurs most commonly in the region of the permanent first molars in older children and adolescents. While the gingiva appear normal, the teeth have excessive mobility. The bone loss can be confirmed radiographically.

Mucocele   A mucocele is a raised, bluish vesicle, most commonly on the lower lip but rarely on the upper lip, palate, tongue, or mucosa. It is caused by the traumatic laceration of a minor salivary gland duct that permits accumulation and blockage of mucus.

Ranula   A ranula is a mucous retention cyst of the sublingual salivary gland. It is a large, soft swelling in the floor of the mouth.

Malignancy   Leukemic infiltration of the gingiva can present with extensive or spontaneous bleeding and extremely shiny, edematous, and boggy tissue.

ED Management

Whether the etiology is *herpes, coxsackievirus, aphthous* or *traumatic ulceration* or *geographic tongue*, the major therapeutic goals are oral hygiene and pain relief so that adequate oral intake can continue.

There are a number of options for pain management, but none is universally successful. Viscous lidocaine (2%) may be swabbed onto lesions with a cotton swab. However, seizures can result if large quantities are absorbed, so use lidocaine only when there are a limited number of lesions, as with aphthous ulcers. Do not use viscous lidocaine as a rinse or for lesions in the posterior pharynx (can numb the gag reflex). A 1:1 diphenhydramine/Maalox or diphenhydramine/Kaopectate solution may be swabbed onto lesions, but large quantities can cause diphenhydramine toxicity. Over-the-counter analgesic sprays (Sucrets, Chloraseptic) and remedies (Debacterol, Kancaid) are often the safest and best-tolerated treatment.

In addition, recommend giving acetaminophen (15 mg/kg q 4 h) or ibuprofen (10 mg/kg q 6 h) 30 min before eating. Instruct the parents to encourage oral intake. Ice cream, milk shakes, and ice pops are often accepted.

Refer a patient with *gingival hyperplasia*, a *mucocele*, or a *ranula* to a dentist. See pp 100–104 for the specific treatment of herpes gingivostomatitis.

Thrush   The treatment of thrush is specific: instill 1 mL of nystatin suspension (100,000 U/mL) into each side of the mouth four times daily. Give the doses after feeding to prolong contact between the medication and infected areas. For persistent lesions, have the parent rub the area with a gauze pad soaked in nystatin. Also, look for a source of reinfection, such as nipples or a pacifier. Immunocompromised patients often require more aggressive therapy (pp 309–311); consult with an infectious disease specialist. If the infection persists after antifungal therapy or recurs rapidly, refer the patient for immunologic and HIV evaluation.

Trench Mouth   Treat trench mouth with oral penicillin (50 mg/kg/day divided qid) or clindamycin (20 mg/kg/day divided qid) and rinsing with chlorhexidine 0.12% or a 1:1 solution of 3% hydrogen peroxide and water three times daily. For pain, recommend ibuprofen (10 mg/kg) and a 1:1 mixture of diphenhydramine and Maalox. Treat the underlying condition and refer the patient to a dentist within 24 h.

Follow-up

- Herpes gingivostomatitis: if severe, daily to assess oral intake until improving, otherwise 2 to 3 days
- Gingival hyperplasia, mucocele, or ranula: dentist in 1 week
- Trench mouth: dentist in 24 h

Indication for Admission

- Dehydration or inability to tolerate oral intake secondary to pain

BIBLIOGRAPHY

Amir J, Harel L, Smetana Z: The natural history of primary herpes simplex type 1 gingivostomatitis in children. *Pediatr Dermatol* 1999;16:259–263.

Sonis A, Zaragoza S: Dental health for the pediatrician. *Curr Opin Pediatr* 2001; 13:289–295.

Steelman R, Weisse M, Ramadan H: Congenital ranula. *Clin Pediatr (Phila)* 1998; 37:205–206.

CHAPTER 5

Dermatologic Emergencies

David E. Bank

Since dermatologic diagnoses are made visually, it is difficult to look up the disease in question if the diagnosis is not already known. Therefore, this chapter begins with definitions of dermatologic terms. Once the eruption is described, Table 5-1 can be used as a guide to the most common diagnoses, grouped by clinical appearance. After the differential diagnosis is narrowed, the individual sections can then be consulted.

Table 5-1 Dermatologic Diagnosis by Type of Eruption

Diaper dermatitis
Acrodermatitis enteropathica
Allergic and irritant contact dermatitis
Atopic dermatitis

Candida
Dermatophyte infection
Histiocytosis X
Perianal streptococcal infection
Psoriasis
Seborrheic dermatitis

Inflammatory papules and nodules
Papules
Cellulitis
Drug reaction
Granuloma annulare*
Insect bite
Miliaria rubra
Viral exanthem

Nodules
Erythema nodosum
Furuncle

Papulosquamous diseases
Atopic dermatitis

Contact dermatitis
Id reaction
Lichen planus
Pityriasis rosea
Psoriasis
Scabies
Seborrheic dermatitis
Secondary syphilis
Tinea†

Pustular eruptions
Acne
Candidiasis
Folliculitis
Gonococcemia
Miliaria pustulosa
Sepsis
Transient neonatal pustular melanosis

Skin-colored papules and nodules
Granuloma annulare*
Molluscum contagiosum‡
Verrucae

Vascular reactions
Nonpurpuric (blanching)
Drug reaction

Table 5-1   *(continued)*

Erythema marginatum	Scabies
Erythema migrans¶	Tinea†
Erythema multiforme	Varicella-zoster
Urticaria	
Viral exanthem	*Bullous*
	Bullous impetigo
Palpable purpura (nonblanching)	Contact dermatitis–poison ivy
Coagulopathy	Erythema multiforme major
Drug reaction	Staphylococcal scalded skin
Henoch-Schönlein purpura	syndrome
Meningococcemia	Toxic epidermal necrolysis
Rocky Mountain spotted fever	
Sepsis	**White lesions**
Subacute bacterial endocarditis	*Patches and plaques*
	Pityriasis alba
Vesicobullous	Postinflammatory hypopigmentation
Vesicular	Tinea versicolor
Dyshydrotic eczema	Verrucae
Erythema migrans¶	
Hand-foot-mouth disease	*Papules*
Herpes simplex	Keratosis pilaris
Miliaria crystallina	Molluscum contagiosum‡

*Granuloma annulare can be either inflammatory or skin-colored.

†Tinea is usually papulosquamous; vesicular presentation is uncommon.

‡Molluscum contagiosum can be skin-colored or white.

¶Erythema migrans is usually nonpurpuric; vesicular presentation is uncommon.

DEFINITION OF TERMS

Macule   A macule is a small area (<1.5–2 cm in diameter) of color change, usually red, brown, yellow, or white. A macule is nonpalpable, so its borders can only be distinguished visually. The surface of a macule is usually smooth, but sometimes a small amount of very fine, nonpalpable scale may be present.

Patch   A patch is a macule with a diameter >2 cm. A patch is usually formed from an enlarging macule or the confluence of several macules. Except for the size, patches are identical to macules.

Papule   A papule is a small, palpable mass <0.5 cm in diameter. By definition, a papule is nonvesicular and nonpustular. A papule may be red, brown, yellow, white, or skin-colored. The surface may be smooth, eroded or ulcerated, or covered by scales, crusts, or a combination of secondary features. A papule may be flat-topped, dome-shaped, or pointed.

Plaque   A plaque is a broad, elevated, flat-topped lesion with a diameter >0.5 cm. A plaque is usually formed by a confluence of several papules. Except for the size, plaques are identical to papules.

Nodule A nodule is a circumscribed, elevated, solid lesion that is between 0.5 and 2 cm in diameter. A nodule is essentially a papule that is enlarged in all three dimensions: length, width, and depth. A nodule may have any of the color changes and surface features described for papules, and it may be dome-shaped or slope-shouldered but not flat-topped.

Wheal A wheal is an edematous papule with a smooth surface. The color ranges from pale pink to red.

Vesicle A vesicle is a sharply circumscribed, elevated, fluid-containing lesion less than 0.5 cm in diameter. A vesicle contains clear fluid and is therefore skin-colored. Vesicles are often very fragile; patients with vesicular diseases may lack intact vesicles and present instead with erosions.

Bulla A bulla is a vesicle >0.5 cm in diameter. A bulla may arise as a single large blister or through the coalescence of several small vesicles. Except for the size, a bulla is identical to a vesicle.

Pustule A pustule is a bright white vesicle filled with polymorphonuclear leukocytes. A pustule is not necessarily infected; there is often no visible difference between sterile and infected pustules. Pustules must be differentiated from cloudy vesicles.

Scale Scale is formed by the accumulation of compact desquamation layers of stratum corneum, resulting from abnormal keratinization and exfoliation of cornified keratinocytes. A scale may be greasy and yellowish, silvery and mica-like, fine and barely visible, or large, adherent, and lamellar.

Crust A crust results from dried serum (yellow), blood or bloody exudate (dark red or brown), or pus or purulent exudate (green or yellowish green) overlying areas of lost or damaged epidermis. The colloquial term for a crust is a *scab*.

Erosion An erosion is a moist, slightly depressed vesicular lesion in which part or all of the epidermis has been visibly lost or denuded. Erosions do not extend into the underlying dermis or subcutaneous tissue, so they heal without scarring.

Ulcer An ulcer involves destruction of the dermis, resulting in a sunk-in appearance, in contrast to the superficial presentation of an erosion. An ulcer may be filled with crust or necrotic skin, or the base may be visible as a moist red surface. The crust can be thick, tough, and black secondary to hemorrhage and necrosis. Ulcers often occur when blood flow to the skin is impaired.

Excoriation An excoriation is a scratch mark. The term refers to a traumatic loss of skin caused by scratching, rubbing, or scrubbing of the cutaneous surface. Excoriations occur in pruritic disorders.

Lichenification   Patients who respond to pruritus with chronic, habitual rubbing develop a peculiar thickening of the skin known as lichenification. There is an accentuation of the normal skin markings accompanied by a mild amount of scaling. Lichenified skin feels tough and leatherlike. Lichenification occurs only in the eczematous diseases and is a pathognomonic feature of atopic dermatitis.

ACNE

Acne vulgaris is a disorder involving the pilosebaceous follicles. It is the most common skin disease of the second and third decades, with onset at puberty and an incidence approaching 100% between the ages of 14 and 17 in females and 16 and 19 in males. Acne can be exacerbated by medications, including diphenylhydantoin, isoniazid, iodides and bromides, and lithium. Neonatal acne is secondary to hormonal stimulation of sebaceous glands that have not yet involuted to a prepubertal immature state. Steroid acne is a folliculitis most commonly caused by the prolonged use of topical or systemic corticosteroids or adrenocorticotropic hormone.

Clinical Presentation

Acne vulgaris primarily involves sites where pilosebaceous glands are most numerous (face, chest, upper back). The initial lesions are the pathognomonic open comedones (blackheads) and closed comedones (whiteheads). As the disease progresses, inflammatory lesions are seen, including papules, pustules, nodules, and cysts. The resolution phase is characterized by postinflammatory hyperpigmentation and scarring. Neonatal acne presents with erythematous papules and pustules, rather than comedones, on the nose and cheeks. The typical lesions of steroid acne are small erythematous papules and pustules, without comedones, primarily located on the back and chest.

Diagnosis

The diagnosis of acne vulgaris is usually straightforward. *Adenoma sebaceum* manifests as pink papules on the face of prepubertal patients with tuberous sclerosis. Other cutaneous manifestations (ash-leaf spots, shagreen patch, periungual fibromas) are generally present. *Verrucae* (warts) and *molluscum contagiosum* cause flesh-colored papules without comedones or an inflammatory response. In an infant, *seborrhea* is often misdiagnosed as neonatal acne. Associated cradle cap and retroauricular scaling distinguish seborrhea.

ED Management

Acne vulgaris is a chronic disease; while treatment may be started in the ED, refer the patient to a primary care setting for ongoing care. The therapeutic measures appropriate for ED use are summarized below.

Benzoyl peroxide (2.5–10%) is an effective keratolytic and antibacterial agent that is useful for comedones and mild inflammatory lesions.

Common side effects are redness, drying, and scaling of the skin. Retinoic acid (tretinoin), derived from vitamin A, is extremely useful for treating comedonal acne. Severe skin irritation, peeling, and photosensitization can result; start treatment on an every-other-day basis, usually at night. To minimize these side effects, instruct the patient to limit face washing and to be sure the face is dry prior to applying retinoic acid. Do not use in females who may be pregnant.

Topical antibiotics are a useful adjunct in mild to moderate inflammatory acne. Clindamycin (1%) and erythromycin (2%) are effective without the risk of side effects associated with oral administration. Systemic antibiotics are reserved for unresponsive acne or benzoyl peroxide sensitivity. A minimum of a 4-week course is usually required before any improvement occurs. Tetracycline or minocycline are most frequently used provided that the patient is more than 8 years of age and not pregnant. Side effects include gastrointestinal upset, photosensitization, and monilial vaginitis. In addition, vertigo can occur with minocycline. Erythromycin is particularly useful for younger patients (under 10 years) or when sun exposure is a concern.

Treat mild comedonal acne with a benzoyl peroxide cleanser (2.5–10%) daily or twice a day, depending on the degree of dryness. Add retinoic acid 0.025% cream every other night and gradually increase to nightly use. This combination is particularly effective, as the tretinoin facilitates absorption of the benzoyl peroxide. Alternatively, use a topical antibiotic (1% clindamycin gel or solution; 2% erythromycin gel or solution) as the second drug every morning.

Treat steroid acne with topical benzoyl peroxide and a topical antibiotic (as described above). Discontinue the steroids if possible. No therapy is required for neonatal acne.

Follow-up

- Primary care follow-up in 1 to 2 weeks

BIBLIOGRAPHY

Keowchuk DP: Managing acne in adolescents. *Pediatr Clin North Am* 2000; 47:841–857.

Leyden JJ: Therapy for acne vulgaris. *N Engl J Med* 1997;336:1156–1162.

Sidbury R, Paller AS: The diagnosis and treatment of acne. *Pediatr Ann* 2000; 29:17–24.

ALOPECIA

Alopecia is the loss of hair. In children, it usually presents as a localized scalp condition. Etiologies include alopecia areata (a presumed autoimmune disorder), tinea capitis (fungal infection), trauma or traction secondary to hair care techniques (braiding, straightening, blow-drying) or friction, trichotillomania (self-induced hair loss), and male-pattern baldness.

Diffuse hair loss is far less common. In most instances, the patient has suffered a significant stress (high fever, crash diet, parturition, convulsion) within the previous few months. Cancer chemotherapeutic agents (cyclophosphamide, vincristine), drugs [propranolol, warfarin (Coumadin)], radiation, toxins (lead, boric acid), endocrinopathies (hyper- and hypothyroidism, hypoparathyroidism), nutritional deficiencies (zinc, vitamin A), secondary syphilis, and systemic lupus erythematosus are other etiologies.

Clinical Presentation

Localized Alopecia

Alopecia Areata   Alopecia areata is characterized by the sudden (possibly overnight) appearance of sharply demarcated round or oval patches of hair loss without associated scalp inflammation or scarring. Regrowth may occur in some areas while the disease progresses elsewhere. In 5 to 10% of cases, the lesions may expand to involve the entire scalp (alopecia totalis) or all the body hair (alopecia universalis). At the margins of active lesions, there are loose, easily plucked, "exclamation point" hairs with shortened bulbs and small stumps. The course is variable, but up to 95% of children have complete regrowth within 1 year. Younger patients and those with extensive involvement have a poorer prognosis.

Tinea Capitis   Tinea capitis (see pp 116–119) causes patchy alopecia with scaling and erythema similar to seborrheic dermatitis. Within the patch, "black dots" (infected hairs that are broken off at the scalp level) may be seen. A minority of cases fluoresce under Wood's lamp exposure. An allergic vesicular and pustular reaction (kerion) can develop acutely. The kerion appears as a sharply demarcated, indurated, boggy lesion that can be associated with fever, leukocytosis, and lymphadenopathy. Look for a pruritic papular eruption (Id reduction) elsewhere.

Traumatic and Traction Alopecia   Traumatic and traction alopecia occur where the hair is being pulled, as from braiding, or on the occiput of a young infant who remains supine all day. Characteristically, hair loss is incomplete; short (1- to 2-cm) hairs are found at the margins or within the affected area. These hairs are firmly rooted in normal-appearing scalp.

Trichotillomania   Trichotillomania primarily occurs in school-age girls. The patches of alopecia are not well demarcated, and there are well-rooted residual hairs of varying length. In some cases the eyebrows and eyelashes are also affected.

Male-Pattern Baldness   Male-pattern baldness is a genetically determined bilateral frontoparietal recession with thinning over the vertex. It can also occur in females taking oral contraceptives.

Diffuse Alopecia

With diffuse disorders of any etiology, the scalp generally has a normal appearance, and hairs are easily plucked from the periphery of areas of alopecia.

Diagnosis

For localized conditions, a careful examination of the scalp facilitates the correct diagnosis. Well-demarcated hair loss with normal-appearing scalp suggests *alopecia areata*. Inflammation and scaling, black dots, or fluorescence under Wood's lamp examination are typical of *tinea capitis*. Although a *bacterial scalp infection* may be mistaken for a kerion, it does not usually cause hair loss. Hair loss in areas of possible trauma with no scalp inflammation is characteristic of *traumatic* or *traction alopecia*. The patient may be an infant; there may be a history of hair braiding or straightening; or the patient may have been observed pulling at his or her hair. In addition, the remaining hairs are firmly rooted in the scalp.

When the diagnosis is in doubt, pluck a few hairs from the periphery of the lesion and examine them under a microscope after mixing with 10 to 20% potassium hydroxide (KOH) and gently heating. Experience is required to interpret KOH preparations, but in tinea infections, chains of spores within or surrounding the hair shaft are seen; "exclamation point" hairs confirm alopecia areata. Placing the hairs on either Sabouraud's agar or dermatophyte test medium (DTM) facilitates the growth of fungi.

A careful history may suggest the stressful incident that caused a diffuse alopecia. If a previously undiagnosed systemic disorder such as *syphilis, thyroid disease, lupus*, or *hypoparathyroidism* is suspected, obtain the appropriate blood tests [VDRL, thyroid function tests, fluorescent antinuclear antibody (FANA), or calcium].

ED Management

Most cases of *alopecia areata* require no treatment other than reassurance. If the lesions persist or become particularly widespread, refer the patient to a dermatologist. A change of hair care techniques or reassurance for an infant's parent is usually all that is necessary for *traction* or *traumatic alopecia*. Refer the patient with *trichotillomania* to a primary care setting for further psychosocial evaluation. See p 118 for the treatment of *tinea capitis*.

Manage *diffuse alopecia* by avoiding the offending agent, drug, or toxin (if possible) or by treating the primary condition (lupus, thyroid disease, etc.). Stress-related hair loss is usually self-limited, with complete regrowth and no need for any specific treatment. Refer the patient to a primary care provider.

Follow-up

- Primary care follow-up in 1 to 2 weeks

BIBLIOGRAPHY

Al Fouzan AS, Nanda A: Alopecia in children. *Clin Dermatol* 2000;18:735–743.

Elewski BE: Tinea capitis: a current perspective. *J Am Acad Dermatol* 2000; 42:1–20.

Vasiloudes P, Morelli JG, Weston WL: Bald spots: remember the "big three." *Contemp Pediatr* 1997;14:76–91.

ATOPIC DERMATITIS

Introduction

Atopic dermatitis is a disease that predisposes the skin to excessive dryness and pruritus. Up to 75% of patients have a family history of allergy, asthma, hay fever, or eczema, and about half of affected children will develop one of these other diseases.

Clinical Presentation

Atopic dermatitis can be categorized into three different age-dependent phases that may or may not follow one another. Pruritus and dry skin are the hallmarks at all ages. The infantile stage occurs between 2 months and 3 years and is characterized by erythema, papules, and vesicles on the face, neck, chest, and extensor surfaces of the extremities. In children 5 to 10 years of age, subacute and chronic papular and scaly lichenified lesions occur on the flexor aspects of the neck, arms, and legs. The antecubital and popliteal fossae are particularly involved. The adolescent and adult forms blend into the childhood phase with marked lichenification and flexural, hand, and foot involvement.

Other manifestations may include nummular eczema (well-demarcated papular coin lesions) and pityriasis alba (discrete hypopigmented macules) in children and adolescents.

At any age, the severe pruritus causes scratching, which can lead to secondary bacterial infection. The superimposed pyoderma can confuse the clinical picture.

Atopic individuals can have a number of associated findings, including accentuated palmar creases, white dermographism (blanching of the skin when stroked), and Dennie's pleat (an extra groove of the lower eyelid). Keratosis pilaris (follicular hyperkeratosis) presents with scaly perifollicular papules with central hairs, resulting in a "chicken skin" appearance.

Diagnosis

The diagnosis of atopic dermatitis is suggested by a family history of atopy, a personal history of allergies or asthma, dry and pruritic skin, and the typical location of the lesions, which blend into the surrounding normal skin. In infants, *seborrheic dermatitis* causes a salmon-colored, greasy eruption of the face and scalp that is not pruritic. The eruption of a *contact dermatitis* has a sharp border with the uninvolved skin, and the history can be suggestive of the offending agent. The lesions of *tinea corporis* usually have central clearing and a raised scaly border. *Bacterial infections* are not preceded by pruritus and are generally more localized than atopic rashes. *Psoriatic lesions* are usually well demarcated with a silvery scale. The lesions of *scabies* do not follow the usual sites of predilection that eczema does, and the family or personal history of atopy may be negative.

ED Management

Atopic dermatitis is a chronic condition that is best managed in the primary care setting, but therapy can be initiated in the ED. The goals of therapy are to hydrate the skin, prevent itching, and treat the inflammation. Instruct the patient to use oatmeal baths or soap substitutes (Cetaphil, Aveeno), to avoid excessive bathing, and to use emollients after bathing (Eucerin, Aquaphor, Lubriderm). Hydroxyzine (2 mg/kg/day divided tid) is an effective antipruritic agent. Finally, use a moderate-potency topical corticosteroid ointment (0.1% triamcinolone, 0.05% fluticasone, 0.1% mometasone, etc.) on the body and extremities, but use only a low-potency ointment (1% hydrocortisone, 0.05% aclomethasone, desonide 0.05%, etc.) on the face. Do not use oral steroids without consulting a dermatologist. Protopic 0.03% and tacrolimus 0.1% are new nonsteroidal immunomodulators that can be used on both the face and body.

Treat acute, oozing lesions with Burow's solution dressings for 20 min four times a day. Oatmeal baths may also be soothing. If there is a secondary bacterial infection, use topical mupirocin tid for localized areas of involvement or 40 mg/kg/day of cefadroxil (divided q 12 h), cephalexin (divided q 6 h), or erythromycin (divided q 6 h) for more extensive infection.

Follow-up

- Primary care follow-up in 1 to 2 weeks

Indication for Admission

- Severe involvement in a patient who cannot be adequately treated at home

REFERENCES

Hanifin JM, Tofte SJ: Update on therapy of atopic dermatitis. *J Allergy Clin Immunol* 1999;104(suppl):123–125.

Paller AS: Use of nonsteroidal topical immunomodulators for the treatment of atopic dermatitis in the pediatric population. *J Pediatr* 2001;38:163–168.

Woodmansee D, Christiansen S: Atopic dermatitis. *Pediatr Ann* 1998;27:710–716.

BACTERIAL SKIN INFECTIONS

Bacterial skin infections, or pyodermas, are most commonly caused by group A *Streptococcus* and *Staphylococcus aureus*. Impetigo, folliculitis, furunculosis, and cellulitis are the usual forms of infection.

Clinical Presentation and Diagnosis

Impetigo The most common type is *impetigo contagiosum,* caused by group A *Streptococcus* or *S. aureus*. The eruption usually appears on the face and extremities. Small erythematous macules develop into vesicles that rupture, leaving a typical honey-colored crust that is easily removed but recurs. Fever and regional lymphadenopathy may also occur. Some cases of impetigo are caused by nephritogenic strains of *Streptococcus*, so that subsequent acute glomerulonephritis occasionally occurs. Impetigo is extremely contagious, spreading by autoinoculation (satellite lesions), close contact, and fomites (towels). It is more common in the warm, humid summer months.

Bullous impetigo is usually caused by phage group II staphylococci. Yellowish vesicles on the face, extremities, and trunk rupture, leaving well-demarcated, erythematous, circular macules with a "collarette of scale." Once again, the infection is highly contagious, and fever and lymphadenopathy may occur.

Folliculitis   Folliculitis is a pyoderma involving the hair follicles, particularly in areas subjected to sweating, friction, scratching, and shaving. Coagulase-positive *Staphylococcus* is the most frequent etiologic agent. Folliculitis presents as pruritic, round-topped pustules most commonly seen on the scalp, face, thighs, and buttocks. If the diagnosis is uncertain, examine the pustule under magnification (otoscope). The hallmark of a folliculitis is the presence of a hair shaft in most lesions.

Furunculosis   Furunculosis is a deep follicular infection usually arising from a preceding folliculitis. Furuncles (boils) are tender, erythematous, 1- to 5-cm nodules that become fluctuant, then suppurate. They are seen in hair-bearing areas that are subject to perspiration and friction, including the face, thighs, buttocks, and scalp. In contrast, an abscess is usually a solitary lesion that is not associated with hair follicles. With recurrent furunculosis, consider associated conditions such as diabetes mellitus, obesity, corticosteroid treatment, immunoglobulin deficiency, neutropenia of any etiology, and defective neutrophils (chronic granulomatous disease, Chédiak-Higashi syndrome).

Cellulitis   Cellulitis, an infection involving the subcutaneous tissues, causes poorly demarcated, tender, erythematous swelling. It is often associated with fever, local lymphadenopathy, and lymphangitic streaking. Sites of infection are areas subjected to superficial trauma, such as the face and extremities. Most common pathogens are coagulase-positive *Staphylococcus* and group A *Streptococcus*. Rarely, in unimmunized children under 5 years of age, *Haemophilus influenzae* type B (HITB) can cause cellulitis, particularly of the facial and periorbital areas, though this is exceedingly rare in the HIB vaccine era. Children with HITB cellulitis may have associated systemic toxicity and high fever, and the lesion may develop a violaceous hue.

Erysipelas   Erysipelas is an uncommon superficial cellulitis caused by group A *Streptococcus*. A tense, erythematous, tender, well-demarcated, rapidly spreading swelling results.

ED Management

Impetigo   Treat with mupirocin ointment (2%) tid. For widespread disease or if mupirocin is unavailable or ineffective, use 40 mg/kg/day of cefadroxil (divided bid), cephalexin (divided qid), or erythromycin (divided qid) for 7 to 10 days; clindamycin (20 mg/kg/day divided qid) and amoxicillin-clavulanate (200/28.5, 400/57 or 875/125) formulations, 45 mg/kg/day of amoxicillin divided bid) are alternatives. Treat weeping lesions with tap water or 5% Burow's solution on open dressings for 10 min tid.

Folliculitis   Folliculitis occasionally responds to 7 to 14 days of treatment with a topical antibiotic (mupirocin 2%, clindamycin 1%). If the response is inadequate, treat with the same oral antibiotics as for impetigo for 7 to 10 days.

Furunculosis and Cellulitis   Treat with the same oral antibiotics as for impetigo. Warm soaks every 2 h are a helpful adjunct to antibiotic therapy. Delineate the margins of the infection with a pen so that the response to therapy can be assessed objectively. However, if there is fever, proximal lymphadenopathy, and lymphangitic streaking, admit the patient and treat with IV antibiotics (nafcillin 100 mg/kg/day divided q 6 h, cefazolin 50 mg/kg/day divided q 8 h, or clindamycin 40 mg/kg/day divided q 6 h).

If HITB cellulitis is suspected, obtain a complete blood count (CBC) and blood culture and perform a lumbar puncture if the patient is irritable. Admit the child for IV therapy with cefuroxime (150 mg/kg/day divided q 8 h), cefotaxime (150 mg/kg/day divided q 6 h), or ceftriaxone (100 mg/kg/ day divided q 12 h).

Treat furunculosis or cellulitis in a child with an *immune deficiency* with IV nafcillin (150 mg/kg/day divided q 6 h). Add cefotaxime (150 mg/kg/day divided q 6 h) if HITB is suspected.

Erysipelas   Treat with penicillin (250 mg qid) for 10 days. Admission for IV therapy may be necessary if there is an inadequate response.

Follow-up

- Impetigo: 2 to 3 days if no improvement
- Folliculitis: primary care follow-up in 1 to 2 weeks
- Furunculosis: 2 to 3 days
- Cellulitis without fever: 1 to 2 days

Indications for Admission

- Suspected HITB cellulitis
- Furunculosis or cellulitis in a patient with an immune deficiency
- Fever, proximal lymphadenopathy, and lymphangitic streaking in association with cellulitis or other deep skin infection
- Inadequate response to outpatient management

BIBLIOGRAPHY

Darmstadt GL: Oral antibiotic therapy for uncomplicated bacterial skin infections in children. *Pediatr Infect Dis J* 1997;16:227–240.

Mancini AJ: Bacterial skin infections in children: the common and not so common. *Pediatr Ann* 2000;29:26–35.

Oumeish I, Oumeish OY, Bataineh O: Acute bacterial skin infections in children. *Clin Dermatol* 2000;18:667–678.

CANDIDA

Candidiasis is caused by the fungus *Candida albicans*, which inhabits the gastrointestinal tract of young infants and the vaginal vault of mature females. Factors that predispose to candidiasis include local heat or moisture, systemic antibiotics, diabetes mellitus, and corticosteroids.

Clinical Presentation

Cutaneous Candidiasis   Cutaneous candidiasis is most frequently found in the intertriginous areas. It is characterized by moist, beefy-red, well-demarcated macules with raised, scaly edges. Satellite vesicles and pustules may be seen near the borders. Primary infection in the diaper region causes a perianal rash, and secondary infection of a diaper rash of any other etiology is very common.

Oral Candidiasis   Oral candidiasis (thrush) presents in the first weeks of life with loosely adherent, cheesy white plaques on the tongue, soft and hard palates, and buccal mucosa. The mucosal surfaces are beefy-red, and the lesions bleed when scraped lightly with a tongue blade. These lesions are often painful, and a marked decrease in oral intake can occur in young infants. Thrush in older patients is usually associated with some underlying condition (immunosuppression, broad-spectrum antibiotics), but it can occur in otherwise healthy infants. Recurrent thrush can be seen in HIV-infected children; esophageal candidiasis occurs in up to 20% of these patients.

Perlèche   Perlèche (angular cheilitis) presents as erythema and fissuring at the corners of the mouth. It may be associated with overbite, braces, poor mouth closure, or lip smacking.

Diagnosis

The typical intense erythema, scaly border, and satellite lesions suggest the diagnosis of cutaneous candidiasis. *Contact diaper rashes* usually do not involve the intertriginous areas, while *seborrheic diaper eruptions* are often associated with cradle cap and postauricular scaling. When the diagnosis is in doubt, scrape the border of the eruption and examine the scale under a microscope after mixing with 10 to 20% KOH and gently heating. Budding yeasts and pseudohyphae are seen with *Candida.*

Thrush is often confused with *milk,* but the latter can easily be scraped from the oral mucosa without causing any bleeding.

Angular cheilitis can resemble *impetigo,* but the characteristic honey-colored crust is not present. The perioral eruption of *herpes simplex* presents with grouped vesicles that are not usually located at the corners of the mouth.

ED Management

Many topical agents are available, including nystatin, miconazole, clotrimazole, and econazole. Apply one of these creams three or four times a day to cutaneous eruptions and perlèche. The "-azoles" are preferred in the inguinal region or when it is difficult to distinguish tinea from monilia. Avoid combination products containing neomycin, which can be sensitizing. Steroid-containing preparations, such as clotrimazole-betamethasone, are beneficial when inflammation or contact dermatitis is present. However, limit the treatment to no more than a 1-week course. If the eruption is particularly inflamed, use 5% Burow's solution soaks three or four times a day. Treat macerated or wet-looking areas with frequent diaper changing and Zeasorb-AF at each diaper change.

For thrush, instill 1 mL of a nystatin oral suspension in each side of the mouth qid, after feedings, until 5 days after the lesions have resolved. Advise the parent to rub persistent lesions with a gauze pad soaked with nystatin suspension and to discard any old pacifiers. Suspect an underlying immunodeficiency in children with persistent or recurrent thrush in the absence of antibiotic use. For these patients, clotrimazole troches or ketoconazole can be used (see "HIV Emergencies," pp 339–352).

Follow-up

- Primary care follow-up in 1 to 2 weeks

BIBLIOGRAPHY

Hoppe JE: Treatment of oropharyngeal candidiasis and candidal diaper dermatitis in neonates and infants: review and reappraisal. *Pediatr Infect Dis J* 1997; 16:885–894.

Lane AT: Cutaneous candidiasis. *Pediatr Dermatol* 1995;12:369.

Wolf R, Wolf D: Diaper dermatitis. *Clin Dermatol* 2000;18:657–660.

CONTACT DERMATITIS

There are two forms of contact dermatitis: primary irritant dermatitis and allergic contact dermatitis. Primary irritant dermatitis is a nonallergic reaction caused by soaps, detergents, acids, alkalis, saliva, urine, and feces. It is more common than allergic contact dermatitis in infants and young children. The strength of the irritant and duration of exposure determine the severity of the eruption.

Allergic contact dermatitis is secondary to a delayed hypersensitivity response that depends on a genetic predisposition and the site and duration of the contact, as well as previous exposure and sensitization. Common causes include clothing, shoes, nickel, cosmetics, and plants of the *Rhus* genus (poison ivy, oak, and sumac).

Clinical Presentation

Acute contact dermatitis presents as an acute eczematous reaction, with erythema, swelling, vesicles, and pustules. Usually the eruption is seen within a few hours (primary irritant) or 8 to 12 h (allergic) of the contact. There is a sharp demarcation between the involved and uninvolved skin. Chronic lesions resemble chronic eczema, with thickening and lichenification.

Contact with *Rhus* antigen involves exposed areas unless there has been fomite spread of the resin (via pets, clothing, etc.). The dermatitis often appears in a linear pattern, as the resin is spread by the plant brushing along exposed skin. The nature of the dermatitis varies according to the sensitivity of the patient and ranges from erythema to papules or bullae. Highly sensitive patients may react within 2 to 3 h of exposure, although most rashes present within 1 to 3 days. If there is no reexposure, the eruption may persist from 1 to 3 weeks. The fluid in bullae is not contagious, despite the common misconception that it can spread the eruption. Although poison ivy is most frequent in the summer, it can also occur in the colder months from contact with the resin on dried twigs.

Diagnosis

Inquire about exposure to possible offending agents (new soap, detergent, shoes, or foods, or playing in the woods) and whether there have been previous similar episodes or there is known sensitivity to a substance. On examination, the presence of an eczematoid eruption either in nontypical locations or in a linear pattern is highly suggestive of contact dermatitis, as are the sharp borders of the rash (atopic eczema blends into neighboring normal skin).

ED Management

The need to avoid further contact is obvious. Treat an acute dermatitis with open wet dressings (tap water, normal saline, 5% Burow's solution) qid, soothing baths (Aveeno, oatmeal) daily, and antihistamines (hydroxyzine 2 mg/kg/day divided tid or diphenhydramine 5 mg/kg/day divided qid). For intense inflammation or pruritus, apply a medium-potency steroid (see Table 5-2). Use prednisone for severely edematous and vesicular dermatitis, particularly if the face or eyelids are involved. Start with 0.5 to

Table 5-2   Potency of Topical Corticosteroids

CHEMICAL NAME	BRAND NAMES
Low Potency	
Alclometasone 0.05%	Aclovate
Desonide 0.05%	Tridesilon
Fluocinolone 0.01%	Synalar
Hydrocortisone 0.25–2.5%	Carmol HC, Cortaid, Eldecort, Hytone, etc.
Medium Potency	
Betamethasone 0.1%	Diprosone
Fluocinolone 0.025%	Synalar
Flurandrenolide 0.05%	Cordran
Fluticasone 0.05%	Cutivate
Hydrocortisone valerate 0.2%	Westcort
Mometasone 0.1%	Elocon
Triamcinolone 0.1%	Aristocort, Kenalog
High Potency	
Do not use without dermatologic consultation	

1.5 mg/kg/day (40 mg/day max), then taper over 10 to 14 days to prevent a rebound in the eruption.

For a chronic dermatitis, use a medium-potency topical corticosteroid along with soothing baths and moisturizers. Tar preparations (Estar gel, Zetar emulsion) may also be effective.

Follow-up
- Two to three days if prednisone is prescribed, otherwise primary care follow-up in 1 week

Indications for Admission
- Severe disease with extensive involvement

BIBLIOGRAPHY

Epstein WL, Guin JD, Maibach HI: Poison ivy update. *Contemp Pediatr* 2000; 17:54–70.
Friedlander SF: Contact dermatitis. *Pediatr Rev* 1998;19:166–172.
Weston WL, Bruckner A: Allergic contact dermatitis. *Pediatr Clin North Am* 2000;47:897–907.

DIAPER DERMATITIS

Diaper rashes can begin as early as the first month of life and may persist or wax and wane over the next 2 or 3 years. *Candida* superinfection commonly occurs with a diaper rash of any other etiology.

Clinical Presentation

Irritant and Allergic Contact Dermatitis   Irritant and allergic contact dermatitis is usually located on the convex surfaces of the buttocks, genitalia, and lower abdomen, sparing the intertriginous folds. Secondary candidal infection is common.

Candida   Candidal infections may be primary, with perianal erythema, or secondary. Beefy-red erythema—with well-demarcated, raised scaly borders and satellite papules, pustules, and vesicles—is seen. Involvement of the intertriginous creases and associated oral thrush are common, and the eruption can spread up the abdomen and down the thighs. The scrotum is often involved in males. Consider secondary candidiasis if a diaper rash does not respond to the usual therapeutic measures. Persistent or frequently recurring diaper candidiasis can occur in HIV-infected children. Although *Candida* is the most common fungus seen in the diaper area, dermatophyte infection can also occasionally present with an annular scaling border to the eruption.

Seborrheic Dermatitis   Seborrheic dermatitis presents as nonpruritic, salmon-colored, greasy scales on a well-demarcated erythematous base. Characteristically, a similar eruption is simultaneously seen on the face, along with scaling of the scalp and retroauricular areas. Involvement of the intertriginous creases is common, and secondary candidiasis can occur.

Atopic Dermatitis   Atopic dermatitis can occasionally cause a moist, erythematous diaper rash in association with a similar eruption on the face, trunk, and extensor surfaces of the extremities. These infants are extremely unhappy because of the intense pruritus. The onset is between 2 and 6 months of age; usually the family history is positive for allergies, eczema, hay fever, or asthma.

Congenital Syphilis   Congenital syphilis usually presents between 2 and 6 weeks of age with macules, papules, and bullae of the anogenital region and palms and soles. Lesions of condylomata lata (pp 119–120) may be seen around the anus, buttocks, skin folds, and angles of the mouth. Hepatosplenomegaly is common.

Langerhans Cell Histiocytosis (Histiocytosis X)   Histiocytosis X may cause a diaper eruption that resembles seborrhea but is more discretely papular. These papules may feel firm or slightly infiltrated or indurated and can appear hemorrhagic or purpuric. Furthermore, ulceration may occur, which is rare in seborrhea or psoriasis.

Acrodermatitis Enteropathica   Acrodermatitis enteropathica in the diaper area can resemble *Candida* or psoriasis. However, there may be a vesicobullous eruption of the perioral area, fingers, and toes. The patient may also have diarrhea, cachexia, and alopecia.

Psoriasis   Psoriasis can occasionally occur in the first few years of life. It is characterized by the presence of well-demarcated red plaques that are often covered with copious amounts of white or silver (micaceous) scales. New lesions are often small, 1- to 3-mm papules that subsequently enlarge and coalesce with adjacent lesions to form large plaques. Other common sites for psoriatic lesions are the elbows, scalp, knees, and lumbosacral region.

Perianal Streptococcal Disease   Perianal group A streptococcal infection is characterized by a persistent, bright red, usually tender eruption that is sharply demarcated from the adjacent normal skin. There can be perianal tenderness and itching and occasionally rectal pain, painful defecation, anal fissures, and secondary stool withholding.

Diagnosis

In general, the clinical presentations are sufficiently different so that there are no difficulties in making the diagnosis. When the picture is not typical, a secondary candidal infection of an irritant, contact, or seborrheic dermatitis has most likely occurred. This can be confirmed, if necessary, by microscopic examination of some scales that have been mixed with 10 to 20% KOH and heated gently. Budding yeasts and pseudohyphae are seen in candidal infections. A dermatophyte infection can also be confirmed (branching hyphae and spores).

   Pruritus is the key to diagnosing *atopic dermatitis*. Consider *congenital syphilis* if there are lesions on the palms and soles or *histiocytosis X* if the eruption is papular. If the infant appears malnourished, with chronic diarrhea and alopecia, consider *acrodermatitis*. *Psoriasis* is suggested by the typical distribution and morphology of the lesions. *Perianal streptococcal infection* can be confirmed by obtaining a bacterial culture if there is intense perianal erythema.

ED Management

Meticulous diaper care is the cornerstone of therapy. Instruct the parents to keep the diaper area dry (with frequent changes and air drying), to use loose-fitting diapers, and to avoid rubber pants. Recommend mild cleansers, such as Cetaphil or Aveeno, instead of soap. Discontinue talcum powder, which may be irritating. Inflammation secondary to irritants, contact dermatitis, seborrhea, or atopic dermatitis responds to a mild topical steroid (see Table 5-2) after diaper changing. If the eruption is particularly moist, soaks with tap water or 5% Burow's solution are helpful.

Many topical agents are available, including nystatin, miconazole, and clotrimazole. Apply one of these creams three or four times a day with diaper changes. The "-azoles" are preferred in the diaper region or when it is difficult to distinguish tinea from *Candida*. Nystatin, which is in Mycostatin and Mycolog, is effective only against *Candida* and other yeast fungi; it is not effective against dermatophyte infections. Add oral nystatin (1 mL to each side of the mouth tid, after feeding) if there is oral thrush or a recurrent candidal diaper rash. If there is concomitant inflammatory or contact dermatitis, use a combination antifungal and steroid (clotrimazole-betamethasone). However, limit the treatment course to no more than 1 week, as this steroid is particularly potent.

Treat *perianal streptococcal infection* with penicillin VK (50 mg/kg/day divided qid) or 40 mg/kg/day divided qid of either cephalexin or erythromycin.

A diaper eruption may be the presenting sign of an underlying systemic disorder (*immunodeficiency, histiocytosis X, acrodermatitis enteropathica, psoriasis*). Therefore, if the rash does not respond to these routine measures or the infant either is not thriving or has recurrent infections, referral to a dermatologist is indicated.

Follow-up

- Perianal streptococcal infection: 2 to 3 days
- Other diaper rashes: primary care follow-up

BIBLIOGRAPHY

Boiko S: Making rash decisions in the diaper area. *Pediatr Ann* 2000;29:50–56.
Kazaks EL, Lane AL: Diaper dermatitis. *Pediatr Clin North Am* 2000;47:909–919.
Wolf R, Wolf D: Diaper dermatitis. *Clin Dermatol* 2000;18:657–660.

DRUG ERUPTIONS

Potentially, any drug can cause a rash. The most common offending agents are the penicillins and sulfonamides, while acetaminophen, antihistamines, digoxin, corticosteroids, theophylline, and thyroid hormones rarely cause an eruption. In general, suspect that a drug given within 1 week of the onset of the rash is the cause; it is unusual for medications that have been administered for long periods of time to be implicated. However, there are many exceptions to these rules, and there are no tests to confirm that an eruption is due to a particular agent. The priority in the ED is the expeditious treatment of an anaphylactic reaction.

Clinical Presentation and Diagnosis

Drugs can cause a range of eruptions, including acne, erythema multiforme minor or major, erythema nodosum, a lupus-like butterfly rash, urticaria and angioneurotic edema, and macular and photosensitivity reactions. For each rash morphology there are certain agents that are most likely to be involved (Table 5-3).

Fixed Drug Eruptions   Fixed drug eruptions recur in the same location each time the agent is administered. The lesions are usually violaceous, round plaques that may have dusky centers with bullae. These are few in number and are most common on the extremities and genitals.

Amoxicillin Rash   Between 5 and 10% of patients taking ampicillin or amoxicillin will have an erythematous, nonpruritic, macular eruption primarily on the trunk, face, and extremities. The typical onset is between days 4 and 8, although the rash can occur after the first or last dose of a

Table 5-3   Causes of Drug Eruptions

TYPE OF ERUPTION	MOST COMMON DRUGS
Acneiform	Corticosteroids, diphenylhydantoin, isoniazid, lithium, oral contraceptives
Erythema multiforme	Sulfonamides, penicillins, barbiturates, phenytoin, carbamazepine
Erythema nodosum	Sulfonamides, phenytoin, oral contraceptives
Fixed drug eruption	Barbiturates, tetracyclines, phenolphthalein, sulfonamides
Lupus-like	Procainamide, hydralazine
Macular eruptions	Sulfonamides, phenytoin, barbiturates, penicillins, gold, erythromycin, tetracyclines, isoniazid, chloramphenicol, thiazides, salicylates
Photosensitivity	Tetracyclines (especially demeclocycline and doxycycline), phenothiazines, thiazides, sulfonamides, coal-tar preparations, soaps and detergents containing salicylanilides (hexachlorophene)
Purpura	Penicillins, sulfonamides, oral contraceptives
Toxic epidermal	Barbiturates, phenytoin, salicylates, penicillins, sulfonamides, other necrolysis antibiotics, tranquilizers, allopurinol
Urticaria	Penicillins, cephalosporins, sulfonamides, codeine, salicylates

course. This is not a true allergy and does not necessitate discontinuing the drug or avoiding penicillins in the future.

ED Management

In most cases, the only treatment required is discontinuing the offending agent. However, in the absence of urticaria, it is not necessary to stop amoxicillin or ampicillin.

Treat pruritus with hydroxyzine (2 mg/kg/day divided tid) or diphenhydramine (5 mg/kg/day divided qid).

Treat *photosensitivity reactions* by avoiding sunlight and using sunscreens with a sun protection factor of 15 or greater.

The treatment of *anaphylaxis* (pp 22–24), *acne* (pp 80–81), *erythema multiforme* (pp 95–96), *erythema nodosum* (pp 97–98), *toxic epidermal necrolysis* (pp 98–99), and *urticaria* (pp 26–28) is discussed elsewhere.

Follow-up

- Erythema multiforme, purpura, urticaria: 2 to 3 days if no improvement

Indications for Admission

- Toxic epidermal necrolysis
- Stevens-Johnson syndrome
- Anaphylactoid reactions

BIBLIOGRAPHY

Morelli JG, Tay Y-K, Roers M, et al: Fixed drug eruptions in children. *J Pediatr* 1999;134:365–367.

Roujeau JC, Stern RS: Severe adverse cutaneous reactions to drugs. *N Engl J Med* 1994;331:1272–1285.

Wolkenstein P, Revuz J: Allergic emergencies encountered by the dermatologist. Severe cutaneous adverse drug reactions. *Clin Rev Allergy Immunol* 1999; 17:497–511.

ERYTHEMA MULTIFORME

Erythema multiforme is considered to be a hypersensitivity reaction, most often to infectious agents including viruses (herpes simplex virus, hepatitis virus, Epstein-Barr virus, adenovirus), bacteria (*Mycobacterium tuberculosis, Staphylococcus, Streptococcus, Neisseria gonorrhoeae*), *Mycoplasma,* and fungi (*Coccidioides, Histoplasma*). Other etiologies are drugs (penicillins, sulfonamides, tetracycline, phenytoin), collagen vascular diseases (lupus, rheumatoid arthritis), pregnancy, poison ivy, and neoplasms (leukemia, lymphoma).

Erythema multiforme is classified as either minor (no bullae; most often caused by infections) or major, also known as the Stevens-Johnson syndrome (bullae; most often caused by drugs).

Clinical Presentation

The disease is seen in all age groups, although it is uncommon in children under 3 years of age. Prodromal symptoms of cough, coryza, sore throat, vomiting, and myalgias may precede the eruption by 1 to 10 days. The typical lesion of erythema multiforme minor is the erythematous iris or target-shaped plaque, occasionally with petechiae within the margins. However, macules, papules, and localized bullae can occur. In mild cases, the eruption is symmetric, predominantly over the extensor surfaces, palms and soles, and mucous membranes.

When the disease progresses to erythema multiforme major (Stevens-Johnson syndrome), there is high fever as well as severe constitutional symptoms with extensive bullous involvement of the mucous membranes (oral, ocular, and genital). Superficial ulceration and hemorrhagic crusting of the mucous membranes also occur. Severe eye involvement can occur, with conjunctivitis and keratitis. Lesions appear in successive crops over 10 to 15 days, after which slow resolution occurs.

Diagnosis

When the characteristic target lesions are present, there is little difficulty in making the diagnosis. However, erythema multiforme is most often confused with *urticaria*, in which the plaques are pruritic. Also, each individual hive lasts less than 24 h; this is the primary differentiating point between the two conditions. In a *vasculitis*, palpable, nonblanching purpuric lesions are characteristic.

ED Management

If an etiology is not apparent (drug history, herpes, hepatitis, pharyngitis, pregnancy, poison ivy eruption) but the patient appears well, a viral infection is the probable cause and workup can be deferred. If the patient appears ill, obtain a heterophile antibody, cold agglutinins, and hepatitis surface antigen (HBsAg), and place a PPD. Also obtain a throat culture if there is a pharyngitis and a chest x-ray if there are lower respiratory tract symptoms.

Appropriately treat any underlying illness (erythromycin for *Mycoplasma,* etc.). In mild cases, all that is needed is acetaminophen (15 mg/kg q 4 h) and wet compresses (normal saline or 5% Burow's solution) tid for localized bullae. Diphenhydramine-Maalox (1:1) rinses may ease the debilitating oral pain of the mucous membrane involvement. Consult an ophthalmologist for any ocular involvement. The use of corticosteroids is controversial for children with erythema multiforme major; admit the patient and consult with a dermatologist.

Follow-up

- Patient with erythema multiforme minor: 2 to 3 days to check PPD and laboratory results

Indications for Admission

- Inability to take liquids adequately, irritability
- Stevens-Johnson syndrome

BIBLIOGRAPHY

Freedberg IM (ed): Fitzpatrick's *Dermatology in General Medicine,* 4th ed. New York: McGraw-Hill, 1993, pp 586–599.

Leaute-Labreze C, Lamireau T, Chawki D, et al: Diagnosis, classification, and management of erythema multiforme and Stevens-Johnson syndrome. *Arch Dis Child.* 2000;83:347–352.

Weston WL: What is erythema multiforme? *Pediatr Ann* 1996;25:106–109.

ERYTHEMA NODOSUM

Erythema nodosum is a hypersensitivity reaction that occurs most commonly in patients with respiratory infections, particularly group A streptococcal pharyngitis and primary tuberculosis. Other associations include fungal infections (coccidioidomycosis, histoplasmosis, dermatophytosis), Lyme disease, infectious mononucleosis, cat-scratch disease, mycoplasma pneumonia, pregnancy, inflammatory bowel disease, sarcoid, lymphoma, leukemia, and drug reactions (bromides, sulfonamides, oral contraceptives). Erythema nodosum is more common in females and in patients over 10 years of age; it is seen more often in the spring and fall.

Clinical Presentation

Erythema nodosum presents with multiple 1- to 5-cm oval, bruise-colored, slightly elevated nodules symmetrically distributed over the anterior tibias. Less commonly, lesions occur on the extensor surfaces of the arms, thighs, face, and neck. Nodules can be warm and extremely tender and frequently are accompanied by arthralgias. Strep-induced erythema nodosum usually appears within 3 weeks of the infection. The eruption then usually disappears without scarring within 6 weeks. There may be recurrences over a period of weeks to months but rarely thereafter.

Diagnosis

Usually the nodules are so characteristic that there is little difficulty in making the diagnosis. *Insect bites* are pruritic and not symmetrically distributed; *bruises* are usually not elevated and resolve over several days; and a *cellulitis* is hot, usually unilateral, not well demarcated, and often associated with lymphangitic streaking or local lymphadenopathy.

Inquire about a history of upper respiratory infection, tick bites, trauma, recent travel, possible tuberculosis exposure, and medication use. Obtain a rapid strep test or a throat culture and place a 5TU PPD. If tuberculosis, sarcoid, or a systemic fungal infection is suspected, also obtain a chest x-ray.

ED Management

The priority is treatment of the underlying disease or elimination of the offending drug. Bed rest, leg elevation, and ibuprofen (10 mg/kg q 6 h) are helpful. Refer atypical, persistent, or recurrent cases to a dermatologist.

Follow-up

- As per the underlying illness

BIBLIOGRAPHY

Brodell RT, Mehrabi D: Underlying causes of erythema nodosum. Lesions may provide clue to systemic disease. *Postgrad Med* 2000;108:147–149.

Kakourou T, Drosatou P, Psychou F, et al: Erythema nodosum in children: a prospective study. *J. Am Acad Dermatol* 2001;44:17–21.

EXFOLIATIVE DERMATOSES

The staphylococcal scalded skin syndrome (SSSS) is a distinctive dermatosis caused by an epidermolytic toxin produced by phage group II strains of staphylococci, types 3A, 3B, 3C, 55, and 71. SSSS must be distinguished from toxic epidermal necrolysis (TEN).

TEN is a severe exfoliative disorder thought to be a more severe variant of erythema multiforme major. The pathogenesis probably involves drug-induced necrosis of the basal cell layer of the epidermis, leading to a subepidermal separation. As the name suggests, TEN is characterized by the rapid onset of widespread epidermal necrolysis. The most common offending agents in children include ibuprofen and other nonsteroidal anti-inflammatory drugs, hydantoins, phenolphthalein, procaine, sulfonamides, penicillin or other antibiotics, barbiturates, tranquilizers, vaccines, salicylates, aminopyrine, allopurinol, phenytoin, and griseofulvin.

Clinical Presentation

SSSS   This dermatosis usually occurs in children under 5 years of age. It begins abruptly with a generalized macular erythema after a period of fever and irritability. There may be a pharyngitis, conjunctivitis, rhinorrhea, or discrete staphylococcal infection. The eruption becomes scarlatiniform (sandpaper-like) and tender, with wrinkling, bullae, sheet-like exfoliation, and a positive Nikolsky's sign (a peeling of normal-appearing skin with light pressure). Crusting radiating out from the orifices (mouth, nose, eyes) is typical, but mucous membrane involvement is rare. Despite the marked skin tenderness and irritability, these patients do not appear toxic. If hydration is maintained, recovery occurs in 1 to 2 weeks.

TEN   This disorder is rare in young children, usually occurring in patients over 10 years of age. It presents with widespread macular erythema and stomatitis. As the erythema progresses, the skin begins to separate between the epidermis and dermis. During this stage, the upper layer of the epidermis may become wrinkled or may be removed by light stroking (Nikolsky's sign). The patient subsequently develops flaccid bullae, then varying degrees of skin exfoliation, from localized to the entire body surface. The mortality rate is high (15–25%) secondary to sepsis and fluid and electrolyte imbalances.

Diagnosis

Early in the course, SSSS may resemble *scarlet fever* (nontender skin, pharyngitis, and strawberry tongue, negative Nikolsky), *Kawasaki disease* (erythema of the conjunctiva, lips, and oral mucosa; strawberry tongue; negative Nikolsky), and *Stevens-Johnson syndrome* (target lesions, mucous membrane involvement, negative Nikolsky). The diagnosis of SSSS is confirmed by isolation of staphylococci from body orifices or rarely the blood.

Suspect *TEN* in an older child who is taking one of the offending agents. In typical cases the diagnosis is evident, although before vesiculation occurs, impending TEN is difficult to distinguish from other morbilliform eruptions. TEN is suggested by the characteristic perioral crusting with prominent involvement of several mucosal sites, generalized or focal erythema with exquisite tenderness, bullae, positive Nikolsky's sign, and large areas of sheet-like exfoliation. When the diagnosis is uncertain, TEN can be differentiated from SSSS by a skin biopsy: separation of the superficial layer of the epidermis subcorneally occurs in SSSS, whereas dermal-epidermal separation is characteristic of TEN.

ED Management

If SSSS or TEN is suspected, obtain a CBC, electrolytes, and blood culture; admit the patient; and consult a dermatologist. For possible SSSS, also obtain cultures of all body orifices (including conjunctivae) and treat with IV antistaphylococcal antibiotics (nafcillin 150 mg/kg/day divided q 6 h). When the diagnosis of SSSS or TEN is not clear, consult a dermatologist, who can make the differentiation with a skin biopsy.

Indications for Admission

- All cases of TEN or SSSS

BIBLIOGRAPHY

Ladhani S, Evans RW: Staphylococcal scalded skin syndrome. *Arch Dis Child* 1998;78:85–88.

Ladhani S, Joannou CL: Difficulties in diagnosis and management of the staphylococcal scalded skin syndrome. *Pediatr Infect Dis J* 2000;19:819–821.

Ringheanou M, Laude TA: Toxic epidermal necrolysis in children—an update. *Clin Pediatr (Phila)* 2000;39:687–694.

GRANULOMA ANNULARE

Granuloma annulare (GA) is a relatively common cutaneous disorder of unknown etiology. Although GA may occur at any age, 40% of the cases appear in children younger than 15 years of age.

Clinical Presentation

The primary lesion of GA is a nonscaling, dome-shaped or slightly flattened papule 3 to 6 mm in diameter. These papules may be skin-colored, pink, or violaceous and are typically arranged in the form of a ring. Ring size may vary from 1 to 10 cm in diameter, and multiple rings are present in about 50% of patients. Granuloma annulare may occur on any part of the body, but it usually begins on the lateral or dorsal surfaces of the feet, hands, and fingers.

Diagnosis

Granuloma annulare must be distinguished from other annular eruptions, particularly *tinea corporis*, which is a scaling disease (GA has no scale). Erythema migrans (*Lyme disease*) can present as a single annular plaque with central clearing. To differentiate these, use low-power magnification (otoscope) to inspect the lesion. With GA, there classically are individual papules that form the ring. In addition, on palpation, the individual papules of GA can be appreciated, as opposed to the continuous ring of erythema migrans. See Table 5-4 for the differential diagnosis of annular lesions.

ED Management

Lesions of granuloma annulare usually disappear spontaneously, often within several months to several years, with no residual scarring. If GA is severe or generalized, consult a dermatologist, who may treat with topical or intralesional corticosteroids.

Follow-up

- One to two weeks

BIBLIOGRAPHY

Hanson SG, Levy ML: Granuloma annulare. *Pediatrics* 1999;103:195–196.
Smith MD, Downie JB, DiCostanzo D: Granuloma annulare. *Int J Dermatol* 1997; 36:326–333.

HERPES SIMPLEX

Herpes simplex infections are caused by two major antigenic types, although the clinical diseases are indistinguishable. Herpes simplex 1 was traditionally responsible for nongenital infections, while type 2 was the agent in sexually transmitted disease. However, this distinction is no longer true.

After primary spread by person-to-person contact, the virus remains latent in sensory ganglia, with reactivation at a later time. Among the possible reactivating stimuli are fever, local trauma, stress, menstruation, and ultraviolet light.

Clinical Presentation

The hallmark of herpes infection is a cluster of vesicles on an erythematous base. In general, recurrent disease is associated with fewer constitutional symptoms, smaller vesicles, closer grouping of lesions, and a shorter clinical course than the primary infection.

Gingivostomatitis and Labial Herpes   Gingivostomatitis and labial herpes are common in infants and young children. With primary infection, fever, malaise, sore throat, salivation, and cervical adenopathy occur in association with vesicles in the oral cavity. These vesicles then ulcerate, while the gingiva are erythematous, swollen, and tend to bleed easily. Decreased oral intake may lead to dehydration in infants. Resolution takes 10 to 14 days.

Table 5-4. Differential Diagnosis of Annular Lesions

DIAGNOSIS	MORPHOLOGY	SIZE	LOCATION	DURATION	ASSOCIATED FINDINGS
Erythema migrans	Rapidly enlarging Round or oval plaques Annular or targetoid	>5 cm	Trunk Peripheral extremities	4–8 weeks	Fever, malaise, headache Arthralgia History of tick bite
Erythema multiforme	Erythematous to violaceous Targetoid plaques	1–5 cm	Symmetric, acral Palms and soles	>7 days	Nonspecific viral URI Streptococcal pharyngitis Herpes infection Infectious mononucleosis
Granuloma annulare	Pink to violaceous Smooth papules and plaques	1–5 cm	Distal extremities	Months–years	Asymptomatic
Nummular eczema	Scaly plaques Excoriations	1–5 cm	Extremities	Weeks–months	Pruritus Follicular prominence
Tinea corporis	Scaly plaques Central clearing	Varies	Anywhere	Weeks–months	Cat or dog exposure
Urticaria	Erythematous and edematous Papules and plaques	Varies	Generalized	Usually <24 hours	Pruritus Angioneurotic edema

Adapted from Nopper A, Markus R, Esterly N: When it's not ringworm: annular lesions of childhood. *Pediatr Ann* 1998;27:136–148.

Recurrent infection is often preceded by burning or tingling in the affected areas for hours to several days. The lesions occur on the cheeks, chin, and vermilion borders of the lips but not in the mouth. The grouped vesicles dry quickly and form a crust. Healing occurs in 5 to 14 days, but secondary impetiginization can occur.

Genital Herpes   In females, primary vulvovaginitis is characterized by malaise, fever, vaginal burning, and severe dysuria. The vesicles and erosions may be superficial or deep; involve the vagina, labia, and perineum; and coalesce into large ulcers. In males, the disease affects the penile shaft, glans, urethra, and scrotum. The lesions are painful single or multiple vesicles that rapidly erode and form a crust. Bilateral tender adenopathy is usually present in both sexes. Recurrent disease affects both sexes and occurs with a prodrome of pain or tingling, followed by the clustered vesicles that rupture and form ulcers. The course is 10 to 14 days, with pain, dysuria, and lymphadenopathy.

Neonatal Herpes   Neonatal disease occurs either as an ascending infection after premature rupture of the membranes or by direct spread to the neonate during passage through an infected birth canal. Neonatal infection can be asymptomatic or present as a local infection or disseminated life-threatening disease. Generally, the infant becomes ill during the first week of life, when oral or cutaneous vesicles are noted, most commonly on the face or scalp. Fever, lethargy, and hepatosplenomegaly can occur; with dissemination, there may be ocular (keratoconjunctivitis), central nervous system (encephalitis), and pulmonary (pneumonia) involvement. Dissemination can also occur in the absence of cutaneous lesions. A similar spectrum of disease can occur in immunocompromised patients.

Keratoconjunctivitis   Primary ocular disease presents as a purulent conjunctivitis with edema, vesicles, and corneal ulcers. In contrast to other etiologies of conjunctivitis, pain and photophobia are common because the cornea is involved. With recurrent disease, keratitis or corneal ulcers occur in association with a vesicular eruption of the conjunctiva, eyelids, periorbital skin, and tip of the nose.

Whitlow   Herpetic whitlow results from inoculation of the virus into the fingers, causing a painful, localized, vesiculobullous eruption with swelling and erythema. It is usually found distally on the finger that the child habitually sucks. The course is 10 to 14 days.

Diagnosis

Always suspect herpes when there are grouped vesicles on an erythematous base. The presumptive diagnosis of a herpetic infection can be made by performing a Tzanck smear: open the vesicle, blot up the fluid, scrape the bottom of the lesion onto a glass slide, and stain with Wright's or Giemsa stain. With herpes, multinucleated giant cells are seen. The diagnosis can be confirmed by culturing the virus from vesicle fluid; this requires 24 to 48 h.

Gingivostomatitis and Labial Herpes   The differential diagnosis of mouth sores is discussed on pp 72–75. *Vincent's angina* is an acute gingivitis, occurring in adolescents and young adults, that resembles herpes without buccal involvement. *Stevens-Johnson syndrome* may be associated with cutaneous lesions, and *hand-foot-mouth disease* is often associated with vesicular lesions on the hands and feet. Recurrent labial herpes is most often confused with *impetigo*, although the crust in impetigo has a typical honey color.

Genital Herpes   Herpes is the major cause of vesicles and ulcers of the genitalia, but confusion with *syphilis* is common. The diagnosis of sexually transmitted diseases is summarized on pp 286–293.

Neonatal Herpes   Neonatal herpes can resemble any of the transplacental *TORCH* infections or *bacterial sepsis*, especially when there are no cutaneous lesions. A complete sepsis workup (including lumbar puncture) and TORCH titers are indicated for infants presenting in this manner. Do not dismiss the possibility of neonatal herpes if the mother claims never to have had herpes or not to have had active disease at the time of delivery.

Keratoconjunctivitis   See pp 495–499 for other etiologies of a "red eye." However, the symptoms of ocular pain and photophobia along with the intense conjunctival involvement do not occur with a routine *viral* or *bacterial conjunctivitis*. In recurrent infection, be suspicious of ocular involvement if a vesicular eruption is noted on the tip of the nose, since the innervation is the same.

Whitlow   A whitlow can resemble a *paronychia* or *bullous impetigo*. In the latter two, the vesicles are deep and filled with yellowish purulent fluid; the pain is not severe. Herpetic vesicles contain clear, opalescent fluid, which gives a whitish appearance.

ED Management

Despite progress in the development of antiviral drugs, the mainstays of therapy for children with herpetic *gingivostomatitis*, *herpes labialis*, and *whitlow* are analgesia (acetaminophen, ibuprofen), soaks (sitz baths, 5% Burow's solution), and patience. On occasion, an infant with severe oral disease can become dehydrated and require intravenous fluids. For patients with significant gingivostomatitis that interferes with adequate intake, swab the lesions with viscous lidocaine (2%). However, use it judiciously, as viscous lidocaine can cause seizures if large quantities are absorbed and cardiotoxicity when it is used as a rinse or for lesions in the posterior pharynx.

Genital Herpes   The treatment is summarized on p 292. In general, treatment of primary or recurrent disease results in faster resolution of the pain and pruritus and decreased formation of new lesions. Also, suppressive therapy can reduce the frequency of recurrences.

Keratoconjunctivitis   Refer any patient with suspected herpetic kerato-conjunctivitis to an ophthalmologist for further evaluation and treatment (acyclovir ophthalmic ointment). Never prescribe ocular corticosteroids, which may facilitate spread of the infection.

Neonates and Immunocompromised Patients   Treat with IV acyclovir (60 mg/kg/day divided q 8 h) for 21 days. Attempt to culture the virus from mucocutaneous lesions, urine, saliva, and cerebrospinal fluid.

Whitlow   Confirm the diagnosis with a Tzanck smear if necessary. Treat symptomatically and avoid any surgical incision.

Follow-up

- Gingivostomatitis and labialis: 1 to 2 days if no improvement
- Keratoconjunctivitis: as per the ophthalmologist
- Whitlow: primary care follow-up in 1 to 2 weeks

Indications for Admission

- Herpetic infection in a neonate or immunocompromised patient
- Poor oral intake and dehydration in an infant with gingivostomatitis

BIBLIOGRAPHY

Annunziato PW, Gershon A: Herpes simplex virus infections. *Pediatr Rev* 1996; 17:415–423.
Sonis A, Zaragoza S: Dental health for the pediatrician. *Curr Opin Pediatr* 2001; 13:289–295.
Whitley RJ, Roizman B: Herpes simplex virus infections. *Lancet* 2001;357:1513–1518.

HYPOPIGMENTED LESIONS

Clinical Presentation

White or hypopigmented lesions are caused by either a decreased number of melanocytes or a decreased amount of melanin within the keratocytes.

Pityriasis Alba   Pityriasis alba presents as one to several dozen small (one to several centimeters in diameter) white patches predominantly on the cheeks, arms, and trunk. The margins are sharply delineated, and there is a fine brawny scale. It is often seen in association with atopic dermatitis. It is most common in children 3 to 10 years of age and in dark-skinned individuals because of the considerable color contrast between involved and uninvolved areas. In light-skinned individuals, the disease is most apparent in the summertime, when tanning heightens the contrast.

Tinea Versicolor   Tinea versicolor (pityriasis versicolor) is a fungal infection that can present with hypopigmented, well-demarcated, scaling, oval macules on the upper trunk and back, proximal arms, and neck. It is more common in the summertime, as the involved areas do not tan.

Postinflammatory Hypopigmentation   Postinflammatory hypopigmentation may follow the involution of a variety of inflammatory skin disorders, particularly burns, bullous disorders, infections, eczematous or psoriatic lesions, and pityriasis rosea. The pattern of hypopigmentation usually fits fairly well with the historical description of the original insult. There may be hyperpigmentation at the periphery of the white patch.

Tuberous Sclerosis   Tuberous sclerosis is an autosomal dominant disease characterized by the triad of seizures, mental retardation, and facial papules (adenoma sebaceum). Among the other cutaneous manifestations are the ash-leaf spots—well-demarcated hypopigmented macules that are found predominately on the trunk. Ash-leaf spots are usually evident from birth, particularly under a Wood's lamp. Other skin findings that may be seen are the shagreen patch and periungual fibromas.

Vitiligo   Vitiligo affects about 1% of the population and appears to be inherited as an autosomal dominant trait with variable penetrance. Although the etiology of vitiligo is unknown, the current hypothesis suggests autoimmune destruction of the melanocytes by circulating autoantibodies. A patient with vitiligo may have another autoimmune disease such as hyperthyroidism, hypothyroidism, Hashimoto's thyroiditis, adrenocortical insufficiency, pernicious anemia, polyendocrine deficiencies, parathyroid abnormalities, or myasthenia gravis. Vitiligo presents with asymptomatic oval or irregular ivory-white macules and patches surrounded by a well-demarcated or hyperpigmented border. These lesions may grow and coalesce to form large, irregularly shaped areas of depigmentation. The distribution includes the face, axillae, and dorsal surface of the hands, usually (but not exclusively) in a bilaterally symmetric manner. No scale is present visually or upon scraping. Vitiligo can occur at any age, but the peak incidence is from late childhood to middle adult life.

Diagnosis

Pityriasis alba, pityriasis versicolor, vitiligo, and postinflammatory hypopigmentation can all present with lesions of similar appearance. The lesions of *vitiligo* are alabaster-white, in contrast to the other conditions, in which the lesions are lighter than normal skin color but not completely white. In addition, vitiligo is classically symmetric. Dermatologic consultation is necessary if the diagnosis remains in doubt.

Pityriasis alba can usually be diagnosed by the typical appearance and distribution in a patient known to have atopic dermatitis. *Postinflammatory hypopigmentation* can often be diagnosed by a history of preceding irritation, inflammation, or other rash. The hypopigmented macules of *tuberous sclerosis* lack the characteristic milk-white appearance of the lesions of vitiligo. Furthermore, in tuberous sclerosis, lesions are present at birth or during the early neonatal period and do not change with age.

The differentiation of *tinea versicolor* from these other conditions is facilitated by scraping the lesions, mixing the scale with 10 to 20% KOH, heating gently, and then examining microscopically. Tinea versicolor has a characteristic "spaghetti and meatballs" appearance. Also, tinea versicolor infections fluoresce under Wood's lamp examination.

Albinism (generalized or partial) may be difficult to distinguish from vitiligo. Albinism, however, is present from birth.

ED Management

Pityriasis Alba   There is no effective treatment, although most children outgrow the disease by early to midadolescence. Occasionally, therapy with a very mild topical steroid (1% hydrocortisone cream bid) and moisturizers may diminish the demarcation between normal and whiter skin. Stress to the family that sun protection is imperative because the affected areas cannot tan normally and may be more susceptible to burning, and tanning accentuates the difference between the normal and hypopigmented skin, worsening the patient's appearance.

Tinea Versicolor   The treatment is discussed on p 118.

Postinflammatory Hypopigmentation   Since the defect is primarily epidermal, postinflammatory hypopigmentation generally improves over time without any therapy.

Tuberous Sclerosis   There is no treatment. Rather, refer the patient to a primary care provider to investigate for other stigmata of the disease.

Vitiligo   The single most important piece of advice is for the patient to use appropriate sun protection, as areas of vitiligo are unable to tan normally and therefore are not protected from the sun.

Follow-up

• Primary care follow-up in 2 to 4 weeks

BIBLIOGRAPHY

Galan EB, Janniger CK: Pityriasis alba. *Cutis* 1998;61:11–13.
Halder RM: Childhood vitiligo. *Clin Dermatol* 1997;15:899–906.
Sunenshine PJ, Schwartz RA, Janniger CK: Tinea versicolor: an update. *Cutis* 1998;61:65–68, 71–72.

LICE

Three varieties of lice—the head louse, the body louse, and the pubic louse—parasitize humans. The head louse is transmitted by direct personal contact, by contact with infected upholstery, and by sharing hats, combs, brushes, and towels. Body and pubic lice are acquired via bedding, clothing, and person-to-person (sexual) contact. The body louse can carry rickettsial disease (typhus and trench fever) and spirochetal disease (relapsing fever).

Clinical Presentation

Pediculosis Capitis (Head Lice)   The patient usually presents with pruritus of the scalp, ears, and neck, which can occasionally be very severe. Nits (eggs) are oval and yellow-white, measuring 0.3 to 0.8 mm in size. They are found close to the scalp, firmly cemented to the hair around the ears and the occiput. They project from the side of the hair shaft and do not surround it. Nits more than 1.25 cm from the scalp are probably no longer viable. Adult lice are usually not seen. Secondary impetigo, folliculitis, or furunculosis is common and may mask the primary disease.

Pediculosis Corporis (Body Lice)   These lice live in the linings and seams of clothing and occasionally emerge to bite the host. Erythematous macules become intensely pruritic papules and urticarial wheals, with secondary eczematization and impetiginization.

Phthirus Pubis (Pubic Lice; "Crabs")   Itching is frequently the initial symptom, but secondary infection is common. Pubic and axillary hair and the eyelashes can be affected. The organisms can be identified as brownish crawling "flecks," and nits may be seen attached to the hair shafts. Lice bites can cause nonblanching gray-blue macules (maculae ceruleae) on the lower abdomen and thighs.

Diagnosis

The diagnosis of lice infestation is based on the history of possible contact, itching, and visualization of the lice or nits. Nits fluoresce under Wood's lamp examination, and microscopic identification of a nit confirms the diagnosis. Infestation with body and pubic lice may resemble *eczema* or *folliculitis*. Body lice can also simulate *scabies*.

ED Management

Pediculosis Capitis   Treat with either a permethrin or pyrethin-based shampoo. Instruct the parents to apply a single 10-min application of permethrin (Nix) after first shampooing and towel-drying the scalp. An equally effective alternative is two 10-min applications of a pyrethrin-based product (A200, Rid) 1 week apart. Treat all contacts at the same time. Recommend that the parents use a fine-toothed comb to remove nits. Instruct the family to wash the clothing and bedding in very hot water [>52°C (125°F)] for 10 min and to place all hats, combs, and headgear in a plastic bag until after the second shampoo. Use lindane shampoo (Kwell) in children older than 2 years if these medications do not eradicate the infestation.

Pubic Lice   Apply a pyrethrin-based product for 10 min, then repeat in 1 week. Use lindane shampoo if the infestation persists. Advise the patient to have all sexual contacts treated.

Body Lice   Frequent bathing and laundering [>52°C (125°F) for at least 10 min] of clothing and bedding are all that is usually necessary. If lice are noted, treat with a pyrethrin or lindane lotion: apply to the entire body from the jawline down, leave on overnight, then wash off in the morning. Treat pruritus with hydroxyzine (2 mg/kg/day divided tid) or diphenhydramine (5 mg/kg/day divided qid).

Eyelash Lice   Treat with petrolatum applied bid for 8 days. Remove any nits mechanically.

Follow-up

• Primary care follow-up in 1 week

BIBLIOGRAPHY

Angel TA, Nigro J, Levy ML: Infestations in the pediatric patient. *Pediatr Clin North Am* 2000;47:921–935.
Burkhart CG, Burkhart CN: An assessment of the topical and oral, prescription and over-the-counter treatments for head lice. *J Am Acad Dermatol* 1998;38: 979–982.
Meinking TL: Infestations. *Curr Probl Dermatol* 1999;11:77–107.

MOLLUSCUM CONTAGIOSUM

Molluscum contagiosum is an eruption caused by a virus of the pox group, spread by direct person-to-person contact and autoinoculation. The disease occurs at any age but is most common between 3 and 15 years.

Clinical Presentation

The lesions start as small papules that typically grow to 3 to 6 mm in diameter, but they can be as large as 2 to 3 cm. They are usually flesh-colored or slightly erythematous and dome-shaped, with a central umbilication. Papules are found on the face, trunk, extremities, and pubic region, either alone or in clusters, and number from one to several hundred. The duration of individual lesions is variable; although most resolve within 9 to 12 months, some may persist for 2 to 3 years. Chronic conjunctivitis or keratitis may occur with eyelid lesions. Particularly severe eruptions with thousands of lesions can occur in patients with atopic dermatitis or depressed cellular immunity. Although molluscum is usually an asymptomatic process, up to 10% of patients develop an eczematoid hypersensitivity reaction around the lesions.

Diagnosis

Although confusion with *warts, bacterial infections, papillomas*, and *acne* can occur, the diagnosis of molluscum is usually easily established by the distinctive appearance of the flesh-colored papules with central umbilication. To verify the diagnosis, spray a lesion with ethyl chloride (Frigiderm) to accentuate the central umbilication or open a papule, smear the contents onto a glass slide, and stain with either methylene blue, Wright's stain, or Gram's stain. The presence of microscopic round-to-oval smooth-walled cytoplasmic masses ("molluscum bodies") resembling a cluster of grapes confirms the diagnosis.

ED Management

Untreated lesions often resolve spontaneously within several months to years. If there are cosmetic concerns or the lesions continue to spread, application of liquid nitrogen or curettage of individual lesions is effective. Curettage is quick but is usually not tolerated by young children. Alternatively, each papule can be pierced with a needle and the contents expressed.

Refer the patient to a dermatologist prior to instituting therapy if the diagnosis is in doubt or if there are either facial lesions or multiple papules.

Follow-up

- Primary care follow-up in 2 to 4 weeks

BIBLIOGRAPHY

Lewis EL, Lam M, Crutchfield CE III: An update on molluscum contagiosum. *Cutis* 1997;60:29–34.
Prasad SM: Molluscum contagiosum. *Pediatr Rev* 1996;17:118–119.

NEONATAL RASHES

Compared with that of a child or adult, the skin of a newborn is thinner, sweats less, and has less hair and fewer melanocytes. As a result, newborn skin appears dry and scaly and is more likely to develop blisters or erosions in response to minor traumas.

Clinical Presentation and Diagnosis

Erythema Toxicum Neonatorum   Erythema toxicum is a self-limited eruption that is very common in the first week of life. It can be present at birth or may not appear until as late as 2 weeks of age. It is characterized by a combination of small (<3 mm) macules, papules, and yellowish pustules on an erythematous base, giving the skin a "flea-bitten" appearance. The lesions can be anywhere on the body, although the palms and soles are usually spared. Despite the appearance, the infant is well, with no other signs of illness. When the diagnosis is in doubt, unroof a pustule and Gram's or Wright's stain the contents. Eosinophils are characteristic of erythema toxicum, in contrast to the neutrophils seen with a *bacterial infection*. In addition, the contents are sterile.

Milia   Milia are tiny (<2 mm), yellowish sebaceous cysts that are commonly seen on the cheeks, nose, chin, and forehead of about 50% of newborns. They typically disappear without treatment within the first few months of life.

Miliaria   Miliaria (heat rash) is a group of disorders caused by keratinous obstruction of the eccrine sweat ducts. Miliaria can occur in any season, often secondary to overdressing an infant. There are two main types of heat rash; miliaria rubra (prickly heat) is the more common type and occurs on covered skin, especially where there is friction from clothing. It is characterized by pruritic, erythematous 1- to 2-mm papules and vesicles that are grouped in clusters with surrounding erythema. Miliaria crystallina (sudamina) is characterized by 1- to 2-mm, clear, thin-walled vesicles on otherwise normal skin. The rash is asymptomatic and occurs primarily in the intertriginous areas. Sunburn can cause this type of miliaria.

Mongolian Spots   Mongolian spots are poorly circumscribed dark brown to blue-black patches that are usually found over the lumbosacral area and buttocks. They are very common in newborns, occurring in more than 90% of African Americans and native Americans, 80% of Asians, and 70% of Hispanics. Mongolian spots are present at birth; some may fade over the first few years of life, while others persist into adulthood. They may be single or multiple and can vary in size from a few millimeters to >10 cm in diameter. Although they can be confused with *ecchymoses*, Mongolian spots do not undergo the color changes seen with bruising or a coagulopathy.

Neonatal Acne   Neonatal acne is secondary to hormonal stimulation of sebaceous glands that have not yet involuted to a prepubertal immature state. It presents at birth or in the first few weeks of life with erythematous papules and pustules exclusively on the face.

Neonatal Herpes   Neonatal disease occurs either as an ascending infection after premature rupture of the membranes or by direct spread to the neonate during passage through an infected birth canal. Neonatal infection can be asymptomatic or present as a local infection or disseminated life-threatening disease. Generally, the infant becomes ill during the first week of life, when oral or cutaneous vesicles are noted, most commonly on the face or scalp. Fever, lethargy, and hepatosplenomegaly can occur; with dissemination, there may be ocular (keratoconjunctivitis), central nervous system (encephalitis), and pulmonary (pneumonia) involvement. Dissemination can also occur in the absence of cutaneous lesions.

Seborrhea   Seborrheic dermatitis is a scaling eruption of unknown etiology generally limited to the areas of the body with the greatest number of sebaceous glands. The disease usually presents between 2 and 8 weeks of age with nonpruritic, dry, erythematous scaling of the scalp (cradle cap), often accompanied by retroauricular scaling and occipital lymphadenopathy. The eruption may progress to involve the forehead and face, with the development of characteristic salmon-colored greasy scales on a well-demarcated erythematous base. In the diaper area, the eruption has a similar appearance, with involvement of intertriginous areas. Secondary candidal infection can occur. These babies are happy and do not appear sick.

Transient Neonatal Pustular Melanosis   Transient pustular melanosis is another self-limited neonatal eruption of unknown etiology. In contrast to erythema toxicum, it is present at birth, occurring in 0.2 to 0.4% of newborns. It is characterized by clusters of vesicles and pustules, found primarily on the chin, forehead, nape, trunk, and lower legs. The lesions rupture easily within 24 to 48 h, with resultant hyperpigmentation that fades over the subsequent 1 to 3 months. As with erythema toxicum, the contents are sterile, but neutrophils will be seen on Gram's or Wright's stain.

ED Management

Reassurance is all that is needed for erythema toxicum, milia, Mongolian spots, neonatal acne, and transient neonatal pustular melanosis.

Miliaria   Management consists of cool baths and avoiding excessive heat and humidity. Parents may overdress an infant, mistakenly attempting to keep the baby's hands and feet warm. Advise them that the proper amount of clothing can be ascertained by feeling the infant's neck or upper back, which should be comfortably warm and not hot and sweaty. Cornstarch will keep intertriginous areas dry.

Seborrhea   Usually, treatment of the infant's scalp also clears the remainder of the eruption. Adherent scale can be removed by gently massaging mineral oil or Baler's P&S Liquid into the scalp and leaving it on for 15 min. Afterward, brush the scalp gently or comb with a fine-toothed comb, then shampoo. For more severe cases, an antiseborrheic shampoo—such as Head & Shoulders, Sebulex, Zetar, or Meted—is effective when used twice weekly. Treat severe facial eruptions with a short course (3–5 days) of 1% hydrocortisone cream bid.

Neonatal Herpes   Neonatal herpes can resemble any of the transplacental *TORCH* infections or *bacterial sepsis*, especially when there are no cutaneous lesions. A complete sepsis workup (including lumbar puncture) and TORCH titers are indicated for infants presenting in this manner. Do not dismiss the possibility of neonatal herpes if the mother denies ever having had herpes or having active disease at the time of delivery. The treatment of neonatal herpes is detailed on p 104.

Follow-up

- Primary care follow-up in 1 to 2 weeks

Indication for Admission

- Suspected neonatal herpes

BIBLIOGRAPHY

Eichenfield LF, Hardaway CA: Neonatal dermatology. *Curr Opin Pediatr* 1999;11: 471–474.
Treadwell PA: Dermatoses in newborns. *Am Fam Physician* 1997;56:443–450.
Wagner A: Distinguishing vesicular and pustular disorders in the neonate. *Curr Opin Pediatr* 1997;9:396–405.

PALPABLE PURPURA

Vascular reactions are categorized as blanching (nonpurpuric) and non-blanching (purpuric). Most vascular reactions involve only dilatation of the blood vessels, with no extravasation of blood, so that the eruption blanches with pressure. That is, when direct pressure is placed on the lesion, it fades completely. Less commonly, in a purpuric eruption, there is extravasation of blood, so that the lesions do not blanch completely. Palpable purpura implies that in addition to not blanching, the lesions are slightly elevated and therefore palpable.

The distinction between palpable and nonpalpable purpura is of critical importance In nonpalpable purpura there are often bruises or ecchymoses caused by trauma or a clotting abnormality. In contrast, palpable purpura almost always signifies some type of vasculitis secondary to a serious disease. Possible etiologies include meningococcemia with coagulopathy, subacute bacterial endocarditis (SBE), systemic lupus erythematosus (SLE), Rocky Mountain spotted fever, Henoch-Schönlein purpura (HSP), and drug reactions. The priority in evaluating a nonblanching vascular process is to rule out or treat sepsis expeditiously.

Clinical Presentation

Palpable purpura presents as elevated, nonblanching, erythematous to violaceous plaques and nodules. Dependent areas, such as the legs and feet, are the most common sites.

Diagnosis

Rapidly obtain a complete history, including medication use, previous illnesses, travel, tick bite, and whether fever, other rashes, headache, or arthralgias have been noted. The priority on physical examination is to suspect sepsis (high fever, lethargy, or toxicity in association with palpable purpura), especially *meningococcemia.*

See the appropriate sections for the evaluation of patients with possible *SLE* (pp 600–601), *HSP* (pp 600–601), *SBE* (pp 55–57), and *Rocky Mountain spotted fever* (pp 377–380). If there is any doubt, assume that the patient has sepsis.

ED Management

If the patient is febrile or appears toxic, treat palpable purpura as *bacterial sepsis* until proven otherwise. Immediately obtain a complete blood count and blood culture and treat with broad-spectrum antibiotics. If meningitis cannot be ruled out clinically, perform a lumbar puncture, but do not delay antibiotic therapy in an ill patient.

Treat a *drug eruption* (pp 93–95) by discontinuing the offending agent. The management of *HSP* is discussed elsewhere (p 601).

Follow-up

- As per the underlying illness

Indication for Admission

- Possible sepsis

BIBLIOGRAPHY

Leung AK, Chan KW: Distinguishing vesicular and pustular disorders in the neonate. *Curr Opin Pediatr* 1997;9:396–405.

Wells LC, Smith JC, Weston VC, et al: The child with a non-blanching rash: how likely is meningococcal disease? *Arch Dis Child* 2001;85:218–222.

PITYRIASIS ROSEA

Pityriasis rosea is a benign, self-limited eruption of unknown etiology but presumed to be viral in origin because of the frequent prodromal symptoms, seasonal clustering, and lifelong immunity that develops in 98% of patients. However, person-to-person transmission has not been confirmed.

Clinical Presentation

Pityriasis rosea occurs predominantly in adolescents and young adults and less commonly in children under 5 years of age. After a variable prodrome of malaise, about 75% of cases present with an initial lesion called a "herald patch." This is a 2- to 5-cm scaling, erythematous plaque with a "collarette of scale" (the scaling forms a circle within the borders of the plaque) seen anywhere on the body. The generalized eruption that follows 2 to 21 days later characteristically consists of small, ovoid papules, also with collarettes of scale. The long axes of these lesions follow the cleavage lines on the back and trunk in a so-called "Christmas tree" pattern. This can be more easily appreciated by having the patient twist his or her spine at the waist and by examining the axillae. In older patients, the rash spares the distal extremities, face, and scalp. In younger children, the head and neck may be affected and papules, vesicles, or pustules may be seen. Lesions continue to occur for up 2 weeks, with clearing in 6 to 10 weeks. Postinflammatory hypo- or hyperpigmentation can result.

Diagnosis

The history of the herald patch and the characteristic nature of the lesions of the generalized eruption usually suffice to confirm the diagnosis of pityriasis rosea. However, the herald patch may resemble a *tinea corporis* infection, although these grow slowly and are not followed by a generalized eruption. The lesions of *erythema migrans* are not scaly, expand more rapidly, and grow to larger dimensions than a herald patch.

Several other diseases are characterized by diffuse erythema and scaling, including *guttate psoriasis, nummular eczema, drug reactions*, and *seborrheic dermatitis*, but the face and distal extremities are often involved and there is no "Christmas tree" pattern. The eruption of *secondary syphilis* can look very similar but may involve the palms and soles. Obtain a VDRL if the patient is sexually active.

ED Management

For most patients no treatment is necessary. Antihistamines (hydroxyzine 2 mg/kg/day divided tid; diphenhydramine 5 mg/kg/day divided qid) alleviate the pruritus. Topical corticosteroids may be useful in very inflammatory cases but generally do not shorten the course of the disease. However, ultraviolet light or sunlight exposure may hasten the resolution of the rash. Refer patients with lesions persisting for more than 12 weeks to a dermatologist.

Follow-up

- Primary care follow-up in 2 to 4 weeks

BIBLIOGRAPHY

Allen RA, Janniger CK, Schwartz RA: Pityriasis rosea. *Cutis* 1995;56:198–202.
Hartley AH: Pityriasis rosea. *Pediatr Rev* 1999;20:266–269.

PSORIASIS

Psoriasis is an inherited disorder of unknown etiology that was previously thought to be uncommon in childhood. However, 27% of patients develop the disease before age 15, 10% before age 10, and 6.5% before age 5. Patients with active lesions present at birth (congenital psoriasis) have also been reported.

Clinical Presentation

Psoriasis is characterized by well-demarcated red plaques that are often covered with copious amounts of white or silver (micaceous) scales. New lesions present as small, 1- to 3-mm papules that subsequently enlarge and coalesce with adjacent lesions to form large plaques. Partial coalescence can result in gyrate or serpiginous plaques. Linear lesions may also occur, reflecting the Koebner phenomenon, whereby psoriatic plaques are induced by local cutaneous trauma. The most common sites for psoriasis are the elbows, scalp, knees, genitalia, lumbosacral region, and extensor surfaces of the arms and legs. In infants, psoriasis may also present in the diaper area. Nail changes are also often present, including nail plate pitting, onycholysis, and yellowish discoloration of the nail plate ("oil drop").

Guttate psoriasis presents with a sudden outbreak of hundreds of small, red, nonconfluent papules. Guttate psoriasis is often triggered by an infection, particularly streptococcal.

Diagnosis

Classic lesions of psoriasis are not difficult to diagnose, especially when there is a positive family history. The only other common disease that exhibits the Koebner phenomenon is *lichen planus*, in which the papules are usually pruritic and limited to a few areas of the body, including the flexor surfaces and oral mucosa. *Pityriasis rosea* can usually be differentiated on the basis of the herald patch and the "Christmas tree" distribution on the torso. A positive KOH preparation confirms the diagnosis of *tinea corporis*. If the diagnosis remains in doubt, consult a dermatologist, who can perform a skin biopsy.

ED Management

If the psoriasis is mild and limited to only a few sites, therapy may be initiated in the ED. Recommend mild soaps or cleansers (Dove or Cetaphil), moisturizers, and mild- to moderate-potency topical steroids. Treat stubborn scalp psoriasis with thick, adherent plaques with P&S liquid, applied with a cotton pledget once or twice a day, followed 6 to 8 h later by an antiseborrheic tar or steroid shampoo. It is important to explain to all patients that psoriasis is a chronic condition that is treated but not cured and that there are often alternating periods of exacerbation and remission.

Refer patients with psoriasis to a dermatologist.

Follow-up

- Dermatology follow-up in 2 to 4 weeks

BIBLIOGRAPHY

Arbuckle HA, Hartley AH: Psoriasis. *Pediatr Rev* 1998;19:106–107.
Morris A, Rogers M, Fischer G, et al: Childhood psoriasis: a clinical review of 1262 cases. *Pediatr Dermatol* 2001;18:188–198.

SCABIES

Scabies is caused by infection with the itch mite. It is acquired by close personal contact, although spread via fomites (clothing, linen, and towels) is possible, as the mite can survive for 2 to 5 days away from humans. The average person is infested with only about 10 to 15 organisms, so pruritus is presumed secondary to an acquired sensitivity to the mite and its feces and eggs.

Clinical Presentation

The usual complaint is generalized pruritus, especially at night. The most common sites of involvement are the interdigital webs, flexor aspects of the wrists, extensor surfaces of the elbows, and nipples, axillae, genitalia, and abdomen. The head, neck, palms, and soles can be infected in infants and young children. The characteristic lesion is the burrow, a short, serpiginous ridge that ends with a vesicle. Other common findings are erythematous, excoriated papules and vesicles, with secondary crusts, eczematization, and bacterial infection. The lesions vary, based on the duration of infection and degree of sensitization of the patient.

Diagnosis

Scabies is a "great imitator" of other pruritic eruptions. The diagnosis is suggested by a history of contact with an infected person, the intense pruritus, and the variable nature of the lesions. *Atopic dermatitis* most commonly occurs on the flexor surfaces; involvement of the interdigital webs is uncommon. The lesions of *pityriasis rosea* are well circumscribed and not on the distal extremities. With *folliculitis*, a hair shaft can be seen in each papule. Since the lesions of scabies can become impetiginized, differentiation can be very difficult, although pruritus is not as intense in *impetigo*.

To confirm the diagnosis, place a drop of mineral oil on a burrow, then gently scrape the top off with a no. 15 scalpel blade. Place the scrapings on a microscope slide, cover with a coverslip, and examine at 10× magnification. The diagnosis is confirmed by finding eggs, mites, or oval brown feces.

ED Management

Permethrin 5% (Elimite cream) is now the drug of choice for scabies. Massage the cream into the skin from the head to the soles of the feet and leave it on for 8 to 14 h. Treat the scalp of infants. Treat all household contacts simultaneously, as it can take up to 30 days for a nonsensitized individual to become symptomatic. Wash the bedclothes and linens or store them away for at least 5 days. Repeat the treatment twice, 2 and 7 days later. If Elimite is unsuccessful, treat patients over 2 years of age with lindane (Kwell).

Follow-up

- Primary care follow-up in 1 to 2 weeks

BIBLIOGRAPHY

Hoke AW, Maibach HI: Scabies management: a current perspective. *Cutis* 1999; 64(suppl):2–16.
Meinking TL: Infestations. *Curr Probl Dermatol* 1999;11:77–107.
Peterson CM, Eichenfield LF: Scabies. *Pediatr Ann* 1996;25:97–100.

TINEA

Superficial dermatophytoses are called tinea, although tinea versicolor is caused by *Pityrosporum orbiculare* (not a dermatophyte). The name of the particular infection is based on the clinical location.

Clinical Presentation

Tinea Capitis   Tinea capitis is caused by infection of the hair shaft. Patchy alopecia with scaling, erythema, and infected hairs that are broken off at scalp level (black dots) are seen. An acute hypersensitivity reaction with a boggy, inflammatory mass (kerion) associated with fever, leukocytosis, and lymphadenopathy can develop.

Tinea Corporis   Tinea corporis, or ringworm, is an infection of the glabrous (nonhairy) skin. Infection occurs via contact with an infected individual, infected animal (kitten or puppy), and fomites. The lesions are well-circumscribed annular patches or plaques, with central clearing and a raised, scaly, papular, or vesicular border.

Tinea Cruris   Tinea cruris, or "jock itch," is an infection of the groin and upper thighs that is rare before puberty. More frequent in hot, humid environments and in obese or very athletic individuals, tinea cruris is exacerbated by tight-fitting, chafing clothing. Sharply demarcated, bilaterally symmetric, scaly erythematous plaques that spare the scrotum and labia are typical. Secondary candidal infection can occur but is rare.

Tinea Pedis   Tinea pedis, or "athlete's foot," is a pruritic eruption that is uncommon in prepubertal children. The findings range from mild scaling to marked erythema, maceration, fissuring, and vesiculation involving the toes and interdigital webs. The infection may spread to the soles and sides of the feet, but the dorsal aspects of the toes are usually spared. An allergic response to the fungus (id reaction) occasionally causes an erythematous vesicular eruption on the trunk, upper extremities, and palms.

Tinea Unguium   Tinea unguium (onychomycosis) is a fungal infection of the nail plate that usually occurs in association with dermatophytosis elsewhere (hands, feet). The infection begins in the tip of the nail, which becomes discolored, lusterless, and friable with subungal hyperkeratosis and separation of the distal nail from the nail bed (onycholysis).

Tinea Versicolor   Tinea versicolor (pityriasis versicolor) is an infection of the upper trunk and back, proximal arms, and neck that is particularly common in warm climates. The causative organism is *Pityrosporum orbiculare*. Hypo- or hyperpigmented, well-demarcated, scaling oval macules with little or no erythema or pruritus are seen. Tinea versicolor is diagnosed more commonly in the summertime, as the involved areas will not tan while the surrounding uninfected skin does.

Diagnosis

The differentiation of fungal infections from other conditions is facilitated by scraping the lesions, mixing the scale with 10 to 20% solution, heating gently, and then examining microscopically. Hyphae or spores are seen in these fungal infections, while tinea versicolor has a characteristic "spaghetti and meatballs" appearance. In addition, if the diagnosis is in doubt, culture the fungus on Sabouraud's agar or dermatophyte test medium (DTM), although tinea versicolor will not grow. Finally, a minority of tinea capitis and all tinea versicolor infections will fluoresce under Wood's lamp examination.

Tinea capitis is the only common etiology of childhood alopecia that causes scalp inflammation; the eruption may fluoresce under a Wood's lamp, and black dots may be seen. The scalp is normal in *alopecia areata, traction alopecia,* and *trichotillomania. Seborrheic dermatitis* causes scaling without hair loss. *Bacterial infections* of the scalp are uncommon; usually there is no hair loss, as with a kerion.

Tinea corporis can resemble *contact dermatitis,* the herald patch of *pityriasis rosea, erythema migrans,* and *nummular eczema.* The characteristic central clearing and raised, well-demarcated scaly border usually suggest the diagnosis.

Tinea cruris can be confused with *contact dermatitis, intertrigo,* and *erythrasma,* a *Corynebacterium* infection that fluoresces coral-red under Wood's lamp examination. In addition, secondary candidal infection can occur and confuse the picture, although the therapy is not altered.

Before the diagnosis of tinea pedis is made in a prepubertal patient, consider *dyshydrotic eczema, atopic dermatitis,* and *contact dermatitis,* which can involve the dorsum of the foot. With these conditions, there may be a history of sleeping in socks or with the feet enclosed in pajamas or in sneakers. The id reaction is characterized by the absence of fungus in the area of the reaction, an identifiable focus of fungal infection (usually on the feet), and spontaneous clearing when the primary fungal infection is eradicated.

Tinea unguium must be confirmed with a positive culture, as *psoriasis, eczema, trauma,* and *congenital ectodermal syndromes* can all give a similar appearance.

Tinea versicolor resembles *pityriasis alba, postinflammatory hypopigmentation, vitiligo, seborrheic dermatitis,* and *secondary syphilis.* However, none of these conditions fluoresces under Wood's lamp examination, and all are KOH-negative.

ED Management

Tinea Capitis   Tinea capitis cannot be treated topically. If possible, obtain a culture (see p 117) prior to treating the patient with oral griseofulvin (15 mg/kg/day microsize; 10 mg/kg/day ultramicrosize) for 6 to 8 weeks. Leukopenia, neutropenia, and hepatotoxicity are uncommon side effects. If therapy extends longer than 8 weeks, obtain biweekly CBCs and liver function tests and discontinue the drug if the absolute neutrophil count drops below $1000/mm^3$ or the liver transaminases exceed $2\frac{1}{2}$ times normal. During the first week of griseofulvin therapy, daily use of a topical antifungal (clotrimazole, miconazole, tolnaftate) or selenium (Selsun) shampoo may decrease the period of infectivity.

Tinea Corporis, Tinea Cruris, Tinea Pedis   Treat with clotrimazole, miconazole, or tolnaftate, two or three times daily, for 4 weeks. In addition, soak inflammatory lesions with normal saline or 5% Burow's solution compresses. Keep affected areas dry; this is particularly important for tinea pedis and tinea cruris, where antifungal powders are helpful. Instruct the patient to wear cotton (instead of synthetic) underwear and socks to help dissipate moisture.

Tinea Unguium   The treatment is oral griseofulvin. However, in view of the long course (6–18 months) of therapy and high recurrence rate, refer the patient to a dermatologist rather than initiating treatment in the ED.

Tinea Versicolor   Treat for 2 weeks with either 2.5% selenium sulfide shampoo or ketaconazole shampoo. Advise the patient to apply the shampoo to the affected skin for 30 min three times a week or daily for 5 min in the shower for 2 weeks. Topical antifungals are also effective but more expensive. Inform the patient that the normal skin pigment will not return until after the treated lesions are exposed to ultraviolet light.

Follow-up
• Primary care follow-up in 2 weeks

BIBLIOGRAPHY

Hubbard TW: The predictive value of symptoms in diagnosing childhood tinea capitis. *Arch Pediatr Adolesc Med* 1999;153:1150–1153.

Stein DH: Tineas—superficial dermatophyte infections. *Pediatr Rev* 1998;19: 368–372.

Suarez S, Friedlander SF: Antifungal therapy in children: an update. *Pediatr Ann* 1998;27:177–184.

VERRUCAE

Verrucae, or warts, occur in 5 to 10% of children between the ages of 10 and 16 years. They are benign tumors of the epidermis caused by a DNA (papilloma) virus that spreads via autoinoculation and person-to-person contact. Local trauma seems necessary to promote infection with the virus, so that lesions are most common on the fingers, hands, elbows, and plantar surfaces. The incubation period is 1 to 6 months, and, while the course is extremely variable, two-thirds of all lesions resolve spontaneously within 2 years. A patient can have from one to several hundred warts.

Clinical Presentation

Common Warts   Common warts (verruca vulgaris) occur predominantly on the dorsal surfaces of the hands and the periungual regions. They usually begin as pinpoint, flesh-colored papules that grow larger (1–10 mm), with roughened surfaces, grayish color, and sharply demarcated borders. Often these lesions are studded with black dots (thrombosed capillaries). Periungual warts most commonly occur in children who bite their nails.

Flat Warts   Flat warts (verruca plana) are tan to flesh-colored, soft, flat, small (2- to 6-mm) papules that occur primarily on the face, neck, arms, and hands. These are particularly common on shaved areas. Contiguous lesions can become confluent and plaque-like.

Plantar Warts   Plantar warts (verruca plantaris) usually occur in weight-bearing areas of the sole of the foot. They are flat with sharp margins, and black dots are seen within the lesions. Pressure forces them into the tissues of the foot, and this leads to marked tenderness when walking. They often coalesce into a single large plaque called a mosaic wart.

Venereal Warts   Venereal warts (condylomata acuminata) are soft, reddish pink, filiform lesions that may coalesce into larger, cauliflower-like clusters. They are located primarily on the genitalia and around the anus. Proctoscopic examination may reveal involvement of the rectal mucosa as well. Condylomata acuminata are usually sexually transmitted, but in one-third of cases they may be associated with warts elsewhere on the body. However, sexual abuse is a concern when venereal warts are found on a young child.

Diagnosis

The diagnosis of common or flat warts can be confirmed by the lack of skin markings over the lesion and by the presence of black dots (thrombosed dermal capillaries) beneath the surface. Gentle paring with a scalpel causes small bleeding points, which represent intact capillaries. Lateral pressure causes pain.

Periungual warts can be confused with the periungual fibromas of *tuberous sclerosis.* However, other cutaneous manifestations of tuberous sclerosis are usually present (adenoma sebaceum, ash-leaf spots, shagreen patches).

Plantar warts may resemble calluses, corns, and black heel (*talon noir*). *Calluses* do not have sharp, well-demarcated margins and no black dots are seen. *Corns* typically occur at the metatarsophalangeal joints, and direct pressure causes pain. There are no black dots, and the overlying skin markings reamin intact. Corns have sharp margins and a characteristic translucent particle at the core. *Black heel* occurs in athletes who make frequent sudden stops, causing blackish pinpoint hemorrhages. The margin is not well demarcated, and paring does not reveal bleeding points.

Condylomata acuminata must be differentiated from the *condylomata lata* of secondary syphilis. The latter are 1- to 3-cm grayish pink nodules occurring in the same regions. Dark-field microscopy or serology (VDRL and FTA) is necessary to confirm the diagnosis.

ED Management

Adjust therapy for the type, location, and duration of the wart and the age of the patient. Consider the high rate of spontaneous resolution and the discomfort to the patient of the treatment. Often benign neglect is the best approach. Keratolytic therapy may be instituted in the ED for a patient with a few lesions. The usual combination is salicylic acid (10–16%) with lactic acid (10–16%) in flexible collodion. Instruct the patient to apply this solution daily after bathing and then cover the wart for 24 h with a waterproof adhesive bandage. Repeat the procedure after paring the wart with the side of a scalpel or rubbing with a washcloth, emery board, or pumice stone. Commercially available salicylic acid plaster is useful for plantar warts. Cut it to fit the lesion, tape it in place for 4 to 5 days, then pare the necrotic tissue and reapply the plaster if necessary. Inform the family that multiple reapplications will likely be necessary.

Refer patients with lesions on the face, multiple hand warts, periungual and subungual warts, large plantar warts, or venereal warts to a dermatologist for other available therapies, which include liquid nitrogen, cantharidin, electrodesiccation and curettage, and podophyllin. See p 547 for the evaluation and management of possible sexual abuse.

Follow-up

- Primary care or dermatology follow-up in 1 to 2 weeks

BIBLIOGRAPHY

Beutner KR: Cutaneous viral infections. *Pediatr Ann* 1993;22:247–252.
Cohen BA: Warts and children: can they be separated? *Contemp Pediatr* 1997; 14:128–149.
Siegfried EC: Warts on children: an approach to therapy. *Pediatr Ann* 1996;25:79–90.

CHAPTER 6

ENT Emergencies

Jeffrey Keller and Ashutosh Kacker

ACUTE OTITIS MEDIA

Acute otitis media (AOM) is a suppurative infection of the middle ear caused by bacteria and viruses. It accounts for up to one-third of acute health care visits by ill children. By 1 year of age, 62% of children will have had one episode; 17% of these will have had three; and another 17% will have had more than six. The incidence is highest during the winter months, secondary to the greater frequency of viral upper respiratory infections (URIs). Children with normal immunity may have multiple episodes in a year. Risk factors for AOM include day care attendance, secondhand smoke exposure, use of a pacifier, bottle feeding, and family history of ear infection.

The most common bacterial etiology identified is *Streptococcus pneumoniae* (30–40%), followed by nontypable *Haemophilus influenzae* (20–30%), *Moraxella catarrhalis* (10–20%), and *Streptococcus pyogenes*. The gram-negative enteric organisms (*Escherichia coli, Klebsiella, Proteus, Pseudomonas*) and *Staphylococcus aureus* are responsible for about 15% of cases in the first few months of life but are exceedingly rare afterward. Viruses are now considered to be frequent pathogens (up to 50% of cases); agents that have been implicated include parainfluenza, respiratory syncytial virus, influenza, adenovirus, and enterovirus. Anaerobes, *Mycoplasma pneumoniae*, and *Chlamydia trachomatis* are not considered to be significant pathogens. About one-third of middle ear cultures are found to be sterile.

Clinical Presentation

AOM is usually preceded by an upper respiratory infection with cough and rhinorrhea. Ear symptoms, usually with fever, begin 2 to 3 days later. In addition to pain, the older child may complain of dizziness, buzzing in the ear, or decreased hearing. In an infant there may be nonspecific symptoms such as irritability, decreased feeding, sleep disturbance, vomiting, or diarrhea. In many cases, the patient has only fever, a

121

persistent upper respiratory infection, or behavioral changes (cranky, not feeding or sleeping well). A young patient may present with ear tugging, but this is an unreliable sign of AOM. Occasionally, there is a history of severe ear pain that resolved abruptly when a bloody or yellowish discharge began to drain from the external canal (tympanic membrane perforation). In summary, clinical history alone is an inaccurate predictor of AOM; therefore, examine the ears of a patient with any of the symptoms mentioned above, even if otoscopy in the previous 24 to 36 h did not reveal an otitis media.

Diagnosis

Examine the tympanic membrane for shape (concave, retracted, bulging), color (pearly gray, injected, erythematous, yellow), the presence of landmarks (light reflex, malleus), and mobility. Redness alone is not sufficient to make the diagnosis, since crying can cause erythema of the drum. Perform pneumatic otoscopy, focusing on the light reflex. Decreased mobility of the tympanic membrane, which can be confirmed by tympanometry (flat tympanogram), is the most sensitive indicator of a middle ear effusion. A combination of erythema, bulging with or without a purulent effusion, loss of normal anatomic landmarks, and decreased mobility are characteristic of an AOM. Tympanic membrane perforation with recent onset of bloody or purulent ear discharge is also diagnostic. The history of a recent URI, complaints of ear pain, and constitutional symptoms such as listlessness and fever are insufficient to make the diagnosis without the typical otoscopic findings.

The optimal position for examination varies with the age of the patient. Infants and young children are best examined supine on the table, restrained by an adult. An older child can be examined seated on the parent's lap, face to face with the examiner. One of the parent's arms can tightly embrace the child while the other holds the patient's head.

In some cases there may be impacted cerumen in the ear canal obstructing the view of the tympanic membrane. Remove it by curetting or irrigating with warm water 10 min after instilling several drops of hydrogen peroxide (if no tympanic membrane perforation is suspected).

Carefully examine the head, neck, teeth, and gums. Other common causes of otalgia include *otitis externa* (pain on traction of the pinna), *acute myringitis* (inflammation of the tympanic membrane with or without bulla formation), *teething* (especially in young children), *serous otitis media* (dark air-fluid level or bubbles behind tympanic membrane, retracted tympanic membrane), and *pharyngitis* (particularly herpangina in younger children). In addition, a *dental abscess* (gum swelling and tenderness), *parotitis* (swelling over the angle of the jaw), and *temporomandibular joint disease* (pain with palpation of the temporomandibular joint, especially upon mouth opening and closing) can present with otalgia.

ED Management

Despite the presence of an otitis media, perform a thorough physical examination to be certain that the patient does not have a more serious

Table 6-1 Antibiotic Doses for Otitis Media and Sinusitis

ANTIBIOTIC	DAILY DOSE	DIVIDED
Amoxicillin (usual dose)	40 mg/kg	tid
Amoxicillin (high dose)	80 mg/kg	tid
Amoxicillin-clavulanate (200/28.5, 400/57, 875/125 forms)		
Usual dose	45 mg/kg of amoxicillin	bid
High dose	80 mg/kg of amoxicillin	bid
Azithromycin		
First day	10 mg/kg	qd
Days 2–5	5 mg/kg	qd
Cefixime	8 mg/kg	qd
Cefpodoxime	10 mg/kg	bid
Cefuroxime	30 mg/kg	bid
Cefprozil		
Otitis	30 mg/kg	bid
Sinusitis	15 mg/kg	bid
Ceftriaxone IM	50 mg/kg	
Clarithromycin	15 mg/kg	bid
Trimethoprim-sulfamethoxazole (TMP-SMX)	15 mg/kg of TMP	bid

infection, such as meningitis. If the patient is toxic-appearing or under 1 month of age, perform a sepsis evaluation and admit for aggressive inpatient parenteral management.

1–2 Months of Age Treat an afebrile, well-appearing infant less than 2 months of age with ceftriaxone (50 mg/kg IM). However, if there is fever [>38.1°C (>100.6°F)], toxicity, irritability, evidence of a systemic infection, a complicated neonatal course, or a previous hospitalization with antibiotic treatment, admit the patient (see "Evaluation of the Febrile Child," pp 335–339), perform an evaluation for sepsis and treat with IV antibiotics.

From 2 Months to 2 Years of Age It has recently been suggested that antibiotics might not be necessary for treating AOM. However, since there are no reliable clinical criteria for distinguishing which patient has a viral versus bacterial etiology for an otitis, treat with a 10-day course of amoxicillin (see Tables 6-1 and 6-2). A patient who attends day care or has received antimicrobial therapy in the last 3 months is at greater risk for a resistant organism. Treat with high-dose amoxicillin, high-dose amoxicillin-clavulanate, cefuroxime, or cefpodoxime.

Older Than 2 Years Treat with a 10-day course of amoxicillin. If the patient is not at risk for a resistant organism (see above), a shorter 5-day

Table 6-2   Antibiotic Treatment of AOM (>2 Months of Age)*

ANTIBIOTICS IN PRIOR MONTH?	DAY 0	CLINICAL TREATMENT FAILURE: DAY 3	CLINICAL TREATMENT FAILURE: DAY 10–28
No	High-dose amoxicillin Usual-dose amoxicillin	High-dose amoxicillin-clavulanate Cefuroxime/cefpodoxime/cefprozil Ceftriaxone IM	Same as day 3
Yes	High-dose amoxicillin High-dose amoxicillin-clavulanate Cefuroxime/cefpodoxime	Ceftriaxone IM Clindamycin/cefprozil Tympanocentesis	High-dose amoxicillin-clavulanate Cefuroxime/cefpodoxime/cefprozil Ceftriaxone IM Tympanocentesis

*See Table 6-1 for antibiotic doses.
Modified from Dowell SF, Butler JC, Giebink GS, et al. *Pediatr Infect Dis J* 1999;18:1–9.

course of oral cefpodoxime, cefprozil, or cefuroxime is a convenient alternative. If it is the parent's preference, it may be reasonable to defer antibiotic treatment for a patient who does not appear toxic and has not been treated with antibiotics in the prior 3 months. The parents must be comfortable with the plan. Ensure that adequate analgesia will be given (see below). If these criteria cannot be satisfied, give antibiotics as above. Instruct the parents to return in 3 to 5 days if the child remains symptomatic (fever, ear pain, decreased hearing) or does not seem to be better. If the tympanic membrane continues to appear infected (erythematous, bulging, loss of landmarks), initiate antibiotic therapy.

At any age, if the patient has significant vomiting or if compliance with a 10-day regimen is unlikely, give a single dose of ceftriaxone (50 mg/kg IM). If the child has recently failed a course of antimicrobial therapy, give a series of three daily injections.

Glycerin with benzocaine analgesic otic drops (one to two drops qid), acetaminophen (15 mg/kg q 4 h), and ibuprofen (10 mg/kg q 6 h) are useful for pain and discomfort. In the ED, instilling a single dose of one to two drops of 2% viscous lidocaine may ameliorate extreme discomfort. Antihistamine-decongestant combinations are not indicated, as there is no evidence of efficacy. Use them only when treatment of a specific symptom (rhinitis) is desired.

The patient should be afebrile within 48 to 72 h after beginning antibiotic therapy; persistence of fever suggests a treatment failure. Reexamine the child, looking for other sources of fever. If none is found and the otitis media persists, give an alternative antibiotic (Table 6-2). Also instruct the parents to return at the completion of therapy if the child remains symptomatic (as above). Change to an alternative antibiotic if the tympanic membrane continues to appear infected and reevaluate the patient in 1 week.

A sterile effusion occurs in more than 40% of children following an acute otitis media. This usually resolves without intervention, although a temporary conductive hearing loss can persist until the effusion resolves.

Tympanocentesis is indicated for systemic toxicity, severe unremitting pain, no response to conventional therapy, or a suppurative complication (facial nerve paralysis, mastoiditis, meningitis, brain abscess) and may be necessary in some immunocompromised patients. Obtain an otolaryngology consult.

Follow-up
- Patient not treated with antibiotics: 3 to 5 days
- Patient treated with antibiotics: 2 to 3 days if still febrile or at the completion of therapy if still symptomatic

Indications for Admission
- Infant less than 2 months of age with temperature over 38.1°C (100.6°F)
- Toxic appearance
- Immunocompromised patient with fever
- Suppurative complication (mastoiditis, meningitis, brain abscess) or seventh nerve palsy

BIBLIOGRAPHY

Dowell SF, Butler JC, Giebink GS, et al: Acute otitis media: management and surveillance in an era of pneumococcal resistance—a report from the Drug-Resistant *Streptococcus pneumoniae* Therapeutic Working Group. *Pediatr Infect Dis J* 1999;18:1–9.

Glasziou PP, Del Mar CB, Hayem M, et al: Antibiotics for acute otitis media in children. *Cochrane Database Syst Rev* 2000;(4):CD000219.

Hoberman A, Paradise JL, Cohen R: Duration of therapy for acute otitis media. *Pediatr Infect Dis J* 2000;19:471–473.

Klein JO: Management of otitis media: 2000 and beyond. *Pediatr Infect Dis J* 2000;19:383–387.

MASTOIDITIS

Although the incidence of mastoiditis has decreased significantly with introduction of antibiotics for otitis media, it continues to occur periodically in all age groups, including young infants. The most common etiologies are group A *Streptococcus*, *Streptococcus pneumoniae*, *S. aureus*, anaerobes, and *Haemophilus influenzae*.

Clinical Presentation

Mastoiditis often takes a few weeks to develop and typically follows an untreated or incompletely treated otitis media. The physical findings include swelling, erythema, and tenderness over the mastoid process behind the ear. The auricle is typically displaced anteroinferiorly because of mastoid swelling; in some cases, a fluctuant collection of purulent material can be palpated on the lateral surface of the mastoid process (e.g., subperiosteal abscess). The ipsilateral tympanic membrane is frequently but not always erythematous and bulging. Edema and sagging of the posterior external auditory canal wall may be seen upon careful examination of the external auditory canal. Fever greater than 38.3°C (101°F) is common.

Diagnosis and ED Management

If mastoiditis is suspected based on clinical findings, obtain an axial/coronal computed tomography (CT) scan of the temporal bones to rule out possible extension of infection beyond the mastoid. Clouding of the mastoid air cells and loss of the intermastoid cell septa secondary to the osteomyelitic process are seen in coalescent mastoiditis. The radiographic findings of fluid in the middle ear and mastoid without the loss of bony septa may be the result of a recent otitis media and do not necessarily indicate acute mastoiditis in the absence of the typical clinical findings. Plain mastoid radiographs are not necessary.

Admit all children with acute mastoiditis, consult an otolaryngologist, and treat with IV ampicillin-sulbactam (150 mg/kg/day divided q 6 h) or cefuroxime (100 mg/kg/day divided q 8 h). Tympanocentesis can be helpful in obtaining fluid for Gram's stain and culture. Surgical drainage is indicated if a subperiosteal or intracranial abscess is seen on CT scan or if the patient does not improve clinically with 24 to 48 h of intravenous antibiotics.

Indication for Admission

- Acute mastoiditis

BIBLIOGRAPHY

Ghaffar FA, Wordemann M, McGracken GH Jr.: Acute mastoiditis in children: a seventeen-year experience in Dallas, Texas. *Pediatr Infect Dis J* 2001; 20:376–380.

Harley EH, Sdralis T, Berkowitz RG: Acute mastoiditis in children: a 12-year retrospective study. *Otolaryngol Head Neck Surg* 1997;116:26–30.

Luntz M, Brodsky A, Nusem S, et al: Acute mastoiditis–the antibiotic era: a multicenter study. *Int J Pediatr Otorhinolaryngol* 2001;57:1–9.

SEROUS OTITIS MEDIA

Serous otitis media (SOM) is the presence of nonsuppurative fluid in the middle ear. Although no overt signs of infection are seen in SOM, bacterial organisms have been documented in 30 to 70% of cultured middle ear fluid.

Clinical Presentation and Diagnosis

Despite adequate treatment, serous otitis frequently follows an episode of acute otitis media. Usually there are no complaints, although an infant may be fussy when recumbent, while an older child may note decreased hearing or mild balance disturbances.

On pneumatic otoscopy, the tympanic membrane appears darkened and retracted without evidence of acute infection (i.e., no erythema). There may be an air-fluid level with bubbles visible behind the drum. Mobility is limited, as can be confirmed by impedance testing (retracted tympanic membrane with negative middle ear pressure).

ED Management

The management of serous otitis is both controversial and unsatisfactory. A short course of antibiotic therapy may lead to resolution of chronic fluid in a small percentage of children; however, watchful waiting is the best treatment option. The empiric use of antihistamine-decongestant combinations (chlorpheniramine or brompheniramine with pseudoephedrine) has been advocated by the manufacturers, although there has been no documentation of any therapeutic value. Also, oral steroids offer only a temporary benefit and therefore are not indicated.

Refer the patient to a primary care provider to assess the frequency of acute infections. Arrange for a hearing evaluation if fluid has been present for more than 3 months. Myringotomy and pressure-equalizing tubes may be indicated for unresponsive, recurrent otitis media or significant conductive hearing loss (hearing threshold greater than 20 dB), especially in a child with speech delay.

BIBLIOGRAPHY

Kubba H, Pearson JP, Birchall JP: The aetiology of otitis media with effusion: a review. *Clin Otolaryngol* 2000;25:181–194.

Patterson M, Paparella MM: Otitis media with effusion and early sequelae: flexible approach. *Otolaryngol Clin North Am* 1999;32:391-400.

Roddey OF, Hoover HA: Otitis media with effusion in children: a pediatric office perspective. *Pediatr Ann* 2000;10:623–629.

OTITIS EXTERNA

Otitis externa, also known as "swimmer's ear," generally occurs in the summertime, when swimming leads to the trapping of excess moisture in the external auditory canal. This results in a mixed infection of fungi (*Aspergillus* and *Candida*) and bacteria (*Pseudomonas, Klebsiella,* and *Enterobacter*).

Clinical Presentation and Diagnosis

Generally there is a history of recent swimming or of manipulation of the external canal with a pointed object or Q-tip. The patient is usually afebrile but complaining of ear pain and itching, with a thick white, yellow, or green discharge from the external canal. Extreme discomfort when pulling the pinna or tragus distinguishes the discharge of otitis externa from that caused by a perforated tympanic membrane. Otoscopy reveals an erythematous canal, which can be so swollen that it prevents visualization of the tympanic membrane. In the absence of a history of swimming or ear canal manipulation, consider a foreign-body impaction.

ED Management

Treat otitis externa with a topical, broad-spectrum antibiotic ear drop. Preparations that contain hydrocortisone often reduce swelling more effectively. Use acetic acid with or without hydrocortisone (3–5 drops tid × 7 days), ciprofloxacin-hydrocortisone (3 drops bid × 7 days), ofloxacin (5 drops bid <12 years, 10 drops bid ≥12 years, × 10 days) or polymyxin B-neomycin-hydrocortisone (3–5 drops tid × 7 days). If a perforated tympanic membrane cannot be ruled out, use a preparation that is less caustic to the middle ear structures, such as polymyxin B-neomycin-hydrocortisone suspension, rather than the solution. Instill the drops either directly into the canal or onto a cotton ear wick, which ensures delivery of the drug throughout the external canal. In addition, keep the canal dry; further swimming is not permitted unless the child wears earplugs. Complete resolution takes 5 to 7 days. If the child is prone to recurrences, use two drops of a prophylactic mixture of half rubbing (isopropyl) alcohol–half water after every swim. If there is no improvement in 2 days, refer the patient to an otolaryngologist for cleaning of the ear canal and possible ear wick placement.

Severe otitis externa with associated cellulitis of the pinna requires admission for systemic antibiotics. Consult an otolaryngologist.

Follow-up

- 48 h if the symptoms do not begin to improve

BIBLIOGRAPHY

Hannley MT, Denneny JC III, Holzer SS: Use of ototopical antibiotics in treating 3 common ear diseases. *Otolaryngol Head Neck Surg* 2000;122:934–940.

Rea P, Joseph T. A GP strategy for otitis externa. *Practitioner* 1998;242:466–471.

Sander R. Otitis externa: a practical guide to treatment and prevention. *Am Fam Physician* 2001;63:927–942.

CERVICAL LYMPHADENOPATHY

Cervical lymphadenopathy can be considered in three broad etiologic categories: reactive, adenitis, or associated with systemic illness.

Reactive   Most enlarged cervical lymph nodes are reactive, found in conjunction with a viral or bacterial infection of the head or neck. Palpable cervical lymph nodes are present in approximately 80 to 90% of preschool and young, school-age children, especially if they have had a recent upper respiratory tract infection. These nodes are generally benign and no workup or specific treatment is necessary.

Adenitis   An adenitis is an infection of the lymph node itself, most commonly (60–85%) caused by *S. aureus* or group A *Streptococcus*, although viral and anaerobic infections have been implicated. Atypical *Mycobacterium* and *Mycobacterium tuberculosis* can result in a node with all the signs of acute infection. Cat-scratch disease may cause cervical, axillary, or inguinal adenitis.

Systemic Disease   Systemic diseases, especially infectious mononucleosis and mono-like syndromes [cytomegalovirus (CMV), toxoplasmosis, leptospirosis, brucellosis, and tularemia], sarcoidosis, Kawasaki syndrome, and HIV can cause cervical as well as generalized lymphadenopathy. The possibility of a malignancy (leukemia, Hodgkin's disease, non-Hodgkin's lymphoma) is always a concern.

Clinical Presentation

Reactive   Most often the presentation of cervical adenopathy reflects the primary illness (URI, sore throat, etc.). Other complaints include a neck mass, stiff neck (unwillingness to move the neck side to side), or torticollis. Reactive nodes are usually multiple, discrete, firm, smaller than 1 to 2 cm in diameter, nontender, and mobile. The overlying skin is neither erythematous nor adherent. In general, reactive adenopathy subsides in 2 to 3 weeks, but it can persist.

Adenitis   With an adenitis, the node becomes enlarged, tender, and fluctuant. The overlying skin is warm, erythematous, and occasionally adherent. The hallmarks of an atypical mycobacterial infection are the presence of skin erythema overlying a nontender lymph node in an afebrile, otherwise well-appearing child. The node often suppurates. Cat-scratch disease is characterized by a papule at the site of the scratch, followed in 5 to 60 days by regional lymphadenitis. Despite the impressive lymphadenopathy, the patient usually appears well, although 30% may have fever.

Systemic Disease   Mononucleosis and mono-like illnesses (pp 352–354) can present with generalized tender lymphadenopathy, sometimes in association with an exudative pharyngitis, macular rash, and hepatosplenomegaly. These nodes are firm and mobile. Kawasaki disease (pp 360–362) and HIV (pp 339-352) are discussed elsewhere.

A malignant node is fixed, hard, and matted. It is frequently supra-clavicular in location. The node(s) may be described as persistent or continuously growing. Weight loss, weakness, pallor, night sweats, fever, petechiae, and ecchymoses are other possible findings.

Diagnosis

Perform a thorough examination of the head, neck, teeth, and gums to find a source of infection draining into the affected node(s). Weakness, fever, rash, hepatosplenomegaly, and generalized lymphadenopathy are all indicative of a systemic disease. Weight loss, pallor, bleeding manifestations, and high fever may be signs or symptoms of a malignancy.

Enlargement of the parotid gland obscures the angle of the mandible. Infectious *parotitis*, usually viral in etiology, may cause unilateral or bilateral swelling with severe tenderness. Intraoral examination may reveal swelling, erythema, or a discharge from the opening of Stensen's duct (opposite the second upper molar).

If there is a stiff neck, the priority is to be certain that the patient does not have meningitis. Other etiologies of meningismus include muscle spasm, neck trauma, peritonsillar cellulitis, cervical osteomyelitis, and other infected neck masses (branchial cleft cyst, thyroglossal duct cyst, hemangioma).

There are seven features of the affected node(s) to consider:

1. *Single or Multiple (Unilateral or Bilateral)* Enlargement of a single node generally occurs in an adenitis, although tuberculous adenitis causes bilateral involvement. Reactive adenopathy and systemic diseases most often result in multiple, bilateral involvement.
2. *Location(s)* The location of a reactive node can suggest the site of the primary infection (preauricular-conjunctiva or external ear canal; occipital-scalp; submental and submandibular-intraoral). Supraclavicular adenopathy is suspicious for a malignancy, while occipital adenopathy suggests a viral illness. Generalized lymphadenopathy most commonly occurs during mononucleosis or a mono-like infection, although leukemia is a possible etiology.
3. *Size* Reactive nodes are typically small (<2 cm). Massive enlargement can occur with an atypical mycobacterial infection.
4. *Rate of Growth* Nodes that slowly enlarge suggest a malignancy, while rapid enlargement occurs in an infected or reactive node.
5. *Mobility* In general, a freely movable node is benign. A node that is fixed to adjacent structures or matted to other nodes suggests a malignancy, mycobacterial infection, or cat-scratch disease.
6. *Consistency* Soft or firm nodes are benign. Fluctuance occurs in adenitis. A rubbery consistency is noted in sarcoidosis, and malignant nodes are usually rock-hard.
7. *Overlying Skin* Bacterial adenitis causes erythema and warmth of the overlying skin. However, adherence occurs in cat-scratch disease and atypical mycobacterial infection. A reactive node does not affect the overlying skin.

ED Management

Reactive   "Benign" reactive nodes found in conjunction with a head or neck infection require treatment of the primary illness only. If the pharynx is erythematous, obtain a throat culture. Benign nodes can be followed without intervention. Reassure the family and arrange for primary care follow-up.

Adenitis   When adenitis is diagnosed, obtain a throat culture and give an oral antibiotic with staphylococcal and streptococcal coverage such as cefadroxil (40 mg/kg/day divided bid) or cephalexin (40 mg/kg/day divided qid). Alternatives are cefprozil (20 mg/kg/day divided bid), cefuroxime (30 mg/kg/day divided bid), or azithromycin (12 mg/kg qd). Warm compresses, applied for 15 to 30 min every 3 to 4 h, are also necessary. Have the patient return in 2 to 3 days. If there is clinical improvement or a positive throat culture, continue the antibiotics for a total of 10 days. If the node has not responded to antibiotics and warm compresses, change to clindamycin (25 mg/kg/day divided qid) or amoxicillin-clavulanate (200/28:5; 400/57; 875/125 formulation 45 mg/kg/day of amoxicillin divided bid) and follow up in 2 more days. If the node becomes fluctuant, arrange for a CT scan of the neck with contrast to determine the location and extent of the abscess.

Admit patients who are toxic or have nodes unresponsive to oral antibiotic therapy for parenteral treatment (nafcillin 150 mg/kg/day divided q 6 h or ceftriaxone 100 mg/kg/day divided q 12 h). Obtain a complete blood count (CBC) with differential, heterophile antibody and blood culture prior to starting intravenous therapy. Indications for a node biopsy include age greater than 10 years, persistent and unexplained weight loss or fever, skin ulceration or fixation to the node, supraclavicular location, or continuously increasing size.

If atypical mycobacterial infection is suspected, surgical curettage/ excision is required, as the infection is frequently resistant to antitubercular medication. Avoid incision and drainage, which can result in a chronic fistula. If tuberculosis is suspected because of possible exposure or travel, place a 5TU PPD.

If the PPD is positive, consider *Mycobacterium* as the cause of the infection. Obtain a chest x-ray and admit the patient for surgical consultation, collection of culture specimens, and institution of antituberculous therapy (pp 383–387).

Systemic Disease
When a mononucleosis syndrome is suspected, obtain a heterophile antibody or Monospot test. Treatment is supportive. Note that the heterophile antibody may be negative early in the disease and in young or immunocompromised patients. If a malignancy is suspected, the initial evaluation includes a chest x-ray and CBC with differential and reticulocyte count prior to hematology consultation.

Treat parotitis with analgesia (acetaminophen 15 mg/kg q 4 h, ibuprofen 10 mg/kg q 6 h), warm compresses, sialogogues (e.g., lemon swabs), and hydration. If there is evidence of duct obstruction, overlying erythema and tenderness, or purulent drainage from Stensen's duct, give antistaphylococcal antibiotics such as cephalexin (40 mg/kg/day divided qid) or amoxicillin-clavulanate (875/125 formulation, 45 mg/kg/day of amoxicillin divided bid). Obtain a CT scan of the neck if the patient has persistent or recurrent parotitis or an abscess, or if an anatomic obstruction (e.g., stone) is suspected.

Follow-up

- Bacterial adenitis: 2 to 3 days
- Parotitis: 2 to 3 days

Indications for Admission

- Cervical adenitis associated with toxicity or inadequate oral intake
- Cervical adenitis unresponsive to outpatient treatment
- Evaluation of a suspected malignancy
- Institution of antituberculous therapy

BIBLIOGRAPHY

Chiu TH, Lin TY: Clinical and microbiological analysis of six children with acute suppurative parotitis. *Acta Paediatr* 1996;85:106–108.
Peters TR, Edwards KM: Cervical lymphadenopathy and adenitis. *Pediatr Rev* 2000;21:399–404.
Weiler Z, Nelly P, Baruchin AM, Oren S: Diagnosis and treatment of cervical tuberculous lymphadenitis. *J Oral Maxillofac Surg* 2000;58:477–481.

EPISTAXIS

Epistaxis usually originates from the anterior nasal septum (Kiesselbach's area). Trauma (nose picking, punch, fall), upper respiratory infections, excessive use of decongestants or topical nasal steroids, an overly dry environment, and foreign bodies are predisposing factors. Rarely, structural abnormalities (hemangioma, telangiectasia, or angiofibroma), a bleeding diathesis (usually thrombocytopenia), or hypertension is involved. While children are often rushed into the ED because of "massive" blood loss, clinically significant bleeding is unusual.

Clinical Presentation

Usually an anterior septal source is evident. It is rare for the bleeding to be bilateral, but blood crossing behind the nasal septum can mimic a bilateral bleed. Sometimes, if the site is posterior or if the child is sleeping, the blood may present as hematemesis.

Diagnosis

Examine the nasal cavity with the child sitting on the parent's lap, using a bright light (otoscope). If a bleeding source is found, the examination may be terminated, as multiple sites are unusual (except in the case of a fractured nasal septum). If the patient has suffered nasal trauma, look for a septal hematoma, which appears as a bluish-black mass on the anterior septum, filling the nasal cavity. Occasionally, a mucosal hemangioma or telangiectasia is seen. If no cause is found but blood is noted trickling down the throat, assume that there is a posterior source.

Examine the skin for hemangiomata or telangiectasias, which may also be present in the nasal cavity. Jaundice, petechiae, purpura, lymphadenopathy, and hepatosplenomegaly may suggest a bleeding diathesis, and pallor, tachycardia, gallop rhythm, or orthostatic changes in vital signs may reflect significant blood loss.

In general, no workup is required for a nosebleed in an otherwise well child with an anterior septal source. Obtain a spun hematocrit if anemia is suspected. Evaluate for bleeding diathesis (pp 302–306) if the patient has any of the physical findings enumerated above, a long history of recurrent nosebleeds, easy bruising, hemarthrosis, multiple subconjunctival hemorrhages, or a family history of excessive bleeding.

ED Management

Most anterior bleeds respond to pressure. Pinch the nares together for a full 5 min with the child sitting upright (to prevent swallowing of blood). If this is unsuccessful, soak a cotton ball with 1:1000 aqueous epinephrine or 0.05% oxymetazoline solution and place it in the nasal cavity. Alternatively, pack the nose with petrolatum-impregnated gauze, Merocel nasal packing, or Gelfoam. After hemostasis is obtained, apply topical anesthesia with 4% lidocaine or benzocaine and cauterize the site for 3 s with a silver nitrate stick, although this is usually reserved for patients with recurrent bleeds. Treat hemangiomata or telangiectasias in the same way, but do not use cautery if a bleeding diathesis is suspected (possible tissue slough). Humidification, saline nose drops during the day, and the application of petrolatum (Vaseline) to the septum at bedtime help to reduce the recurrence of nosebleeds. If a nasal septal hematoma is suspected, consult an otolaryngologist for immediate drainage so as to prevent a septal abscess and subsequent nasal deformities.

If routine measures are ineffective or the source is posterior, use a posterior pack, most frequently placed by an otolaryngologist. Topically anesthetize the nose, insert a posterior nasal balloon pack (Epistat or Rhinostat), blow up the posterior balloon, pull anterior until it fits snugly in the nasopharynx, and then inflate the anterior balloon until the bleeding stops. Fill both balloons with saline solution. If nasal balloon packs are not available, pass an uninflated Foley catheter through the nose into the pharynx, inflate the balloon, then pull the catheter back until it fits snugly posteriorly in the nose. Fill the nose with petrolatum-impregnated gauze up to the balloon and place a clamp across the catheter where it exits the nose. If an anterior or posterior nasal pack is placed, give the patient broad-spectrum antibiotics to prevent an acute sinusitis (see Table 6-3). Otolaryngologic consultation is indicated.

Follow-up

- Unilateral anterior pack: 48 h for pack removal

Indications for Admission

- Bilateral anterior pack
- Posterior pack
- Bleeding diathesis or significant blood loss

Table 6-3   Antibiotic Treatment of Acute Bacterial Sinusitis in Children*

SEVERITY	ANTIBIOTICS IN PAST 4-6 WEEKS?	INITIAL THERAPY	SWITCH OPTIONS IF THERE IS NO IMPROVEMENT OR WORSENING AFTER 72 H
Mild	No	Amoxicillin-clavulanate Amoxicillin Cefpodoxime *or* cefuroxime	Reevaluate patient Amoxicillin-clavulanate *or* cefixime *or* cefpodoxime Amoxicillin-clavulanate *and* clindamycin
	If beta-lactam-allergic:	Azithromycin *or* clarithromycin Trimethoprim-sulfamethoxazole	Reevaluate patient/combination[†] Reevaluate patient/combination
Mild *Or*	Yes	Amoxicillin-clavulanate Amoxicillin	Reevaluate patient Amoxicillin-clavulanate *or* cefixime *or* cefpodoxime
Moderate	No	Cefpodoxime *or* cefuroxime	Amoxicillin-clavulanate *and* clindamycin
	If beta-lactam-allergic:	Azithromycin or clarithromycin Trimethoprim-sulfamethoxazole Clindamycin	Reevaluate patient/combination Reevaluate patient/combination Reevaluate patient/combination
Moderate	Yes	Amoxicillin-clavulanate Amoxicillin-clavulanate *and* clindamycin	Reevaluate patient/combination Reevaluate patient/combination
	If beta-lactam-allergic:	TMP-SMX *and* clindamycin	Reevaluate patient/combination

*See Table 6-1 for antibiotic doses.
†Combination: Amoxicillin-clavulanate or clindamycin *and* second antibiotic based on culture and sensitivity.
Modified from Sinus and Allergy Health Partnership: Antimicrobial treatment guidelines for acute bacterial rhinosinusitis. *Otolaryngol Head Neck Surg* 2000;123:5–31.

134

BIBLIOGRAPHY

Chopra R: Epistaxis: a review. *J R Soc Health* 2000;120:31–33.
Pond F, Sizeland A: Epistaxis. Strategies for management. *Aust Fam Physician* 2000;
29:933–938.
Tan LK, Calhoun KH: Epistaxis. *Med Clin North Am* 1999;83:43–56.

FOREIGN BODIES

Foreign bodies found in the nose or ear commonly include inanimate objects (toys, earrings, etc.), vegetable material, and insects. The nose is the most common site of foreign-body impaction in children under 3 years of age, and the ear is the most frequent site in patients between 3 and 8 years of age. Unfortunately, the signs and symptoms of a foreign body may be subtle, and there may be no clear history of insertion.

Clinical Presentation and Diagnosis

Aural   A foreign body in the ear can cause pain, tinnitus, and—as in the case of a live insect—extreme discomfort. Recurrent otitis externa raises the possibility of an aural foreign body. Although this is usually a benign condition, inexpert attempts at removal can push the object further into the canal, perforate the eardrum, and cause bleeding and swelling of the canal.

Nasal   A nasal foreign body presents with a unilateral foul-smelling discharge with unilateral obstruction. Usually the object can be seen anteriorly in the nose, but swelling of the mucosa can obscure visualization.

Esophageal   An esophageal foreign body is an unusual but potentially serious problem. Most objects pass into the stomach. However, possible sites for lodging include the inferior margin of the cricoid cartilage, the level of the aortic arch, and the area just superior to the diaphragm. Symptoms may include pain, dysphagia, vomiting, and dyspnea (secondary to laryngeal compression), although a patient may be asymptomatic. Subsequent edema can cause esophageal obstruction (dysphagia and drooling), upper airway obstruction, and possible perforation leading to mediastinitis.

ED Management

Aural   Usually, a foreign body in the external auditory canal is easily removed with suction or a wire loop, curette, or small alligator forceps. Irrigation can be used for nonvegetable objects. Prior to attempting to remove a live insect, drown it with mineral oil, a solution of 1% lidocaine with 1:1000 epinephrine, or 95% alcohol. Do not instill any solution if a tympanic membrane perforation is suspected (blood in the canal in association with ear pain). Arrange for otolaryngology consultation if the object cannot be removed.

Nasal   Most nasal foreign bodies become impacted between the anterior nasal septum and the inferior turbinate. Prior to attempting to remove the foreign body, restrain the child with the head immobilized. Next, anesthe-tize the nasal mucosa with 4% lidocaine spray and suction any nasal dis-charge with a Frazier-tip suction to enhance visualization. Use a nasal speculum with either a curette or an alligator forceps to remove the object. Routine use of topical decongestants is not recommended, as it may allow the object to migrate further posteriorly and result in aspiration. Antibi-otics are not required after successful removal of the foreign body. Con-sult with an otolaryngologist if removal is unsuccessful or if the object is in the posterior nasal cavity.

Esophageal   Most esophageal foreign bodies, whether round, irregular, or sharp, will pass without difficulty. However, drooling, dysphagia, stri-dor, or substernal pain or fullness suggest that the object may be lodged in the esophagus. Obtain anteroposterior and lateral soft tissue neck x-rays to determine the presence and number of radioopaque foreign bodies and whether the object(s) is in the esophagus or trachea. An esophageal for-eign body typically aligns in a coronal orientation, while a laryngeal or tracheal foreign body lies in the sagittal plain. If it is not clear whether the foreign body is radioopaque, obtain a searching image x-ray by placing an identical object in a cup of water next to the patient.

A patient with minimal symptoms can be monitored for 12 to 24 h to see if the object passes spontaneously. However, if the patient is sympto-matic, arrange for removal, under general anesthesia, through rigid eso-phagoscopy. If a disk battery or sharp object is identified in the esophagus, consult an otolaryngologist to arrange expeditious removal under general anesthesia. The National Button Battery Ingestion Hotline (202-625-3333; TDD 202-362-8563) available 24 h per day for questions.

Follow-up

- Sharp foreign body that has passed into the stomach: obtain a follow-up abdominal x-ray in 1 week.
- Blunt foreign body that has passed into the stomach: return at once if vomiting or abdominal pain occurs.
- Button battery that has passed in to the stomach: 24 h for x-ray and then every 3 to 4 days.

Indications for Admission

- Esophageal foreign body that has been present longer than 12 to 24 h
- Symptomatic patient

BIBLIOGRAPHY

Friedman EM: Tracheobronchial foreign bodies. *Otolaryngol Clin North Am* 2000;
33:179–185.
Koempel JA, Holinger LD: Foreign bodies of the upper aerodigestive tract. *Indian J Pediatr* 1997;64:763–769.
Messner AH: Pitfalls in the diagnosis of aerodigestive tract foreign bodies. *Clin Pediatr (Phila)* 1998;37:359–365.

NECK MASSES

Although the majority of neck masses in children are benign enlarged lymph nodes, the possibility of a malignancy is often a concern. In general, neck masses can be considered in four categories: lymph nodes (pp 129–132), congenital masses, benign tumors, and malignancies.

Clinical Presentation and Diagnosis

Congenital Masses
Branchial Cleft Cyst   A branchial cleft cyst is often not diagnosed until late childhood or early adulthood (average age, 13 years), when it becomes infected. At that time a discrete, erythematous, tender, fluctuant mass is noted in the lateral neck, typically anterior to the sternocleidomastoid muscle. On occasion, there is a fistula anterior to the muscle with an orifice that drains mucus and retracts with swallowing. If the acute infection is properly treated with antibiotics, the cyst shrinks, but it may reexpand during subsequent upper respiratory infections.

Thyroglossal Duct Cyst   A thyroglossal duct cyst usually presents as an asymptomatic midline neck mass at or below the level of the hyoid bone. The sexes are affected equally, and 50% of cases present prior to age 10 years. These frequently become infected and respond to antibiotics, only to reemerge during the next upper respiratory infection. In between, the mass is cystic or solid, nontender, and mobile. The pathognomonic feature is elevation of the mass when the tongue is protruded. Occasionally, the cyst contains ectopic thyroid tissue.

Congenital Muscular Torticollis   Congenital muscular torticollis or fibromatosis colli presents at 1 to 2 weeks of age as a hard, nontender mass within the body of the sternocleidomastoid. Characteristically, the head is tilted to the affected side, the baby faces away from the lesion, and there can be flattening of the unaffected side of the head. The family may report that the baby looks in one direction only.

Benign Tumors
Cystic Hygroma   A cystic hygroma usually presents as an irregular, soft, painless, compressible, lateral neck mass that transilluminates and can increase in size during straining. About 50% are present at birth and 90% are noted during the first 2 years of life. Massive enlargement can cause obstruction of the airway or the esophagus. Typical locations are the submental, preauricular, and submandibular areas.

Hemangioma   Hemangiomas are more frequently present at birth, and all are seen during the first year of life. Unlike the case with cystic hygromas, there is a 3:1 female preponderance. Most are of the cavernous type, often located within the parotid gland in the preauricular area. Infection or hemorrhage can cause acute enlargement, and the mass becomes bluish in color when the infant is crying or straining.

Dermoid Cyst   A dermoid cyst typically is an asymptomatic, cystic mid-line mass located in the submental region. A teratoma has a similar presentation, but calcifications or teeth are often seen on x-ray.

Malignant Tumors

About one-quarter of all the malignancies of childhood occur in the neck and more than half of these are either *Hodgkin's disease* or lymphosarcoma (p 311). Hodgkin's disease usually (80%) presents in the upper neck as a painless, hard or firm, fixed, slowly enlarging unilateral node. Most patients are over 5 years old. Forty percent of *lymphosarcomas* present extranodally in the neck throughout the pediatric age range, and the disease is often (40%) bilateral. A slowly growing, hard or rubbery, fixed mass is seen. Weight loss and hepatosplenomegaly are features of both diseases.

A *rhabdomyosarcoma* can originate in the nasopharynx or ear; symptoms are determined by the site. A nasopharyngeal mass presents as chronic adenoidal hypertrophy, with adenoidal facies, snoring, mouth breathing, serous otitis, and a serosanguineous nasal discharge. There may also be extension to the base of the skull with cranial nerve deficits. A mass in the ear causes chronic otitis, ear discharge, and mastoiditis. Weight loss can occur with a mass in either location. Other rare neck malignancies include *fibrosarcoma* (mandible most common site), *thyroid cancer* (history of neck irradiation), and both primary (causing Horner's syndrome) or metastatic (located in orbit, nasopharynx) *neuroblastoma.*

ED Management

Congenital Masses   Treat an infected *branchial cleft cyst* or *thyroglossal duct cyst* with 40 mg/kg/day of cephalexin (divided qid) or cefadroxil (divided bid) and warm soaks every 2 h. Since these lesions have a tendency to become reinfected, refer the patient to an otolaryngologist so that elective excision can be performed. A neck ultrasound or thyroid scan is a prerequisite for thyroglossal duct excision, as the cyst may contain all of the patient's thyroid tissue. Instruct the parents of a child with a *sternocleidomastoid tumor* and torticollis to perform stretching exercises four times a day: Straighten the head into a midline position, then rotate the head to the affected side and hold for 10 s.

Benign Tumors   If there are no signs or symptoms of airway compromise, refer patients with massive enlargement of a *cystic hygroma* or *hemangioma* or extreme disfigurement to an otolaryngologist. On occasion, a dermatologist or plastic surgeon should see the child so that cosmetic reconstruction can be planned. *Dermoids* and *teratomas* require elective excision.

Malignant Tumors   If a malignancy is suspected (hard, nontender, slowly growing mass; systemic signs and symptoms; a clinical picture consistent with a mass in the ear or nasopharynx), obtain a CBC, reticulocyte count, and a chest x-ray to rule out mediastinal or hilar node enlargement. Admit the patient and consult an oncologist.

Follow-up

- Infected branchial cleft cyst or thyroglossal duct cyst: 48 to 72 h

Indications for Admission

- Airway or esophageal obstruction
- Suspected malignancy

BIBLIOGRAPHY

Connolly AA, MacKenzie K: Paediatric neck masses—a diagnostic dilemma. *J Laryngol Otol* 1997:111:541–545.

McGuirt WF: The neck mass. *Med Clin North Am* 1999;83:219–234.

Swischuk LE, John SD: Neck masses in infants and children. *Radiol Clin North Am* 1997:35:1329–1340.

SINUSITIS

The paranasal sinuses develop as outpouchings of the nasal chamber. They enlarge as the child grows, so that the importance of a particular sinus varies with the age of the patient. The maxillary and ethmoid cells are present at birth, while the sphenoid and frontal sinuses are not aerated until approximately 2 and 7 years of age, respectively.

Acute sinusitis is a bacterial infection lasting less than 30 days. The organisms responsible for most cases of acute sinusitis are similar to those implicated in acute otitis media and include *S. pneumoniae,* nontypable *H. influenzae, M. catarrhalis,* and *S. aureus.* Chronic sinusitis is predominately caused by anaerobes, *S. aureus,* alpha *Streptococcus,* and nontypable *H. influenzae.*

Clinical Presentation

The most common signs and symptoms of acute sinusitis are dry cough (daytime but possibly worse at night), persistent (>7–10 days) nasal discharge, and fever. Children over 5 years of age may complain of a headache that is accentuated by leaning forward. Younger patients (<5 years) may have malodorous breath in the absence of a pharyngeal or dental infection. Facial pain and swelling occur, but are not as common as in adults.

Diagnosis

Sinusitis is usually diagnosed on clinical grounds alone. Suspect sinusitis if a patient has a nasal discharge that persists longer than expected for the typical URI (>7–10 days), especially if there is fever, headache, and cough. Radiographic confirmation is not necessary in children 6 years of age and younger. Confirmatory radiographs in older children are rarely needed; however, plain sinus films (Caldwell and Waters views) detect acute maxillary, frontal, and ethmoid sinusitis. Plain films are not adequate for identifying sphenoid disease. Reserve axial/coronal CT scans of the paranasal sinuses for patients suspected of having an orbital or intracranial complication. Transillumination and ultrasound are of limited value.

Various combinations of headache, cough, fever, and nasal discharge can occur with viral *URIs, influenza,* or *pneumonia.* Malodorous breath may be secondary to a *dental abscess, pharyngitis,* or *nasal foreign body. Cough variant asthma* may also present with a nocturnal cough.

ED Management

The treatment of suspected acute sinusitis is summarized in Table 6-3 (antibiotic doses are in Table 6-1); prescribe a 14- to 21-day course (or treat 7 days after the patient is symptom-free). Amoxicillin (40 mg/kg/day divided tid) is the first-line choice. Risk factors for resistance to amoxicillin include (1) day care attendance, (2) antibiotics within the previous 90 days, and (3) age <2 years. For children with any of these risk factors, use high-dose amoxicillin, amoxicillin-clavulanate, or the alternative medications listed in Table 6-2. Data are lacking on the usefulness of adding oral decongestants or topical nasal vasoconstrictor therapy to antibiotics.

Drainage, irrigation, and culture of the paranasal sinuses are indicated for patients who are immunocompromised, unresponsive to medical therapy, toxic, or suffering from one of the rare intracranial complications (brain abscess, subdural empyema, cavernous sinus thrombosis) or an orbital cellulitis. Nasal cultures are of limited value, as they do not accurately predict the pathogen responsible for acute sinusitis.

Admit a patient with acute frontal sinusitis if there is an air-fluid level and moderate to severe pain and treat with IV antibiotics because of the increased risk of intracranial spread. Also admit a patient with sphenoid sinusitis.

Follow-up

- Acute sinusitis: 48 to 72 h. If symptoms persist, change to an alternative medication or consult an otolaryngologist for possible parenteral antibiotics and sinus drainage.

Indications for Admission

- Acute frontal sinusitis with an air-fluid level and moderate to severe pain
- Sphenoid sinusitis
- Systemic toxicity
- Unremitting headache or incapacitating symptoms
- Orbital cellulitis or intracranial complication

BIBLIOGRAPHY

American Academy of Pediatrics, Subcommittee on Management of Sinusitis and Committee on Quality Improvement: Clinical practice guideline: management of sinusitis. *Pediatrics* 2001;108:798–808.

McAlister WH, Kronemer K: Imaging of sinusitis in children. *Pediatr Infect Dis J* 1999;18:1019–1020.

Sinus and Allergy Health Partnership: Antimicrobial treatment guidelines for acute bacterial rhinosinusitis. *Otolaryngol Head Neck Surg* 2000;123:5–31.

PERIORBITAL AND ORBITAL CELLULITIS

The orbital septum is a fibrous membrane running from the periosteum of the orbital bones to the tarsal plates. It separates the skin and subcutaneous tissues from intraorbital structures. Although the clinical pictures are similar, differentiation of periorbital (preseptal) cellulitis from orbital (postseptal) cellulitis is critical.

Clinical Presentation and Diagnosis

Both periorbital and orbital cellulitis present with warm, tender, erythematous lid swelling, usually associated with fever and regional adenopathy.

Periorbital Cellulitis   Periorbital cellulitis can be divided into two types. The infection may be preceded by an obvious break in the skin (insect bite, laceration, impetigo), with the causative agents being *S. aureus* or group A *Streptococcus*. More commonly, the infection occurs as a result of local spread from an ethmoid sinusitis with *M. catarrhalis*, pneumococcus, or (rarely) *H. influenzae* type B (HITB) infection. In a sinusitis-related case, the patient may have a history of a persistent nasal discharge, and the upper eyelid may be affected first, with subsequent spread to the lower lid. With either type of periorbital cellulitis, mild to moderate conjunctival swelling and hyperemia with a mucoid to purulent discharge may be present.

Orbital Cellulitis   The hallmarks of a postseptal infection are proptosis, chemosis, and decreased extraocular mobility in association with fever and toxicity. Decreased visual acuity may also occur late in the course.

Distinguishing periorbital from orbital cellulitis is critical because more aggressive medical and surgical intervention may be required with the latter. Passively open the eyelids to examine the eyes. Look for conjunctival injection, discharge, proptosis, chemosis, and decreased extraocular mobility and check the visual acuity. If the distinction between periorbital and orbital infection is not clear on clinical grounds, obtain a noncontrast axial/coronal CT scan of the orbit and sinuses. If orbital cellulitis is suspected or confirmed, promptly consult both an otolaryngologist and an ophthalmologist.

Lid erythema and swelling may be caused by a *conjunctivitis* (viral or bacterial), in which marked palpebral conjunctival injection is seen, or an *insect bite*, in which a punctum may be identified. An *allergic reaction* and the *nephrotic syndrome* can cause lid swelling (generally bilateral) in the absence of erythema, tenderness, or fever. Proptosis can be secondary to an *orbital tumor,* although the signs of infection are usually absent, while *hyperthyroid exophthalmos* can be confused with proptosis.

ED Management

As mentioned above, when the distinction between a periorbital and an orbital infection is not clear, radiologic studies can be helpful. Since an orbital cellulitis can be a life-threatening illness, always err on the side of overdiagnosing a postseptal infection.

Periorbital Cellulitis   A child with mild preseptal cellulitis secondary to a break in the skin may be treated as an outpatient with cefadroxil (40 mg/kg/day), cephalexin (40 mg/kg/day divided qid), amoxicillin-clavulanate (200/28.5, 400/57, or 875/125 formulation, 45 mg/kg/day of amoxicillin divided bid), or cefuroxime (30 mg/kg/day divided bid). If the infection is sinusitis-related, give a topical nasal decongestant (oxymetazoline bid) and amoxicillin-clavulanate or cefuroxime (as above). Also recommend warm compresses four times a day.

Admit the patient if there is a fever greater than 39.4°C (103.0°F), significant eyelid edema, decreased extraocular mobility, inability to tolerate oral antibiotics, or signs of systemic toxicity and treat with IV antibiotics (ampicillin-sulbactam 150 mg/kg/day divided q 6 h or cefuroxime 100 mg/kg/day divided q 8 h) and a topical nasal decongestant. Obtain a CBC and blood culture.

HITB Cellulitis   If HITB periorbital cellulitis cannot be ruled out because of a history of inadequate immunization, admit the patient and treat with IV or IM ceftriaxone 100 mg/kg/day divided q 12 h or IV cefuroxime 100 mg/kg/day divided q 8 h or ampicillin-sulbactam 150 mg/kg/day divided q 6 h. Obtain a CBC and blood culture, and if the child is lethargic or has meningeal signs, perform a lumbar puncture prior to initiating therapy.

Orbital Cellulitis   The IV antibiotic treatment is the same as for a preseptal cellulitis (see above). As mentioned above, obtain an axial/coronal CT scan of the paranasal sinuses and orbits and both otolaryngology and ophthalmology consultations early in the evaluation of the patient. Abscess drainage is indicated if there is extreme toxicity, evidence of intracranial spread (focal neurologic findings), decreased visual acuity, or no response to 24 h of antibiotics. However, treat small subperiosteal abscesses with 24 to 48 h of IV antibiotics prior to surgical intervention.

Follow-up

- Preseptal cellulitis: 24 to 48 h. Instruct the family to return immediately for IV therapy if symptoms worsen.

Indications for Admission

- Preseptal cellulitis associated with fever or toxicity or unresponsive to 24 to 48 h of oral antibiotics
- Suspected *H. influenzae* type B periorbital cellulitis
- Orbital cellulitis

BIBLIOGRAPHY

Ambati BK, Ambati J, Azar N: Periorbital and orbital cellulitis before and after the advent of *Haemophilus influenzae* type B vaccination. *Ophthalmology* 2000; 107:1450–1453.

Pond F, Berkowitz RG: Superolateral subperiosteal orbital abscess complicating sinusitis in a child. *Int J Pediatr Otorhinolaryngel* 1999;48:255–258.

Powell KR: Orbital and periorbital cellulitis. *Pediatr Rev* 1995; 16:163–167.

UPPER RESPIRATORY INFECTIONS

Upper respiratory infections are generally mild illnesses caused by numerous organisms. However, if a URI does not resolve within 3 to 4 days, consider the possibility of a more serious illness (otitis, sinusitis, pneumonia, etc.).

Clinical Presentation

Most often, the patient is afebrile or has a low-grade temperature, with watery or mucoid rhinorrhea. Sneezing, coughing, and conjunctival injection are other features. Infants may have noisy breathing or decreased ability to feed.

Diagnosis

Inquire about fever, cough, appetite, vomiting, diarrhea, treatments given at home, and whether anyone else at home is ill. Perform a complete examination, looking for evidence of bacterial infection such as nasal discharge (*sinusitis, allergic rhinitis*), otitis media, *pharyngitis*, and nuchal rigidity (*meningitis*). Auscultate the lungs for decreased breath sounds or rales (*pneumonia*) or wheezing (*asthma* or *bronchiolitis*).

ED Management

Although there are myriad over-the-counter cold remedies, there are few data proving efficacy. Antihistamine-decongestant combinations have been shown to have little effect on the common cold. Recommend rest, fluids, and acetaminophen (15 mg/kg q 4 h). For infants, give normal saline nose drops (two drops in one nostril at a time), followed by gentle aspiration with a bulb syringe. A vaporizer may be helpful for all age groups.

Follow-up

- Return to primary care provider if symptoms worsen [toxicity, fever >39.4°C (103°F), ear pain] or do not resolve within 3 to 4 days.

BIBLIOGRAPHY

Abramowicz M (ed): Over-the-counter (OTC) cough remedies. *Med Lett Drugs Ther* 2001;43:23–25.
Katcher ML: Cold, cough, and allergy medications: uses and abuses. *Pediatr Rev* 1996;17:12–17.
Turner RB: Treating the common cold. *J Pediatr* 1997;131:501–502.

PHARYNGOTONSILLITIS

Pharyngitis is most often caused by viral infections (adenovirus, parainfluenza, rhinovirus, coronavirus, CMV, Epstein-Barr virus, coxsackie A virus). Approximately 20 to 30% of cases are caused by group A beta-hemolytic *streptococci* ("strep throat"). Other rare etiologies include *Mycoplasma*, group C and G *Streptococcus*, toxoplasmosis, *Chlamydia*, *Neisseria gonorrhoeae*, tularemia, and diphtheria (very rare).

Clinical Presentation and Diagnosis

The older child usually complains of pain or difficulty with swallowing. The toddler may act cranky or irritable, refuse food or fluids, and have sleep disturbances. Other findings may include drooling or difficulty handling secretions, fever, otalgia, and tender anterior cervical lymphadenopathy. Infection of the pharynx causes erythema of the tonsils and tonsillar pillars with or without tonsillar enlargement. In older patients *epiglottitis* may present with severe dysphagia.

Viral Infections   Low-grade fever [<38.3°C (101°F)] associated with conjunctivitis, rhinitis, or cough suggests a viral etiology. Tonsillar exudate, toxicity, and severe difficulty swallowing are unusual findings in the common viral infections. However, adenovirus can cause a severe pharyngitis with exudate and ulceration. Thick gray mucus covering the tonsils can be seen in infectious mononucleosis and mono-like syndromes (CMV, toxoplasmosis, tularemia). Generalized lymphadenopathy, hepatosplenomegaly, an erythematous maculopapular rash, fever [>38.3°C (101°F)], periorbital edema, urticaria, upper airway obstruction secondary to lymphoid hyperplasia, and severe, prolonged lethargy are other manifestations of infectious mononucleosis, especially in the adolescent (pp 352–354). Herpangina (coxsackieviruses) causes a vesicular eruption in the posterior pharynx.

Streptococcal Infection   Streptococcal infection is suggested by whitish yellow exudate on the tonsillar surface, palatal petechiae, a red uvula, tender anterior cervical lymphadenopathy, halitosis, headache, and fever greater than 38.3°C (101°F). On occasion, associated severe abdominal pain can mimic acute appendicitis. Marked dysphagia, with drooling and difficulty breathing, occurs less frequently. An erythematous sandpaper-like scarlatiniform rash with perioral pallor may develop. Other findings are a "strawberry" tongue, accentuation of the rash in the flexion creases (Pastia's lines), and, late in the course, periungual desquamation.

Peritonsillar Abscess   Occasionally, a bacterial pharyngitis can evolve over several days into a peritonsillar abscess. This usually occurs in an adolescent who has not been treated with antibiotics, although adequate antimicrobial coverage does not always prevent this complication. Virtually all cases of peritonsillar abscess are caused by group A beta-hemolytic streptococci, although uncommonly *S. aureus* and anaerobes are implicated.

A peritonsillar abscess causes severe sore throat and toxicity, with difficulty opening the mouth (trismus), drooling, a "hot potato" muffled voice, and swelling of the uvula with deviation to the unaffected side. The tonsil is markedly erythematous and covered with a whitish exudate. Anterior and superior to the tonsil there is soft palate swelling, which is sometimes fluctuant. The head may be tilted to the unaffected side, and tender cervical adenopathy is usually prominent on the same side as the abscess.

Retropharyngeal Abscess   A retropharyngeal abscess is a complication of streptococcal pharyngitis or trauma or an extension of a vertebral osteomyelitis (most often caused by *S. aureus*). The patient presents with drooling, respiratory distress (stridor), and hyperextension of the neck. Torticollis may also be present. On examination, the posterior pharyngeal wall can be seen bulging anteriorly. A soft tissue lateral neck x-ray reveals an increase in prevertebral soft tissue; a neck CT scan with IV contrast will confirm the retropharyngeal abscess.

ED Management

Clinical evaluation alone is an inaccurate method for diagnosing strep throat. Streptococcal infection may be diagnosed either by a throat culture on 5% sheep's blood agar or by a rapid agglutination test, which is useful for early diagnosis. False-negative results, although rare, are possible with all the rapid strep tests, so a throat culture is indicated if the rapid test is negative.

Treat pharyngitis symptomatically, with gargles, lozenges, and acetaminophen (15 mg/kg q 4 h) or ibuprofen (10 mg/kg q 6 h). If a rapid strep test or throat culture is positive for beta-hemolytic streptococci, treat with antibiotics to prevent rheumatic fever as well as to shorten the course of the acute pharyngitis. Therapy consists of 10 days of oral antibiotics: penicillin VK (25 mg/kg/day divided tid), cefadroxil (20 mg/kg qd), or, for penicillin-allergic patients, erythromycin ethyl succinate (40 mg/kg/day divided bid or tid) or clindamycin (25 mg/kg/day divided tid). Alternatively, azithromycin 12 mg/kg/day can be used for 5 days. If compliance is not assured, give one dose of intramuscular benzathine penicillin G mixed with procaine penicillin [600,000 U of benzathine <27 kg (60 lb); 1,200,000 U of benzathine >27 kg (60 lb)]. At least 20% of group A beta-hemolytic streptococci are resistant to tetracycline, while sulfonamides (including trimethoprim-sulfamethoxazole) do not reliably eradicate acute streptococcal infections and therefore are not appropriate therapy.

Treat a *peritonsillar abscess* with intravenous penicillin G (50,000–100,000 U/kg/day divided q 6 h) and incision and drainage by an otolaryngologist. However, discharge a patient who is able to drink liquids adequately after the procedure. Prescribe amoxicillin-clavulanate (200/28.5, 400/57 or 875/125 formulation, 45 mg/kg/day of amoxicillin divided bid) or, if penicillin-allergic, clindamycin (20 mg/kg/day divided qid), and pain medication (ibuprofen, 10 mg/kg q 6 h; acetaminophen with codeine 1 mg/kg q 6 h, 30 mg maximum). A tonsillectomy may be indicated on an elective basis to prevent recurrences.

Treat a *retropharyngeal abscess* with IV ampicillin-sulbactam (150 mg/kg/day divided q 6 h) and admit for drainage in the operating room under general anesthesia. If the patient is allergic to penicillin, use IV clindamycin (40 mg/kg/day divided q 6 h).

When the clinical picture is suggestive of *infectious mononucleosis* or if the patient has been suffering an unusually prolonged or severe sore throat, an evaluation for mononucleosis is indicated. Obtain a CBC with differential to look for atypical lymphocytosis and a Monospot test or heterophile antibody. If there is upper airway obstruction, insert a nasopharyngeal airway and give prednisone (pp 352–354). Advise the patient to avoid contact sports for several months.

Follow-up
- Strep throat: primary care in 1 week, or sooner if symptoms worsen
- Peritonsillar abscess (drained): 2 to 3 days
- Mononucleosis: primary care follow-up in 2 weeks to assess for splenomegaly or sooner if respiratory symptoms develop.

Indications for Admission
- Severe dysphagia preventing oral intake
- Patient not taking adequate oral fluids, status–post incision and drainage of a peritonsillar abscess
- Retropharyngeal abscess
- Any evidence of respiratory distress

BIBLIOGRAPHY

Dajani AS: Current therapy of group A streptococcal pharyngitis. *Pediatr Ann* 1998; 27:227–280.

Gerber MA: Diagnosis of group A streptococcal pharyngitis. *Pediatr Ann* 1998; 27:269–273.

Lee SS, Schwartz RH, Bahadori RS: Retropharyngeal abscess: epiglottitis of the new millennium. *J Pediatr* 2001;138:435–437.

Schraff S, McGinn JD, Derkay CS: Peritonsillar abscess in children: a 10-year review of diagnosis and management. *Int J Pediatr Otorhinolaryngol* 2001;57: 213–218.

CHAPTER 7

Endocrine Emergencies

Holly Schachner and Miriam Silfen

ADRENAL INSUFFICIENCY

The adrenal cortex is divided into three zones: the outermost glomerulosa, which produces aldosterone; the middle fasciculata, which produces cortisol and androgens; and the innermost reticularis, which produces androgens. Hypothalamic corticotropin-releasing hormone stimulates the secretion of pituitary adrenocorticotropic hormone (ACTH), which, in turn, stimulates adrenal glucocorticoid secretion.

Lesions of the hypothalamus, pituitary, or adrenal cortex may cause adrenal insufficiency. In children, failure of the adrenal cortex (primary adrenal insufficiency) accounts for the majority of cases. Congenital adrenal hyperplasia (CAH), an inherited defect in steroid biosynthesis, is the most common cause. Other etiologies include autoimmune adrenalitis (Addison's disease), fulminant infections (adrenal hemorrhage in meningococcemia), trauma, HIV infection, tumor, infiltrative disease, tuberculosis, and bilateral adrenalectomy.

The causes of central (hypothalamic or pituitary) adrenal insufficiency are central nervous system (CNS) tumors, trauma, and idiopathic causes. The most common etiology is exogenous steroid administration; a patient receiving supraphysiologic doses for more than 1 to 2 weeks is at risk for adrenal insufficiency and acute adrenal crisis.

Acute adrenal crisis (Addisonian crisis) is a life-threatening emergency caused by relative or absolute deficiencies of cortisol and aldosterone. Crisis occurs when the adrenal gland fails to respond to stress with up to a tenfold increase in cortisol secretion. This rise in cortisol secretion is dependent on increased ACTH release. Crisis may be precipitated by bacterial or viral infections or dental or surgical procedures. Prompt recognition of the presenting symptoms and immediate treatment is imperative.

Clinical Presentation

The initial complaints are often nonspecific, so that the key to making the diagnosis is to suspect it. The presentation may be gradual, with subtle

147

complaints such as weakness, fatigue, malaise, anorexia, and weight loss. Salt craving may be reported, and the blood pressure may be normal or low. Alternatively, there may be an acute presentation, with fever, weakness, lethargy, abdominal pain, nausea, vomiting (possibly bilious), guarding and rebound tenderness, dehydration, hypotension, and/or shock. Seizures, secondary to hypoglycemia, may also occur. The presentation may also be fulminant, and sudden death can occur.

A subtle physical examination finding is skin hyperpigmentation, most often on the lips and buccal mucosa, nipples, groin, palmar or axillary creases, and areas of old scars or friction (knees, elbows, knuckles). Skin hyperpigmentation is a sign of increased ACTH secretion in primary adrenal insufficiency; it does not occur in hypothalamic/pituitary adrenal insufficiency. Other possible signs include petechiae and purpura (overwhelming sepsis, usually meningococcemia), hypoglycemic seizures (glucocorticoid insufficiency), midline craniofacial malformations (e.g., septooptic dysplasia, cleft lip/palate, holoprosencephaly), and micropenis (hypopituitarism). Central adrenal insufficiency is often associated with other hypothalamic/pituitary hormone deficiencies, which may manifest as growth failure, delayed pubertal progression, micropenis, and, in the case of CNS lesions, diabetes insipidus.

A patient on glucocorticoid therapy with signs of Cushing's syndrome (hypertension, moon facies, central obesity, purple striae, acne) is likely to have adrenal suppression. Clinical adrenal insufficiency or acute adrenal crisis can occur upon withdrawal of steroids or when there is physiologic stress (surgery, infection, trauma) without an appropriate increase in the glucocorticoid dose.

A female infant with CAH is usually diagnosed soon after birth because of ambiguous genitalia, ranging from mild clitoromegaly to male appearance with bilateral cryptorchidism. A male infant with CAH usually has normal external genitalia and is therefore often not diagnosed in the immediate newborn period. The patient may present at 1 to 3 weeks of life with fatigue, poor feeding, and vomiting, resembling the clinical picture of sepsis. Alternatively, there may be a fulminant presentation with dehydration, shock, or sudden death. A family history of consanguinity, CAH, or neonatal deaths may be elicited. On physical examination, hyperpigmentation (as described above) may be noted.

Diagnosis

The key to diagnosing acute adrenal crisis is to maintain a high degree of suspicion, especially in a previously well infant who has mild to moderate illness but deteriorates quickly. The prominent gastrointestinal symptoms of adrenal crisis can resemble *gastroenteritis* (diarrhea is frequent), an *acute abdomen* (involuntary guarding and rebound tenderness), and *intestinal obstruction* (bilious vomiting).

If impending or acute adrenal crisis is suspected, do not delay treatment while waiting for confirmatory laboratory tests. Initiate diagnostic testing and treatment simultaneously. Obtain blood for a complete blood count (CBC), electrolytes, glucose, and serum cortisol while establishing IV access.

Acute adrenal insufficiency may cause hyponatremia, hypochloremia, and hyperkalemia with a serum sodium/potassium ratio <28 (although dysrhythmias due to hyperkalemia are rare). Hypoglycemia and neutropenia [white blood cell count (WBC) <5000/mm³] can occur, although these can also be signs of *sepsis*. In addition, there is increased plasma renin, increased urinary excretion of sodium if the patient is aldosteronedeficient (i.e., salt-wasters), and decreased urinary excretion of potassium.

Generally, patients in shock have an elevated serum cortisol level; with adrenal insufficiency, the serum cortisol is inappropriately low. An ACTH stimulation test (250 µg Cortrosyn IV with 0- and 60-min cortisol levels) is often needed to confirm the diagnosis of adrenal insufficiency. A 60-min cortisol level >25 mg/dL or more than twice the 0-min level suggests normal adrenal reserves. The usefulness of ACTH stimulation testing is limited in central adrenal insufficiency.

ED Management

Once the diagnosis is suspected, therapy includes aggressive fluid management and steroid replacement. If needed, definitive assessment of adrenal function can be done after the acute emergency has passed.

Acute Crisis

1. *Fluid Management:* Clinical assessment tends to underestimate the severity of the hypovolemia. Consider the patient to be at least 10% dehydrated. Start an IV and give 20 mL/kg of normal saline over 30 min. Repeat the boluses until the patient becomes normotensive. Once the blood pressure is normal, continue with D_5 NS for patients with salt-losing adrenal insufficiency. Change non–salt losers to $D_5^{1/2}$ to $^{2/3}$NS if the electrolytes are normal.

   Total fluid requirements are in the range of 1.5 to 2 times maintenance; reassess as therapy continues. Add potassium (10–20 mEq/L) once the patient voids; cortisol administration will rapidly induce kaliuresis and a fall in the serum potassium. If the patient is hypoglycemic, give 1 mL/kg D_{50}, check the blood sugar hourly until stable, and increase the dextrose to D_{10} or $D_{12.5}$, as needed, to keep the blood glucose >60 mg/dL.

2. *Corticosteroid Replacement:* Give a stat dose of hydrocortisone (Solu-Cortef) IV push or IM (infant: 25 mg; small child: 50 mg; larger child or adolescent: 100 mg) followed by 25 mg/m² (or 1 mg/kg) IV or IM q 6 h.

3. *Shock:* If shock persists despite the crystalloid boluses, give a plasma expander, such as Plasmanate (20–40 mL/kg), or a vasopressor, such as dopamine (see "Shock," pp 18–22). Vasopressors may be ineffective unless preceded by adequate cortisol replacement.

4. *Mineralocorticoid Replacement:* Mineralocorticoid replacement is not necessary during the acute ED treatment because high-dose glucocorticoids with mineralocorticoid activity are given with normal saline (steps 1 and 2). Once the patient is stable and can take oral fluids, give 9α -fluorocortisol (Florinef) 0.1 to 0.2 mg PO qd to salt-wasters.

5. *Underlying Pathology:* Identify and treat any underlying cause of the stress. Infection is the most common precipitating factor.
6. *Complications:* ICU monitoring may be necessary, especially if the patient remains comatose or hypotensive or the underlying pathology takes a fulminant course (sepsis). Complications of excessive fluid, salt, or steroid replacement include hypernatremia, hypokalemia, pulmonary edema, congestive heart failure, and hypervolemia.

Minor Illness or Stress in Adrenal Insufficiency

1. *Patient Taking Maintenance Corticosteroids* (e.g., a patient with CAH or Addison's disease): For a minor illness, such as low-grade fever [<38.8°C (102°F)], double the daily dose of hydrocortisone. For a moderate illness, such as fever >102°F (>38.8°C) and/or a bacterial infection, triple the total daily dose and divide into a q 6 h dosing regimen. If the patient cannot tolerate oral medications, give the same dose IM or IV.
2. *Patient Taking Pharmacologic Doses of Steroids* [for asthma, nephrotic syndrome, immune thrombocytopenic purpura (ITP), leukemia, collagen vascular diseases, etc.]: Most pharmacologic doses are greater than physiologic doses. If the steroid dose is not already twice the maintenance dose of hydrocortisone (20–30 mg/m^2/day), double the dose (to 40–60 mg/m^2) when the stress is trauma or surgery. If the stress is a serious infection, with an etiology that may be adversely affected by high-dose steroids (such as fungal infection in a patient with cystic fibrosis), consult with pediatric infectious disease and endocrine specialists and lower the dose to 30–50 mg/m^2/day divided q 6 h. If a patient receiving a tapering dose of corticosteroids develops symptoms of adrenal insufficiency, increase the dose to the most recent dose at which he or she was asymptomatic, then initiate a more gradual taper after consulting with a pediatric endocrinologist.
3. *Patient Who Has Recently Completed a Steroid Course:* A patient who within the past 6 months has completed a 10- to 14-day (or longer) course of corticosteroids is at risk for developing adrenal insufficiency. If the patient has symptoms of adrenal insufficiency, perform an ACTH stimulation test (see above); if testing reveals adrenal insufficiency, start maintenance hydrocortisone at 10 to 15 mg/m^2/day divided q 8 h, although a larger dose may be needed. If the patient shows symptoms of an acute adrenal crisis, treat as above. A reevaluation of the patient's adrenal reserve may be indicated approximately 6 months after the last steroid course; normal results eliminate unnecessary future stress steroid doses.

For all of the above scenarios, continue the oral stress dose (double or triple) of hydrocortisone for the duration of the stress and then taper quickly, over 4 to 7 days, to the previous or maintenance dose. In addition, advise the family of a steroid-dependent child to obtain and have the child wear a Medic Alert bracelet and to carry a card that indicates the current steroid dose, indications, and doses for stress as well as the prescribing physician's name and contact numbers.

Follow-up

- Stress doses of hydrocortisone required: daily, until the stress has resolved

Indications for Admission

- Addisonian crisis
- Vomiting, inadequate oral intake, or postural vital sign changes in a patient known to be at risk for adrenal insufficiency
- Uncertain medication compliance at home

BIBLIOGRAPHY

Krasner AS: Glucocorticoid-induced adrenal insufficiency. *JAMA* 1999;282: 671–676.
Oelkers W: Adrenal insufficiency. *N Engl J Med* 1996;335:1206–1212.
Pang S: Congenital adrenal hyperplasia. *Endocrinol Metab Clin North Am* 1997; 26:853–891.

DIABETES INSIPIDUS

Diabetes insipidus (DI) is a syndrome characterized by an inability to concentrate urine. Central diabetes insipidus is defined by a deficiency of antidiuretic hormone (ADH, vasopressin). A variety of acquired hypothalamic lesions can cause central DI, including tumors, basilar skull fractures, neurosurgical complications, granulomatous diseases, vascular lesions, meningitis, and encephalitis. In approximately 50% of cases, however, no primary etiology can be found (idiopathic, congenital defect).

Nephrogenic DI is caused by renal unresponsiveness to ADH. The defect may be congenital or secondary to hypercalcemia, hypokalemia, drugs (lithium, amphotericin), or chronic renal disease, including ureteral obstruction, polycystic kidney disease, renal medullary cystic disease, or sickle cell disease.

Clinical Presentation

DI causes renal loss of water, which can lead to enormous urine output and acute thirst. Water loss is compensated by increasing intake, so that dehydration is unusual in an awake patient. However, infants, children with altered mental status, and patients whose thirst centers are affected by the primary process (hydrocephalus, postconcussive syndrome) are at increased risk for hypernatremic dehydration.

An infant is usually irritable but eager to suck, often exhibiting a distinct preference for water over milk. An older child presents with the abrupt onset of polyuria and polydipsia, followed by enuresis, vomiting, and constipation. Nocturia and a preference for ice water are common. Unexplained fever and failure to thrive are other presentations.

CNS abnormalities such as irritability, altered consciousness, increased muscle tone, convulsions, and coma occur secondary to hypernatremia. These findings correlate with the degree and rapidity of the rise in serum sodium.

Diagnosis

The cardinal diagnostic features are as follows:

- A high rate of dilute urine flow (urine output >4 mL/kg/h)
- Clinical signs of dehydration
- Mild to marked degree of serum hypernatremia (>150 mEq/L)
- Hyperosmolality (>300 mosm/L)
- Low urine osmolality and specific gravity despite a normal or elevated serum osmolality

If the dehydration is mild, the urine osmolality is less than the serum osmolality. However, if there is severe dehydration or a low glomerular filtration rate, urine output decreases and urine osmolality increases above that of the serum; this may temporarily obscure the diagnosis.

Other causes of polyuria, including *psychogenic water drinking* (nocturia unusual), *organic polydipsia* (hypothalamic lesion), and osmotic diuresis (*diabetes mellitus, IV contrast administration, chronic renal insufficiency*), can be distinguished by the history, electrolytes, blood urea nitrogen (BUN), and creatinine. With a *urinary tract infection* (pp 613–616), there will be symptoms such as urgency, frequency, and dysuria. A large urinary volume can lead to bladder distention, which can then mimic *obstructive uropathy.*

ED Management

If DI is suspected, obtain urine for routine analysis as well as osmolality, sodium, potassium, and culture. Obtain blood for electrolytes, calcium, BUN, creatinine, osmolality, and ADH level. The diagnosis is confirmed if hypernatremia and serum hyperosmolality are documented in association with large volumes of dilute urine (specific gravity ≤1.005, urine osmolality ≤ serum) that is negative for glucose.

In addition, perform a complete neurologic examination with evaluation of visual fields and obtain a CT scan of the head. If the etiology is not clear, admit the patient.

If the patient is dehydrated, hyperpyrexic [>38.3°C (101°F)], or has a depressed level of consciousness, start treatment in the ED. Give antidiuretic therapy (vasopressin SQ/IM/IV or DDAVP intranasal/SQ/IV) according to the guidelines below.

Vasopressin

SQ (20 U/mL): Give 0.05 to 0.1 U/kg per dose q 4–6 h. Titrate the dose to the desired effect. This route is preferred for a patient with new-onset DI, one who is dehydrated or has an altered mental status, or a DI patient who must undergo neurosurgery or prolonged surgery of any type.

Aqueous Pitressin drip (10 U/0.5 mL): Dilute to 0.01 U/mL by adding 5 U (0.25 mL) to 500 mL NS or D_5W. Give 0.003 to 0.012 U/kg/h. Start with the lowest dose, then, after 30 to 60 min, titrate rapidly to the desired effect (double the IV rate).

DDAVP

IV or SQ (4 mg/mL): Dilute with NS (1 mL DDAVP with 9 mL NS = 0.4 μg/mL) and give 0.01 to 0.03 μg/kg per dose qd or bid.

Intranasal [10 μg/0.1 mL (spray); 250 μg/2.5 mL (rhinal tube)]: Give 5 to 20 μg per dose qd or bid (start with lower dose and titrate to the desired effect).

Pay meticulous attention to fluid management. Use a flow sheet to document fluid input and output, replacement of urine output and insensible losses, vital signs, urine specific gravity, and serum electrolytes.

Indication for Admission

- New-onset or symptomatic DI

BIBLIOGRAPHY

Al-Agha AE, Thomsett MJ, Ratcliffe JF, et al: Acquired central diabetes insipidus in children: a 12-year Brisbane experience. *J Paediatr Child Health* 2001;37: 172–175.

Bichet DG, Oksche A, Rosenthal W: Congenital nephrogenic diabetes insipidus. *J Am Soc Nephrol* 1997;8:1951–1958.

Maghnie M, Cosi G, Geovese E, et al: Central diabetes insipidus in children and young adults. *N Engl J Med* 2000;343:998–1007.

DIABETIC KETOACIDOSIS

Diabetic ketoacidosis (DKA) may be the initial presentation of a new diabetic or a complication in a previously diagnosed patient. Infection is the most common precipitating factor, but trauma, pregnancy, emotional stress, and noncompliance are other causes. An absolute or relative insulin deficiency is present, along with increased levels of counterregulatory hormones (glucagon, cortisol, growth hormone, and catecholamines), leading to deranged metabolism, hyperglycemia, osmotic diuresis, hypertonic dehydration, and finally ketoacidosis. In ketoacidosis, the acidosis is secondary to ketonemia with beta-hydroxybutyric acid and acetoacetate, its redox partner.

Clinical Presentation

The patient usually presents with abdominal pain, nausea, vomiting, dehydration, and hyperpnea. Vomiting in the absence of diarrhea can also be a presentation of DKA. The history often reveals polydipsia, polyuria, nocturia, enuresis, and, with new-onset diabetes, recent weight loss or lack of weight gain in a growing child. Characteristic Kussmaul breathing (deep sighing breathing) can be present, but respirations may be depressed if the patient is severely acidotic (pH ≤6.9).

Mild DKA   DKA is considered mild if there is ketonemia with a compensated metabolic acidosis, normal pH, and minimal signs of dehydration. The vital signs may be normal except for possible hyperpnea.

Moderate DKA   In moderate DKA, the arterial pH is >7.2, but there are signs of moderate to severe dehydration, including dry mucous membranes and decreased skin turgor. Ketonemia is present as well.

Severe DKA   Severe DKA is defined as a pH <7.2 with ketonemia and severe dehydration as well as evidence of intravascular volume depletion (poor capillary refill, tachycardia, weak peripheral pulses, hypotension, orthostatic changes in vital signs).

Diagnosis

In the known diabetic, consider DKA when the patient complains of abdominal pain, vomiting, or malaise. The diagnosis may be more difficult to make in a patient presenting for the first time (see Table 7-1). In addition to acidosis and ketonemia, significant hyperglycemia (>500 mg/dL) is common, although DKA can occur with a glucose of 200 to 300 mg/dL. In fact, the glucose level is more indicative of the sugar content of what the patient has been drinking while attempting to maintain hydration than the severity of the DKA.

In DKA, sodium stores are depleted, but serum sodium may be low, normal, or high, depending on the water balance. The measured sodium is lower than the true value because of the shift of water into the extracellular space (sodium decreases 1.6 mEq/L for each 100 mg/dL rise in glucose over 100 mg/dL) and the increase in serum lipid and protein levels (pseudohyponatremia). In addition, the low sodium level may reflect water retention secondary to increased secretion of ADH.

Table 7-1   Differential Diagnosis of Diabetic Ketoacidosis

Metabolic Acidosis	*Polyuria, Nocturia,*
Severe gastroenteritis	*Abdominal Pain*
with hypovolemia	UTI
Salicylate poisoning	
Other ingestions	*Hyperglycemia*
Ethanol	Salicylate poisoning
Methanol	(glucose <300 mg/dL)
Ethylene glycol	Iron toxicity
Isoniazid	Hypernatremia
Iron	Stress
	Sepsis
Coma	
Hypoglycemia	*Ketonuria (without hyperglycemia)*
Sedative hypnotic or	Fasting states
narcotic overdose	Gastroenteritis with vomiting
Lactic acidosis	Anorexia of any etiology
Nonketotic hyperosmolar coma	Salicylate poisoning
CNS trauma, infection, bleeding	

While there is usually a total body potassium deficit, the initial serum potassium concentration may be normal or elevated because of hemoconcentration, insulin deficiency, and the shifting of potassium into the extracellular space secondary to the metabolic acidosis. The measured potassium rises 0.6 mEq/L for every 0.1 drop in the pH, so that a low initial potassium level (<3.5 mEq/L) is an unusual and ominous finding.

Finally, in the absence of infection, the white blood cell (WBC) count may be elevated (18,000–20,000/mm^3) in a patient with DKA secondary to the increase in circulating catecholamines and hemoconcentration.

ED Management

After a rapid evaluation of the patient's status, initiate therapy to correct fluid deficits, electrolyte imbalances, acidosis, and hyperglycemia. Avoid overly vigorous management, which can cause excessively rapid changes in glucose, osmolality, and pH and may therefore contribute to the development of complications. Treat any concomitant pathology or complications [sepsis, increased intracranial pressure (ICP), or coma].

Assessment
History   Determine the duration of the current illness and any precipitating factors such as infection, trauma, or stress. If the patient is a known diabetic, document the current insulin regimen (and adherence) and the time of the last injection.

Physical Examination   Note the vital signs (including the presence of Kussmaul respirations), degree of dehydration, level of consciousness, funduscopic exam, and focus of infection. If possible, weigh the patient and try to determine his or her premorbid weight.

Initial Laboratory Evaluation   Obtain blood for STAT electrolytes, BUN, osmolality, glucose, calcium, phosphorus, pH (venous or arterial), CBC, and a bedside fingerstick glucose measurement. Also, obtain a urinalysis and an electrocardiogram (ECG; check for peaked T waves). Prior to beginning insulin therapy for a patient with new-onset diabetes, save an additional 7 mL of blood in a red-top tube for insulin, C-peptide, and relevant autoantibodies [insulin autoantibodies (IAA), islet cell antibodies (ICA), and glutamic acid decarboxylase antibodies (GAD)] and 2 mL in a lavender-top tube for an HgbA1$_C$ level.

Treatment
Start and maintain a flow sheet. Within the framework of the following guidelines, assess each case individually. In general, however, the goals are slow, steady rehydration over a minimum of 48 h, a decrease in the serum glucose of 100 mg/dL/h, and a stable corrected sodium while the measured sodium increases. Use a slower rate of fluid replacement for a small child or if there is severe acidosis, an elevated corrected sodium, significant hyperosmolality (>300), or a long prodromal illness.

In severe DKA (pH <7.2), monitor the pH and electrolytes every 1 to 2 h until the pH is >7.2, then every 2 to 4 h. Check the glucose every hour via fingerstick. Perform a brief neurologic evaluation every 1 to 2 h.

Reassess the fluid management every 4 h, or more often if the patient's clinical progress is not satisfactory. In general, an older child tends to appear more dehydrated than he or she is, whereas an infant tends to appear less dehydrated. Aim to admit the patient within 2 h.

For the first 2 h, while calculating the fluids and checking laboratory results, keep the patient NPO.

1. *Fluid Resuscitation:* Give an IV bolus of normal saline (20 mL/kg) over the first hour to establish adequate intravascular volume and tissue perfusion.

   Continue with normal saline if the corrected sodium is <140 mEq/L with an osmolality >310 mEq/L (high blood sugar). To calculate the corrected sodium, add 1.6 mEq/L to the measured sodium for every 100 mg/dL of glucose over 100 mg/dL: Corrected sodium = measured + [1.6 × (serum glucose − 100)/100]. Use normal saline until the sodium rises to near normal levels as the blood sugar falls. However, if the corrected sodium is >160 mEq/L, consult with a pediatric endocrinologist and use a lower sodium concentration in the IV fluid.

2. *Deficit Fluids:* Once intravascular volume has been restored and adequate perfusion is established, calculate the fluid deficit as 1 L/kg of body weight lost and plan to replace it using normal saline over 24 h. Replace the deficit over 48 h if the osmolality is >320. However, avoid excessive hydration (>4 L/m^2/day), which has been associated with cerebral edema and a poor outcome. Subtract the initial IV resuscitation fluids and the insulin infusion volume from the total fluid volume.

3. *Maintenance Fluids:* Calculate the daily maintenance fluids as 100 mL/kg for the first 10 kg of premorbid body weight, 50 mL/kg for the next 10 kg, and 20 mL/kg for every kilogram above 20 per 24 h and give as ½NS. Replacement of ongoing losses may be necessary, especially if there is polyuria (>4 mL/kg/h). For a polyuric patient, measure the urinary losses every 4 to 8 h, then replace half of this volume over the next 4 to 8 h with ½NS in a separate "piggyback" line. Also replace the volume of vomitus with ½NS in this line.

4. *Sodium:* Usually, the volume of NS and ½NS used to replace the deficit, run the insulin infusion, replace excess urine losses, and provide maintenance fluids will also provide the calculated sodium requirement. Replace one-half of the sodium deficit in the first 12 h and the remainder over the subsequent 36 h.

5. *Potassium:* DKA is associated with a marked depletion of total body potassium, while correction of the acidosis will also cause hypokalemia.

   a. Add potassium once urine output is documented, the serum potassium is <5.0 mEq/L, and the T waves are not peaked on the ECG.

   b. Generally, use 40 mEq/L of KCl, although the calculated potassium needs are greater. If the serum potassium is <3.5, use 40 mEq/L of KCl and 20 mEq/L of K phosphate.

    c. There is also a depletion of total body phosphate. However, IV phosphate is indicated only if there has been prolonged illness or it is expected that the patient will be NPO for more than 24 h. In such a case, if the phosphate is <3 mEq/L, give half of the potassium replacement as K phosphate.

    d. If hypocalcemia develops, stop the IV K phosphate and replace it with KCl.

    e. Measure the phosphorus and calcium every 4 to 6 h and repeat the ECG (looking for peaked T waves secondary to a high potassium level) every 2 to 4 h.

6. *Insulin and Glucose:* An insulin drip provides a therapeutic serum insulin level while facilitating rapid dose changes if needed. After the initial fluid resuscitation, the goal is to decrease the blood sugar by 100 mg/dL/h; avoid a more rapid drop. Start the insulin infusion within the first 2 h of treatment but do not give an insulin bolus.

    a. Add 100 U (1 mL) of regular insulin to 500 mL of normal saline. Therefore, there will be 0.2 U/mL.

    b. Prior to running the drip, allow 50 mL of the mixture to flow through the IV in order to saturate insulin binding sites in the tubing.

    c. Run the IV at an hourly rate of 0.5 mL/kg/h. This gives an initial dose of 0.1U/kg/h.

    d. Start at 0.05 U/kg/h if the patient is markedly hyperglycemic (glucose >1000 mg/dL), is <2 years of age, is hyperosmolar (>320–350), or has recently received a subcutaneous dose of insulin.

    e. Add D_5W to the replacement solution when the glucose drops below 200 mg/dL.

    f. Continue the infusion until the ketonemia is cleared or clearing. Adjust the rate of the drip to maintain a blood glucose of 120 to 180 mg/dL. However, do not decrease the drip rate below 0.03 U/kg/h. If the patient is becoming hypoglycemic at this rate, increase the dextrose in the IV solution to $D_{7.5}$ or D_{10}. Calculate the glucose requirement per unit of insulin; most patients require 3 to 5 g of glucose per unit of insulin.

7. *Bicarbonate:* Do not use sodium bicarbonate unless the pH <7.0 or the serum bicarbonate is <5 mEq/L. The dose is 0.5 to 1 mEq/kg by IV infusion over 1 h, *not as an IV push.*

8. *Laboratory Assessments:*

    a. Repeat the glucose hourly.

    b. Obtain electrolytes, BUN, and creatinine every 2 h until the trend is normalizing, then every 4 h until normal.

    c. Calculate the corrected sodium with each set of laboratory values.

    d. Obtain calcium and phosphorus levels every 4 to 6 h until the DKA is resolving.

    e. Measure the pH (ABG or VBG) every 1 to 2 h if the DKA is not severe.

    f. Obtain an ECG every 2 to 4 h, looking for peaked T waves (hyperkalemia).

Even with meticulous care, a patient with DKA is at risk for developing cerebral edema, especially if the serum sodium does not rise as expected when the serum glucose falls. Signs and symptoms of increased ICP (pp 468–470) classically occur 6 to 18 h into treatment and include headache, vomiting, lethargy, disorientation, funduscopic changes (absent venous pulsations, blurring of optic disk margins), decorticate or decerebrate posturing, and pupillary changes. Any neurologic signs at presentation, prior to treatment, reflect the patient's hyperosmolality. If the patient complains of headache and becomes lethargic during treatment but has a normal funduscopic exam, obtain a stat CT scan of the head. If the patient is unresponsive, posturing, has pupillary changes, or has milder symptoms with funduscopic abnormalities, immediately treat for increased ICP with intubation, elevation of the head to 30 degrees, mild hyperventilation to a Pco_2 of 30 to 35mmHg 0.5 to 1 g/kg of mannitol (over 15–30 min) if needed, and consult a pediatric neurosurgeon.

Also observe the patient for other problems associated with therapy for DKA, such as fluid overload with edema or congestive heart failure (CHF).

Management of Mild DKA (pH >7.2)
Give fluid resuscitation if needed, as above. If the patient is not dehydrated, give ½NS at a maintenance rate plus deficit (based on clinical exam and recent weight loss). Give the known diabetic subcutaneous regular insulin (usually 0.1 U/kg). In the case of a new-onset diabetic not in DKA, treat with appropriate hydration and consult with a pediatric endocrinologist. Do not treat with insulin until after consultation, as such a patient is particularly sensitive to exogenous insulin. Obtain baseline measurements of serum insulin, C peptide, HgbA1$_c$, IAA, ICA, GAD, and thyroid function tests.

Hyperglycemia during Stress
Hyperglycemia may occur in response to stress, such as sepsis or corticosteroid administration, although most patients with stress do not become hyperglycemic. Diabetes cannot be definitively diagnosed during another illness, but the patient requires close follow-up. Obtain IAA, ICA, and GAD to evaluate the risk of type I diabetes, which is greater in a child with positive antibodies, with or without known relatives with diabetes. Refer a patient with any positive antibody test to a pediatric endocrinologist in about 6 weeks for evaluation of glucose tolerance.

Type II Diabetes
Type II diabetes is increasing in frequency among children, though it is more commonly an incidental finding than the cause for an ED visit. It is characterized by insulin resistance and relative insulin hyposecretion. It can present with polydipsia, polyuria, and polyphagia and infrequently with weight loss but rarely with ketosis and/or acidosis unless the patient presents with a significant infection. Alternatively, glucosuria or hyperglycemia may be noted as incidental findings. A patient with type II diabetes is usually obese and frequently has acanthosis nigricans, most commonly on the posterior neck, but lesions may also be found on the anterior neck, in the axillae, and

in the groin. The blood sugar is >200 mg/dL, and the fasting glucose is >125 mg/dL. Management depends on the severity of presentation; a dehydrated patient requires IV fluid (see pp 21–22), and a ketotic patient needs insulin. Also give insulin to a patient who remains hyperglycemic after a bolus of normal saline. Consult with a pediatric endocrinologist to determine whether treatment with oral agents is appropriate.

Follow-up

- Mild DKA in a known diabetic: 1 to 2 days
- Stress hyperglycemia with positive antibody test: endocrinology follow-up in 6 weeks

Indications for Admission

- Newly diagnosed diabetes
- Moderate or severe ketoacidosis
- Known diabetic with an intercurrent illness which limits oral rehydration or therapy (nausea and vomiting)

BIBLIOGRAPHY

Glaser N, Barnett P, McCaslin I, et al: Risk factors for cerebral edema in children with diabetic ketoacidosis. *N Engl J Med* 2001;344:264–269.

Kaufman FR, Halvorson M: The treatment and prevention of diabetic ketoacidosis in children and adolescents with type I diabetes mellitus. *Pediatr Ann* 1999;28:576–582.

White NH: Diabetic ketoacidosis in children. *Endocrinol Metab Clin North Am* 2000;29:657–682.

Shehadeh N, On A, Kessel I, et al. Stress hyperglycemia and the risk for the development of type 1 diabetes. *J Pediatr Endocrinol Metab* 1997;10:283–286.

HYPERCALCEMIA

Hypercalcemia is defined as a serum calcium >11 mg/dL. Etiologies include increased bone resorption (primary hyperparathyroidism, parathyroid hormone–secreting tumors, skeletal metastases, sarcoid, immobilization, thyrotoxicosis), increased gastrointestinal absorption (vitamin D intoxication, milk-alkali syndrome, idiopathic hypercalcemia of infancy), and decreased renal calcium clearance (thiazide use). Traumatic vaginal delivery of large infants can cause subcutaneous fat necrosis, with resultant transient hypercalcemia.

Clinical Presentation

A patient with hypercalcemia usually has a nonspecific presentation, with weakness, listlessness, irritability, gastrointestinal complaints (nausea, vomiting, constipation, abdominal pain), and neurologic symptoms (confusion, depressed consciousness). Hypotonia is a striking finding in the newborn, whereas older children may present with failure to thrive. Hypercalcemia can cause a renal concentrating defect, with resultant polyuria, polydipsia, and dehydration. Long-standing hypercalcemia may lead to band keratopathy, nephrocalcinosis, renal stones, and renal failure with hypertension. Idiopathic hypercalcemia of infancy is associated with Williams syndrome: elfin facies (upturned nose, long philtrum, hypotelorism, receding chin), full lips, stellate pattern of the iris with blue eyes, strabismus, medial flare of the eyebrows, supravalvular aortic stenosis, and mental retardation.

Diagnosis

The diagnosis is confirmed by documenting elevated serum calcium, usually in association with decreased phosphorus, normal or increased alkaline phosphatase, and hyperchloremic acidosis. Radiographs may reveal generalized bone demineralization, lytic skull lesions ("salt and pepper" pattern), nephrocalcinosis, or renal stones.

ED Management

If hypercalcemia is suspected, obtain blood for calcium (total and ionized), phosphorus, alkaline phosphatase, BUN, electrolytes, magnesium, total protein, albumin, 25-OH and 1,25-OH vitamin D, vitamin A, parathyroid hormone, thyroid-stimulating hormone (TSH), and T_4. If the serum calcium is ≥ 11.0 mg/dL or the patient is symptomatic, begin treatment immediately to prevent CNS or renal damage:

1. Increase calciuresis by giving IV normal saline at two to three times maintenance rates, along with furosemide (1 mg/kg IV q 6 h). Ensure adequate hydration before furosemide is given, otherwise the hypercalcemia can worsen.
2. Check that there is no calcium in the patient's IV solution.
3. Decrease calcium absorption by giving corticosteroids (prednisone 2 mg/kg/day divided bid or hydrocortisone 10 mg/kg/day divided qid). However, steroids may not be effective for 4 to 5 days, and rebound hypercalcemia can occur if treatment is discontinued abruptly.
4. Consult a pediatric endocrinologist to institute therapy to inhibit bone resorption. Options include calcitonin (4 U/kg/12 h SQ), which may be effective for the pain; bisphosphonates (pamidronate), which are not yet approved for children by the U.S. Food and Drug Administration; and mithramycin (25 µg/kg over 4–6 h).
5. Reserve dialysis for a patient in renal failure.

Indication for Admission

- Treatment required for hypercalcemia

BIBLIOGRAPHY

Marks KH, Kilav R, Naveh-Many T, et al: Calcium, phosphate, vitamin D, and the parathyroid. *Pediatr Nephrol* 1996;10:364–367.

Nishiyama J: Hypercalcemia in children: an overview. *Acta Paediatr Jpn* 1997;39:479–484.

Rodd C, Goodyer P: Hypercalcemia of the newborn: etiology, evaluation, and management. *Pediatr Nephrol* 1999;13:542–547.

HYPERNATREMIA

Hypernatremia is defined as a serum sodium level ≥150 mEq/L. Hypernatremia occurs when there is a relative excess of sodium compared to water. Normally, hypertonicity stimulates both the secretion of antidiuretic hormone (ADH) and an extremely powerful compensatory thirst, which can keep up with as much as 15 to 20 L of pure water loss.

Regardless of the etiology, acute hypernatremia has a mortality of 10 to 70%. CNS morbidity has been reported in up to two-thirds of patients, although it is unclear whether this is a result of the primary disease or the treatment.

There are three categories of hypernatremia:

1. *Low Total Body Sodium (TBNa); Lower Total Body Water (TBW):* Most often, this occurs in the setting of hypernatremic dehydration in infants, usually secondary to gastrointestinal losses (particularly during rotavirus infection). Osmotic diuretics (mannitol, glucose, urea) can also cause water loss in excess of salt loss.
2. *Normal TBNa; Low TBW:* Central and nephrogenic DI cause excessive renal water loss. In central DI caused by trauma, hydrocephalus, or neoplasia there may be a concomitant derangement in the thirst mechanism, further predisposing to hypernatremia. Increased insensible losses (hypermetabolic states with fever) and tachypnea can also result in hypernatremia, while restricted access to water (infants, developmentally impaired children, bedridden patients) may put a patient at increased risk.
3. *Increased TBNa (Uncommon):* Primary hyperaldosteronism, Cushing's syndrome, and salt poisoning (inappropriately mixed infant formula, salt tablet ingestion, iatrogenic sodium bicarbonate administration) result in excess body sodium. Except in the case of salt poisoning, very high serum sodium levels are unusual.

Clinical Presentation

The clinical signs and symptoms result from the physiologic response to serum hypertonicity. Most conscious patients will exhibit a voracious thirst and, if given the opportunity, will drink water. If ADH and oral intake do not compensate, serum hypertonicity occurs and the brain cells shrink, leading to CNS signs and symptoms. Lethargy alternating with irritability and a high-pitched cry (infants) occur early; followed by tremors and ataxia; then muscle twitching, tonic spasms, and seizures (both focal and generalized); and ultimately leading to coma.

Physical signs may include altered mental status, hypertonia, hyperreflexia, and nuchal rigidity (secondary to hypertonia). Since intracellular fluid shifts extracellularly, the intravascular volume is maintained, so that signs of intravascular volume depletion are late findings. Chvostek's sign may be elicited occasionally, and a smooth, velvety, or doughy feel to the skin may be noted. Localizing neurologic findings suggest the possibility of CNS hemorrhage as a sequela of brain shrinkage.

In a patient with DI (pp 151–153), signs of intravascular depletion and dehydration may be absent if the thirst mechanism and access to water are preserved. Salt poisoning may cause pulmonary edema (tachypnea, hepatomegaly, rales) and acute CNS pathology without signs of intravascular depletion. An infant exposed to extreme heat and humidity is at risk for hypernatremic dehydration; consider child abuse or neglect in such cases.

Diagnosis

Hypernatremia is usually discovered incidentally when electrolytes are obtained because of gastroenteritis, fever, altered mental status, seizures, polyuria, or polydipsia. In general, since the presentation of hypernatremia is nonspecific, early diagnosis requires a high index of suspicion. Consider hypernatremia if the skin has a velvety, doughy feel or if the clinical history fits the common etiologies.

If increased total body sodium from improper feeding technique is suspected, obtain some of the infant formula from the home and send it to the company and/or laboratory for evaluation. Also, watch how the caregiver prepares powdered formula and/or dilutes concentrated formula.

Once hypernatremia is documented, use the urine osmolality and urine sodium to categorize the patient (Table 7-2).

ED Management

Be judicious in the fluid management of any patient with an electrolyte abnormality, as rapid correction carries its own risks, such as cerebral edema. If there are signs of intravascular depletion (resting tachycardia,

Table 7-2   Diagnosis of Hypernatremia

TBNA*	TBW†	URINE OSMOLALITY	URINE SODIUM
Low	*Lower*		
	GI losses (>800 mosm/L)	Hypertonic	<10 mEq/L (low)
	Osmotic diuresis	Hypertonic	>20 mEq/L (high)
Normal	*Low*		
	Diabetes insipidus	Isotonic/ hypotonic	Variable
	Insensible losses	Hypertonic	Variable
Increased	*Low/high*		
	Salt poisoning	Isotonic/ hypertonic	>20 mEq/L (high)

*Total body sodium.
†Total body water.

orthostatic changes in vital signs, weak peripheral pulses, poor capillary refill), give repeated boluses of 20 mL/kg of isotonic crystalloid (normal saline, Ringer's lactate) until perfusion is normalized. Hypernatremia is not a contraindication to using isotonic fluids, as these are hypotonic relative to the patient's serum; the hypernatremia will not be exacerbated.

Hyperglycemia and hypocalcemia often accompany hypernatremia. Once the intravascular volume has been restored, obtain a CBC, electrolytes, Dextrostix test, calcium, creatinine, urinalysis, urine sodium and osmolality, and any other laboratory tests pertinent to the patient's presentation.

TBNa and TBW Depletion   In hypernatremic dehydration, the key to therapy is restoration of isotonicity without causing rapid fluid shifts into the brain cells. Otherwise, cerebral edema can ensue. First, give normal saline boluses until perfusion is normalized (as above). Then, replace the deficit over 48 h, using D_5 ½NS with one ampule of 10% calcium gluconate added per 500 mL of replacement fluid; add 40 mEq/L of potassium acetate after adequate urinary output is established. The goal is a slow fall in the serum sodium of 0.5 to 1.0 mEq/h. Increase the sodium in the replacement fluid if the sodium fall is too rapid. Measure the sodium and glucose hourly to document the rate of sodium correction, and follow the calcium and potassium every 2 to 4 h until normal levels are documented or the replacement is nearly complete. If hyperglycemia occurs, do not use insulin unless there are signs of glucose intolerance (glycosuria), as the glucose will generally correct with hydration alone. Increase the calcium infusion if hypocalcemia occurs (pp 164–165).

TBNa Normal; TBW Depleted   Give maintenance fluids along with one-half of the excess urine output as D_5W. Treat central DI with vasopressin (pp 151–152).

Increased TBNa/Salt Poisoning   Treat with peritoneal dialysis if the serum sodium >200 mEq/L or the patient has seizures or is comatose. Otherwise, give normal saline at a maintenance rate with furosemide (1 mg/kg) to achieve a net loss of sodium in excess of water.

Hypertension may be the presenting sign of a patient with hyperaldosteronism. Consult a pediatric endocrinologist.

Indications for Admission

- Symptomatic hypernatremia
- New-onset DI

BIBLIOGRAPHY

Mishkin MB, Simonet M, Lawrence C, et al: Hypernatremia in infancy. *Curr Opin Pediatr* 1998;10:156–160.

Moritz ML, Ayus JC: The changing pattern of hypernatremia in hospitalized children. *Pediatrics* 1999;104:435–439.

Palevsky PM: Hypernatremia. *Semin Nephrol* 1998;18:20–30.

HYPOCALCEMIA

Hypocalcemia is defined as a total serum calcium <7.0 mg/dL or an ionized calcium <3.5 mg/dL. However, mild symptoms can occur with a total serum calcium of 7.5 mg/dL in neonates and 8.5 mg/dL in older children.

In the ED, most cases are secondary to hyperventilation-induced alkalosis, which causes increased calcium binding to protein, thereby decreasing the serum ionized calcium. Other, less common etiologies include hypoparathyroid conditions (idiopathic, pseudo-, transient neonatal, post-thyroid surgery, hemochromatosis), renal failure, massive transfusion, hypomagnesemia, hyperphosphatemia, and vitamin D deficiency or defective metabolism.

Clinical Presentation

Clinical manifestations of hypocalcemia primarily involve the nervous system. Mild hypocalcemia may cause nonspecific hyperreflexia, but more serious decreases in the ionized calcium lead to muscle cramps and paresthesias of the hands, the feet, and the perioral region. Hypocalcemic tetany causes flexion at the wrists and metacarpophalangeal joints, extension at the interphalangeal joints, and adduction of the thumb into the palm (carpopedal spasm). In the extreme situation, seizures and life-threatening laryngospasm can occur.

Nonspecific symptoms include lethargy, emotional lability, irritability, impaired cognition, vomiting, and diarrhea. The newborn may present with poor feeding, vomiting, lethargy, and cyanosis.

Characteristic physical findings include the Chvostek's sign (facial muscle twitching elicited by tapping the facial nerve just anterior to the ear) and Trousseau's sign (carpopedal spasm elicited by maintaining a blood pressure cuff at just above systolic pressure for 2–3 min).

Typically, the hyperventilating adolescent presents with hypocalcemic symptoms in addition to anxiety, tachypnea, and labored breathing. There may be a history of recent emotional upset or past psychiatric disorders.

Findings in patients with long-standing hypocalcemia may include cataracts, metastatic calcifications, dry and brittle hair and nails, and dry, coarse skin.

Diagnosis

Hyperventilation   Suspect hyperventilation-induced hypocalcemia in an older child or adolescent who presents with tachypnea, anxiety, and carpopedal spasm. If the presentation is not typical for hyperventilation or the patient has hyperpnea rather than tachypnea, obtain an arterial blood gas (ABG). An increased pH, decreased P_{CO_2}, and normal P_{O_2} confirm the diagnosis and rule out other causes of hyperventilation, such as *hypoxia* or a *metabolic acidosis.*

Other Etiologies   Immediately obtain an ECG to determine the corrected QT (QTc) interval, which is prolonged with hypocalcemia. In addition, obtain blood for total or ionized calcium, electrolytes, phosphorus, magnesium, and alkaline phosphatase. The diagnosis of hypocalcemia is confirmed by either a low serum total calcium (<7 mg/dL) or ionized calcium (<3.5 mg/dL).

The phosphorus is elevated (>6 mg/dL in young child; >5 mg/dL in older child) in *hypoparathyroidism,* but low in *vitamin D deficiency.* Alkaline phosphatase is generally normal in hypoparathyroidism, but elevated in *vitamin D deficiency.*

Candidiasis or increased skin pigmentation suggests *autoimmune hypoparathyroidism,* while a round face, stocky build, mental retardation, and short fourth and fifth metacarpals and metatarsals occur in *pseudohypoparathyroidism.*

ED Management

Hyperventilation   Instruct the patient to breathe slowly in and out of a paper bag or a face mask with a reservoir attached and the side ports taped shut. This causes rebreathing of CO_2, leading to a decreased serum pH and thus an increased ionized calcium. Occasionally sedation is required. Use either hydroxyzine (1 mg/kg) or diphenhydramine (1–2 mg/kg) or a more rapid-acting anxiolytic, such as IV lorazepam (0.03 mg/kg) or diazepam (0.05–0.2 mg/kg). Once the hyperventilation has stopped, try to discover the precipitating cause and reassure the patient and the family as to the benign nature of the episode.

Other Etiologies   Give symptomatic patients (seizures, laryngospasm, tetany) 10% calcium chloride, 5 to 7 mg/kg of elemental calcium (0.2–0.25 mL/kg) slowly IV, while continuously monitoring the ECG. Cessation of the symptoms, along with shortening of the QTc interval, is the endpoint of ED therapy. A continuous IV infusion or repeated boluses may be required, in an intensive care setting. Treat asymptomatic patients with oral calcium (75 mg/kg/day of elemental calcium, divided q 6 h).

Follow-up

- Hyperventilation as a manifestation of anxiety: primary care follow-up within 1 week for evaluation and possible psychiatric referral.

Indications for Admission

- Symptomatic patient unless the etiology is hyperventilation
- Asymptomatic patient with a first episode of hypocalcemia

BIBLIOGRAPHY

Langman CB: New developments in calcium and vitamin D metabolism. *Curr Opin Pediatr* 2000;12:135–139.

Marks KH, Kilav R, Naveh-Many T, et al: Calcium, phosphate, vitamin D, and the parathyroid. *Pediatr Nephrol* 1996;10:364–367.

HYPOGLYCEMIA

Hypoglycemia occurs when there is failure to maintain glucose homeostasis secondary to defects in substrate, enzymes, or hormones. The def-

Table 7-3   Etiologies of Hypoglycemia

Decreased glucose intake	*Liver disease*
Fasting	Fructosemia
Malnutrition	Fulminant hepatitis
Malabsorption	Galactosemia
Hormone deficiencies	Glycogenoses (type I, II)
Growth hormone	Reye's syndrome
Cortisol	*Ingestions*
Glucagon	Alcohol
Thyroid disease	Oral hypoglycemic agents
Other	Propranolol
Islet cell adenoma	Salicylates
Ketotic hypoglycemia	
Sepsis	

inition of hypoglycemia depends upon the age of the patient and the method by which the specimen was obtained: consider hypoglycemia to be a whole blood glucose <50 mg/dL in a full-term newborn infant and <60 mg/dL in a child or adult.

Although there are many etiologies of hypoglycemia (Table 7-3), it is most commonly seen in diabetics having an "insulin reaction" secondary to insulin overdose, skipped or late meals, or exercise without an adjustment in food intake or insulin dosage. In a nondiabetic <8 years of age, ketotic hypoglycemia is the most common cause. Prolonged fasting, gastroenteritis, hyperinsulinemia, hormone deficiencies (panhypopituitarism, growth hormone, ACTH, cortisol), or a ketogenic diet may also lead to hypoglycemia.

Hypoglycemia in the newborn period may be transient or persistent. Transient neonatal hypoglycemia can be seen in an infant who was born prematurely, is small for gestational age, has erythroblastosis fetalis, has sustained birth trauma, or is the infant of a diabetic mother.

Clinical Presentation

A neonate presents with jitteriness, irritability, poor feeding, apnea, perioral cyanosis, irregular respirations or tachypnea, hypothermia, hypotonia, seizures, and an abnormal cry. An infant or older child can have gastrointestinal symptoms (hunger, nausea, abdominal pain) or neurologic complaints (headache, speech and vision disturbances, weakness, anxiety, behavior changes, short attention span, ataxia, seizures, coma). These symptoms may occur with or without the signs of catecholamine excess (sweating, pallor, tachycardia).

A patient with hypoglycemia secondary to hormone deficiencies, such as growth hormone deficiency (GHD) or panhypopituitarism, may have a microphallus or undescended testes. An infant or child with a metabolic defect may present with metabolic acidosis, hepatosplenomegaly, increased uric acid and lactic acid levels, and positive urine or serum ketones.

Ketotic Hypoglycemia Ketotic hypoglycemia presents in a young child with the typical signs of hypoglycemia, usually in the early to late morning hours. The patient typically has a history of fasting, poor or late food intake, or gastroenteritis. There are ketones in the urine.

Diagnosis

If hypoglycemia is suspected or the patient has an altered mental status or seizures, obtain a Dextrostix test. Confirm a low glucose level with a whole blood glucose value. Obtain a birth history, prenatal history, and family history, which may be positive for other infants with hypoglycemia or metabolic acidosis.

If the patient is not a known diabetic, prior to any treatment, obtain blood for cortisol, growth hormone, and insulin in addition to liver function tests, alanine (decreased in *ketotic hypoglycemia*), lactate (increase suggests an *inborn error of metabolism*), electrolytes, serum ketones (negative in *hyperinsulinism;* positive in *ketotic hypoglycemia*), venous pH, and thyroid function tests. Test the urine for ketone bodies (positive in *ketotic hypoglycemia*) and reducing substances (*disorders of galactose, fructose,* and *tyrosine metabolism*).

If the symptoms followed a meal, determine whether fructose or galactose was the sole sugar consumed. Ask about possible ingestion of *alcohol* or an *oral hypoglycemic agent.* Vomiting suggests *acidosis, gastroenteritis, food poisoning,* or *acute liver disease.*

Short stature, microphallus, and midline defects (cleft palate, single maxillary central incisor) suggest *hypopituitarism.* Increased skin pigmentation may indicate compensatory ACTH release (*primary adrenal insufficiency*). Hepatomegaly occurs in *glycogen storage diseases, inborn errors of carbohydrate metabolism,* and *liver disease,* but not in *ketotic hypoglycemia.*

ED Management

Regardless of etiology, the treatment of hypoglycemia is glucose. Encourage an alert child to drink a carbohydrate-containing solution (orange juice, apple juice, soft drink with sugar). If the patient is unconscious, vomiting, or unable to take fluids orally, give a bolus of 0.5 to 1.0 g/kg of glucose IV. Give an older child 1 to 2 mL/kg of D_{50} and a young child 2 to 4 mL/kg of D_{25}. Treat a neonate with a smaller bolus (0.25–0.5 g/kg) of D_{25} (1–2 mL/kg). Follow bolus therapy with a continuous infusion of 10% glucose, with maintenance electrolytes, at a maintenance rate. If the blood glucose falls below 40 mg/dL, change to a 15 or 20% glucose solution.

If the hypoglycemia persists (*hyperinsulinemia*), give glucagon (30–50 µg/kg, up to 1 mg IV, IM, or SQ), then 1 h later give IV hydrocortisone (Solu-Cortef 100 mg/m^2 for infants; 3 mg/kg for children). However, since a glycemic response to these hormones requires adequate amounts of substrates, continue the glucose continuous infusion. Diazoxide (5–20 mg/kg/day PO) is the drug of choice for hyperinsulinism.

Instruct the family of a child with *ketotic hypoglycemia* that the child must not miss meals. Treat hypoglycemia and/or ketonuria with carbohydrate-containing beverages, as above. Discharge the patient if the glucose normalizes, oral intake is adequate, and close follow-up is arranged.

Follow-up

- Ketotic hypoglycemia: primary care follow-up in 1 week

Indications for Admission

- Hypoglycemic episode in a nondiabetic unless patient is known to have ketotic hypoglycemia and the glucose normalizes
- Hypoglycemia in a diabetic if the cause is unclear or self-destructive behavior is likely

BIBLIOGRAPHY

Cornblath M, Ichord R: Hypoglycemia in the neonate. *Semin Perinatol* 2000;24: 136–149.

Leteif AN, Schwenk WF: Hypoglycemia in infants and children. *Endocrinol Metab Clin North Am* 1999;28:619–646.

Verrotti A, Fusilli P, Pallotta R, et al: Hypoglycemia in childhood: a clinical approach. *J Pediatr Endocrinol Metab* 1998;11(suppl 1):147–152.

HYPONATREMIA

Hyponatremia is defined as a serum sodium concentration <130 mEq/L. Hyponatremia may be associated with hypovolemic, euvolemic, or hypervolemic states.

Hypovolemia   Hypovolemic hyponatremia is caused by loss of sodium in excess of water. Most often this is secondary to extrarenal losses, especially gastrointestinal, but sweating (cystic fibrosis) and "third spacing" from burns, trauma, peritonitis, effusions, ascites, and pancreatitis are other etiologies. Renal salt wasting is seen in diuretic abuse, osmotic diuresis, salt-wasting nephropathy, renal tubular acidosis (types 2 and 4), and adrenal insufficiency.

Euvolemia   The most common cause is the inappropriate secretion of ADH (SIADH) secondary to CNS pathology (meningitis, trauma) or pulmonary disease (pneumonia, tuberculosis). Drugs—such as nicotine, morphine, barbiturates, isoproterenol, antineoplastic agents, carbamazepine, and acetaminophen—have been implicated as "antidiuretic" agents. Other etiologies are hypothyroidism and water intoxication. Glucocorticoid deficiency can cause euvolemic or hypovolemic hyponatremia.

Hypervolemia   Hypervolemic hyponatremia is characterized by edema formation, as in congestive heart failure, cirrhosis, nephrotic syndrome, and renal failure.

Clinical Presentation

The clinical presentation of hyponatremia is determined by the absolute concentration and rate of fall of the serum sodium and the intravascular volume.

Hypovolemia   With depletion of the intravascular space, signs of hypovolemia predominate. There may be tachycardia, orthostatic vital sign changes, and poor capillary refill.

Euvolemia   Clinical findings are related to the serum sodium level. A rapid decrease to the range of 120 to 125 mEq/L may cause gastrointestinal symptoms such as anorexia, nausea, and vomiting, with agitation, headache, muscle cramps, seizures, and coma. Other neurologic signs (decreased deep tendon reflexes, pathologic reflexes, Cheyne-Stokes respiration, and pseudobulbar palsy) can be present, especially when the level is <120 mEq/L. The patient may be asymptomatic, with a sodium <120 mEq/L, if the fall in the serum sodium occurred slowly, over days to weeks.

Hypervolemia   In hypervolemia, there may be signs of fluid excess, including tachycardia, hypertension, edema, headache, pulmonary rales, and hepatomegaly.

Diagnosis

Hyponatremia is usually discovered incidentally, when electrolytes are obtained because of vomiting, dehydration, altered mental status, or seizures. Once hyponatremia is reported, rule out *pseudohyponatremia* as a result of increased serum proteins or lipids; usually the plasma has a milky appearance. Next, consider *dilutional hyponatremia* secondary to the presence of excess solutes, such as glucose or mannitol, which cause intracellular fluid to shift to the extracellular space. In a diabetic, for every 100 mg/dL increase in glucose over 100 mg/dL, the serum sodium is lowered by 1.6 mEq/L.

The urinary sodium level can help distinguish among the various etiologies of hyponatremia. The urine sodium is <20 mEq/L in hypovolemic states secondary to extrarenal diseases and most hypervolemic states; a urine sodium >20 mEq/L suggests *renal salt wasting, SIADH,* and other euvolemic conditions. With *renal failure,* the urine sodium may be >40 mEq/L except in acute *glomerulonephritis* (when it is typically low).

ED Management

Immediately treat symptomatic hypovolemia (poor peripheral pulses, delayed capillary refill, orthostatic changes) without waiting for the laboratory confirmation of hyponatremia. Give 20 mL/kg boluses of isotonic crystalloid (normal saline, Ringer's lactate) until adequate perfusion is established. Obtain blood for serum electrolytes, BUN, and creatinine and urine for urinalysis, sodium, creatinine, and osmolality. Begin definitive therapy once the initial serum and urine studies confirm the diagnosis. If there are severe neurologic symptoms secondary to a serum sodium level <125 mEq/L, give hypertonic saline [3% (513 mEq/L) or 5% (855 mEq/L)] to raise the sodium above 125 mEq/L. Replace this deficit over 4 h using the following formula:

$$\text{mEq sodium needed} = (125 - \text{patient's sodium}) \times (0.6) \times (\text{body weight in kg})$$

Raise the serum sodium to 135 mEq/L over the subsequent 24 h. Do not exceed a rate of correction of 1.5 to 2.0 mEq/L/h. Measure the serum sodium every 2 h until it is >135 mEq/L and all symptoms have resolved. Subsequent treatment then depends on the initial assessment of the intravascular volume status.

In an asymptomatic patient, the sodium can be corrected much more slowly, with a goal of no more than a 1.0 mEq/L/h increase if concentrated sodium is used. Rapid correction can lead to central pontine myelinolysis—characterized by somnolence, disorientation, and aphasia, which may progress over a few weeks to quadriplegia.

Hypovolemia   Replace volume with NS or D_5NS. In adrenal insufficiency, sodium deficits are difficult to replace without corticosteroid replacement (pp 149–150).

Euvolemia   Limiting the water intake to two-thirds maintenance, including all fluids (e.g., IV medications), may be all that is required. Immediately begin treatment of the cause of SIADH.

Hypervolemia   If the patient is edematous, restrict fluids to two-thirds maintenance; give furosemide (1 mg/kg IV) if there is pulmonary edema and respiratory compromise.

Indications for Admission

- Symptomatic hyponatremia
- Hyponatremia of undetermined etiology

BIBLIOGRAPHY

Gross P: Correction of hyponatremia. *Semin Nephrol* 2001;21:269–272.
Gross P, Reimann D, Henschkowski J, et al: Treatment of severe hyponatremia: conventional and novel aspects. *J Am Soc Nephrol* 2001;12(suppl 17):S10–S14.
Miller M: Syndromes of excess antidiuretic hormone release. *Crit Care Clin* 2001;17:11–23.

THYROID DISORDERS

Hyperthyroidism primarily affects children >6 years of age. The most common cause is diffuse toxic goiter (Graves' disease). Other etiologies include thyroiditis with hyperthyroidism, thyroid adenoma, and exogenous overdosage.

Thyrotoxicosis is the clinical manifestation of hyperthyroidism without the severe cardiovascular, thermoregulatory, gastrointestinal, and neurobehavioral symptoms associated with thyroid storm or crisis, a life-threatening complication rarely seen in children. In 50% of episodes of thyroid storm there is an identifiable precipitating factor (stress, infection, surgery, childbirth).

Hypothyroidism is a very rare emergency, but time is critical, as a delay in therapy is associated with decreased IQ. Thyroid screening, either TSH or T_4, is part of the newborn screen in every state. Patients with the highest percentile of TSH or the lowest percentile of T_4 from a certain day are recalled. Therefore, false-positives occur, but this is necessary to ensure that all truly hypothyroid newborns are identified.

Clinical Presentation

The onset of hyperthyroidism is gradual, with complaints of palpitations, sweating, heat intolerance, weight loss despite increased appetite, tremor, nervousness, increased frequency of bowel movements, and emotional lability. Short attention span, inability to concentrate, deteriorating school performance, attacks of dyspnea, and easy fatigability may occur. Oligomenorrhea and irregular menses may result in the postmenarchal female. Newborns may exhibit irritability, inability to feed (breast or bottle), and inadequate weight gain. Hyperthyroidism in the newborn can be difficult to diagnose; however, expeditious diagnosis and treatment are critical.

On examination, almost all hyperthyroid patients (except in the case of exogenous overdose) have a goiter, and a characteristic bruit may be heard over the thyroid. The skin is warm and moist, and tachycardia (particularly increased resting pulse rate), increased systolic blood pressure, and widened pulse pressure are common. Eye signs, when present, include lid retraction, staring, lid lag, and exophthalmos (not as common as in adults). Ophthalmoplegia is rarely seen, but when present could represent severe exophthalmos and nerve entrapment (or myasthenia gravis, a rare coexisting disease). There may be proximal muscle weakness, brisk deep tendon reflexes, and fine tremors of the eyelids, fingers, or tongue.

Thyroid storm often starts abruptly with the sudden onset of severe thyrotoxic symptoms and fever, often up to 41.1°C (106°F). There may be cardiovascular symptoms (tachycardia, arrhythmia, heart failure, shock), neurologic findings (agitation, tremor, psychosis, stupor, coma), and gastrointestinal complaints (abdominal pain, vomiting, diarrhea, hepatomegaly, jaundice).

Diagnosis

The differential diagnosis of hyperthyroidism includes *anxiety attack, sepsis, pheochromocytoma, gastroenteritis,* and *congestive heart failure.* Other possible midline neck masses include *thyroglossal duct cyst, dermoid cyst, cystic hygroma,* and *neuroblastoma* (with Horner's syndrome). Exophthalmos or ophthalmoplegia can be confused with a *neuroblastoma, intraorbital tumor,* and *orbital cellulitis.* The typical gradual onset of hyperthyroidism makes the early diagnosis difficult. However, the presence of a goiter or bruit along with other symptoms of hyperthyroidism usually suggests the diagnosis.

If a newborn is brought to the ED with documentation of a failed thyroid screen, consult a pediatric endocrinologist and obtain blood for TSH, free and total T_4, and thyroxine-binding globulin.

ED Management

Hyperthyroidism
If there are mild to moderate symptoms of thyrotoxicosis, obtain a thyroid hormone profile [TSH, free T_4, T_3RIA, thyroid antibodies (antithyroid microsomal, antithyroglobulin), and thyroid-stimulating immunoglobu-

lin]. Typical findings are elevated free T_4, total T_4 or T_3, and FT_4I, with a suppressed (low) TSH. Antibodies (thyroid-stimulating, and/or antithyroglobulin antimicrosomal antibodies) may be present. Treatment can be deferred until these values are known unless the symptoms are severe, in which case give propylthiouracil (5–7 mg/kg/day PO divided q 8 h) and propranolol (1–2 mg/kg/day PO divided q 6 to 8 h), or if thyroid storm is suspected.

Thyroid Storm
Thyroid storm requires *immediate treatment.* After obtaining blood for T_3, T_4, and TSH, cortisol, CBC, electrolytes, and LFTs, the goals are to decrease the thyroid hormone levels acutely and block their peripheral effects. Call for an immediate pediatric endocrinology consult and initiate therapy using the following modalities:

Propranolol   Treat the symptoms of hyperthyroidism with propranolol, although it has no effect on the cause. Give a child 0.5 to 2.0 mg/kg/day divided q 6 h (60 mg/day maximum) and an older adolescent 20 to 40 mg q 6 h. If gastrointestinal symptoms preclude oral treatment, give 0.025 mg/kg IV over 10 min. The dose may be repeated three to four times, but consult a pediatric cardiologist. Possible side effects include hypotension, hypoglycemia, bronchospasm, and heart block.

Thionamides   Thionamides treat hyperthyroidism by blocking the synthesis of T_3 and T_4. Propylthiouracil (PTU) also blocks conversion of T_4 to T_3. Use PTU 5 to 7 mg/day divided q 8 h, maximum 1200 mg/day, or methimazole (Tapazole), 0.5 to 0.7 mg/kg/day divided q 8 h. These drugs can be given either PO or via a nasogastric tube.

Oral Iodide (Lugol's Solution)   Lugol's solution is 5% iodine and 10% potassium iodide (126 mg iodine/mL, or 8 mg iodine per drop). Give children and adolescents 10 drops (80 mg iodine) PO tid after the thionamides. Alternatively, use potassium iodide (1 g/mL), 150 to 200 mg PO tid for infants <1 year of age; 300 to 500 mg PO tid for children and adolescents. However, propranolol is so effective in blocking the beta-adrenergic effects that iodides are often unnecessary.

Dexamethasone   Dexamethasone (1–2 mg q 6 h) may be used in extreme cases, as in a patient with heart failure, arrhythmias, or shock.

Temperature Regulation   Use antipyretics (acetaminophen 15 mg/kg; ibuprofen 10 mg/kg), cooling blankets, and muscle relaxants as needed. However, do not give aspirin, which may elevate the T_4 level.

Hypothyroidism
Treat with thyroxine. Newborns require a higher dose than older children, 8 to 10 µg/kg/day. The goal is to maintain the T_4 in the high range of normal for newborns (10 to 13 mg/dL).

Follow-up

- Hyperthyroidism without thyroid storm: 2 to 3 days
- Neonatal hypothyroidism: pediatric endocrinology follow-up in 1 to 3 days

Indications for Admission

- Thyroid storm
- Hyperthyroidism with heart failure, arrhythmias, shock, or psychosis

BIBLIOGRAPHY

Polak M: Hyperthyroidism in early infancy: pathogenesis, clinical features and diagnosis with a focus on neonatal hyperthyroidism. *Thyroid* 1998;8:1171–1177.

Raza J, Hindmarsh PC, Brook CG: Thyrotoxicosis in children: thirty years' experience. *Acta Paediatr* 1999;88:937–941.

Zimmerman D: Fetal and neonatal hyperthyroidism. *Thyroid* 1999;9:727–733.

CHAPTER 8

Environmental Emergencies

Anthony J. Ciorciari
  • Katherine J. Chou (Contributor—Hyperbaric Oxygen Therapy)

BURNS

Each year 450,000 children are evaluated for burn injuries. Approximately 50% of major burns occur in patients under 20 years of age, and nearly one-third occur in children under 10 years of age. In the United States, burns are the third most common cause of pediatric injury-related mortality.

Common types of burn injuries are thermal (scald and flame), chemical (acids and alkalis), electrical, and radiation (sunburn). Scald burns are the most frequent type in children under 5 years of age, while flame burns are most common between 5 and 13 years of age.

Approximately 10% of child abuse cases involve burns, accounting for 15 to 20% of all childhood burns. The most common mechanism is scalding. Other causes include burns from appliances, matches, and tobacco products.

Clinical Presentation

The presentation and severity of a thermal injury are determined by the type and temperature of the agent causing the burn and the duration of exposure to the agent.

Determining the surface area and depth of tissue involved are priorities in evaluating the extent of a burn injury. The "rule of nines" used in older children and adolescents requires modification for infants and young children, because the percent of the total body surface area (BSA) represented by the various body parts changes with age. Use the patient's own hand (including the fingers) as the standard: the area of the palmar surface equals 0.8 to 1% of the BSA. Depth can be difficult to estimate, since the injury is usually not uniform in all affected areas and the depth may progress over time. Scald burns other than those caused by immersion tend to be superficial, while chemical burns tend to be deep. Electrical burns (pp 182-185) can cause tissue damage that is deeper than suspected during the initial examination.

First-Degree Burns   Sunburn is the most common example of a first-degree burn. First-degree burns involve only the superficial epidermal layers. The area appears pink or light red and blanches with pressure; there are no blisters, and the burn is dry. Healing generally takes place within 6 days without scarring.

Second-Degree Burns   Second-degree burns are also known as partial-thickness burns. They are subdivided into superficial and deep types. Superficial partial-thickness burns involve the papillary layer of the dermis. They present with blisters and bullae and are typically bright red or mottled in color. They have a moist surface, and the superficial skin can be wiped away. These burns are extremely painful. With proper care, they heal within 10 to 20 days. Deep partial-thickness burns involve the reticular layer of the dermis. The skin may appear yellow-white or dark red (nonblanching), with a dry or mildly moist surface. There is sensation to pressure only. These injuries may be difficult to distinguish from third-degree burns and may require more than 21 days for healing, with residual scar formation.

Third-Degree Burns   Third-degree, or full-thickness, burns are usually caused by flame, hot grease or oil, chemicals, or prolonged immersion. All skin elements are lost, with coagulation of blood vessels. The skin is dry or leathery, grayish-white, and waxy. Thrombosed superficial veins may be visible. The patient has sensation to deep pressure only. Wound closure requires resurfacing and grafting, because the burned surface will not support the migration of normal epithelium from the unburned periphery.

Fourth-Degree Burns   Fourth-degree burns have the same etiologies as third-degree burns. They involve the subcutaneous layer, fascia, tendon, muscle, and/or bone. The extensive amount of necrotic tissue can produce systemic toxicity from tissue breakdown products and deep infection.

Diagnosis

The evaluation of any burn injury includes determination of the cause, location, and depth of the burn. Look for evidence of inhalation injury or other associated injuries, and note any preexisting illness. Always consider child abuse when the patient presents with burns to the buttocks or burns with a sharp delineation from immersion or the application of a hot object to the skin.

Burns can be classified as minor, moderate, or major based on the severity of the burn and the involved BSA. *Minor* burns are first- and second-degree injuries encompassing less than 10% of the total BSA. *Moderate* burns include partial-thickness burns that cover 10 to 20% of the total BSA. Full-thickness injuries covering <10% of the total BSA are also considered moderate. *Major* burns include partial-thickness burns involving more than 20% of the BSA and third-degree burns involving more than 10% of the BSA, as well as burns of the hands, face, eyes, ears, feet, and perineum.

ED Management

First-Degree Burns   Treat pain with aspirin (15 mg/kg q 4 h) or ibuprofen (10 mg/kg q 6 h). Hydrocortisone cream (1%) may help reduce the pain and swelling of severe sunburn, especially if the eyelids and face are involved, but do not apply steroids to higher-degree burns. Cool showers and baths are also helpful. Severe itching can occur after a few days and persist for more than 1 week; treat with hydroxyzine (2 mg/kg/day divided tid, 50 mg per dose maximum) or diphenhydramine (5 mg/kg/day divided qid, 50 mg per dose maximum).

Second-Degree Burns   Immediately remove any clothing that is hot or soaked with chemical. Mineral oil mixed with cool water can remove substances like tar. To decrease the burning process, apply sterile gauze pads soaked with slightly cooled [12°C (53.6°F)] or room-temperature saline. To be effective in preventing microvascular changes, the cooling must occur within 30 minutes of the burn.

Before the burn is cleaned, parenteral analgesia, such as IM or IV morphine sulfate (0.10 to 0.15 mg/kg q 15–60 min, as needed), may be required. Do not attempt IV access in a burned area. Gently clean the burned surface with chlorhexidine solution (Hibiclens) and rinse thoroughly. Debride devitalized tissues using aseptic technique. Remove blisters if they are broken, cloudy, or expected to break (>2.5–3 cm in diameter or on flexor surfaces). Otherwise, do not needle-aspirate intact blisters.

Silver sulfadiazine (SSD, Silvadene) has both gram-positive and gram-negative activity and provides good prophylactic antibiotic coverage. It also facilitates debridement. However, do not use silver sulfadiazine on the face, on children with hypersensitivity to sulfonamides, or on infants under 2 months of age (bacitracin ointment is an acceptable alternative). Use a sterile tongue depressor to apply a 2-mm layer and cover with either a nonadherent or petrolatum-impregnated dressing; then wrap with gauze.

If the hand and fingers are involved, dress each finger individually and place the hand in a "position of function" (wrist flexed 20–30 degrees, metacarpals flexed 60–90 degrees, interphalangeal joints as close to 0 degrees as possible). Use a sling to elevate the extremity above the level of the heart.

Clean and dress the burn daily. At each dressing change, remove the silver sulfadiazine completely, as it loses its antibacterial activity.

Biobrane (Woodruff Laboratories, Santa Ana, CA), a biosynthetic dressing coated with collagen peptides, is indicated for superficial second-degree burns (those with no chance of becoming third-degree burns). Apply directly to a cleaned burn area, then cover with an absorbent dressing; this should be changed every 24 hours. The Biobrane will separate on its own in 1 to 2 weeks. Apply it to flat surfaces only.

Third-Degree Burns   If the burn encompasses less than 2% of the total BSA, with no involvement of the face, hands, feet, or perineum, the care is the same as for second-degree burns. If more than 2% of the total BSA is involved, admit the patient to a burn unit.

General Approach to the Burned Child

1. Stop the burning process by removing burned clothing and copiously lavaging all chemical burns. Apply cool or room-temperature soaks to reverse the thermal gradient and relieve pain (second-degree burns), but avoid hypothermia.

2. Assess and maintain ventilation. Check for signs of inhalation injury (pp 194-196); if any are present, measure the oxygen saturation and immediately perform fiberoptic laryngoscopy to rule out involvement of the upper airway. Obtain a carboxyhemoglobin level if the patient was in a closed-space fire.

3. Initiate IV fluid therapy for patients with partial- or full-thickness burns over more than 20% of the BSA. Immediately place a large-bore IV catheter in either a central or peripheral vein found in an unburned area. Treat signs of hypovolemia with a 20 mL/kg bolus of normal saline (NS) or lactated Ringer's solution. Use dopamine (5–20 μg/kg/min) if poor perfusion persists. For patients not in shock, administer NS or lactated Ringer's solution, 2 to 4 mL/kg per percent of total BSA burned over the first 24 h. Give one-half of the calculated total over the first 8 h (starting from the time of the burn incident) and the remainder over the next 16 h. For children weighing less than 30 kg, add the estimated daily maintenance fluid requirement. Patients weighing more than 30 kg do not need the maintenance fluids added as part of the fluid replacement. The goal is a urine output of at least 1 mL/kg/h in a young child and 0.5 mL/kg/h in an adolescent.

   Insert an indwelling urinary catheter using aseptic technique in any burn victim needing IV fluids. Discard any urine obtained when the catheter is inserted, as this may have been in the bladder before the burn injury. Check the urine (with a dipstick) for hemoglobin or myoglobin; if positive, obtain a microscopic urinalysis to differentiate hematuria from myoglobinuria (rhabdomyolysis). If myoglobin is present, increase the fluid rate to maintain a brisk urine output (2 mL/kg/h).

4. Take a careful history. Inquire about the cause of the burn, preexisting illnesses, chronic medications, and allergies. Suspect child abuse if the accident occurred when the child was reportedly alone, the injury is attributed to a sibling, the history varies from one interview to another, there is a previous history of accidental trauma, the history is incompatible with the observed injury, or there was delay in seeking medical attention.

5. Ascertain the tetanus immunization status; give 0.5 mL of tetanus toxoid booster if the last immunization was more than 5 years ago. If the patient has received fewer than three tetanus toxoid boosters, give 0.5 mL of tetanus immune globulin as well as 0.5 mL of tetanus toxoid booster.

6. Perform a careful physical examination. Check for corneal injury with fluorescein staining if the lids are burned, the eyelashes have been singed, or eye damage is suspected. Evaluate the patient for associated injuries, especially fractures and head trauma, and signs of child abuse. Nonaccidental burn injuries include pattern burns; sharply

demarcated burns of the hands, feet, buttocks, and perineum; and stocking-glove burn injuries.

7. Insert a nasogastric tube and attach it to suction if the burn exceeds 20% of the total BSA or if there is nausea, vomiting, or abdominal distention. An ileus is common as a result of splanchnic vasoconstriction.

8. Give pain medication as needed (IM or IV morphine sulfate, 0.1 to 0.15 mg/kg q 15–60 min).

9. Perform the initial burn wound care as described above.

10. Examine the patient for circumferential injuries. Remove all rings, bracelets, and restrictive clothing. Look carefully for signs of impaired circulation, including cyanosis, impaired capillary refill, changes in sensation, deep tissue pain, or paresthesias. If circulatory impairment is a possibility, call a burn surgeon or a plastic surgeon, as an escharotomy may be necessary.

Follow-up

- First-degree burns: Return at once if blisters form.
- Second- and third-degree burns: Return at once if there are any signs or symptoms of impaired circulation (numbness, tingling, or color change distal to the bandage) or infection (fever, vomiting, poor feeding, or change in mental status). Otherwise, follow up with a primary care provider or burn specialist (depending on extent and depth of burns) in 3 or 4 days.

Indications for Admission

- First-degree burns: Total body involvement or if the patient is at risk for dehydration.
- Second-degree burns: >5% of the total BSA in infants, >10% in children, >15% in adolescents, or when the burns involve critical areas such as the face, hands, feet, or perineum.
- Third-degree burns: >2% of the total BSA or involvement of the face, hands, feet, or perineum.
- Circumferential burns.
- Comorbidity (diabetes, immunodeficiency), multiple trauma.
- Electrical burns from a current of 220 V or more.
- Patients with any size burn whose family seems unable to cope with recommendations for care and follow-up.
- Transfer the patient to a special burn treatment facility if the total burn is >20% total BSA or if there are third-degree burns covering >10% of the total BSA.

Guidelines for Transferring the Burn Victim

In addition to the usual considerations when any patient is being transferred to another institution, there are several special concerns in transferring a burn victim:

1. The patient's airway must be securely protected. An accidental extubation in a burn victim with a swollen airway can prove fatal. A physi-

cian who is able to perform an emergency intubation and/or emergency cricothyroidotomy must accompany the patient.

2. Just prior to transport, remove all saline-soaked dressings and replace them with sterile dry gauze dressings to prevent hypothermia.

3. Treat the patient with adequate sedation and analgesia to minimize pain and agitation.

BIBLIOGRAPHY

Hansbrough JF, Hansbrough W: Pediatric burns. *Pediatr Rev* 1999;20:117–123.
Kao CC, Garner WL: Acute burns. *Plast Reconstructr Surg* 2000;101:2482–2493.
Monafo WW: Initial management of burns. *N Engl J Med* 1996;335:1581–1586.

DROWNING AND NEAR-DROWNING

Drowning is death from asphyxia while submerged or within 24 h of submersion. Near-drowning is a submersion episode of sufficient severity to warrant medical attention for the victim. Up to 60% of drowning deaths occur in individuals less than 20 years of age. Drowning is the fourth leading cause of fatal injuries in childhood and is most common among patients under 4 years of age. The true incidence of near-drowning is estimated to be 2 to 20 times greater than what is reported. Approximately 6% of drownings are believed to be secondary to child neglect or abuse.

Drowning and near-drowning can be classified pathophysiologically as either "wet" or "dry." Some 80 to 90% of cases are wet drownings, in which aspiration has occurred. The other 10 to 20% are categorized as dry drownings, in that aspirate entering the upper airway causes laryngospasm and subsequently asphyxia. Death may be caused directly by laryngospasm or by cerebral hypoxia, carbon dioxide narcosis, or cardiac arrest.

Aspiration of either salt water or fresh water results in hypoxemia. As little as 1 to 3 mL/kg of water can cause pulmonary vasoconstriction and pulmonary hypertension. In saltwater drownings, intrapulmonary shunting and decreased compliance occur, and ventilation/perfusion mismatch soon follows. In freshwater drownings, pulmonary surfactant is either washed out or altered, leading to noncardiogenic pulmonary edema and the adult respiratory distress syndrome (ARDS).

Hypothermia is the double-edged sword of drowning. Although cold water may be beneficial in that it decreases metabolic demands and shunts blood from nonvital to vital organs, adverse effects such as dysrhythmias (sinus bradycardia, atrial and ventricular fibrillation, asystole) and exhaustion often occur.

Clinical Presentation and Diagnosis

The history virtually always provides the diagnosis. Inquire about the site and duration of submersion, water temperature, possibility of trauma or physical abuse, drug or alcohol use, and past medical history.

A drowning victim's mental status may range from fully alert to comatose. The patient may have no signs of respiratory distress or may present with tachypnea, nasal flaring, and/or retractions. Auscultation of the lungs may reveal adventitious sounds, and any type of dysrhythmia may be seen on the electrocardiogram (ECG). Among adolescents, inquire about drinking or drug use prior to the event.

Trauma is often involved in near-drowning. Pay particular attention to the possibility of injuries to the head or cervical spine. Consider internal injuries to the chest or abdomen, especially if the patient does not respond appropriately to resuscitation interventions. Electrolyte imbalance and blood volume disturbances usually do not occur unless a significant amount (22 mL/kg) of water has been aspirated. Blood volume disturbances can also be present when significant trauma has occurred. Renal failure is uncommon.

ED Management

Handle the patient carefully because of the possibility of cervical spine injury (pp 641–644). Place a rectal temperature probe to confirm the core temperature, rapidly assess the airway and breathing, and provide 100% oxygen. Indications for assisted ventilation via bag-valve-mask apparatus and endotracheal intubation are apnea or an oxygen saturation less than 90% while inspiring 100% oxygen or signs of neurologic deterioration. The patient may require positive end expiratory pressure (PEEP) if there is an inadequate response to the initial ventilator settings. Treat bronchospasm with nebulized albuterol (0.03 mL/kg in 5 mL NS) and repeat as needed. There is no evidence that steroids are beneficial in aspiration-induced bronchospasm.

Assess the cardiac status and continuously monitor the ECG. If the patient is pulseless, start basic life support, then advanced life support as warranted by the ECG rhythm and clinical status. However, most resuscitation drugs are not effective in a severely hypothermic patient and are therefore contraindicated during rewarming (see hypothermia, pp 192–194). One exception is glucose; give 0.5 to 1 g/kg (1–2 mL/kg D_{50}; 0.25–0.5 mL/kg D_{25}) to any patient with altered mental status. Also give naloxone (2.0 mg IV or 4.0 mg ET) to adolescents if there is any suggestion by history of a narcotic overdose.

Start at least one large-bore IV with normal saline or lactated Ringer's solution. However, give fluids cautiously, since these patients are at risk for pulmonary and cerebral edema, and warm the fluids if the patient is hypothermic. Initial laboratory studies include a complete blood count (CBC), electrolytes, blood urea nitrogen (BUN), creatinine, glucose, creatine phosphokinase (CPK), arterial blood gas (ABG), serum pregnancy test (for female patients of childbearing age), serum osmolality, and blood type and cross match (if there is any suspicion of trauma). Also obtain an ECG and a chest radiograph. Other tests, such as additional x-rays or computed tomography (CT) scans, are dictated by the history of the event and serial assessments.

An initially well-appearing child may rapidly develop both pulmonary and neurologic complications any time within the first 24 h. However, most asymptomatic children may be discharged after 8 h of observation if the physical examination, initial chest x-ray, and all tests are normal; the physician is assured that the family is reliable; and adequate follow-up is arranged. Poor prognostic signs include a submersion duration of greater than 9 min, prolonged apnea, or coma.

Follow-up

- At once if pulmonary (cough, tachypnea, dyspnea) or neurologic (altered mental status) symptoms develop, otherwise primary care follow-up in 2 to 3 days

Indications for Admission

- History of prolonged submersion
- Respiratory or neurologic symptoms
- An abnormal chest x-ray; admit for at least 24 h

BIBLIOGRAPHY

Orlowski JP, Szpilman D: Drowning. Rescue, resuscitation, and reanimation. *Pediatr Clin North Am* 2001;48:627–646.
Sachdeva RC: Near drowning. *Crit Care Clin* 1999;15:281–296.
Zuckerman GB, Conway EJ Jr: Drowning and near drowning: a pediatric epidemic. *Pediatr Ann* 2000;29:360–366.

ELECTRICAL INJURIES

Small children, especially toddlers, frequently sustain low-voltage electrical injuries when they insert objects (pins or keys) into household sockets or chew on electrical cords. Older children are more likely to sustain high-voltage electrical injuries by contacting live third rails or power lines when climbing.

Most of the harmful effects from electrical injuries are due to the heat generated, which is directly related to current, tissue resistance, and duration of contact. Serious electrical injuries are uncommon but carry a mortality risk of approximately 40%.

Electrical injuries are usually categorized in terms of high- (greater than 1000 V) or low- (less than 1000 V) voltage injuries. Household current is low-voltage (110 V). Because voltage is directly related to current, high-voltage injuries are usually more serious, although a low-voltage contact applied to areas of low resistance can also cause serious injury.

Clinical Presentation and Diagnosis

A child who has had contact with electric current can present with first-, second-, or third-degree burns of the skin, as well as entrance and exit burns (which are usually third-degree). There may also be burns at flexor creases of the fingers and at the oral commissure. Commissure burns may be associated with delayed labial artery bleeding 2 to 21 days later.

If the electric current takes a vertical path, cardiac involvement is more likely. Cardiac complications include all forms of dysrhythmias, ranging from occasional ectopic atrial and/or ventricular premature contractions

(VPCs) to first-, second- and third-degree atrioventricular (AV) blocks, ventricular tachycardia, and ventricular fibrillation. Common ECG abnormalities include accelerated sinus rhythm and nonspecific ST–T-wave changes. These are usually evident upon initial ED evaluation. Pulmonary involvement can include pulmonary contusion, hemothorax, pneumothorax, and/or ventilatory arrest.

Central nervous system involvement may be due to the electrical injury itself or the subsequent fall after the event. The patient can present with any type of mental status change. Other neurologic symptoms, such as paralysis, can occur immediately or can be delayed for up to several days. Both upper- and lower-motor-neuron findings may appear on examination. Electric current can cause tetany of skeletal muscle. This can lead to all types of musculoskeletal injury, from strains to fractures and/or dislocations.

Vascular injuries can include hemorrhage, either immediate or delayed, in addition to thrombosis. Renal complications can include renal failure, which may be due to either hypovolemia or rhabdomyolysis.

High-Voltage Injuries   The patient may present with a variety of complications involving a number of organ systems. Asystole, respiratory arrest, and hypoxia-induced ventricular fibrillation are the most common causes of immediate death. These injuries are associated with hemolysis, rhabdomyolysis, direct burns of the lung or viscera, cardiac dysrhythmias, neurologic injuries, renal failure, and fractures or ruptured viscera secondary to falls.

Low-Voltage Injuries   Most low-voltage injuries initially present with a small, localized, painless, white parchment-like patch of skin. However, within a few hours of biting on an electric cord or exposed household wire, there can be considerable edema of the lips, tongue, and gums. Rarely, severe intraoral edema may result in airway obstruction. If the child conducts electricity, muscle paralysis and ventricular dysrhythmias may occur. Fortunately, conduction with low voltage is rare, so these are usually limited injuries.

Flash Burns   These are thermal injuries in which an arc of electricity passed from a voltage source to ground. Electrons do not pass through the body, but proximity to the superheated air produced by the flash may cause cutaneous burns.

ED Management

High-Voltage Injuries   Rapidly assess the adequacy of the airway. Use the chin-lift maneuver without hyperextension to maintain patency if there is the possibility of a cervical spine injury, either directly from the electrical injury or from resulting trauma (e.g., fall from a tree or ladder). If the patient is not breathing, ventilate with a bag-valve-mask resuscitator and prepare for intubation. If respirations are adequate, administer 100% oxygen via a nonrebreather mask.

Assess the cardiovascular status, obtain an ECG, and secure a large-bore IV. If the patient is pulseless and the ECG monitor reveals ventricular fibrillation or pulseless ventricular tachycardia, defibrillate with an energy level of 2 J/kg (see Ventricular Fibrillation, pp 41–42).

If the patient presents with signs of inadequate tissue perfusion, give a fluid bolus of 20 mL/kg of NS and repeat as needed. If the child remains hemodynamically unstable, continue rapid intravenous hydration and start a dopamine drip at 2 to 5 µg/kg/min (see Shock, pp 21–22). However, inadequate tissue perfusion may be due to an associated thoracic, abdominal, or long-bone injury sustained after the electrical insult. Always consider major trauma in patients presenting in shock after an electrical injury.

If the patient has a normal pulse rate and blood pressure, give IV hydration with $D_5\frac{1}{2}NS$ at a rate of 1½ to 2 times maintenance. Aim for a urine output of at least 2 to 3 mL/kg/h, but do not add potassium for the first 24 h unless the patient has documented hypokalemia. The presence of rhabdomyolysis (hemoglobin or myoglobin on urine dipstick and/or an elevated CPK-MM) indicates significant deep tissue injury and predicts renal failure unless a brisk urine output is quickly established. To prevent precipitation of pigment in the renal tubules, give sodium bicarbonate, 1 mEq/kg IV bolus over 20 min, followed by a drip of 1 mEq/kg over 30 min to maintain a urine pH of 7 to 8. Use mannitol (0.5 g/kg) only if urine output remains inadequate after large volumes of IV fluid have been given.

Initial laboratory tests include blood for an ABG, CBC, electrolytes, glucose, BUN, creatinine, prothrombin time (PT) and partial thromboplastin time (PTT), serum osmolality, pregnancy test (for adolescent females of childbearing age), a urinalysis, and a 12-lead ECG. CPK-MB and troponin may be useful if the patient has suffered a cardiac contusion. If the injury occurred in a closed-space fire, obtain a carboxyhemoglobin level.

Perform a secondary survey to check for surface thermal burns, orthopedic injuries, or evidence of compartment syndrome. If the patient presents with an altered mental status, evidence or suspicion of an intoxicant, or distracting injury, clear the cervical spine radiographically. However, computed tomography (CT) of the head is also indicated for continued altered mental status after electrical injury.

Categorize and treat surface thermal burns in the usual fashion (see Burns, p 177). If there are no signs of systemic involvement secondary to an electrical burn and the surface burns are considered minor, discharge the patient after a 6- to 8-h period of observation.

Low-Voltage Injuries   Quickly assess the patency of the airway, especially if there are burns of the mouth. Perform a careful physical examination, looking for evidence of both an entrance and an exit wound. For the common electrical burn of the mouth, local wound management includes oral hygiene and direct wound care with topical bacitracin. If localized tissue charring is present and there is any suggestion of injury to underlying structures, immediate surgical consultation is necessary. When significant portions of the lips are involved (especially the oral commissure), consult a plastic surgeon or oral surgeon. Warn the parents of the risk of bleeding 2 to 21 days after the injury, as the burned tissue begins to separate. This bleeding can be controlled by local pressure but occasionally requires suture ligation in the ED.

Burns that are sustained by placing a metal object into a wall socket can usually be managed with routine local burn care only. Cardiovascular and neurologic complications are rare; therefore if the vital signs (particularly the pulse) and mental status are normal and in the absence of a history of loss of consciousness, tetany, wet skin, or evidence of current flow across the head, an ECG and cardiac monitoring are not necessary.

Follow-up

- Immediate for any signs or symptoms of impaired circulation (numbness, tingling, color change distal to the bandage) or infection (fever, vomiting, poor feeding, change in mental status). Otherwise, primary care follow-up in 3 to 4 days

Indications for Admission

- The presence of both an entrance and an exit wound
- Any neurologic or cardiovascular instability
- Mouth burns in a child unwilling or unable to take adequate fluids by mouth
- All high-voltage electrical burns

BIBLIOGRAPHY

Bailey B, Gaudreault P, Thivierge RL, et al: Cardiac monitoring of children with household electrical injuries. *Ann Emerg Med* 1995;25:612–617.

Jain S, Bandi V: Electrical and lightning injuries. *Critl Care Clin* 1999;15: 319–331.

Maryinez JA, Nguyen T: Electrical injuries. *South Med J* 2000;93:1165–1168.

FROSTBITE

Frostbite occurs when ice crystals form within the soft tissues as a consequence of exposure to cold. For this to occur, the soft tissues have to be cooled to -4 to $-2.2°C$ (24.8–28°F). Low ambient temperatures and high wind velocity quicken the freezing process. The tissue temperature is influenced by the circulation in the extremity and the cold stress, which in turn depends on the environmental temperature, wind chill, moisture, and protective insulation. Circulation in the extremity, which influences the tissue's internal heat flow, is affected by constrictive garments, the position of the extremity, local pressure, and vasospasm. The most severe damage occurs to tissues that freeze, thaw, and then refreeze. Factors that predispose to cold injury include inadequate nutrition, smoking, alcohol and drug use, fatigue, and tight clothing.

Clinical Presentation and Diagnosis

Frostbite most commonly involves distal, relatively poorly perfused regions of the body, such as fingertips, toes, earlobes, and the nose. In children, areas that have poor heat-generating ability and insulation, including the cheeks and chin, are also at high risk for frostbite. However, any area of skin that is exposed to prolonged cold can be affected.

Initially, frostbite presents with a painful cold feeling and skin blanching. This is followed by numbness, while the involved area becomes waxy, white, and firm. Deeply frostbitten skin feels hard and appears white with a yellow to blue tint. Superficially frostbitten skin also feels firm but will indent when pressure is applied. All patients experience a sensory deficit (touch, pain, temperature) in the involved region that may extend just proximal to the line of demarcation of the frostbite.

Upon thawing an area of superficial frostbite, there is a throbbing pain followed by a tingling sensation. Deeper injuries become mottled-blue, swollen, and extremely painful upon warming. Edema occurs within 3 h after thawing; vesicles and bullae form in more severe cases after 6 to 48 h. Immediately following thawing, findings such as sensation to pinprick, good color, warm tissue, and large, clear, nonhemorrhagic blebs—which, if the digits are involved, extend completely to the tips—suggest a relatively favorable prognosis for tissue viability. Poor prognostic signs include the late occurrence of small, dark hemorrhagic blebs that do not extend to the tips of the extremities, cyanosis, and the absence of edema.

ED Management

The goal of therapy, prevention of further soft tissue destruction, is accomplished via rapid rewarming. Thaw the frozen part by immersion in water heated to 37.8 to 42°C (100–108°F); do not use warmer water, which may cause burns. A whirlpool is ideal for an extremity, as thawing time is decreased when water is circulated. Carefully monitor the temperature; as the bath cools, add hotter water to maintain the desired temperature range. Avoid rubbing or massaging the frostbitten area.

The warming usually takes 30 to 45 min; remove the extremity after thawing has occurred. The endpoint is when the affected area becomes soft, develops a purple-red color, and sensation starts to return. While in the last stages of rewarming, the patient may experience severe pain and require analgesia (morphine sulfate 0.10 to 0.15 mg/kg IV).

After thawing, inspect the wound. Debride any ruptured blebs, apply an antibiotic ointment such as bacitracin, and cover with bulky sterile dressings. Place cotton between affected fingers or toes. Again, the use of a potent analgesic such as morphine may be necessary, but prophylactic antibiotics are not indicated. Obtain plastic surgery consultation early in the course of treatment. An escharotomy is indicated if the digits are not freely mobile. Give tetanus toxoid (0.5 mL) if the last immunization was more than 5 years ago.

Follow-up

- Daily follow-up until injured areas are healing well

Indication for Admission

- Frostbite of hands and/or feet

BIBLIOGRAPHY

Murphy JV, Banwell PE, Roberts AH, et al: Frostbite: pathogenesis and treatment. *J Trauma* 2000;48:171–178.

Raboid M: Frostbite and other localized cold-related injuries, in: Tintinalli JE, Ruiz E, Krome RL (eds): *Emergency Medicine: A Comprehensive Study Guide,* 4th ed. New York: McGraw-Hill, 1996, pp 846–850.

Reamy BV: Frostbite: review and current concepts. *J Am Board Fam Pract* 1998;11:34–40.

HEAT-EXCESS SYNDROMES

Most cases of heat illness occur during the summer months. Environmental conditions that increase the risk of heat-excess injuries include the lack of air conditioning and enclosure in a small, unventilated space such as an automobile. Extreme physical activity, underlying illness, alcohol abuse, inadequate fluid intake, and drugs such as cocaine, salicylates, amphetamines, phenothiazines, antihistamines, or anticholinergics—coupled with any of the predisposing environmental factors—place a person at a high risk for developing hyperthermic injury.

Children are less efficient thermoregulators than adults. They exhibit a slower speed of acclimatization, have a lower sweating rate, and produce more metabolic heat per kilogram of body weight, placing a greater strain on thermoregulatory mechanisms. Children also have a higher set point (the change in core temperature when sweating starts) than adults.

Clinical Presentation

Heat Cramps   Heat cramps are painful muscle cramps that are probably caused by electrolyte depletion in association with insufficient blood supply to an exercising muscle. Large muscle groups, such as the hamstrings and the gastrocnemius, are most likely to be involved. Clinically, the affected muscles are contracted. However, the onset may be delayed, occurring when the patient is showering after exercise or resting. The patient has a normal mental status and normal vital signs, but the core temperature may be slightly elevated. There may or may not be sweating.

Heat Exhaustion   Heat exhaustion is caused by excessive sweating associated with inadequate intake of water and salt in a hot environment. Symptoms include headache, dizziness, fatigue, syncope, visual disturbances, nausea, vomiting, malaise, myalgias, and muscle cramps. The patient is usually diaphoretic, tachycardic, and tachypneic and may have orthostatic changes in vital signs. The rectal temperature is typically 38 to 40°C (100.4–104.0°F).

Heat Stroke   Heat stroke is a *life-threatening emergency* that occurs when the core body temperature exceeds 40.5°C (104.9°F). The estimated mortality is greater than 50%. It is associated with acute neurologic changes, including irritability, aggression, and emotional instability. Heat stroke has been classified as either classic or exertional. *Classic heat stroke* occurs in an infant secondary to poor water intake. It has a relatively slow onset, with the insidious development of anorexia, nausea, vomiting, headaches, dry skin, and progressive deterioration of mental function. Sweating is usually absent and rhabdomyolysis and hypoglycemia are uncommon. *Exertional heat stroke* usually occurs in a patient who engages in prolonged physical activity. It presents with the rapid onset of severe prostration, headache, syncope, tachycardia, tachypnea, and hypotension. Lactic acidosis is common and rhabdomyolysis, hypoglycemia, and hypocalcemia are often present. These patients may have dry or wet skin. The most important prognostic sign is the duration, not the degree, of the hyperthermic state.

Diagnosis

The differential diagnosis of heat cramps includes electrolyte abnormalities (*hyponatremia, hypocalcemia*) and *black widow spider envenomation.* Consider *neuroleptic malignant syndrome, meningitis, sepsis, thyrotoxicosis, salicylate ingestion, malaria,* and *Rocky Mountain spotted fever* in the differential diagnosis of heat exhaustion and heat stroke.

ED Management

Heat Cramps   Treat heat cramps by placing the patient at rest in a cool environment. In mild cases, replace salt with a salt-containing oral rehydration solution. For severe cases, start an IV and give the patient 20 mL/kg of normal saline. Obtain blood for a CBC and electrolytes (including calcium and magnesium). The patient may be discharged after clinical improvement (well hydrated, no cramps).

Heat Exhaustion   Immediately place the patient in a cool environment, remove any excess clothing, and sponge with lukewarm tap water. Then increase the heat dissipation by placing fans directed to blow air across the patient. Assess the airway and breathing and administer 100% oxygen. Start a large-bore IV, give 20 mL/kg of NS, then reassess the patient's hydration status and response to fluids. Obtain a CBC, electrolytes, and urinalysis. Discharge the patient after cooling and volume replacement if vital signs are normal and symptoms have resolved.

Heat Stroke   Rapidly assess airway and breathing and intubate a patient who is comatose, seizing, or has an oxygen saturation less than 90% while breathing 100% oxygen. Obtain vital signs including a rectal temperature (use a rectal probe), and monitor the cardiac rhythm. Undress the patient completely and start the cooling process by spraying with lukewarm tap water, then positioning fans to blow air across the body. It is estimated that the evaporation of 1 g of water transfers seven times as much heat as melting 1 g of ice. Use ice packs to the axillae, neck, and groin as supplemental treatment. Continue this aggressive cooling at a rate of approximately 0.1°C (0.2°F) per minute until the core temperature reaches 39°C (102.2°F). Prevent shivering, which generates body heat, with IV lorazepam (0.1 mg/kg IV). Alcohol baths are contraindicated due to the potential for alcohol intoxication. Acetaminophen and ibuprofen have no role in the treatment of heat stroke.

Start two large-bore IVs, immediately give 0.5 to 1 g/kg dextrose (1–2 mL/kg D_{50}; 2–4 mL/kg D_{25}), give two 20-mL/kg boluses of NS, then reassess the circulatory status. If the patient remains in shock after the second bolus of crystalloid, consider severe vasodilatation. Use central venous pressure (CVP) monitoring to guide further fluid therapy, since continued boluses may cause pulmonary edema. If the CVP is low, continue to give fluid boluses. If the CVP is normal, start dopamine at a rate of 2 to 5 μg/kg/min. Insert a Foley catheter and carefully monitor intake and output.

Initial laboratory studies include CBC, PT/PTT, electrolytes, BUN, creatinine, glucose, CPK, serum osmolality, salicylate level, pregnancy test (for females of childbearing age), urinalysis, and an ECG. Reassess the patient frequently to identify complications such as brain cell injury, liver and pulmonary injury, rhabdomyolysis, and disseminated intravascular coagulation.

Follow-up

- Heat cramps: primary care follow-up in 1 to 2 weeks
- Heat exhaustion: next day

Indication for Admission

- Heat stroke

BIBLIOGRAPHY

Hett HA, Brechtelsbauer DA: Heat-related illness. Plan ahead to protect your patients. *Postgrad Med* 1998;103:107–120.

Khosla R, Guntupalli KK: Heat related illnesses. *Crit Care Clin* 1999;15:251–263.

Waters TA: Heat illness: tips for recognition and treatment. *Cleve Clin J Med* 2001;68:685–687.

HYPERBARIC OXYGEN THERAPY

Hyperbaric oxygen therapy (HBOT) involves the administration of oxygen under increased ambient pressure. While the indications for HBOT are controversial, the most common emergency conditions that appear to benefit from HBOT are decompression sickness, air embolism, and carbon monoxide (CO) poisoning. Other indications for HBOT are listed in Table 8-1.

Table 8-1   Indications for Hyperbaric Oxygen Therapy

TRADITIONAL INDICATIONS	NEWER INDICATIONS
Decompression sickness	Cyanide poisoning
Acute air embolism	Wound healing
Carbon monoxide poisoning	Necrotizing soft tissue infections
Gas gangrene	Acute traumatic ischemia
	Osteoradionecrosis
	Thermal burns
	Compromised skin grafts and flaps

Adapted from Weiss LD, Van Meter KW: The applications of hyperbaric oxygen therapy in emergency medicine. *Am J Emerg Med* 1992;10:558–567, with permission.

Decompression Sickness and Air Emboli

Decompression sickness occurs when nitrogen in the blood comes quickly out of solution, resulting in bubble formation in the circulation and tissues. Air emboli result from leakage of air bubbles into the circulation and may cause circulatory obstruction. This may be iatrogenic (cardiovascular procedures, central line placement, lung biopsies, hemodialysis) or may result from uncontrolled ascents in scuba diving.

In treating both these disorders, HBOT relies upon two basic laws of physics: Boyle's law (the pressure of a gas is inversely proportional to its volume), and Henry's law (the amount of gas dissolved in solution is directly proportional to its partial pressure). HBOT causes a reduction in the size of the trapped bubbles and forces them back into solution from the circulatory system and tissues.

Carbon Monoxide Poisoning

Carbon monoxide competes with oxygen for hemoglobin and cytochrome binding sites. Toxicity results from direct hypoxic damage to tissues, inhibition of cellular respiration by disruption of the cytochrome system, and lipid peroxidation in the central nervous system. Signs and symptoms of carbon monoxide poisoning include fatigue, nausea, vomiting, and neurologic abnormalities ranging from headache to personality deficit to frank coma.

HBOT increases the oxygenation of the tissues, decreases the half-life of carboxyhemoglobin (COHb) from approximately 320 min (range of 128–409 min) at sea level (1 atm) in 21% oxygen to approximately 15 to 30 min at 3 atm in 100% oxygen, and prevents lipid peroxidation in the brain.

Since the serum (either venous or arterial) COHb level may not reflect tissue COHb levels and often does not correlate with the degree of toxicity, the signs and symptoms of toxicity are equally important in determining the need for therapy for CO poisoning. HBOT is recommended for a patient with a history of unconsciousness after exposure to CO regardless of COHb level, a history of or continued mental status change or other neurologic deficit, cardiac dysfunction or ischemia, a COHb level >25% regardless of symptoms, or for any pregnant woman with a history of CO exposure (regardless of COHb level). The only absolute contraindication to HBOT is an untreated pneumothorax. Patients to be treated cautiously include those with chronic obstructive lung disease, significant upper respiratory infections, fever, seizure disorder, diabetes, or a history of chest surgery or pneumothorax. Also, unstable patients who have had a cardiac arrest and/or require pressors for support may experience little improvement in clinical symptoms after HBOT because of other ongoing medical problems, and they are difficult to resuscitate inside the hyperbaric chamber. A patient who has suffered a cardiac arrest has a very poor prognosis and may not experience enough benefit from HBOT to warrant the risks.

Initial ED Management and Preparation for HBOT

Initial priorities include addressing the ABCs (airway, breathing, and circulation), providing 100% oxygen via a tight-fitting nonrebreather mask or endotracheal tube, and obtaining a COHb level from venous or arterial blood using a heparinized 1-mL syringe. If the patient is in respiratory distress or requires ventilatory support, secure an IV and obtain an ABG, ECG, and chest x-ray. Other tests may be indicated, including serum electrolytes, liver function tests, and creatinine. In addition, assess the patient for other traumatic injuries, smoke inhalation, or cyanide poisoning. These conditions must be fully addressed before the patient is taken into the hyperbaric chamber.

Once it is determined that HBOT is indicated, prepare the patient for the chamber. If the patient is intubated with a cuffed endotracheal tube, replace the air in the cuff with saline or water, since fluids do not compress under pressure. Change glass IV bottles, which may implode under pressure, to flexible plastic IV bags. Adjust IV drip rates manually with pressure bags. Open the nasogastric tube (if inserted) to gravity to allow for equalization of pressure between the stomach and the atmosphere. Make sure that the patient's clothing is made of cotton or flame-retardant material, and remove any fire hazards—including matches, lighters, jewelry, watches, alcohol, cosmetics, lubricants, hairsprays, and newspapers—from the patient and keep them out of the chamber.

Sedate and paralyze (pp 6–8) intubated patients to minimize the risk of extubation, and consider restraints for patients with altered mental status who may improve and awaken during treatment and injure themselves or chamber personnel. Optional considerations include performing needle myringotomies to prevent tympanic membrane rupture in intubated patients and prophylactic administration of a decongestant (pseudoephedrine 1 mg/kg) to an awake patient to help prevent middle ear and sinus barotrauma.

One current treatment protocol for CO poisoning involves administering 100% O_2, via tight-fitting mask or endotracheal tube, at 2.8 atmospheres absolute (ATA) for two 23-min periods interrupted by a 5-min interval on 21% oxygen.

HBOT may result in barotrauma to any air-filled cavity that cannot equilibrate with ambient pressure. The middle ear and/or sinuses are most commonly affected. Rarely, barotrauma may cause a pneumothorax or air embolus.

Oxygen toxicity to the central nervous system (CNS) may occur with prolonged exposure to 100% oxygen. Additionally, the seizure threshold may be lowered and autonomic regulation of respiration may be affected. However, neurotoxicity is very unusual with the low-pressure, short-duration treatments used in most clinical situations.

Pulmonary toxicity may occur with 100% inspired oxygen at increased pressure for prolonged exposures. Although pulmonary toxicity will occur after 6 h of continuous exposure to 100% O_2 at 2 ATA, no HBOT protocol requires this length of treatment.

Other side effects include accelerated cataract growth, temporary worsening of myopia or improved presbyopia, claustrophobia, and fatigue. Technical complications of HBOT include a fire risk within the chamber where oxygen is being used and the inadequacy of equipment and personnel to perform prolonged resuscitation on a patient while pressurized within the chamber.

Follow-up

- Asymptomatic patient: next day

Indication for Admission

- Any patient treated with HBOT who has continued significant respiratory, cardiovascular, or neurologic compromise

BIBLIOGRAPHY

Caplan ES: Hyperbaric oxygen. *Pediatr Infect Dis J* 2000;19:151–152.
Liebelt EL: Hyperbaric oxygen therapy in childhood carbon monoxide poisoning. *Curr Opin Pediatr* 1999;11:259–264.
J Sheridan RL, Shank ES: Hyperbaric oxygen treatment: a brief overview of a controversial topic. *J Trauma* 1999;47:426–435.

HYPOTHERMIA

Hypothermia, a core temperature less than or equal to 35°C (95°F), is usually caused by accidental exposure. At less than 35°C (95°F), the human body loses its ability to generate sufficient heat to maintain bodily functions. Below 30°C (86°F), the body assumes the temperature of the surrounding environment.

Children are at particular risk because of their large body surface area, lack of fat insulation, inadequate shivering, and inability to escape a cold environment. Prolonged out-of-hospital resuscitation and cold-water immersion are common causes of hypothermia. Predisposing factors include malnutrition, hypoglycemia, major trauma, hypothyroidism, Addison's disease, and drug use or abuse (alcohol, sedatives, antidepressants). Although most cases of accidental exposure are seen in winter, hypothermia may occur in the spring and fall during wet, windy weather. Hypothermia may develop acutely within minutes in a victim of cold water immersion or insidiously over days in a neonate in a poorly heated home.

Clinical Presentation

Initially there is vasoconstriction with shivering, chattering teeth, dysarthria, and clumsiness. Below 32.2°C (90°F), shivering ceases, the patient is apathetic and disoriented, the pulse and blood pressure fall, and there may be arrhythmias (atrial fibrillation and sinus bradycardia are most common). Lethargy and a depressed gag reflex combined with cold-induced bronchorrhea and capillary damage predispose to aspiration pneumonia. Below 30°C (86°F), stupor and coma ensue, along with unreactive pupils, absent doll's eyes, areflexia, and imperceptible vital signs.

Diagnosis

Consider a patient with cold skin, altered mental status, and bradycardia to be hypothermic until proved otherwise. In addition, any severe injury or illness can be associated with hypothermia. Since the diagnosis of hypothermia rests on measuring the core temperature, use a thermocouple probe inserted 3 to 5 cm into the rectum.

A "J" or Osborne wave may be observed on the ECG of a hypothermic patient. This is a hump at the J point immediately after the QRS complex; it is seen in up to 80% of cases. Other ECG findings include prolonged PR, QRS, and/or QT intervals.

Investigate for precipitating and complicating factors such as *alcohol* or *drug intoxication* (barbiturates, phenothiazines), *near-drowning, head trauma, sepsis*, or *hypoglycemia*. Consider other causes of hypothermia, including *hypothyroidism* and *Addison's disease*, when a patient fails to respond to rewarming measures with a rise in core temperature of at least 1°C per hour.

ED Management

Classify the hypothermia as mild (32.2–35.0°C; 90.0–95.0°F), moderate (28.0–32.2°C; 82.4–90.0° F), or profound (<28.0°C; 82.4°F).

Passive rewarming is satisfactory for mild hypothermia. Remove all wet or cold clothing, place layers of blankets on the patient, give warm IV fluids (normal saline at maintenance), and administer warmed (47°C; 116.6°F) humidified oxygen.

A patient with moderate hypothermia requires active external rewarming, as with electric warming blankets, hot water bottles, heating pads, or a warming bed. However, IV access must have already been obtained and fluid therapy initiated before active rewarming is started; otherwise, as vasodilatation occurs during warming, the patient can become acutely hypotensive and develop a fatal cardiac arrhythmia.

Treat severe hypothermia with active core rewarming; use warmed nasogastric, peritoneal, or pleural lavage. For peritoneal dialysis, use a commercial dialysate, normal saline, or lactated Ringer's solution heated to 45°C (113°F). Place two trocars (one for infusion and one for drainage) into the peritoneal cavity to achieve a flow rate of 4 to 6 L/h.

Because of the very low threshold for cardiac arrhythmias, handle a victim of hypothermia as gently as possible. Rapidly assess airway and breathing. Intubate if the patient requires a protected airway or has an oxygen saturation less than 90% on warmed, humidified oxygen.

Monitor the cardiac rhythm and obtain the rectal core temperature with a low-reading thermometer. A tympanic thermometer is unreliable. If the patient is hypotensive, give a 20-mL/kg fluid challenge of normal saline through a large-bore IV. If peripheral vasoconstriction interferes with obtaining venous access, insert a central femoral line, but avoid catheters that enter the heart, since they may induce cardiac dysrhythmias. After obtaining access and before initiating IV fluids, obtain blood for CBC, electrolytes, BUN, creatinine, calcium, magnesium, amylase, osmolality, and PT and PTT. If the patient has altered mental status, give glucose [0.5–1.0 g/kg (1–2 mL/kg of D_{50}) IV] and naloxone (0.02 mg/kg). Treat hypotension unresponsive to fluid boluses with a dopamine drip (start at 2–5 μg/kg/min). Place a Foley catheter and send urine for dipstick and microscopic analysis.

Ventricular fibrillation and asystole (not bradycardia) are the only indications for chest compressions, since external cardiac massage can induce fatal ventricular arrhythmias in profound hypothermia. Ventricular fibrillation may occur spontaneously when the core temperature is below 28°C (82.4°F). If ventricular fibrillation or pulseless ventricular tachycardia is present, attempt defibrillation (2 J/kg first attempt; 2–4 J/kg second attempt; 4 J/kg third attempt), although electrical defibrillation/unsynchronized cardioversion is unlikely to be successful at core temperatures below 28 to 30°C (82.4 to 86°F). If the rhythm is refractory to electrical conversion, administer lidocaine (1 mg/kg IV bolus), which can be repeated at the same dose in 5 to 15 minutes. Alternatively, give amiodarone (5 mg/kg bolus) followed by defibrillation/unsynchronized cardioversion (4 J/kg). Amiodarone can be repeated twice (to 15 mg/kg). Follow each dose of lidocaine or amiodarone with defibrillation/unsynchronized cardioversion (up to 3 times at 4 J/kg) within 30 to 60 seconds of delivery of the medication. Most atrial arrhythmias are benign and disappear with rewarming.

Because of the difficulty in distinguishing between hypothermia and death, continue all resuscitative measures until the patient's core temperature is greater than 32°C (89.6°F).

Indication for Admission

• Hypothermia

BIBLIOGRAPHY

Giesbrecht GG: Prehospital treatment of hypothermia. *Wilderness Environ Med* 2001;12:24–31.
Hanania NA, Zimmerman JL: Accidental hypothermia. *Crit Care Clin* 1999;15: 235–249.
Lloyd EL: Accidental hypothermia. *Resuscitation* 1996;32:111–124.

INHALATION INJURY

Inhalation injuries account for up to 50% of fire-related deaths in the United States. Such injuries comprise three distinct clinical entities: thermal burns of the upper airway, smoke inhalation, and carbon monoxide poisoning. The clinical presentations, treatments, and prognoses differ, and serious, life-threatening complications can occur insidiously or rapidly.

Thermal Injury   Thermal burns from inhalation injuries almost never involve the lungs or lower airways because of the poor heat-carrying capacity of air and the excellent heat-dissipating capacity of the upper airway. Thermal injury above the glottis is very common and probably the most immediate life-threatening problem in a patient with inhalation injury. However, lower parenchymal injury can occur with steam burns.

Smoke Inhalation   Many of the chemical components in smoke (aldehydes and organic acids), as well as soot and particulate matter, cause direct parenchymal injury when inhaled, resulting in acute pulmonary insufficiency, pulmonary edema, and bronchopneumonia.

Carbon Monoxide Poisoning   Carbon monoxide (pp 190–191) is a colorless, odorless, tasteless gas produced by incomplete combustion of carbon-containing materials (wood, fuel, paper). CO poisoning is the most common cause of fire-related deaths. CO binds to hemoglobin with an affinity approximately 250 times greater than that of oxygen, resulting in displacement of oxygen from hemoglobin, and causing cellular anoxia affecting all organ systems.

Clinical Presentation and Diagnosis

Thermal Injury   Thermal injury of the upper airway causes laryngeal edema and laryngospasm, which can occur at any time within the first 24 h and lead to total airway obstruction within minutes. Clinically, there is a history of exposure to smoke or fire in an enclosed space in association with cough, tachypnea, hoarseness, stridor, or carbon-tinged sputum. Burns on the head, face, or neck and singed nasal hairs may also be present.

Smoke Inhalation   A patient with flame burns, the smell of smoke on his or her clothing, or a history of being in an enclosed smoke-filled room is at high risk for developing pulmonary injury from smoke inhalation. Hoarseness, wheezing, rales, or soot-tinged sputum may be early evidence of pulmonary insufficiency. However, the absence of these signs does not rule out parenchymal damage, since a child who appears symptom-free 1 to 2 h postinhalation may go on to develop significant respiratory problems within a matter of hours. In general, pulmonary insufficiency with bronchospasm occurs in the first 12 h postinhalation, pulmonary edema occurs 6 to 72 h postinhalation, and bronchopneumonia occurs more than 60 h postinhalation. The ABGs and chest x-rays may not deteriorate until 12 to 24 h postinhalation. Therefore if there is a suspicious history, evaluate and treat the patient for smoke inhalation.

Carbon Monoxide Poisoning   The measured level of carboxyhemoglobin (COHb) correlates only moderately with the clinical picture and degree of CO poisoning. At COHb levels of 10 to 15%, patients are fatigued and may have decreased exercise tolerance. At 15 to 25%, nausea and headaches occur. Levels of 30% cause confusion and weakness. The patient loses consciousness at 40%, and levels >60% may be fatal. The COHb level may not accurately reflect the degree of CO poisoning at the cellular level. Therefore rely on the history and clinical presentation in assessing and managing an inhalation victim for CO poisoning.

ED Management

Thermal Injury   Mental status changes, cough, tachypnea, hoarseness, stridor, carbon-tinged sputum, singed nasal hairs, or burns on the head, face, or neck are absolute indications for immediate direct visualization of the mouth and upper airway. This can be done in the ED with either a fiberoptic bronchoscope or a laryngoscope, but ensure that the personnel and equipment to perform an emergency intubation or tracheostomy are at the bedside. Upon visualization of the airway, the presence of erythema, edema, dried mucosa, or small blisters on the hard palate or mucosa of the upper airway are clear indications for elective early intubation. All the other signs and symptoms mentioned above are relative indications for elective intubation. Expectant observation of a patient with a history of smoke exposure or any of the typical signs or symptoms is appropriate only in a facility where emergency intubation and/or tracheostomy can be performed immediately. If intubation is required, sedate the patient if necessary. Keep the patient intubated for 2 to 5 days until the laryngeal edema subsides and an air leak is noted around the endotracheal tube. Steroids are contraindicated in the victim of smoke inhalation with concomitant burns and are ineffective in patients with isolated thermal injuries of the upper airway. Elective tracheostomy significantly increases the morbidity and mortality of patients with smoke inhalation and is never indicated.

Smoke Inhalation   Provide humidified 100% oxygen either by a tight-fitting nonrebreather face mask or through an endotracheal tube (ETT) after intubation. As with thermal injury of the upper airway, fiberoptic bronchoscopy is the standard diagnostic procedure for pulmonary injury. Treat wheezing with nebulized albuterol (0.03 mL/kg), and follow the progression of the pulmonary disease with serial ABGs and chest x-rays. Prophylactic antibiotics and steroids are contraindicated in treating inhalation injury. Good pulmonary toilet, bronchodilators, and humidified oxygen are the mainstays of treatment.

Carbon Monoxide Poisoning   The management of CO poisoning is discussed in detail elsewhere (see Hyperbaric Oxygen Therapy, pp 189–192). However, defer hyperbaric treatment if the patient has severe burns, needs positive end-expiratory pressure (PEEP) for oxygenation, or requires pressors to maintain blood pressure. In centers that do not have a hyperbaric chamber, contact the local poison control center for information as to the location of the nearest available hyperbaric center. If a hyperbaric chamber is not available, provide 100% oxygen to patients with severe CO poisoning for at least 24 h, regardless of the COHb level. Obtain serial ABGs to follow and correct any acid-base derangements.

Indications for Admission

- Documented thermal injury of the upper airway
- Severe CO poisoning
- Smoke inhalation with upper or lower airway injury
- History of significant smoke or fire exposure in an enclosed area

BIBLIOGRAPHY

Kimmel EC, Still KR: Acute lung injury, acute respiratory distress syndrome and inhalation injury: an overview. *Drug Chem Toxicol* 1999;22:91–128.
Lee-Chiong TL: Smoke inhalation injury. *Postgrad Med* 1999;105:55–62.
Lentz CW, Peterson HD: Smoke inhalation is a multilevel insult to the pulmonary system. *Curr Opin Pulm Med* 1997;3:221–226.

LEAD POISONING

Lead poisoning in children is usually the result of chronic ingestion. Young children are at risk of lead exposure through pica (ingestion of lead-based paint chips), lead-contaminated dust or dirt along heavily traveled roads, and water carried by outdated lead pipes. In addition, exposure to lead can occur through burning of automobile battery casings, improperly home-glazed ceramics, or certain folk medicines (e.g., the Mexican remedies *azarcon* and *greta*). Despite widespread lead screening programs, children who frequent inner-city EDs may have disproportionately elevated lead levels.

Clinical Presentation

The majority of patients are asymptomatic but are brought to the ED because they have been observed eating paint chips or have an elevated microsample lead level. Otherwise, the signs and symptoms of early plumbism are vague and nonspecific. Anorexia, abdominal pain, constipation, intermittent vomiting, listlessness, and irritability are common. With increasing levels, encephalopathy develops, with persistent vomiting, drowsiness, clumsiness, and frank ataxia. Kidney damage results in a spectrum ranging from slight aminoaciduria to a full Fanconi syndrome. High lead levels are also associated with a microcytic anemia.

A mildly elevated blood lead level (<25 μg/dL) is associated with decreased intelligence and impaired development. A lead level of 25 to 60 μg/dL may cause headache, irritability, and anemia. With a lead level of 60 to 80 mg/dL, there are gastrointestinal symptoms and subclinical renal effects. With a level >80 mg/dL, there may be overt intoxication, with encephalopathy, increased intracranial pressure, and seizures.

Diagnosis

The risk of lead exposure is primarily determined by the patient's home environment. In most cases the nonspecific presentation may be mistaken for a *viral syndrome*. However, consider lead poisoning in a patient who lives in pre-World War II housing, has a history of pica or iron-deficiency anemia, or has a family history of lead poisoning. Clinical features suggesting plumbism include persistent vomiting, listlessness, irritability, clumsiness, or loss of acquired developmental skills. Although rare, severe lead poisoning can present as an acute encephalopathy, afebrile seizures, or signs of increased intracranial pressure. Also consider lead poisoning if there is evidence of child abuse or neglect.

Nonspecific laboratory findings include anemia (normocytic or microcytic), basophilic stippling, and the presence of radioopaque chips on abdominal x-ray.

ED Management

If lead poisoning is suspected (based on symptoms) or the patient has an elevated screening microsample, obtain a whole blood lead level, CBC, and, if there is a history of pica or the child was seen with paint chips in its mouth, an abdominal radiograph. If the radiograph is positive (radioopaque particles in the intestinal tract), give a pediatric hypertonic phosphate enema, then repeat the x-ray. The management of acute encephalopathy (pp 332–335), seizures (pp 470–476), and increased intra-cranial pressure (pp 468–470) are discussed elsewhere.

Chelation Therapy
Asymptomatic and Lead Level 45 to 69 μg/dL   Arrange for outpatient chelation, preferably with oral dimercaptosuccinic acid (succimer), 350 mg/m^2 q 8 h for 5 days, then q 12 h for 14 days.

Symptomatic Patient or Lead Level >69 μg/dL   Admit the patient and treat with two drugs, oral dimercaptosuccinic acid (as above) and CaNa$_2$EDTA (edetate), 1000 to 1500 mg/m^2/day by IV infusion. Obtain pretreatment electrolytes, calcium, creatinine, and a urinalysis.

Encephalopathy   Give IM British antilewisite (BAL, or dimercaprol) 300 to 500 mg/m^2/day divided q 4 h for 3 to 5 days, followed 4 h later by CaNa$_2$EDTA (as above).

Follow-up
- Asymptomatic patient with a lead level <19 μg/dL: repeat blood lead test in 1 month
- Asymptomatic patient with a lead level 20 to 44 μg/dL: repeat blood lead test in 1 week
- Asymptomatic patient with a lead level 45 to 69 μg/dL: repeat blood lead test in 48 h

Indications for Admission
- Any symptoms of lead poisoning
- Lead level of 70 μg/dL or greater

BIBLIOGRAPHY

Berlin CM Jr: Lead poisoning in children. *Curr Opin Pediatr* 1997;9:173–177.
Etzel RA (ed): *Handbook of Pediatric Environmental Health.* Elk Grove Village, IL: American Academy of Pediatrics, 1999, pp 131–144.
Markowitz M: Lead poisoning. *Pediatr Rev* 2000;21:327–335.

LIGHTNING INJURIES

Lightning is a direct current estimated to be up to 200,000 amps and 1 billion volts. There are about 1500 human lightning strikes each year, the mortality is approximately 30%, and nearly three-fourths of survivors have permanent sequelae. The incidence of lightning strikes is highest in the summer months, with the majority of cases occurring in the afternoon.

Lightning causes injury by direct strike, ground strike, splash, and blunt trauma. Direct strike is considered the most serious, as the patient absorbs the entire charge. It most often occurs when the victim is in the open or in contact with metal objects. Ground strike occurs when the lightning strikes the ground near a person; the closer the patient is to the ground strike, the more likely it is that injury will ensue. Splash injury occurs when lightning jumps from the primary site through the air to a person. Blunt injury is estimated to occur in one-third of lightning strikes. It is the result of the expansion and explosion of rapidly cooling air.

Electrical energy follows the path of least resistance. Blood vessels and nerves have the lowest resistance, followed by tendon, skin, and muscle. Bone and fat have the highest resistance. However, skin resistance, and therefore the extent of injury, depends on whether the skin is wet (decreased skin resistance, less penetration of deep tissues) or dry (increased skin resistance, more penetration of deep tissues).

Clinical Presentation

Lightning injuries frequently affect multiple organ systems. Cutaneous burns may range from minor first-degree to severe third-degree burns. Dermal ferning, or feathering burn, is a reddish erythema that appears within several hours of the injury and disappears in several days. It is characteristic of lightning injuries. Burns may also present in a linear or punctate fashion, but discrete entrance and exit burns are rare.

Signs of CNS involvement include mental status changes, amnesia, paralysis, and seizures. Many types of brain injury have been documented, such as subdural and epidural hematoma and intraventricular hemorrhage.

Dysrhythmias, including ventricular fibrillation, ventricular tachycardia, asystole, and nonspecific ST–T-wave changes, may occur but usually resolve within 24 h. Myocardial infarction is uncommon. Vascular instability may ensue but resolves after several hours.

Possible pulmonary injuries include pulmonary contusions and hemopneumothorax. Muscle injury can result in rhabdomyolysis and myoglobinuria. Approximately one-half of lightning victims have an eye injury, including cataracts, retinal detachment or hemorrhage, or optic nerve injury. Cataracts are most frequently unilateral and may occur immediately after the lightning strike or as late as 2 years thereafter. Otologic injuries include tympanic membrane rupture, which occurs in over 50% of victims, and middle ear hematoma. Hearing loss may be a late sequela.

Psychiatric effects are a special late consequence among children. These include anxiety, sleep disturbances, separation anxiety, and secondary enuresis.

ED Management

The management of lightning strikes is basically the same as that for electrical injuries (pp 182–185). This includes basic and advanced life support, a full trauma examination, and neurologic, renal, and dermatologic assessment. Pay special attention to the possibility of otologic and ophthalmologic injuries, common to lightning strikes.

Follow-up

- Ophthalmologic and otologic follow-up in 2 to 3 days
- Psychiatric follow-up within 1 month

Indication for Admission

- Cardiovascular, neurologic, or renal injury (by history or direct observation in the ED)

BIBLIOGRAPHY

Fahmy FS, Brinsden MD, Smith J, et al: Lightning: the multisystem group injuries. *J Trauma* 1999;46:937–940.

Jain S, Bandi V: Electrical and lightning injuries. *Crit Care Clin* 1999;15:319–331.

Lederer W, Wiedermann FJ, Cerchiari E, et al: Electricity-associated injuries II: outdoor management of lightning-induced casualties. *Resuscitation* 2000;43: 89–93.

CHAPTER 9

Gastrointestinal Emergencies

Jeremiah J. Levine and Toba A. Weinstein

ASSESSMENT AND MANAGEMENT OF DEHYDRATION

The most common causes of dehydration in children are vomiting (pp 212–215) and diarrhea (pp 217–222).

Clinical Presentation and Diagnosis

Dehydration is classified by the percentage of total body water lost: mild (<5%), moderate (5–10%), and severe (>10%). A variety of signs and symptoms and ancillary data help to distinguish the degree of dehydration (Table 9-1). A mildly dehydrated child has dry mucous membranes and decreased urinary output, with a urine specific gravity under 1.020. If the child is moderately dehydrated, there are additional signs and symptoms of dehydration, such as tachycardia, orthostatic changes in heart rate and

Table 9-1   Assessment of Degree of Dehydration

SIGNS/SYMPTOMS	MILD (<5%)	MODERATE (5–10%)	SEVERE (>10%)
Tachycardia	+/–	+	+
Dry mucous membranes	+	+	+
Depressed fontanelle	–	+	+
Sunken eyeballs	–	+	+
Abnormal skin turgor	–	+/–	+
Decreased urine output	+/–	+	+
Capillary refill time > 2 s	–	+/–	+
Weak peripheral pulses	–	–	+
Hypotension	–	–	+
Hyperpnea	–	–	+
Altered mental status	–	+/–	+
Urine specific gravity	Normal/high	Normal/high	High
Serum acidosis	–	+/–	+

blood pressure, and a depressed fontanelle in an infant. Urine specific gravity is generally greater than 1.030. A severely dehydrated child appears ill and listless and has prolonged capillary refill (>2 s), tachypnea or hyperpnea, sunken eyeballs, and abnormal skin turgor (tenting). The urine specific gravity is greater than 1.035 and there is a metabolic acidosis.

ED Management

The management priorities are stabilization of the patient's vital signs, replenishment of the intravascular volume, and correction of electrolyte abnormalities. Assess the degree of dehydration and check for orthostatic changes in a patient old enough to cooperate. Measure the pulse and blood pressure with the patient supine for 5 min and again after the patient has been standing or sitting upright for 2 min. A pulse increase >20 bpm and/or a fall in systolic blood pressure (BP) >20 mmHg are positive orthostatic findings. If the patient complains of weakness or dizziness while sitting, the test is positive. Do not have the patient stand.

Severe Dehydration

IV fluid restoration is necessary for severe dehydration, shock, or if the patient is unable to take fluids orally or has an altered mental status.

Initial Intravascular Restoration
Give fluid resuscitation with a 20-mL/kg bolus of normal saline (NS) or lactated Ringer's solution over 20 to 30 min. Patients with renal or cardiac disease are at risk for developing congestive heart failure, and patients with sickle cell disease are at risk for acute chest syndrome; be extremely careful in assessing their fluid status. Obtain blood for electrolytes, blood urea nitrogen (BUN), creatinine, and glucose. Also obtain a urinalysis; if the urine contains large ketones or if the child is hypoglycemic, add 2 mL/kg of D_{25} (0.5 g/kg of glucose) to the bolus solution. After the first bolus, reevaluate the patient using parameters such as vital signs, the presence or correction of orthostatic changes, and capillary refill. If there is a poor response to the initial bolus, repeat the infusion. If there is a poor response to two IV boluses, consider other associated organ disease or the need for central venous monitoring before giving a third bolus. Following the restoration of adequate intravascular volume, assess the need for replacement of fluid and electrolyte deficits.

Replacement of Fluid and Electrolyte Deficits
Isotonic Dehydration   In isotonic dehydration, the serum sodium is normal. Estimate the percent of dehydration either by physical signs and symptoms or more accurately if a recent premorbid weight is known, although the accuracy of scales varies. Multiply the percent of dehydration by the weight of the child to calculate the fluid deficit (e.g., 10% dehydration × 20 kg child = a deficit of 2 L). Administer maintenance fluid requirements plus half of the deficit over the first 8 h and the second half over the following 16 h. In general, either $D_5\frac{1}{2}NS$ (>2 years of age) or $D_5\frac{1}{3}NS$ (<2 years of age) is an adequate solution. After the patient has voided, add potassium chloride (20 mEq/L) to the IV bag.

Hypotonic Dehydration   Hypotonic dehydration occurs when salt losses exceed water losses or when water intake exceeds required salt intake. By definition, the serum sodium is less than 130 mEq/L. Use the following formula to calculate the sodium deficit to be added to the replacement fluids (see Hyponatremia, pp 168–170):

$$\text{mEq sodium required for replacement} = (125 - \text{measured sodium}) \times (\text{premorbid body weight in kg}) \times 0.6$$

Give the sodium replacement over 4 h but do not exceed a rate of correction of more than 1.5 to 2.0 mEq/h.

Hypertonic Dehydration   Hypernatremia is defined as a serum sodium greater than 150 mEq/L. It occurs when water losses exceed salt losses or in the setting of excessive salt intake. The degree of dehydration is more difficult to determine in these patients because the extracellular fluid space is preserved. Calculate the free water deficit:

$$\text{Free water (mL)} = (\text{measured sodium} - 145) \times 4 \text{ mL/kg} \times (\text{premorbid weight in kg})$$

Because of the potential for neurologic complications, *correct the serum sodium and free water deficit slowly over 48 h*, with a daily sodium decrease of 10 to 15 mEq/L. In general, $D_5\frac{1}{2}NS$ is an appropriate solution. Add one ampule of 10% calcium gluconate to each 500 mL of replacement fluid. Also, add 40 mEq/L of potassium acetate after the patient voids (see Hypernatremia, pp 161–163).

Mild and Moderate Dehydration

A patient with mild or moderate dehydration can be orally rehydrated if willing and able to tolerate fluids.

Vomiting
If the child has been vomiting, wait 1 h after the last vomiting episode to initiate oral fluids. For infants and toddlers, use a rehydration or maintenance solution containing 45 to 50 mEq/L of sodium and 25 to 30 g/L of glucose (Pedialyte, Infalyte, etc.). Treat an older child with an oral electrolyte solution, sweetened weak tea, decarbonated soda, or dilute fruit juice. Give an infant (<1 year of age) 30 to 50 mL/kg over 4 h in small (5 to 10 mL) aliquots and an older child small volumes of fluid (10–20 mL) every 15 to 20 min over the next hour. Reassess the hydration status. If the patient looks well and has not vomited, discharge him or her with written instructions on how to advance the diet. Instruct the parent to double the volume every hour until the child is taking 60 mL every 20 min without vomiting. If the patient vomits at home, instruct the parents to wait an hour and then begin again with 10 to 20 mL every 15 min and advance every hour. A second episode of vomiting at home requires a return to the ED or prompt contact with the primary care provider. When the child is tolerating 60 mL every 20 min, the liquid diet can be liberalized. Restrict the diet to clear liquids for 12 to 24 h.

Once it is clear that the child can take fluids, instruct the parents to give breast milk or full-strength formula to infants and to offer a BRAT diet (bananas, rice, applesauce, toast) if the child eats solid food. An infant eating solid foods may be given bananas and other fruit, cereals (mixed with formula or water), and starchy vegetables. An older patient may have rice or noodles, toast with jelly, fruits, vegetables, crackers, clear soup, and chicken in addition to the above foods. If the child continues to feel well after 48 h, milk and other foods may be added to the diet.

Diarrhea

Start oral rehydration with an electrolyte solution (Pedialyte, Infalyte, etc.), giving a total volume of 30 to 50 mL/kg over a 3- to 4-h period in small aliquots (15–30 mL) while doing hourly reassessments of hydration status. Failure of oral rehydration (inability to take adequate volume PO, excessive ongoing losses) is an indication for IV rehydration. Once the initial rehydration is tolerated, resume giving milk to an infant, whether breast- or formula-fed. An infant who has large, watery stools can have the milk feedings supplemented with feedings of oral electrolyte solution. For older infants and toddlers already taking solid foods, recommend an electrolyte solution, clear soup, or decarbonated soda with a low-fat complex-carbohydrate diet, such as bananas and other fruits, rice, pasta, potatoes, bread with jam, and crackers. Milk can usually be successfully reintroduced. Antidiarrheal compounds and antimotility agents have no role in the management of acute diarrhea.

No Dehydration

If the patient is not vomiting, is less than 5% dehydrated, and appears well, give clear fluids as tolerated. Allow a breast-fed infant to continue to nurse. Make sure all infants and children are drinking prior to discharge.

Follow-up

- Mild or moderate dehydration: primary care follow-up the next day or return to the ED if unable to tolerate oral fluids

Indications for Admission

- Significant ongoing fluid losses and/or inability to tolerate oral fluids
- Severe dehydration
- Hypotonic or hypertonic dehydration

BIBLIOGRAPHY

American Academy of Pediatrics: Practice parameter: the management of acute gastroenteritis in young children. *Pediatrics* 1996;97:424–436.

Burkhart DM: Management of acute gastroenteritis in children. *Am Fam Physician* 1999;60:2555–2563.

Murphy MS: Guidelines for managing acute gastroenteritis based on a systematic review of published research. *Arch Dis Child* 1998;79:279–284.

Murray KF, Christie DL: Vomiting. *Pediatr Rev* 1998;19:337–341.

ABDOMINAL PAIN

Abdominal pain can be due to intra- and extraabdominal causes as well as systemic illnesses. The etiologies can range from minor viral illnesses to urgent surgical conditions; therefore a systematic approach is required.

Clinical Presentation and Diagnosis

Spasm or distention of an abdominal organ usually causes poorly localized, ill-defined visceral pain that can be accompanied by nausea and vomiting. Upper gastrointestinal tract (GI) pathology causes epigastric discomfort; distal small bowel and proximal colonic diseases are perceived as periumbilical pain; and distal colonic pain is referred to the hypogastrium. Stimulation of the parietal peritoneum causes localized and defined somatic pain, often associated with reflex muscle spasm and aggravated by movement or cough.

Ask about the duration, quality, intensity, location, and radiation of the pain and the response to defecation, urination, meals, and change in position. Inquire about associated symptoms.

Determine whether there is upper or lower GI bleeding, fever, vomiting or diarrhea associated with pain, night or early morning awakening, weight loss, or growth failure and whether the pain or tenderness is away from the umbilicus. These findings argue against a benign intraabdominal condition.

Conversely, a history of isolated chronic recurrent periumbilical pain in an otherwise healthy, well-appearing school-age child with no vomiting, diarrhea, fever, or weight loss and a normal physical and rectal examination is likely to be one of several benign conditions such as *functional abdominal pain, irritable bowel syndrome, lactose intolerance,* or *constipation.* Evaluation and treatment of these conditions can be deferred to the primary care setting.

Although a definitive diagnosis is not always possible, a primary goal is the early recognition of surgically correctable emergencies. Begin the examination with the nonthreatening and painless components, leaving the abdominal and rectal examinations to the end. In infants, suspect an intraabdominal surgical emergency such as *malrotation with midgut volvulus* or *intussusception* whenever there is a history of bilious or projectile vomiting and/or bleeding. The signs may be preceded or accompanied by irritability, poor feeding, and lethargy. Suspect a surgical condition if the physical examination reveals abdominal distention, a scaphoid abdomen, localized abdominal tenderness or guarding, a mass, high-pitched or absent bowel sounds, or an ill-appearing patient.

The diagnosis of surgical conditions in verbal children and adolescents is facilitated by a more reliable pain history and a greater degree of cooperation. In this age group, common surgical conditions are *appendicitis* (pp 206–209), *torsion of a testicle* (pp 265–269), *tuboovarian abscess* (p 289), and *ectopic pregnancy* (pp 282–286).

The next priority is the recognition of nonsurgical causes of abdominal pain, such as *infectious gastroenteritis* (pp 217–222), *urinary tract infection* (pp 613–616), *pneumonia* (pp 591–595), *hepatitis* (pp 225–229), and *pelvic inflammatory disease* (pp 286–293). These conditions are differentiated by their associated symptoms. Pneumonia may cause abdominal pain, fever, and mild tachypnea with very little else in the way of respiratory symptoms. A urinary tract infection (UTI), particularly in young children, may present with vague pain, diarrhea, or vomiting as the predominant or sole complaint. In younger children, *viral URIs* (p 143) and *streptococcal pharyngitis* (pp 143–146) may cause vague abdominal pain.

Constipation (pp 236–238) is one of the most common causes of abdominal pain throughout childhood; it is underdiagnosed because physicians mistakenly believe that it can be ruled out by a history of daily bowel movements.

In children with unexplained abdominal pain, consider *physical or sexual abuse* (pp 543–550). Significant trauma to internal abdominal organs can occur (e.g., *splenic hematoma, liver laceration, renal contusion, pancreatic pseudocyst*) without visible evidence on the abdominal wall. Many other conditions can cause abdominal pain in childhood, including *peptic disease, inflammatory bowel disease, pancreatitis* (pp 209–211), *biliary disease* (pp 229–231), *obstructive uropathy or urolithiasis, intraabdominal malignancy,* and genetic or metabolic disorders (*sickle cell, diabetic ketoacidosis, type I hyperlipidemia*). Consider *Henoch-Schönlein purpura* (pp 600–601) in a child with purpura rash and/or arthralgias, and the *hemolytic-uremia syndrome* in a patient with lower GI bleeding, pallor, oliguria, and hypertension. These conditions are recognized by associated symptoms.

If the etiology of severe or chronic abdominal pain is not diagnosed but there is no suspicion of a surgical condition, obtain a complete blood count (CBC), erythrocyte sedimentation rate (ESR), electrolytes, amylase, lipase, urinalysis, and stool guaiac. If these are normal and the child appears well, defer further workup to the primary care setting. Patients with severe or focal pain associated with vomiting or blood in the stool require hospitalization or further ED observation and consultation.

Follow-up

- No suspicion of a surgical condition, patient appears well, initial laboratory tests normal: primary care follow-up within 1 week

Indications for Admission

- Suspected surgical abdomen
- Dehydration or inability to take fluids
- Significant blood loss (tachycardia, orthostatic hypotension)

BIBLIOGRAPHY

Ashcraft KW: Consultation with the specialist: acute abdominal pain. *Pediatr Rev* 2000;21:363–367.

Ross AJ III: Abdominal pain, in Walker WA, Duries PR, Hamilton JR, et al (eds): *Pediatric Gastrointestinal Disease.* Philadelphia: Decker, 2000, pp 129–149.

Scholer SJ, Pitiuch K, Orr DP, et al: Clinical outcomes of children with abdominal pain. *Pediatrics* 1996;98:680–685.

APPENDICITIS

Appendicitis is the most common childhood illness requiring emergency surgery, with a peak incidence between 15 and 24 years. It begins with obstruction of the appendiceal lumen, often secondary to a fecalith. Necrosis of the wall of the appendix ensues, followed by perforation and spillage of stool into the peritoneal cavity with subsequent peritonitis. Early diagnosis is therefore of paramount importance.

Clinical Presentation

In uncomplicated appendicitis (prior to rupture), there is a short history (usually <36 h) of pain, anorexia, nausea, and vomiting in up to 90% of cases. Early in the course, colicky or persistent periumbilical pain is typical. The pain then shifts to the right lower quadrant, where it is constant and severe. Low-grade fever (<38.3°C, 101°F) is common, and a change in stool pattern occurs in about 15% of patients. Other symptoms may include dysuria or labial, testicular, or penile pain. However, maintain a high index of suspicion, as many patients do not have a "classic" presentation.

On physical examination tenderness is greatest over McBurney's point, one-third of the distance along a line from the anterosuperior iliac spine to the umbilicus. There may be positive psoas (pain on passive hip hyperextension) and/or obturator (pain on passive internal rotation) signs. While the examiner is palpating the left lower quadrant, discomfort may be elicited in the right lower quadrant (Rovsing's sign). Involuntary guarding (muscle spasm that persists when the abdomen is palpated with the hips flexed) is common. Rebound tenderness can be elicited by shaking or percussing the abdomen or asking the patient to cough, jump down from the table, or hop. Rectal examination may reveal right-sided tenderness. In the case of a retrocecal appendix, maximum tenderness and rigidity may remain in the periumbilical area or the right flank.

Perforation of the appendix occurs in 20 to 40% of children with appendicitis. If the patient has a ruptured appendix, the pain has usually been present for longer than 36 h. There may be frequent vomiting, dyspnea secondary to elevation of the diaphragm, and a temperature over 38.5°C (101.3°F). A diffusely tender and rigid abdomen indicates peritonitis.

Perforation occurs in 90% of infants with appendicitis because of the difficulty in making the diagnosis. There is a few-hour history of anorexia, vomiting, and lethargy, and the physical examination reveals an ill infant with a distended and rigid abdomen.

Diagnosis

Careful physical examination is the key to diagnosing appendicitis. Save the abdominal and rectal examinations for last, after the rest of the physical examination has been performed. Gently palpate the abdomen, starting away from the right lower quadrant. Try to elicit rebound tenderness. Since appendicitis is a rapidly progressive disease, increasing abdominal pain, tenderness, and rigidity on serial physical examinations are highly suggestive of the diagnosis.

Acute Gastroenteritis   In acute gastroenteritis, vomiting appears either simultaneously with or preceding the onset of abdominal pain; while in appendicitis, the periumbilical pain almost always precedes the vomiting. In gastroenteritis, the pain tends to be crampy and periumbilical and is relieved by diarrhea or vomiting. Bacterial gastroenteritis is often associated with a guaiac-positive stool and fecal leukocytes. Viral gastroenteritis may be associated with a preceding upper respiratory infection. High-volume diarrhea and the absence of signs of peritoneal inflammation suggest gastroenteritis.

Pneumonia   Right-lower-lobe pneumonia may present with pain referred to the abdomen. Tachypnea, pulmonary rales, and a positive chest radiograph confirm the diagnosis.

Urinary Tract Infection   UTIs are distinguished by the presence of frequency, urgency, dysuria, flank pain, suprapubic tenderness, and significant pyuria [>10 white blood cells (WBCs) per high-power field (hpf)], in addition to the fever and abdominal pain that occur with appendicitis.

Constipation   Constipation (pp 236–238) may cause nonmigratory periumbilical, right-lower-quadrant, or left-lower-quadrant pain that is relieved upon defecation. Note that a history of a daily bowel movement does not rule out constipation. There is no fever, vomiting, or laboratory signs of inflammation. On rectal examination, the ampulla is frequently filled with stool.

Functional Abdominal Pain   Functional abdominal pain occurs in the school-age child and is defined as recurrent attacks of abdominal pain that are not associated with fever, vomiting, or weight loss. The chronic nature of this condition differentiates it from appendicitis.

Other Etiologies of Abdominal Pain   The differential diagnosis also includes *hepatitis* (pp 225–229), *pancreatitis* (pp 209–211), *lead poisoning* (pp 196–198), *urolithiasis, diabetic ketoacidosis* (pp 153–159), *Crohn's disease* with involvement of the terminal ileum, *Meckel's diverticulum,* and *Yersinia enterocolitica* infection. In the adolescent female, *pelvic inflammatory disease* (pp 286–293), *ectopic pregnancy* (pp 283–286), *threatened abortion,* or a *twisted ovarian cyst* can mimic acute appendicitis, but the pain is usually lower in the abdomen and there may be vaginal bleeding or discharge.

ED Management

When the diagnosis is evident from the history and physical examination, make the patient NPO, start maintenance IV hydration with $D_5\frac{1}{2}NS$, obtain a CBC and type and cross-match, and consult a surgeon. If there is evidence of intravascular depletion (orthostatic changes in vital signs, delayed capillary refill, hypotension), give the patient a bolus of 20 mL/kg of NS or lactated Ringer's. If perforation is suspected, give the first dose of antibiotics [(ampicillin 100 mg/kg/day divided q 6 h *and* clindamycin 40 mg/kg/day divided q 6 h *and* gentamicin 6 mg/kg/day divided q 8 h) *or* (cefotaxime 150 mg/kg/day divided q 8 h *and* clindamycin 40 mg/kg/day divided q 6h)].

When the diagnosis is uncertain, an abdominal x-ray may be useful, since identification of a fecalith (found in 10% of cases) confirms appendicitis, while a soft tissue mass or focal ileus in the right lower quadrant is suggestive. A focused computed tomography (CT) scan with rectal contrast can *rule out* an appendicitis if the appendix fills, but reserve this test for children in whom the diagnosis remains uncertain after a thorough clinical evaluation. Conversely, an ultrasound can *rule in* appendicitis if a fluid-filled, noncompressible, distended tubular mass >6 mm is found. Sonography is rapid, well tolerated by children, does not involve ionizing radiation, and is extremely useful if an inflamed appendix, periappendiceal abscess, or gynecologic pathology is found, but it is highly operator-dependent. Obtain a chest x-ray if tachypnea, rales, or other pulmonary signs or symptoms are present. An elevated WBC >18,000/mm^3 suggests rupture or another bacterial process (pneumonia, bacterial gastroenteritis). Do not delay surgical evaluation if the WBC is normal in a patient with a clinical picture that is suggestive of appendicitis.

Serum electrolytes may be helpful in patients with abdominal pain and dehydration. A low serum sodium (<130 mEq/L) may reflect third spacing of fluids from the ileus associated with appendicitis. A urinalysis is necessary to rule out DKA (glycosuria and ketonuria) or a UTI (pyuria). There can be WBCs in the urine with an appendicitis. A pelvic examination and pregnancy test are usually necessary for postmenarcheal females with abdominal pain. An abdominal or transvaginal ultrasound can help to identify an adnexal mass or intrauterine pregnancy.

When appendicitis cannot be excluded, obtain a surgical consult and admit the patient for IV hydration and observation (NPO).

Follow-up

- If appendicitis seems highly unlikely, have the patient return in 6 to 8 h (still symptomatic) or sooner if the symptoms intensify. Prescribe a clear liquid diet and no analgesics.

Indication for Admission

- Suspected appendicitis

BIBLIOGRAPHY

Lund DP, Folkman J: Appendicitis, in Walker WA, Durie PR, Hamilton JR, et al (eds): *Pediatric Gastrointestinal Disease*. Philadelphia: Decker, 2000, pp 821–829.

Nance ML, Adamson WT, Hedrick HL: Appendicitis in the young child: a continuing diagnostic challenge. *Pediatr Emerg Care* 2000;16:160–162.

Peña BMG, Mandl KD, Kraus SJ, et al: Ultrasonography and limited computed tomography in the diagnosis and management of appendicitis in children. *JAMA* 1999;282:1041–1046.

ACUTE PANCREATITIS

Acute pancreatitis is a rare but serious cause of significant abdominal pain. Inflammation may be acute, chronic, necrotic, hemorrhagic, or hereditary. The etiologies of acute pancreatitis fall into four groups:

1. *Infections* associated with pancreatitis include mumps, rubella, Epstein-Barr virus, measles, coxsackie B, hepatitis A and B, influenza, and *Mycoplasma*. In addition, pancreatitis can be precipitated by shock, sepsis, peritonitis, inflammatory bowel disease, collagen vascular diseases, Reye's syndrome, Henoch-Schönlein purpura, and hemolytic-uremic syndrome.

2. The leading *mechanical* and/or *structural* cause is blunt abdominal trauma. Other structural causes include common duct obstruction by stones, tumors, or ascaris worms; penetrating ulcers; and congenital anomalies such as choledochal cysts and pancreas divisum.

3. *Metabolic* precipitants include severe diabetic ketoacidosis, severe hypertriglyceridemia (triglyceride >1000 mg/dL), hyperlipidemia, and hypercalcemia.

4. *Toxins* and *drugs* have been associated with pancreatitis in children. Examples include ethanol, methanol, organophosphate insecticides, and heroin. Implicated drugs include amphetamines, furosemide, tetracyclines, sulfonamide, valproic acid, didanosine, 6-mercaptopurine, l-asparaginase, and lamivudine.

Clinical Presentation

The classic symptoms of acute pancreatitis are abdominal pain (which is typically acute in onset and increasing in intensity over several hours), nausea, vomiting, and anorexia. The pain may be located in the epigastrium, right upper quadrant, or periumbilical area. In one-third of patients, the pain may radiate to the back, anterior chest wall, or other areas of the abdomen. The pain and vomiting may be worsened by eating.

On physical examination, the patient may have fever, tachycardia, and hypotension. Tenderness is frequently found in the upper abdomen and the patient may refuse to lie supine. There may be guarding, rebound, distention, and decreased bowel sounds, which may mimic an acute surgical abdomen. With severe hemorrhagic pancreatitis, serosanguinous fluid may track through fascial planes, resulting in blue discoloration of the flanks (Grey Turner sign) or the umbilicus (Cullen sign).

Diagnosis

Pancreatitis may be confirmed by finding elevations of the serum amylase and lipase to three to four times the upper limits of normal. Acute pancreatitis may occur with a normal amylase, and the amylase may be elevated in a large number of other conditions (Table 9-2). The serum half-life of lipase is longer than that of amylase, so it is more sensitive in diagnosing pancreatitis in cases that present 3 to 4 days after the onset of pain. Lipase is also more specific than amylase, because almost all lipase originates from the pancreas. In severe pancreatitis, hypocalcemia, hypomagnesemia, and hyperglycemia may occur. Because of the severe abdominal pain, an abdominal x-ray is frequently obtained that may reveal an ileus with colonic dilatation and a sentinel loop of dilated small bowel suggestive of pancreatitis. Radiologic confirmation requires either abdominal ultrasound or a CT scan. Ultrasound can document the presence of a pan-

Table 9-2   Causes of Amylase Elevation

Pancreatic	*Intestinal*
Acute or chronic pancreatitis	Appendicitis
Pancreatic tumor	Perforated peptic ulcer
Pancreatic ductal obstruction	Intestinal obstruction
Salivary	
Parotitis	*Miscellaneous*
Salivary duct obstruction	Burns
Trauma	Diabetic ketoacidosis
	Macroamylasemia
Biliary	Pregnancy (ruptured ectopic)
Cholecystitis	Renal insufficiency
Biliary duct obstruction	

creatic pseudocyst, dilated ducts, cholelithiasis, abscesses, and ascites. Abdominal CT scan is helpful in suspected traumatic pancreatitis and can also detect associated injury to the liver, spleen, and duodenum.

ED Management

When the diagnosis is suspected, obtain a CBC, electrolytes, glucose, calcium, magnesium, amylase, lipase, and liver-related enzymes. Order an ultrasound or abdominal CT in a patient with an elevated amylase and/or lipase.

The management is largely supportive and includes putting the pancreas to rest by making the patient NPO. Start an IV and aggressively treat signs of hypovolemia with IV fluid boluses of isotonic crystalloid or whole blood (see Shock, pp 18–22), followed by maintenance fluids. Insert a nasogastric tube if there is vomiting or ileus (absent bowel sounds) and request a surgical consult if the precipitating cause is ductal obstruction or abdominal trauma. Admit the patient and give an IV H_2 blocker (ranitidine 1–2 mg/kg q 8 h, 50 mg maximum) to help prevent stress ulceration. Admission to an intensive care unit (ICU) is indicated for severe complications such as shock, impending renal failure, hypoxia, or significant metabolic derangements. Supplemental calcium and magnesium may be needed, and occasionally insulin is required to control the hyperglycemia.

Indications for Admission

- Acute pancreatitis
- Inability to tolerate oral liquids

BIBLIOGRAPHY

Pietzak MM, Thomas DW: Pancreatitis in childhood. *Pediatr Rev* 2000;211: 406–412.

Steinberg W, Tenner S: Acute pancreatitis. *N Engl J Med* 1994;330:1190–2010.

Uretsky G, Goldschmeidt M, James K: Childhood pancreatitis. *Am Fam Physician* 1999;59:2507–2512.

VOMITING

Vomiting is the expulsion of intestinal contents through the mouth. It may be a symptom of a gastrointestinal illness or a systemic process that is not primarily gastrointestinal in origin. Vomiting may have a protective function in eliminating ingested toxins and infectious agents. Protracted vomiting may lead to complications such as dehydration, metabolic alkalosis, esophagitis, Mallory-Weiss tears, malnutrition, and dental problems. Bilious vomiting is always a worrisome symptom.

Clinical Presentation

Vomiting is distinguished from regurgitation by the presence of forceful abdominal contractions. Children can present with nonbilious or bilious emesis; the latter may indicate a surgical process.

Vomiting may be associated with fever, abdominal pain, nausea, diarrhea, hematemesis, or other systemic complaints. There is a large differential diagnosis for vomiting, which is listed in Table 9-3.

Table 9-3   Etiologies of Vomiting in Childhood

Infections	*Gastrointestinal diseases*
Food poisoning	Cholecystitis
Gastroenteritis: viral, bacterial, parasitic	Food allergy
	Gastroesophageal reflux
Meningitis/encephalitis	Hepatitis
Pharyngitis	Inflammatory bowel disease
Respiratory tract infection	Pancreatitis
Sepsis	Peptic ulcer disease
Urinary tract infection	
	CNS conditions
Abdominal surgical conditions	Increased intracranial pressure
Appendicitis	Malignancy
Bezoar	Migraine
Incarcerated hernia	Trauma (obvious or occult)
Intussusception	
Malrotation/volvulus	*Endocrine/metabolic*
Meckel's diverticulum with obstruction	Congenital adrenal hyperplasia
	Diabetic ketoacidosis
Pyloric stenosis	Hypercalcemia
Testicular/ovarian torsion	Uremia
Trauma (intestinal hematoma)	
	Miscellaneous
Drugs/toxins/ingestions	Bulimia
Caustic	Cyclic vomiting
Alcohol	Disturbed mother-infant relationship
Carbon monoxide	Motion sickness
Ethylene glycol	Postnasal drip/swallowed mucus
Foreign body	Posttussive vomiting
Heavy metals (lead)	Pregnancy
Ipecac	Psychogenic vomiting
Iron	Reye's syndrome
Salicylates	
Theophylline	

Infectious   Viral gastroenteritis is the most common cause of vomiting. Children typically present with associated fever, diarrhea, and abdominal pain. Viral gastroenteritis is especially common in the winter months, with *Rotavirus* the most likely viral pathogen in infants. Bacterial enteritis is typically associated with high fever. UTIs, central nervous system infections, otitis media, sepsis, pneumonia, and pharyngitis can all present with emesis.

Food Poisoning   Food poisoning syndromes associated with vomiting are most frequently caused by the ingestion of food contaminated with *Staphylococcus aureus* or *Bacillus cereus*. These are characterized by the acute onset of vomiting and abdominal cramps 1 to 6 h after ingestion of the contaminated food. Diarrhea also occurs in one-third of these cases. Typically, the patient is afebrile, the illness is brief (<12 h), and other exposed individuals may be sick.

Respiratory Disease   Children with respiratory infections and asthma may present with posttussive emesis, when vomiting occurs after bouts of coughing. Young children with upper respiratory tract infections may also vomit if they have swallowed large amounts of mucus.

Metabolic Disorders   During infancy, several metabolic disorders may present with vomiting. There may be an antecedent history of "poor feeding" or intermittent vomiting after feeds. Vomiting may be associated with lethargy, hypotonia, tachypnea secondary to metabolic acidosis, apnea, and/or seizures. Other clues that a metabolic disease may be causing the vomiting in an infant are an unusual odor, unexplained acidosis (organic acids), hypoglycemia, liver disease, or hyperammonemia. There may also be a history of siblings with unexplained death in the neonatal period.

Food Sensitivity   Celiac disease, which is gluten sensitivity, may present with emesis and poor weight gain. Allergic enteropathy can present with emesis with or without associated peripheral eosinophilia and hypoalbuminemia.

Surgical Conditions   Several surgical conditions present with vomiting. Suspect malrotation with midgut volvulus in a lethargic neonate with bilious vomiting; pyloric stenosis in a young infant if there is recurrent projectile vomiting; and intussusception in an infant or toddler whose vomiting occurs with acute bouts of pain, a change in mental status, or bloody stools. An incarcerated inguinal hernia and testicular torsion may also present with vomiting. Consider adhesions and obstruction in any child with a history of prior surgery.

Increased Intracranial Pressure (ICP)   Although rare, vomiting may be caused by increased ICP due to hydrocephalus, central nervous system (CNS) infection, tumor, pseudotumor cerebri, or trauma, which may be occult. Headache, blurred vision, irritability, change in mental status, a bulging fontanelle, and projectile vomiting suggest increased ICP.

Psychological   Rumination in a toddler or older child is seen most often in neurologically impaired children. Bulimia, which presents as binge eating followed by self-induced emesis, occurs in adolescents.

Cyclic Vomiting   This designation refers to recurrent, self-limited attacks of vomiting punctuated by completely asymptomatic intervals in an otherwise well child. Onset is typically in the preschool or school-age years but can occur from 6 months to 18 years of age. Such vomiting often begins in the night or early morning, and the interval between attacks tends to be uniform in 70 to 80% of affected children.

Miscellaneous   Vomiting can occur following accidental and deliberate drug overdoses (e.g., acetaminophen, ethanol, iron, salicylates, theophylline), foreign body or caustic ingestions, or exposure to environmental toxins such as carbon monoxide. Patients with uremia, diabetic ketoacidosis, and pancreatitis may also present with vomiting. Accidental and nonaccidental trauma to the abdomen may present with vomiting (duodenal hematoma, pancreatic pseudocyst). Always consider pregnancy in any adolescent female who presents to the ED with unexplained nausea and vomiting.

Regurgitation   Unlike vomiting, regurgitation is not accompanied by nausea or forceful abdominal contractions. It is most common in young infants who appear well, are afebrile, and continue to feed normally. Most episodes are due to gastroesophageal reflux (GER), in which gastric contents pass into the esophagus during transient periods of lower esophageal sphincter relaxation. Mild GER is common and without sequelae; severe GER may lead to failure to thrive, esophagitis, and pulmonary disease.

Diagnosis

Differentiate vomiting from *regurgitation* by the lack of nausea, diarrhea, fever, and forceful abdominal contractions in the latter. Inquire about the feeding pattern, frequency of burping, and history of GER. Document the duration and frequency of the vomiting and whether it is projectile. Projectile vomiting is seen in *pyloric stenosis, ulcer disease, sepsis, pyelonephritis, urinary tract obstruction, CNS disease*, and some *metabolic diseases*.

Establish whether the vomiting is bilious. Persistent bilious vomiting suggests intestinal obstruction beyond the ampulla of Vater (*malrotation, intussusception, duodenal hematoma*). Repeated forceful vomiting in the absence of obstruction may be bilious because of reverse peristalsis of small intestine contents.

Inquire about associated fever, abdominal pain, or diarrhea. Vomiting that occurs in the morning suggests *increased intracranial pressure, uremia*, and *pregnancy*. Ask about headache, diplopia, ophthalmoplegia, personality changes, and, in infants, irritability or lethargy. These findings suggest a *CNS lesion*.

ED Management

Vomiting   Assess the patient's hydration status and compare the current and premorbid weights if available. Assess vital signs and hemodynamic status and perform thorough physical and neurologic examinations. If intestinal obstruction is suspected, obtain an upright or decubitus abdominal x-ray. Decompress a patient with bilious emesis with a nasogastric tube and make him or her NPO. Give appropriate IV fluid resuscitation (see pp 202–203) and consult a pediatric surgeon.

Gastroenteritis usually responds to small sips of sugar-containing clear liquids (oral electrolyte solution, sweetened weak tea, decarbonated soda, fruit juice). (See pp 203–204).

Regurgitation   Most infants and children with regurgitation do not require acute treatment in the ED if there are no associated symptoms. In infancy, the majority of infants with GER improve by 6 months of age. Instruct the parents to give the infant frequent small feeds and to keep the baby upright after feeds. Thickening the formula with one level tablespoon of rice cereal for every 2 oz may be helpful. Infants and children with GER and associated failure to thrive, pulmonary disease, anemia, or esophagitis require further evaluation; consult a gastroenterologist.

Follow-up

- Mild or moderate dehydration: primary care follow-up the next day or return to the ED if unable to tolerate clear fluids at home

Indications for Admission

- Significant ongoing fluid losses and/or inability to tolerate oral fluids
- Severe dehydration or altered mental status
- Suspected surgical abdomen

BIBLIOGRAPHY

Murray KF, Christie DL: Vomiting. *Pediatr Rev* 1998;19:337–341.
Pearl RH, Irish MS, Caty MG, et al: The approach to common abdominal diagnoses in infants and children. Part II. *Pediatr Clin North Am* 1998;45: 1287–1326.
Sondheimer JM: Vomiting, in Walker WA, Durie PR, Hamilton JR, et al (eds): *Pediatric Gastrointestinal Disease*. Philadelphia: Decker, 2000, pp 97–102.

PYLORIC STENOSIS

Pyloric stenosis must always be considered in an infant with vomiting, especially if there are signs of dehydration and/or poor weight gain. It is five times more common in boys than in girls, usually occurs in full-term infants, and in about 5 to 7% of cases there is a positive family history in a parent or sibling.

Clinical Presentation

The mean age of onset is 3 weeks. Although symptoms may begin any time after birth, they rarely occur after the fourth month. The characteristic nonbilious, projectile vomiting is intermittent at first. As more complete obstruction develops, vomiting occurs after every feeding. Peristaltic gastric waves, traveling from the left upper quadrant to the right lower quadrant, may be seen during feeding. As the vomiting progresses, dehydration, malnutrition, hyperbilirubinemia, and constipation may develop.

Diagnosis

The diagnosis can be confirmed by palpating a small mobile mass ("olive") slightly above and to the right of the umbilicus. The olive-sized pylorus is best felt after the stomach is emptied and the abdominal wall relaxed. The olive is appreciated in about half of the cases, but patience and experience are needed.

Radiologic studies are unnecessary when the pyloric tumor is palpated. Ultrasound is useful as a screening test in suspected cases and is diagnostic when a hypertrophied pyloric mass is identified (pyloric muscle width >4 mm; pyloric channel length >16 mm). If the ultrasound is negative or unavailable but the clinical picture is suggestive of pyloric stenosis, obtain an upper GI radiographic contrast study. A dilated stomach with outlet obstruction and/or a narrowed, elongated pyloric channel that swings upward (string sign) confirms the diagnosis.

Because the obstruction is proximal to the ampulla of Vater, recurrent vomiting causes a hypokalemic, hypochloremic metabolic alkalosis. The electrolytes are often normal early in the course. The electrocardiogram (ECG) may reflect the hypokalemia (prolonged QT interval, U waves, depression and broadening of the T waves). Elevated hemoglobin and hematocrit levels are secondary to hemoconcentration. Indirect hyperbilirubinemia may also be secondary to decreased glucuronyl transferase activity.

Antral web or *atresia* may cause gastric outlet obstruction, but symptoms occur earlier in life and the radiographic picture is diagnostic. The lack of bile rules out more distal lesions such as *duodenal stenosis, annular pancreas*, and *volvulus*. There is no gastric outlet obstruction in *gastroesophageal reflux*, but this condition may sometimes accompany pyloric stenosis. *Improper feeding practices* (large nipple hole, failure to burp the infant, etc.) and some medical conditions—such as *sepsis, UTIs, neurologic disorders,* and *congenital adrenal hyperplasia*—can present with recurrent vomiting but usually are easily distinguished from pyloric stenosis.

ED Management

If an olive is palpated, make the patient NPO, insert a nasogastric tube, order a urinalysis, and obtain blood for a CBC, electrolytes, and type and hold. Start an IV and give a 20-mL/kg bolus of NS if the infant is markedly volume-depleted. Otherwise, infuse $D_5\frac{1}{4}$ to $D_5\frac{1}{2}$NS at a rate appropriate to the patient's weight and hydration status. When the patient is voiding well, add 20 mEq/L of KCl. Delay surgery until any fluid and electrolyte imbalances are corrected.

If an olive is not appreciated and the patient is well hydrated, observe the parent feeding an oral electrolyte maintenance solution. A patient who does not vomit can be discharged, with daily follow-up. If the patient vomits the feed or appears dehydrated, obtain an ultrasound and admit the infant to the hospital for further evaluation. Obtain a urine culture, blood culture, and venous pH in addition to the laboratory tests outlined above.

Follow-up

- Pyloric stenosis ruled out and patient can tolerate oral fluids: follow up the next day

Indications for Admission

- Suspected pyloric stenosis
- Inability to tolerate oral feedings

BIBLIOGRAPHY

Dinkevich E, Ozuah PO: Pyloric stenosis. *Pediatr Rev* 2000;21:249–250.
Hulka F, Cambell TJ, Cambell JR, et al: Evolution in the recognition of infantile hypertrophic pyloric stenosis. *Pediatrics* 1997;100:E9.
Irish MS, Pearl RH, Caty MG, et al: The approach to common abdominal diagnoses in infants and children. *Pediatr Clin North Am* 1998;45:729–772.

DIARRHEA

Gastroenteritis is second only to respiratory illness as a cause of childhood morbidity worldwide. In the United States, acute gastroenteritis is responsible for 4% of all outpatient visits and up to 10% of hospitalizations among children under 5 years of age.

In developed countries with a temperate climate, most gastroenteritis is caused by viral infection; bacterial, parasitic, and protozoal illnesses are less frequent but not uncommon. In viral infection, diarrhea is noninflammatory and results from an enteropathy in which the death of mature villus-tip cells (responsible for disaccharide digestion and monosaccharide absorption) causes an osmotic diarrhea due to the malabsorption of sugars. The pathophysiology of bacterial diarrhea involves a combination of impaired water absorption due to the inflammatory process and often a secretotoxin elaborated by the bacteria. Invasive bacterial disease in the colon results in frequent small, bloody, often mucoid stools, or dysentery. Occasionally, both toxic and inflammatory processes are operative.

Clinical Presentation

The symptoms and signs of gastroenteritis are vomiting, abdominal pain, and diarrhea, typically with fever.

Rotavirus This is the most common cause of acute noninflammatory gastroenteritis in infants and toddlers. Although the illness is most common in the winter months, it is present year-round. Peak age incidence is 3 to 24 months. Symptoms include fever followed by vomiting in 60 to 90% of patients. The diarrhea caused by disaccharide or monosaccharide malabsorption is watery and nonbloody; it lasts from 3 to 7 days. A similar illness is caused by astroviruses, enteric adenoviruses, and caliciviruses.

Norwalk Virus   This is a calicivirus that causes epidemic outbreaks of gastroenteritis characterized by fever, vomiting, diarrhea, and often malaise and myalgias. Norwalk virus affects school-age children, adolescents, and adults. The illness is brief, lasting from 12 to 48 h.

Salmonella   Nontyphoidal *Salmonella* causes a variable clinical illness that depends on the strain of *Salmonella* as well as on host factors. Symptoms include fever, vomiting, and malaise. *Salmonella* may cause grossly bloody diarrhea. In infants under 1 year of age, bacteremia occurs in 5 to 10% of cases. Infection can be acquired from contaminated food (meat, eggs, poultry) and animals (reptiles such as snakes, turtles, and iguanas) and by person-to-person spread.

Enterohemorrhagic Escherichia coli   In the United States enterohemorrhagic *E. coli* 0157:H7 is the organism most frequently isolated from individuals with bloody diarrhea. Although only 5 to 10% of infected individuals subsequently develop hemolytic uremic syndrome (HUS), *E. coli* 0157:H7 is responsible for 90% of HUS occurring in the United States. Infection with *E. coli* 0157:H7 has a summer predominance, and peak attack rates occur in children less than 5 years old. It has a bovine reservoir and is acquired by ingestion of undercooked meat (especially raw hamburger) or unpasteurized milk or cider or from other infected individuals. The clinical illness is characterized by a watery nonbloody diarrhea that progresses to grossly bloody diarrhea with severe abdominal pain. Severe hematochezia occurs in one-third of patients. Fever, typically low-grade, occurs in one-third of patients. HUS (see pp 602–605) occurs 3 to 12 days after the onset of diarrhea and is characterized by a triad of microangiopathic hemolytic anemia, thrombocytopenia, and oliguria or anuria. Clinically the child is pale, irritable, edematous, and oliguric.

Enterotoxigenic E. coli   This is a noninvasive *E. coli* responsible for a self-limited episode of watery diarrhea. It is the major cause of traveler's diarrhea.

Shigella   The clinical symptoms of *Shigella* vary from a mild illness to the classic form of *Shigella* infection, characterized by the rapid onset of high fever and systemic toxicity, with either large-volume watery stools or dysentery. Seizures can occur early in the illness and often precede the diarrhea. Bloody diarrhea occurs in 50% of affected children.

Campylobacter and Yersinia enterocolitica   Neither *Campylobacter* nor *Yersinia enterocolitica* can be distinguished on clinical grounds from other bacterial diarrheas. Both can cause a mild, self-limited gastroenteritis or severe disease with toxicity and/or dysentery. *Yersinia* most commonly causes enterocolitis but is also known to cause a syndrome of fever, abdominal pain, and minimal diarrhea that may mimic appendicitis or inflammatory bowel disease. *Campylobacter* may cause bloody stools in infants and prolonged symptoms imitating inflammatory bowel disease in older children. *Campylobacter* contaminates poultry, but human infection has also been epidemiologically linked to puppies.

Giardia lamblia   This organism can cause acute watery diarrhea in children, not associated with fever or eosinophilia. Chronic malabsorption may also occur. *Giardia* may contaminate water and has appeared in outbreaks at day care centers.

Antibiotic-Related Diarrhea   This type of diarrhea is most often mild and not complicated by pseudomembranous colitis (PMC). PMC is caused by *Clostridium difficile*. Consider PMC in any child with significant antibiotic-related diarrhea, especially if associated with fever, toxicity, abdominal pain, and bloody or purulent stools.

Chronic Nonspecific (Toddler's) Diarrhea   Suspect this condition in a healthy, well-appearing toddler with normal growth and appetite who has large stools containing food particles. There may be a history of an acute viral or diarrheal illness several weeks or months before. Stool evaluation reveals normal bacterial flora without parasitic infection. Toddler's diarrhea may be exacerbated by excessive intake of fluids and juices.

Diagnosis

Inquire about the onset and duration of symptoms (acute diarrhea lasts <2 weeks), the frequency and volume of vomitus and diarrhea, the appearance of the stool, and associated symptoms such as fever and vomiting. Determine what and how much the child has been eating and drinking. The sorbitol in apple and grape juice may exacerbate diarrhea. Ask about the child's urine output and general activity level.

If there is a history of persistent (>5 days) or bloody diarrhea, test the stool for fecal leukocytes and blood (see Table 9-4) and obtain a stool culture if the tests are positive or the illness suggests a bacterial etiology. *Viral diarrhea* is nonbloody and nonmucoid; malabsorbed sugars are present either as reducing substances or converted to acids; and fecal leukocytes are absent. If indicated (i.e., cohorting of patients during an epidemic, diagnosis unclear, unusually sick patient), send a stool sample for rapid enzyme immunoassay for rotavirus. If the stools are grossly bloody, obtain a culture for bacterial pathogens (*E. coli* 0157:H7, *Salmonella, Shigella, Yersinia, Campylobacter, C. difficile* toxin). Obtain a CBC with platelet count, BUN, creatinine, and electrolytes if the patient has proven *E. coli* 0157:H7 infection or is clinically suspected of having HUS.

In infancy, the differential diagnosis of acute gastroenteritis includes diarrhea associated with other infections such as *urinary tract infection, otitis media, sepsis,* and *pneumonia. Allergic colitis of infancy* presents in the first 3 months of life with mucoid, bloody stools. Despite the name "allergic," peripheral eosinophilia is not a sensitive indicator of colitis. Allergic colitis can occur in infants fed cow's milk, soy formula, or breast milk. All stool cultures are negative, and typically the bleeding stops after switching to an elemental formula (Nutramigen, Alimentum) or eliminating cow's milk from the mother's diet (breast-fed infant). In 20 to 40% of cases, there is cross-reaction with soy formula.

Consider *neuroblastoma* and *ganglioneuroma* in children who have persistent watery diarrhea. Consider *inflammatory bowel disease* in children who have either persistent or bloody diarrhea or diarrhea in con-

Table 9-4   Stool Studies

	FINDINGS	IMPLICATIONS
Gross Examination	Blood, mucus, pus	Bacterial infection
Microscopic Examination Add 1–2 drops of methylene blue to stool mucus, cover with a coverslip, then look for WBCs under high-dry power.	>5 WBC/hpf	Bacterial infection
Chemical Examination *Stool pH* Extract water from diaper and check with urine dipstick.	pH ≤ 5	Viral infection Carbohydrate malabsorption
Stool-reducing substances In a test tube, mix 2 drops of stool water with 10 drops of tap water. Add Clinitest tablet and check for reducing substances (compare with accompanying chart in Clinitest box).	+ Reducing substances	Viral infection Carbohydrate malabsorption

junction with constitutional symptoms, fever, weight loss, oral ulcers, arthralgia, or uveitis. Bulky, greasy, foul-smelling stools are associated with *cystic fibrosis, celiac disease, Schwachmann-Diamond syndrome,* and other forms of *pancreatic insufficiency.*

ED Management

The goals of management include (1) recognition, treatment, and prevention of dehydration; (2) prescription of dietary therapy that maximizes nutrient retention; (3) recognition of invasive or potentially invasive infection; and (4) management of the public health aspects of acute gastroenteritis.

Determination of hydration status is the first priority. Use the patient's premorbid weight, vital signs, and clinical characteristics (Table 9-1) to estimate the degree of dehydration. See pp 201–203 for the management of severe dehydration.

Continue to feed milk to an infant with nondehydrating gastroenteritis, whether breast- or formula-fed. Guidelines for the use of soy formula in acute infantile gastroenteritis do not exist. However, it is reasonable to prescribe a switch to soy formula for an infant less than 6 months of age who develops dehydration, is malnourished (less than fifth percentile weight for height), has a significant underlying medical condition, or has diarrhea that does not improve on cow's milk formula after 5 days of illness.

Empiric antibiotic treatment of suspected bacterial gastroenteritis is rarely necessary and may prolong *Salmonella* excretion. More importantly, antibiotic treatment has been epidemiologically linked to HUS and a worse outcome in *E. coli* 0157:H7 infection.

Treat proven *Shigella* with trimethoprim-sulfamethoxazole (8 mg/kg/day of TMP divided bid) for 5 days and *Campylobacter* with erythromycin (40 mg/kg/day divided tid or qid) for 5 to 7 days. Guidelines for treating *Salmonella* in infants are presented in Table 9-5. Do not treat uncom-

Table 9-5   Management of Infants Less Than 1 Year with Diarrhea Not Requiring Hospitalization at Initial Visit

	AGE	MANAGEMENT
I. First Evaluation		
A. Colitis (dysentery, fecal leukocytes)	0–12 months	Stool culture CBC and blood culture if <3 months or if patient appears ill
B. No colitis or diarrhea <5 days	0–12 months	No stool culture Evaluate for nonbacterial causes
C. History of exposure to *Salmonella*	0–3 months	Stool and blood cultures, CBC
II. Follow-up evaluation		
A. Diarrhea ≥5 days	0–12 months	Stool culture
B. Stool and blood cultures positive*	0–12 months	Admit[†] and treat with antibiotics[‡]
C. Stool culture positive*/ blood culture negative		
1. Toxic, ill, immunocompromised	0–12 months	Admit[†] and treat with antibiotics[‡]
2. Febrile, well-appearing	≤3 months	Admit[†] and treat with antibiotics[‡]
3. Febrile, improving	3–12 months	Blood culture TMP-SMX[§] pending blood culture results
4. Afebrile, improving	≤3 months	Oral antibiotics[¶]
	3–12 months	Reexamine and observe at home
D. Stool culture positive*/ blood culture not obtained at first visit		See category IIC CBC and blood culture

*Stool culture positive for *Salmonella*.
[†]Includes evaluation for focal infection of meninges, bone, urinary tract, and other sites.
[‡]Cefotaxime or ceftriaxone.
[§]8 mg/kg/day of TMP divided bid.
[¶]Oral/TMP-SMX pending sensitivities. If <1 month of age, consult an infectious disease specialist.
Adapted from *Pediatr Infect Dis J* 1988;7:620, with permission.

plicated, noninvasive *Salmonella* infections unless the patient is less than 3 months of age, is immunocompromised, has chronic gastrointestinal disease (inflammatory bowel disease, celiac disease), or has severe colitis.

Treatment of *E. coli* 0157:H7 infection is supportive; consult a nephrologist in the event that HUS develops.

Treat *C. difficile*–associated pseudomembranous colitis for 7 days with oral vancomycin (40 mg/kg/day divided qid) or PO or IV metronidazole (35 mg/kg/day divided qid).

Have all family members practice meticulous hand washing during a diarrheal illness. Report enteric pathogen infection to the public health authorities. Exclude from day care children with diarrhea that overflows the diaper, those with bloody stools until treated or resolved, and patients with *Shigella* or *E. coli* 0157:H7 until stool cultures are negative.

Follow-up

- Mild or no dehydration: contact primary care provider in 2 to 3 days

Indications for Admission

- >5% dehydration
- Failure of oral rehydration
- Inability to take fluids orally
- Febrile infant less than 3 months of age with suspected or proven *Salmonella* enteritis or any child with *Salmonella* bacteremia
- Hemolytic-uremic syndrome complicating *E. coli* 0157:H7 infection
- Severe infection with clinical toxicity caused by any enteric pathogen

BIBLIOGRAPHY

American Academy of Pediatrics: Practice parameter: the management of acute gastroenteritis in young children. *Pediatrics* 1996;97:424–436.

Armon K, Stephenson T, MacFaul R, et al: An evidence and consensus based guideline for acute diarrhoea management. *Arch Dis Child* 2001;85:132–142.

Committee on Infectious Diseases, American Academy of Pediatrics: *Report of the Committee on Infectious Diseases,* 25th ed. Elk Grove, IL: American Academy of Pediatrics, 2000, pp 196–198, 243–247, 493–495, 501–506, 510–514, 638–643.

Pickering LK, Cleary TG: Approach to patients with gastrointestinal tract infections and food poisoning, in Feigin RD, Cherry JD (eds): *Textbook of Pediatric Infectious Disease,* 4th ed. Philadelphia: Saunders, 1998, pp 567–601.

JAUNDICE

The goals of the ED evaluation of the icteric child include rapid diagnosis of the acutely treatable causes of icterus (sepsis, obstruction, metabolic disease), identification of patients in acute or impending liver failure (pp 231–233), prophylaxis of susceptible contacts when icterus is caused by viral hepatitis, and reassurance when jaundice is physiologic or related to breast feeding.

Clinical Presentation

Neonates and Infants
Unconjugated Hyperbilirubinemia   Unconjugated hyperbilirubinemia is characterized by elevation of the indirect bilirubin fraction. The direct

bilirubin is less than 15% of the total, bilirubin is absent from the urine, and the stool color is unaffected. Full-term, well-appearing neonates with unconjugated hyperbilirubinemia are likely to have physiologic jaundice. Bilirubin levels peak at 3 days and then start to decrease, typically resolving by 10 days of life. The total bilirubin generally does not exceed 12 mg/dL at any time, and the direct bilirubin is less than 2 mg/dL. Breast-fed infants may have prolonged unconjugated hyperbilirubinemia lasting several weeks. These infants have no evidence of blood group incompatibility, hemolytic disease, or infection.

Unconjugated hyperbilirubinemia that does not fit the pattern of physiologic or breast-milk jaundice and is not due to hemolytic disorders may be caused by dehydration, polycythemia, hypothyroidism, infection (particularly UTI), Crigler-Najjar syndrome, and pyloric stenosis.

Conjugated Hyperbilirubinemia   In conjugated hyperbilirubinemia, the total bilirubin is elevated, the direct bilirubin is greater than 15% of the total, bilirubin is found in the urine, and the stools may be acholic. Conjugated hyperbilirubinemia is never physiologic. Cholestasis is an indication of hepatocellular dysfunction, biliary obstruction, or a metabolic disorder. In infants, biliary atresia and neonatal hepatitis are the most common etiologies.

Children and Adolescents
Unconjugated Hyperbilirubinemia   The most common causes of unconjugated hyperbilirubinemia are hemolytic disorders. Gilbert's syndrome, typically found in postpubertal children, is characterized by mild, fluctuating unconjugated hyperbilirubinemia with levels between 2 and 5 mg/dL. Children with this disorder have normal liver function and transaminases with no evidence of hemolysis.

Conjugated Hyperbilirubinemia   Toxin-induced or viral hepatitides are the most common etiologies. Clinically apparent icteric hepatitis is most commonly caused by hepatitis A (HAV), hepatitis B (HBV), or hepatitis C (HCV) (see Acute Hepatitis, pp 225–229). Occasionally jaundice may be the initial presentation of a chronic liver disease such as Wilson's disease or autoimmune hepatitis.

Hepatotoxins   The most common hepatotoxic medications are acetaminophen, amiodarone, anticonvulsants, antineoplastics, aspirin, erythromycin, estrogens, haloperidol, halothane, immunosuppressives, isoniazid, ketoconazole, penicillins, retinoids, sulfonamides, and zidovudine. Exposure to environmental toxins such as hydrocarbons, arsenic, and *Amanita* mushrooms can also cause hepatitis.

Diagnosis

Differentiate true icterus from carotenemia—a nonpathologic accumulation of dietary carotene that causes yellow skin color in infants and toddlers without scleral icterus. In the jaundiced child, scleral icterus can be appreciated at a total serum bilirubin concentration of approximately 3.0 mg/dL, so that icterus is often noted before jaundice is appreciated. In newborns, jaundice progresses in a cephalocaudal manner with increasing concentrations of total serum bilirubin.

ED Management

If an infant is jaundiced, obtain total and direct bilirubin levels. Calculate the indirect or unconjugated bilirubin level by subtracting the direct bilirubin from the total bilirubin. Infants with physiologic jaundice may be sent home. The Subcommittee on Hyperbilirubinemia of the American Academy of Pediatrics has published guidelines for the management of hyperbilirubinemia in term infants and recommends that phototherapy be considered in levels >12 mg/dL in a 48-h-old neonate and >15 mg/dL in a 72-h-old neonate (Table 9-6).

If the infant has conjugated hyperbilirubinemia, obtain blood for culture, albumin, hepatic profile, prothrombin time (PT), partial thromboplastin time (PTT), CBC, and hepatitis serologies and urine for culture, urinalysis, and reducing substances. Consult with a gastroenterologist and admit the patient to facilitate the evaluation.

As discussed above, the diagnostic approach to the older child with suspected viral hepatitis is outlined elsewhere. There is no specific therapy for acute viral hepatitis. See the section on liver failure (pp 231–233) if the patient has coagulopathy, hypoglycemia, or encephalopathy or returns to the ED with progressive jaundice.

Table 9-6   Management of Hyperbilirubinemia in the Healthy Term Newborn

	TOTAL SERUM BILIRUBIN LEVEL, MG/DL(μMOL/L)			
AGE (h)	CONSIDER PHOTOTHERAPY*	PHOTOTHERAPY	EXCHANGE TRANSFUSION IF INTENSIVE PHOTOTHERAPY FAILS†	EXCHANGE TRANSFUSION AND INTENSIVE PHOTOTHERAPY
<24‡	—	—	—	—
25–48	>12 (170)	>15 (260)	>20 (340)	>25 (430)
49–72	>15 (260)	>18 (310)	>25 (430)	>30 (510)
>72	>17 (290)	>20 (340)	>25 (430)	>30 (510)

*Phototherapy at these total serum bilirubin levels is a clinical option. It is available and may be used on the basis of individual clinical judgment.

†Intensive phototherapy should produce a decline of total serum bilirubin of 1 to 2 mg/dL within 4 to 6 h, and the total serum bilirubin level should continue to fall and remain below the threshold level for exchange transfusion. If this does not occur, it is considered a failure of phototherapy.

‡Term infants who are clinically jaundiced at <24 h are not considered healthy and require further evaluation.

From American Academy of Pediatrics, Provisional Committee for Quality Improvement and Subcommittee of Hyperbilirubinemia: Practice parameter: management of hyperbilirubinemia in the healthy term newborn. *Pediatrics* 1994;94:558–562, with permission.

Follow-up

- Breast-milk or physiologic jaundice: primary care follow-up the next day

Indications for Admission

- Newborn requiring phototherapy
- Infant with conjugated hyperbilirubinemia
- Fulminant hepatitis, with hypoglycemia, coagulopathy, encephalopathy, or vomiting precluding adequate oral intake

BIBLIOGRAPHY

Dennery PA, Seidman DS, Stevenson DK: Neonatal hyperbilirubinemia. *N Engl J Med* 2001;344:581–590.

Provisional Committee for Quality Improvement and Subcommittee on Hyperbilirubinemia: Practice parameter: management of hyperbilirubinemia in the healthy term newborn. *Pediatrics* 1994;94:558–565.

Whitington PF: Chronic cholestasis in infancy. *Pediatr Clin North Am* 1996; 43:1–26.

HEPATITIS

Viral hepatitis is most commonly caused by the hepatitis A, B, or C viruses. Since 1992, universal vaccination of all infants has been recommended for hepatitis B. Hepatitis A vaccination is also available and is recommended for high-risk individuals.

Hepatitis C (HCV) accounts for approximately 90% of what was formerly known as non-A non-B hepatitis. Intravenous drug use is the major risk factor for acquiring HCV. Patients who have received blood products or tattoos or are undergoing hemodialysis are also at risk. Sexual and perinatal transmission can also occur. As with all forms of hepatitis, HCV occurs in the absence of identifiable risk factors.

Hepatitis D (delta hepatitis) only occurs in patients infected with hepatitis B. Hepatitis E is clinically similar to A but is not endemic in the United States. Consider it only in travelers returning from endemic areas, such as Asia, Africa, and Mexico.

Other infections can cause acute hepatitis. These include Epstein-Barr virus, cytomegalovirus, varicella, *Toxoplasma*, and *Leptospira*. Both icteric and nonicteric hepatitis may also complicate HIV infection.

Clinical Presentation

Anicteric hepatitis is the most common form of hepatitis (more than 90% of cases), and patients may be completely asymptomatic. Clinically apparent icteric hepatitis is most commonly caused by HAV or HBV. During the prodromal phase, viral hepatitis may resemble a flu-like illness or gastroenteritis, with fever, lethargy, anorexia, nausea, vomiting, and right-upper-quadrant abdominal pain for about 1 week. The spleen is usually not palpable except in infectious mononucleosis. In general, the symptoms of HAV, HBV, and HCV are the same. In HBV infection, urticaria, purpura, papular acrodermatitis (Gianotti-Crosti syndrome), arthralgias, or

Table 9-7   Clinical and Epidemiologic Characteristics
of HAV, HBV, and HCV

CLINICAL FEATURES	HAV	HBV	HCV
Peak pediatric incidence	1st decade	2nd decade/ neonatal	2nd decade/ neonatal
Route	Fecal-oral	Parenteral/sexual/ perinatal	Parenteral/sexual/ perinatal
Incubation	15–50 days	40–180 days	15–180 days
Onset	Acute	Subacute	Subacute
Fever > 38.3°C (101°F)	Common	Less common	Rare
Anorexia	Severe	Moderate	Moderate
Nausea/vomiting	Common	Less common	Less common
Rash	Rare	Common	Rare
Arthralgias/arthritis	Rare	Common	Rare
Epidemiologic features			
Common source epidemic (food, water)	Yes	No	No
Day care center contact	Yes	No	No
IV drug use	No	Yes	Yes
Blood, blood products, dialysis	No	Yes	Yes
Homosexuality	?	Yes	Yes

arthritis may also occur. These symptoms resolve rapidly and are followed by the onset of jaundice associated with an enlarged tender liver, dark urine, and pale stools. Lymphadenopathy is not a feature of HAV, HBV, or HCV. The epidemiologic and clinical characteristics are summarized in Table 9-7.

Most young children with hepatitis A are without icterus or jaundice. In hepatitis B the icteric phase lasts 1 to 4 weeks, with complete recovery in most cases. A prolonged cholestatic form is rare in children. In about 0.1 to 1% of all cases, a fulminant hepatitis results in hepatic coma and possibly death. Although infection with HAV is not associated with long-term sequelae, both HBV and HCV hepatitis can progress to chronic liver disease and cirrhosis. Acute hepatitis C can progress to chronic disease in up to 70% of patients, and end-stage liver disease occurs in 10%. There is also a carrier state for HBV that can be asymptomatic or associated with chronic liver disease.

Infectious mononucleosis may manifest itself as isolated hepatitis or a syndrome that includes pharyngitis and splenomegaly. Lymphadenopathy occurs in Epstein-Barr, CMV, and HIV infections.

Diagnosis

If hepatitis is suspected, obtain a CBC, differential, albumin, hepatic profile, PT, PTT, electrolytes, glucose, and an acute hepatitis serology panel [hepatitis B surface antigen (HBsAg), surface antibody (anti-HBs), core antibody (anti-HBc), IgM anti-HAV and anti-HCV, and heterophile antibody]. In general, transaminases [AST (SGOT), ALT (SGPT)] increase during the prodromal period and return to normal after the appearance of jaundice. Conjugated hyperbilirubinemia predominates during the icteric stage, and bilirubin levels may be extremely high if there is associated renal disease or hemolysis. Alkaline phosphatase is elevated, but albumin is normal. Leukopenia with atypical lymphocytes may be seen during the prodrome. Abnormalities of clotting factors occur, and a prolonged PT (>5 s over control) is a poor prognostic sign.

Suspect HAV if the patient is in day care, has just returned from travel to an endemic area, or has a history of possible exposure to contaminated food or shellfish. The presence of anti-HAV IgM confirms HAV infection within the previous 4 weeks, while anti-HAV IgG implies that infection (or successful immunization) occurred more than 4 weeks prior to testing.

The most commonly used test for diagnosing HBV is the surface antigen HBsAg, which appears in the blood 4 to 6 weeks after exposure but 1 week to 2 months before any elevation of the transaminases. HBsAg usually disappears 1 to 13 weeks after the onset of clinical disease. Persistence beyond 6 months defines chronic carriage or chronic hepatitis. Anti-HBs is protective, lasts indefinitely, and implies recovery from infection and absence of infectivity. It does not appear until after resolution of the clinical hepatitis and is usually not measurable until several weeks after the disappearance of HBsAg. There can be a serologic "gap" when both HBsAg and anti-HBsAg are absent from the blood. This gap is filled by core antibody anti-HBc, which is not protective. HBV serology is summarized in Table 9-8.

During the prodromal phase, viral hepatitis may be confused with a flu-like illness or *gastroenteritis*. A tender, enlarged liver, hyperbilirubinuria, and increased transaminases suggest the correct diagnosis. During the icteric stage, consider other causes of jaundice such as *biliary obstruction* (right-upper-quadrant colicky pain and mass), *toxins,* and *drugs. Caroten-*

Table 9-8   Hepatitis B Serology

STAGE OF DISEASE	HBsAg	anti-HBs	anti-HBc
Incubation	+	−	−
Acute illness	+	−	+
Early convalescence (serologic gap)	−	−	+
Resolved infection (<6 months ago)	−	+	+
Postrecovery (infection >6 months ago)	−	+	+
Chronic carrier	+	−	+
Postvaccination	−	+	−

emia occurs in infants and is confirmed by the absence of scleral icterus and a normal serum bilirubin. Other causes of elevated transaminases include *alpha₁-antitrypsin deficiency, Budd-Chiari syndrome, congestive heart failure, Wilson's disease, autoimmune hepatitis,* and *steatohepatitis.* In the neonate, intrauterine infections (TORCH; i.e., toxoplasmosis, other agents, rubella, cytomegalovirus, herpes simplex), metabolic disease (*galactosemia*), *biliary atresia,* and a *choledochal cyst* are the major differential diagnostic problems.

ED Management

The diagnostic approach to a child with suspected viral hepatitis is outlined above. There is no specific therapy for acute viral hepatitis. Intravenous hydration may be necessary for patients with severe vomiting. Corticosteroids are contraindicated. See the section on liver failure (pp 231–233) if the patient has coagulopathy, hypoglycemia, or encephalopathy, or returns to the ED with progressive jaundice.

Postexposure Hepatitis Prophylaxis

In the situation where the serologic status of the source of the exposure is unknown, promptly test the source for acute viral hepatitis serologies (HA IgM, HBsAg, IgM anti-HBc, heterophile) and proceed with prophylaxis for hepatitis A or B if indicated.

Hepatitis A Prophylaxis   Give 0.02 mL/kg IM (3 mL maximum in each buttock for an infant or small child; 5 mL maximum in each buttock for an older child or adolescent) of immune globulin (IG) to all household and sexual contacts of patients with HAV. IG is not effective once there is clinical onset of the disease or if the time from exposure is more than 2 weeks. School contacts and health care personnel attending to a patient with HAV require only good handwashing and stool precautions, not IG prophylaxis. When the index patient is known to be infected with HAV, serologic testing of contacts before IG administration is not necessary. Guidelines for managing outbreaks at day care centers have been developed by the Committee on Infectious Diseases of the American Academy of Pediatrics (see Bibliography).

Hepatitis B Prophylaxis   Postexposure HBV prophylaxis is recommended for known HBV exposure in the following settings: perinatal, sexual, and accidental percutaneous or permucosal exposures. In these circumstances give IM hepatitis B immune globulin (HBIG) and HBV vaccination (at time 0, 1 month, and 6 months). HBIG and vaccination must be given as soon as possible (preferably within 24 h) after exposure. The efficacy of postexposure prophylaxis more than 7 days after an acute exposure is questionable except in sexual exposures, where prophylaxis is recommended for up to 14 days. Doses of HBIG and hepatitis B vaccine vary by the patient's age and by the product (Recombivax and Engerix); consult the product insert.

For household exposures to an acute case of hepatitis B, immunoprophylaxis with both HBIG and hepatitis B vaccine are recommended if there has been an identifiable blood or mucosal exposure (e.g., shared razor or toothbrush); also give prophylaxis to infants (0–12 months of age) if the index case is the infant's mother or primary caregiver. In household exposures without the above circumstances, offer vaccination; prophylaxis with HBIG is not necessary.

Guidelines for percutaneous blood exposures to an unknown and unavailable source and for persons who have been previously vaccinated with hepatitis B vaccine may be found in the *Report of the Committee on Infectious Diseases* (see below).

Follow-up

- Suspected viral hepatitis: primary care follow-up in 2 to 3 days
- After HAV or HBV prophylaxis given: primary care follow-up in 2 to 4 weeks

Indication for Admission

- Fulminant hepatitis with hypoglycemia, coagulopathy, encephalopathy, or vomiting precluding adequate oral intake

BIBLIOGRAPHY

Committee on Infectious Diseases, American Academy of Pediatrics: *Report of the Committee on Infectious Diseases,* 25th ed. Elk Grove, IL: American Academy of Pediatrics, 2000, pp 280–306.

D'Agata D, Balistreri WF: Evaluation of liver disease in the pediatric patient. *Pediatr Rev* 1999;20:376–388.

Jonas MM: Viral hepatitis, in Walker WA, Durie PR, Hamilton JR, et al (eds): *Pediatric Gastrointestinal Disease.* Philadelphia: Decker, 2000, pp 939–964.

GALLBLADDER AND GALLSTONE DISEASE

Three types of gallbladder disease occur in children and adolescents: calculous cholecystitis, acalculous cholecystitis, and acute hydrops of the gallbladder. Transient obstruction of the cystic duct may lead to a brief episode of biliary colic without subsequent cholecystitis.

Calculous Cholecystitis   Calculous cholecystitis occurs when a gallstone obstructs the cystic duct or, less commonly, the common duct. This results in swelling and inflammation of the gallbladder. Factors predisposing to gallstone formation are chronic hemolytic disorders, total parenteral nutrition, chronic liver disease, obesity, pregnancy, malabsorption, a history of abdominal surgery, and a family history of gallstone disease. In younger children there may be no predisposing factors.

Acalculous Cholecystitis   This condition is marked by an acutely distended, inflamed gallbladder in the absence of an obstructing gallstone. It occurs as a postoperative complication or as a result of sepsis or systemic infection, Rocky Mountain spotted fever, typhoid fever, shigellosis, and viral gastrointestinal or respiratory infections. In 50% of cases, acalculous cholecystitis is idiopathic.

Hydrops   Acute hydrops of the gallbladder is an acute swelling of the gallbladder without gallstones. It is primarily recognized as a complication of Kawasaki disease (5–20% of patients) but is also seen in viral hepatitis, streptococcal pharyngitis, staphylococcal infection, Henoch-Schönlein purpura, nephrotic syndrome, mesenteric adenitis, and Sjögren's syndrome.

Clinical Presentation

Calculous Cholecystitis   Biliary colic and acute cholecystitis both present with the sudden onset of noncrampy pain that rapidly becomes severe. In biliary colic the severe pain lasts for 1 to 3 h and then moderates into a dull ache over 30 to 90 min. With cholecystitis, the severe pain persists for more than 6 to 12 h. Most commonly, the pain is in the right upper quadrant or epigastrium. The pain may also be periumbilical or diffuse. In one-third of patients the pain radiates to the back, scapula, shoulder, or arm. There may be anorexia, nausea, vomiting, and low-grade fever. As the gallbladder inflammation progresses, there may be local peritoneal inflammation with associated peritoneal pain.

On physical examination the gallbladder is appreciated in one-third of cases, and there is often guarding of the right upper quadrant. Murphy's sign (inspiratory arrest with deep palpation of the right upper quadrant) and Boas' sign (tenderness or hyperesthesia over the right scapula) may be appreciated. Only 15 to 20% of patients develop jaundice. Two-thirds of cases of acute cholecystitis resolve spontaneously over the course of 2 to 3 days, although there may be progression to gallbladder necrosis and perforation with either localized abscess formation or peritonitis.

Acalculous Cholecystitis and Hydrops   Acalculous cholecystitis and acute hydrops of the gallbladder have a clinical presentation that is indistinguishable from that of gallstone disease. In younger patients, the presentation is nonspecific, with right-sided pain, vomiting, and sometimes fever. There may be a palpable mass at the right costal margin.

Diagnosis

Obtain blood for a CBC, hepatic profile, amylase, lipase, and electrolytes. Only 15 to 20% of patients with gallbladder disease will have jaundice or an abnormal hepatic profile. The differential diagnosis for gallbladder disease includes *retrocecal appendicitis* (fever more likely), *peptic ulcer disease* (pain may be relieved by eating), *pancreatitis* (elevated amylase and lipase), and a *choledochal cyst* (found on ultrasound).

ED Management

If gallbladder disease is suspected, make the patient NPO, secure an IV, obtain the blood tests mentioned above, and obtain an ultrasound. The ultrasound will detect stones, gallbladder or ductal distention, and changes in the gallbladder wall and pancreas; it is usually sufficient to make the diagnosis. In questionable cases, obtain a cholescintigraphic

(HIDA) scan or oral cholecystogram. Nonfilling of the gallbladder is diagnostic of cholecystitis.

If cholecystitis or hydrops is diagnosed, obtain a surgical consultation and defer the administration of any pain medications until the surgeon has seen the patient. Urgent surgery is indicated for peritonitis, perforation, or progression of symptoms with worsening pain and fever while under observation. Do not use ceftriaxone in suspected gallbladder disease, as it may cause sludging of the gallbladder contents.

Indication for Admission

- Suspected cholecystitis or hydrops of the gallbladder

BIBLIOGRAPHY

Lobe TE: Cholelithiasis and cholecystitis in children. *Semin Pediatr Surg* 2000;9: 170–176.

McEvoy CF, Suchy FJ: Biliary tract disease in children. *Pediatr Clin North Am* 1996;43:75–98.

Shaffer EA: Gallbladder disease, in Walker WA, Durie PR, Hamilton JR, et al (eds): *Pediatric Gastrointestinal Disease*. Philadelphia: Decker, 2000, pp 1291–1311.

ACUTE LIVER FAILURE

Acute liver failure is rare in childhood. It results from massive hepatic necrosis or hepatic dysfunction. Early recognition and management are critical in order to prevent irreversible complications (particularly cerebral edema) and to allow for possible liver transplantation. The hepatitis viruses are responsible for 80% of cases of childhood acute liver failure beyond the first month of life.

In neonates, the next most frequent cause is metabolic disease (galactosemia, tyrosinemia, hereditary fructose intolerance, hemochromatosis). In older children, the next most frequent cause is toxin exposure (acetaminophen, valproate, isoniazid, halothane, *Amanita* mushrooms). Wilson's disease must always be considered in a child above 6 years of age who presents with acute liver failure. Acute liver failure may also complicate congenital heart disease, cardiac surgery, myocarditis, congestive heart failure, anoxic events, and malignancies.

Clinical Presentation

Acute liver failure may develop over days or weeks, but in all patients the onset is within 8 weeks of the first symptoms. Hepatic encephalopathy, the hallmark symptom, is present in all patients and is divided into four stages: (1) cognitive impairment, disturbance of sleep-wake cycle, no change in level of consciousness; (2) drowsiness, agitation, and confusion, often with mood swings, asterixis, and hyperreflexia; (3) stuporous but arousable, asleep most of the time, and hyperreflexia; (4) coma, no verbal response, and decerebrate or decorticate posturing to painful stimuli.

Complications of acute liver failure include cerebral edema, coagulopathy, hypoglycemia, renal failure, infection, and electrolyte abnormalities.

Diagnosis

Inquire about possible exposure to hepatitis through blood products, travel, and sexual activity. In the case of infants, also ask about exposure to herpes and cytomegalovirus and obtain a dietary history, concentrating on galactose and fructose. Ask about ingestion of toxic medications (isoniazid, acetaminophen, valproate, propylthiouracil, halothane, ferrous sulfate), cocaine use and glue sniffing, mushroom ingestion (*Amanita*), and exposure to industrial chemicals, chlorinated hydrocarbons, and phosphorus. Ask about previous infections and risks for HIV, as immunodeficient patients are at risk for severe hepatitis.

On physical examination, assess the patient for the presence of jaundice, scleral icterus, viral skin lesions, and purpura or petechiae. Perform a careful abdominal examination, assessing both liver and spleen size, and a meticulous neurologic exam, looking for alterations in mental status and signs of increased intracranial pressure (increased muscle tone, hyperventilation, unequal or dilated pupils with sluggish response to light, focal seizures, papilledema, trismus, posturing or loss of brainstem reflexes). Test for asterixis (a forward flapping of the hand) when the patient's arms are extended and the wrists are dorsiflexed. Smell the breath for fetor hepaticus, which is a musty, sweet, or fecal odor to the breath. Some forms of liver failure occur without marked jaundice, and the liver size may be increased, normal, or small.

Usually there are substantial liver-related enzyme abnormalities. Typically (but not always) the transaminase concentrations are 1000 to more than 80,000 U/L, total bilirubin is >15 mg/dL, the PT is >5 s over control, and the serum albumin is <2.5 g/dL. There can be associated hypoglycemia requiring IV fluids with dextrose concentration >5% and an elevated ammonia level.

ED Management

The priorities in the ED are the prompt recognition of acute liver failure and early management of potential complications, of which cerebral edema is the most acutely life-threatening.

Obtain a CBC with differential, electrolytes, BUN, creatinine, and hepatic profile (AST, ALT, CPK, LDH, alkaline phosphatase, bilirubin, total protein, albumin, PT, PTT, and ammonia). Insert an IV and infuse a 10% dextrose solution at a maintenance rate. Monitor the glucose frequently (every 1 to 2 h) and maintain a serum glucose level of at least 40 to 60 mg/dL. Give fresh frozen plasma and vitamin K (5 mg IM) if the PT is >18 s or there is bleeding.

Admit the patient to an intensive care unit (ICU), where the multisystem complications of acute liver failure can be managed. Treat cerebral edema promptly in the ED. Contact the regional liver transplant center to discuss the possibility of immediate liver transplant.

Indication for Admission

- Acute hepatic failure (encephalopathy, coagulopathy, hypoglycemia)

BIBLIOGRAPHY

Rodés AM: Fulminant liver failure. *Lancet* 1997;349:1081–1085.

Treem WR: Hepatic failure, in Walker WA, Durie PR, Hamilton JR, et al (eds): *Pediatric Gastrointestinal Disease*. Philadelphia: Decker, 2000, pp 179–225.

Whittington PF: Fulminant hepatic failure in children, in Suchy FJ (ed): *Liver Disease in Children*. St. Louis: Mosby, 1994, pp 180–213.

HEPATOMEGALY

It is not unusual to palpate the liver below the costal margin in infants and young children. A liver edge more than 3.5 cm below the costal margin in infants and more than 2 cm below the costal margin in children suggests hepatomegaly. Normal liver spans determined by percussion and palpation are 4.5 to 5 cm at 1 week of age, 7 to 8 cm for 12-year-old boys, and 6 to 6.5 cm for 12-year-old girls.

Clinical Presentation and Diagnosis

Apparent liver enlargement may be caused by downward displacement secondary to *intrathoracic conditions* (hyperinflation, pneumothorax), *subdiaphragmatic* or *retroperitoneal masses,* and *thoracic deformities.*

True liver enlargement results from inflammation, storage disorders, infiltrative processes, congestion, and obstruction. The most common cause of hepatomegaly is *infectious mononucleosis* or a mono-like syndrome (*CMV, toxoplasmosis*). Malaise, weakness, fever, pharyngitis, generalized lymphadenopathy, and splenomegaly are associated findings. Other common causes include *viral hepatitis* (vomiting, jaundice, dark urine, acholic stools), *cirrhosis* and *chronic liver disease* (jaundice, spider angiomata, splenomegaly, ascites, hemorrhoids), hemolytic anemias such as *thalassemia* (peculiar facies, jaundice), and *congestive heart failure* (tachypnea, rales, cardiomegaly, edema).

Serious but less common diseases include *leukemia* (pallor, bleeding, fever), *cystic fibrosis* (failure to thrive, recurrent pulmonary illnesses), and *Reye's syndrome* (vomiting, neurologic dysfunction). Rare etiologies include storage disorders (*Pompe's disease, Tay-Sachs disease, tyrosinemia, von Gierke's disease, galactosemia*), drugs (*acetaminophen overdose, carbon tetrachloride, methotrexate, chlorambucil*), *Wilson's disease, alpha$_1$-antitrypsin deficiency, hepatoma, liver hemangiomatosis, malaria,* and liver abscesses. In the newborn, consider congenital *TORCH* infection, *neonatal hepatitis*, and obstructive conditions (*biliary atresia, choledochal cyst*).

ED Management

If the patient does not appear seriously ill or jaundiced, a mono-like illness is most likely. Obtain a CBC with differential, heterophile antibody, hepatic profile, and hepatitis screen. If the diagnosis remains uncertain, refer the patient for further evaluation.

Jaundice, excessive vomiting, altered mentation, failure to thrive, and abnormal bleeding demand an immediate workup. In addition to the laboratory tests mentioned above, obtain a PT, PTT, and glucose. Further evaluation is dictated by the clinical picture and may include bone marrow aspiration, an abdominal CT scan, liver-spleen scan, liver ultrasound, sweat chloride, alpha$_1$-antitrypsin assay, and/or liver biopsy.

Follow-up

- Hepatomegaly without jaundice or ill appearance: primary care follow-up within 1 week

Indications for Admission

- Signs and symptoms of hepatic failure
- Severe vomiting that prevents adequate oral intake
- Suspicion of serious disease (leukemia, heart failure, cirrhosis, etc.)

BIBLIOGRAPHY

Wolf AD, Lavine JE: Hepatomegaly in neonates and children. *Pediatr Rev* 2000;21:303–310.

COLIC

Colic (paroxysmal fussing of infancy) is a well-accepted entity whose etiology and pathogenesis are poorly understood.

Clinical Presentation

Typically, at 2 or 3 weeks of age, an otherwise well baby begins to become fussy, with periods of prolonged crying after feedings. The behavior peaks at 2 months and typically resolves by 3 months of age, although in 30% of cases the symptoms extend into the fourth and fifth months of life.

In mild cases, the fussiness occurs only in the evening or has some other regular diurnal pattern. There may be associated rhythmic kicking, grimacing, and flatus. Vomiting, diarrhea, constipation, and failure to thrive are not features of colic and, between episodes, the infant appears comfortable and alert. The crying may not respond to the parents' attempts at comforting or may stop only to resume when the infant is put down. Notably, the physical and neurologic examinations are normal. In the ED, the parents are concerned about the baby being ill or are exhausted and want relief.

Diagnosis

The key to making the diagnosis of colic is the parents' statement that the infant is perfectly fine between paroxysms. Perform a complete physical examination. If the baby cries during the examination, have him or her suck on a gloved finger or nipple. If this does not stop the crying, place the infant in the prone position or over your shoulder. When distracted, the colicky baby will appear alert and will suck vigorously on a nipple or pacifier. Upon gentle palpation, the abdomen is soft and nontender.

Systemic infections (*sepsis, meningitis, urinary tract infection, septic arthritis, osteomyelitis, pneumonia*), *supraventricular tachycardia, heart failure, congenital glaucoma*, and *infantile spasms* can present with nothing more than fussiness. With these illnesses, however, the infant may be lethargic, be feeding less vigorously, or have fever, vomiting, diarrhea, or constipation. Also, a diurnal pattern of fussiness will be absent. Colic is less likely if the parents describe an overall change in the baby's behavior.

Diarrhea (*gastroenteritis*) or *constipation* may be associated with crampy abdominal pain that may mimic colic. However, the diagnosis of colic cannot be made if either of these symptoms is present. Other considerations include allergy presenting as *allergic colitis* (guaiac-positive stools) and *gastroesophageal reflux* with esophagitis (regurgitation, irritability related to feeds).

Volvulus or *intussusception* may initially present with crampy pain. However, vomiting quickly ensues, followed by signs of intestinal obstruction and rectal bleeding.

Other causes of constant crying include *incarcerated hernia, corneal abrasion*, and *hair tourniquet syndrome* (pp 685–688).

ED Management

The goal of the ED examination is to rule out other conditions that can present with colicky pain. Perform a complete physical examination, including a rectal exam with stool for guaiac. Once the diagnosis is made, reassure the parents that the infant is not seriously ill and that colic is a self-limited phenomenon among well infants. There is no definite cure or universally accepted therapy for colic. Instead, the lack of a recognized etiology has led to the existence of a number of controversial remedies. Dispel any of the commonly held myths about colic, including the idea that medications are beneficial, that infants are "spoiled" by excessive holding, and that colic is caused by parental inexperience and anxiety. Reassure the parents and offer them suggestions that may mitigate a crying attack, such as increased holding and rocking of the baby, more frequent feeding, use of a pacifier, and environmental changes (stroller ride, infant swing, car ride). Avoid antispasmodics, which have not proved effective and may have side effects. Encourage the parents to burp the infant frequently during and after the feeding if they are not already doing so.

If there is suspicion of cow's milk allergy (blood or mucus in stool), change to an elemental formula. Do not advise a nursing mother to discontinue breast feeding but have her try a dairy-free diet for several days.

Follow-up

- Primary care follow-up within the week
- Arrange for psychosocial support if the family can no longer cope with the crying

BIBLIOGRAPHY

Barr RG: Colic and crying syndromes in infants. *Pediatrics* 1998;102:1282–1286.
Friedman EH: Infantile colic. *Arch Pediatr Adolesc Med* 1996;150:770–771.
Wade S, Kilgour T: Extracts from "clinical evidence": infantile colic. *BMJ* 2001;
    323:437–440.

CONSTIPATION

Despite the nonemergent nature of constipation, it is a common cause of ED visits. Constipation may be a transient disturbance precipitated by a brief illness, an anal fissure, a traumatic toileting experience, or a period of poor diet. A very small number of patients have an organic disorder causing their constipation, such as Hirschsprung's disease, hypothyroidism, hypo- or hypercalcemia, neuromuscular dysfunction related to a spinal cord lesion, or medication-related constipation (iron, anticonvulsants, anticholinergics). The majority of children suffer from functional or idiopathic constipation.

Clinical Presentation

In infancy, stools tend to be pasty or "mustard-like" in consistency. More than 90% of infants in the first 4 to 5 months of life have between one and seven bowel movements (BMs) per day, although the frequency in breast-fed infants ranges from a small stool with each feeding to one soft stool every 7 days. In addition, it is common for infants to strain and grunt with defecation and passage of soft stools; this is not considered constipation. Rather, stool consistency (hard, pellet-like, or adult-like formed stools), not frequency, defines constipation in infancy.

In contrast, children over 2 years of age may develop an impaction with overflow or chronic incomplete evacuations. Therefore neither a history of soft stool consistency (overflow) nor daily BMs (incomplete evacuation) rules out constipation. However, after infancy, the most common presentation of constipation is hard, infrequent, large, or painful stools. After the child is toilet trained, constipation is frequently not recognized until it causes other symptoms. The toddler may begin to voluntarily withhold large hard stools. The parents of these children may not recognize "stool withholding" behavior or may confuse the behaviors (stiffening, crying out, clinging to parents, hiding, dancing around) with abdominal pain. In school-age children, constipation may be associated with acute or chronic abdominal pain. The pain may be so intense that it may mimic appendicitis or intussusception.

Encopresis (fecal soiling) is frequently encountered in the ED. This is rarely deliberate but occurs secondary to fecal seepage around an impaction and/or chronic incomplete eliminations. Because diminished rectal sensation is usual in this condition, the patient usually presents with a complaint of diarrhea rather than constipation and stool overflow.

Diagnosis

Always ask about the onset and duration of symptoms, whether there was delay in passing meconium (>24 h) at birth (*Hirschsprung's disease*), and whether there were symptoms in the neonatal period. Obtain a complete dietary history, including fluid intake, toileting history, and medication use (including prior therapy for constipation). Establish whether there are associated symptoms such as abdominal distention, vomiting, poor weight gain and growth (*Hirschsprung's disease*), or the recent onset of gait abnormalities, urinary incontinence, or lower extremity weakness (neurologic signs of a *lower spinal lesion*).

On physical examination, always assess growth by plotting the child's weight and height on a growth chart. On the abdominal examination, determine whether there is distention or palpable retained stool in the abdomen. Before performing a rectal examination, inspect the sacrum for signs of a hair tuft or deep dimple that may indicate an underlying *dysraphism* or *lipoma*. Perform a careful neurologic examination of the lower extremities, focusing on tone, strength, reflexes, sensation, and gait. Inspect the perineal tissues and anus for local inflammation, fissures, and fecal soiling. Assess placement of the anus relative to the tip of the coccyx and the vaginal fourchette or base of the scrotum. Markedly anterior placement of the anus can cause constipation by creating a shelf at the perineum that obstructs the exit of stool.

Perform a rectal examination. Assess anal sphincter tone, rectal size, and the size and consistency of stool in the rectum. A properly done rectal examination should not be painful or traumatic to the child. If the child has signs or symptoms of constipation but has a normal rectal examination, obtain an abdominal flat plate to assess radiographically whether there is fecal retention proximal to the rectum.

Functional or *idiopathic constipation* is strongly suggested by a normal physical examination with normal rectal tone and often an enlarged rectal vault with a retained large or hard stool mass.

Consider *Hirschsprung's disease* if there is a history of delayed meconium passage in the first 24 h of life. Patients who are not diagnosed in the first year of life typically have refractory constipation with distention, vomiting, and growth failure. Typically, a narrow, empty rectum is noted on digital examination. An explosive stool may follow the removal of the examiner's finger.

Hypothyroidism is characterized by coarse features, growth failure, weakness, and developmental delay. *Denervating lesions* of the lower spine are characterized by overflow incontinence or soiling and are often associated with other neurologic symptoms such as lower extremity weakness, areflexia, sensory loss, and urinary symptoms.

Other rare organic causes of constipation include *infant botulism, hypo-* or *hypercalcemia, hypokalemia, diabetes insipidus*, and *congenital muscle disease*. These disorders all have other clinical features that distinguish them from functional constipation.

ED Management

The ultimate goals of treatment are to establish dietary and behavioral patterns in the child and family that compensate for a tendency to constipation. Dietary alterations must include adequate fluid intake; behavioral changes must include toileting that utilizes the gastrocolic reflex. In addition, medical management is often necessary to relieve a fecal impaction, stimulate gastrointestinal motility, or hydrate stool while dietary and behavioral adjustments are made. Medications for constipation have a large therapeutic range, and therapeutic failures due to inadequate dosing occur frequently.

For an infant <6 months old, advise the parents to add 5 to 10 mL of malt extract or dark Karo syrup to the formula three times daily. The dosage may be doubled or halved depending on the infant's response. Do not substitute honey owing to the associated risk of infantile botulism. An infant 6 to 12 months of age requires dietary manipulation in addition to the therapy outlined above. Add barley cereal, prunes, and prune juice to the diet and avoid rice cereal and bananas.

Toddlers and children >10 kg with an impaction require cleaning out with up to two hypertonic phosphate enemas (3 mL/kg/dose) daily until no hard stool is produced, for up to a total of 3 days. Children who weigh >40 kg can have an adult enema. Hypertonic enemas are contraindicated in congestive heart failure and impaired renal function. In addition, initiate therapy with mineral oil (2 mL/kg bid, mixed with fluids) while making dietary adjustments, such as increasing fluids and decreasing dairy intake (particularly milk). Do not use mineral oil if the patient is <2 years of age, neurologically impaired, or has a diminished gag reflex, as there is a risk of aspiration. Add senna syrup (Senokot) ½ to 1 tsp PO bid (maximum 5 mL bid, 1–5 years; 10 mL bid, 5–15 years) to stimulate defecation. Arrange primary care follow-up.

The treatment of encopresis requires an organized, ongoing commitment to the child and family. If there is no evidence of obstruction and the child cannot be cleaned out as an outpatient, admit the patient for continuous polyethylene glycol (25–40 mL/kg/h to 1.2–1.8 L/h until 4 L are administered) via a nasogastric tube, pending clinical response. The required volume requires hospitalization for appropriate administration in a young child. An older child may take the polyethylene glycol electrolyte solution orally (25–40 mL/kg/h until 4 L are administered) until the fecal effluent is free of large fecal masses. Instruct the parents to give a clear liquid diet concomitantly. Arrange follow-up with the primary provider so that the patient can be placed on an appropriate maintenance laxative regimen.

Follow-up

- Constipation without impaction: primary care follow-up in 1 to 2 weeks
- Impaction: 2 days
- Encopresis: at completion of clean-out phase

Indications for Admission

- Severe constipation requiring disimpaction
- Serious underlying disorder (Hirschsprung's disease)

BIBLIOGRAPHY

Abi-Hanna A, Lake AM: Constipation and encopresis in childhood. *Pediatr Rev* 1998;19:23–31.

Loening-Baucke V: Encopresis and soiling. *Pediatr Clin North Am* 1996;43: 279–298.

Youssef NN, DiLorenzo C: Childhood constipation: evaluation and treatment. *J Clin Gastroenterol* 2001;33:199–205.

INTUSSUSCEPTION

Intussusception is the most frequent cause of intestinal obstruction in infants beyond the immediate newborn period. It can occur at any age, although approximately two-thirds of cases are seen in the first year of life. Although the most common type is an ileocolic intussusception, intussusception may occur at any level of the GI tract.

In the majority of cases, no etiology for the intussusception is identified. However, a lead point such as a polyp, lymphoma, or Meckel's diverticulum is seen in 5 to 10% of cases, especially in patients >6 years of age. Mesenteric venous engorgement due to compression between the layers of the intussuscepted bowel causes mucous secretion and blood seepage, leading to the typical currant jelly stools. Later, necrosis of the bowel with subsequent perforation and peritonitis can occur.

Clinical Presentation

Intussusception occurs primarily in healthy, well-nourished infants. Occasionally there is a history of a recent upper respiratory infection, diarrheal illness, or Henoch-Schönlein purpura. Characteristically, intermittent bouts of colicky pain occur more or less regularly at 10- to 15-min intervals. During these paroxysms, the baby may cry out, draw up its legs, and appear extremely uncomfortable. Between episodes, the child may initially appear well but eventually becomes lethargic and apathetic. Vomiting follows the pain and the vomit may contain bile, suggesting an intestinal obstruction. Classic currant jelly stools are present early in only 10% of cases but are eventually seen in 90% of infants and 65% of older children. In some cases, a currant jelly stool is found only with a rectal examination. Constipation, nonspecific diarrhea, and fever may also occur. With recurrent intussusception and spontaneous reduction, symptoms may be subacute or chronic over a period of a few days to weeks.

Initially the abdomen is soft between episodes of pain, but later it becomes distended and tender. In 85% of cases a sausage-like mass can be palpated in the right lower quadrant or upper abdomen. When the intussusception has progressed into the transverse colon, there may be absence of palpable viscera in the right lower quadrant (Dance's sign). An abdominal mass may be appreciated on rectal examination, and blood on the examining finger is occasionally the first sign of the diagnosis. Bowel sounds are initially hyperactive and then become hypoactive or absent.

Occasionally lethargy will be the most prominent presenting sign. A history of crampy abdominal pain and vomiting demands a careful physical examination for an abdominal mass and rectal bleeding. Consider the possibility of intussusception in any child with acute onset of encephalopathy.

ED Management

If intussusception is suspected, immediately notify a pediatric surgeon and radiologist. Insert a nasogastric tube and an IV. Obtain a CBC with differential, type and cross-match, and serum electrolytes. A WBC of 10,000 to 18,000/mm^3 is common, while a higher leukocyte count suggests bowel necrosis. Initiate fluid resuscitation if the child is dehydrated, but do not allow this to delay definitive treatment.

Obtain an abdominal x-ray, which may show dilated small bowel loops, absence of air distal to the obstruction, and a soft tissue mass, usually in the transverse colon. Normal films, however, do not exclude the diagnosis. Ultrasound, in experienced hands, has high diagnostic accuracy. The characteristic ultrasound appearance of an intussusceptum viewed transversely is the target sign. When ultrasound is unavailable, barium enema remains the diagnostic study of choice with barium trickling around the intussusceptum, revealing the level of obstruction and a typical coiled spring appearance. In 70 to 80% of cases, nonoperative hydrostatic reduction occurs during the diagnostic barium enema. In some institutions, fluoroscopically monitored pneumatic (air) reduction is the standard procedure, with an 85 to 90% success rate and low rate of perforation. Prior to the procedure, sedate the patient with IV morphine (0.1 mg/kg).

If there are clinical signs of perforation or shock, pneumatic or hydrostatic reduction is absolutely contraindicated. Give IV antibiotics [ampicillin (100 mg/kg/day divided q 6 h), gentamicin (7.5 mg/kg/day divided q 8 h) and clindamycin (40 mg/kg/day divided q 6 h)] and arrange for surgery. Surgery is also indicated if pneumatic or hydrostatic reduction is unsuccessful.

Indication for Admission

- Suspected intussusception

BIBLIOGRAPHY

Brandt ML: Intussusception, in McMillan JA, DeAngelis CD, Feigin RD, Warshaw JB (eds): *Oski's Pediatrics.* Philadelphia: Lippincott Williams & Wilkins, 1999, pp 1652–1654.
DiFiore JW: Intussusception. *Semin Pediatr Surg* 1999;8:214–220.
Shiels WE II: Childhood intussusception: management perspectives in 1995. *J Pediatr Gastroenterol Nutr* 1995;21:15–17.

UPPER GASTROINTESTINAL BLEEDING

Upper gastrointestinal (UGI) bleeding is always concerning and occasionally life-threatening. By definition, the source of an UGI bleed is proximal to the ligament of Treitz.

Clinical Presentation

A patient with an UGI bleed may present with any or a combination of the following: (1) hematemesis, which is vomiting of bright-red blood or coffee-ground material; (2) melena, which is a tarry black stool; (3) hematochezia, which is bright-red blood per rectum seen in severe and rapid UGI bleeding; and (4) hemodynamic instability (dizziness, dyspnea, shock).

Etiologies of UGI bleeding include peptic disease such as esophagitis, gastritis, duodenitis, and ulcers (esophageal, gastric, duodenal) as well as Mallory-Weiss tears and esophageal varices. The remaining causes, including foreign body and caustic ingestion, gastric outlet obstructions, and inflammatory bowel disease, are listed in Table 9-9.

Table 9-9   Etiologies of Upper Gastrointestinal Bleeding

Newborn/infant

Swallowed maternal blood	Upper GI obstruction
Peptic disease	Foreign body or caustic ingestion
Gastritis	Hemorrhagic disease of the newborn
Ulcer (gastric, duodenal)	Coagulopathy
Esophagitis	Esophageal varices
Duodenitis	

Child

Peptic disease	Foreign body or caustic ingestion
Gastritis	Esophageal or gastric tumors
Ulcer (esophageal, gastric, duodenal)	Vascular malformation
Duodenitis	Hemobilia
Esophagitis	Swallowed blood
Mallory-Weiss tear	Pulmonary hemorrhage
Esophageal varices	Trauma (duodenal hematoma)
Crohn's disease	Munchausen by proxy
Coagulopathy	

Diagnosis

The presence of blood must be confirmed. Red-colored foods or medications can easily be mistaken for blood in patients who present with presumed hematemesis. When the only evidence of bleeding is melena, the diagnosis of a UGI bleed must be confirmed by passing a nasogastric tube and aspirating the stomach contents. Test the material with guaiac, Gastrocult, or Hemoccult.

On physical examination, focus on the vital signs (including orthostatic changes) and signs of shock (skin color and temperature, capillary refill). Examine the nose and pharynx carefully for a source of bleeding. Note any petechiae or purpura suggesting a *coagulopathy*. On abdominal examination, look for splenomegaly, hepatomegaly, or caput medusae (*varices*). Note that in acute variceal bleeding the spleen (now decompressed) may assume a normal size.

Hematemesis may result from *swallowed blood from a nasal, pharyngeal, dental,* or *pulmonary source*. Always ask about epistaxis, pharyngitis, recent dental work, orofacial trauma, and hemoptysis. A neonate may vomit *maternal blood* swallowed during delivery; this is differentiated from fetal blood by the Apt test. In addition, a breast-fed infant may also present with hematemesis due to maternal *mastitis*.

Always ask about recent medication use, including over-the-counter products that may contain *aspirin* or other *nonsteroidal anti-inflammatories*. Other medications associated with UGI bleeding include *anticoagulants, tolazoline,* and *steroids*. Consider *alcoholic gastritis* in adolescents.

In a newborn who has had an anoxic event, stressful delivery, or serious infection, suspect *hemorrhagic gastritis* or *stress ulcers*. Also in this age group, UGI bleeding may complicate *gastric outlet obstruction* and *pyloric stenosis*. *Gastric volvulus* is associated with pain, abdominal distention, and retching. *Coagulopathy* causing UGI bleeding is suggested by petechiae, purpura, or other sites with oozing blood. Infants with *peptic disease, esophagitis, gastritis,* and *ulcers* present with nonspecific signs and symptoms, including regurgitation, vomiting, irritability, and poor feeding.

Suspect an *esophageal foreign body* or *caustic ingestion* when there is an antecedent choking event, drooling, or refusal to swallow. *Esophageal varices* may occur as a result of portal vein thrombosis secondary to umbilical vein catheterization, omphalitis, or congenital anomalies or as a consequence of liver disease. Suspect varices when UGI bleeding is voluminous and/or painless. An antecedent history of splenomegaly or prematurity also raises the possibility of varices.

In young children, *peptic disease* is difficult to diagnose. Both the typical ulcer pain and the history of pain relief with eating may be absent. More often there is generalized abdominal pain. Nocturnal or early morning pain and pain related to meals (food may either exacerbate or relieve pain) are suggestive of peptic disease. Adolescents may have more classic symptoms. Always ask if there is a family history of peptic ulcer disease, *Helicobacter pylori,* or inflammatory bowel disease. When hematemesis follows forceful or repeated vomiting or retching, suspect a *Mallory-Weiss tear.*

ED Management

Unstable Patient

The priority is the recognition and treatment of shock. Begin fluid resuscitation if the patient has orthostatic changes, tachycardia, prolonged capillary refill, and/or altered sensorium. Elevate the patient's legs, administer oxygen, start two large-bore IVs, and give a fluid bolus with 20 mL/kg of NS or Ringer's lactate. Obtain a stat CBC with platelets and type and cross-match. If coagulopathy or liver disease is suspected, obtain a PT, PTT, albumin, and liver-related enzymes. Correct coagulation defects, if present, with vitamin K (5 mg IM), fresh frozen plasma (10 mL/kg), or platelets. Have packed RBCs available and give a transfusion if there is brisk bleeding associated with anemia and hemodynamic compromise (see Bleeding, pp 302–306). Pass a nasogastric tube and lavage with 3 to 5 mL/kg of *room temperature* NS. This will reduce the volume of blood loss but does not stop the bleeding. However, a UGI bleed is not always detected with lavage. Assess continued bleeding by repeated lavages. In the rare instance when persistent UGI bleeding is brisk enough to require ongoing transfusions, consult a pediatric surgeon or gastroenterologist for vasopressin or octreotide therapy or to arrange for emergent measures to control the bleeding.

Stable Patient

If the patient is hemodynamically stable, obtain the same laboratory studies, pass a nasogastric tube, and lavage to detect acute ongoing bleeding. Treat ongoing bleeding with lavage and an H_2 antagonist (ranitidine 1 mg/kg IV q 8 h). Upper endoscopy is indicated for ongoing bleeding, UGI bleeding accompanied by peptic symptoms, and a significant drop in hematocrit regardless of the presence of active bleeding. Continue antacid therapy and/or an H_2 antagonist such as ranitidine 1 to 2 mg/kg IV q 8 h (50 mg maximum) pending endoscopy.

A hemodynamically stable patient who presents with hematemesis without peptic symptoms may be discharged if not actively bleeding. Observe the patient for several hours and document that the hematocrit is normal, stool guaiac is negative, and gastric lavage is clear.

Follow-up

- Hemodynamically stable patient without active bleeding: 1 to 2 days

Indication for Admission

- UGI bleeding, unless hemodynamically stable without ongoing bleeding or peptic symptoms

BIBLIOGRAPHY

Ament ME: Diagnosis and management of upper gastrointestinal tract bleeding in the pediatric patient. *Pediatr Rev* 1990;12:107–116.

Squires RH Jr: Gastrointestinal bleeding. *Pediatr Rev* 1999;20:95–101.

LOWER GASTROINTESTINAL BLEEDING

Lower gastrointestinal (LGI) bleeding is a common complaint during childhood. Most LGI bleeds are minor and not hemodynamically significant. Although severe LGI bleeding is rare, it demands a careful, coordinated approach.

Clinical Presentation

Patients with an LGI bleed may present with hematochezia, melena, or occult blood loss without gross blood. Hematochezia is bright- or dark-red blood per rectum and is usually indicative of colonic or rectal bleeding but can be seen with a severe, rapid upper GI bleed. Melena is tarry jet-black stool that is characteristically malodorous. Melena implies blood loss of 50 to 100 mL/day, usually from an upper GI source. Melena can also be seen with bleeding from the small intestine or ascending colon.

The most common etiologies of LGI bleeding are discussed below and summarized in Table 9-10.

Table 9-10 Etiologies of Lower Gastrointestinal Bleeding

Anal fissure (most common)	Inflammatory bowel disease
Coagulopathy	Intussusception
Colitis	Massive upper GI bleeding
Allergic (infancy)	Meckel's diverticulum
Infectious	Polyp
Inflammatory	Swallowed blood (newborn)
Pseudomembranous	Vascular malformations
Hemolytic uremic syndrome	Volvulus
Henoch-Schönlein purpura	

Anal Fissure   Anal fissures are the most common cause of LGI bleeding, particularly in infants. A small amount of blood is passed following defecation or the stool is streaked with blood. Typically there is a history of constipation or the passage of a painful, firm stool. On examination, a tear in the rectal mucosa or a sentinel skin tag is noted. The patient usually appears well.

Colitis   This is the passage of frequent bloody, mucoid stools. Infectious colitis can present with abdominal pain, tenesmus, and blood and mucus admixed with the stool. Bacterial etiologies include *Salmonella, Shigella, Yersinia, Campylobacter,* and *E. coli.* Infection with *E. coli* 0157:H7 has been associated with the hemolytic uremic syndrome and can present as severe hemorrhagic colitis. Pseudomembranous colitis secondary to *Clostridium difficile* can occur if the patient was recently treated with antibiotics. Cow's milk protein allergy is the most common cause of rectal bleeding in an infant but can also occur in a breast-fed infant if the mother is ingesting milk. An infant with Hirschsprung's enterocolitis usually has a history of constipation.

Inflammatory Bowel Disease   Inflammatory colitis secondary to ulcerative colitis or Crohn's disease may present at any age. Children with ulcerative colitis or Crohn's disease typically have a history of fever, diarrhea, weight loss or poor weight gain or growth, abdominal pain, skin rash, and/or joint pain.

Polyps   Many cases of LGI bleeding in children over 1 year of age are due to polyps. The patient presents with an episode of painless bright-red rectal bleeding or a recurrent pattern of blood in the stool. The physical examination is typically unremarkable unless the polyp is seen protruding from the rectum or palpated on digital examination. Most cases involve a single polyp. There is no associated diarrhea, severe pain, or weight loss. Severe bleeding due to a polyp is unusual and raises the possibility of other diagnoses. There are several syndromes with multiple polyps and cutaneous findings, such as Peutz-Jeghers (perioral pigmentation), Gardner's (bony and soft tissue tumors), and Cronkhite-Canada (alopecia, dystrophic nails) syndromes.

Intussusception   Intussusception classically causes the triad of intermittent colicky abdominal pain, currant jelly stools, and vomiting. It is most common in children 3 months to 3 years of age, with two-thirds of cases occurring in infants <1 year of age. Older children are likely to have a tumor (lymphoma), Meckel's diverticulum, or polyp, which acts as a lead point. The most common presentation is that of a well child who suddenly draws up his or her legs and cries out in pain. The discomfort subsides and the cycle begins again. Occasionally lethargy will be the most prominent presenting sign. A tender, sausage-shaped mass may be noted in the right upper quadrant, while the right lower quadrant feels empty.

Volvulus   A midgut volvulus causes bright-red or maroon LGI bleeding in an infant or toddler. Bilious vomiting can occur secondary to intestinal obstruction and an abdominal mass may be noted. Malrotation with midgut volvulus is a surgical emergency.

Meckel's Diverticulum   The most frequent cause of voluminous LGI bleeding in an otherwise healthy child is a Meckel's diverticulum. There is painless massive bleeding without hematemesis and the physical examination is unremarkable. Anemia may occur due to repeated bleeding episodes.

Henoch-Schönlein Purpura   Henoch-Schönlein purpura may present with colicky abdominal pain and LGI bleeding with or without arthralgias and hematuria. The characteristic symmetric purpuric rash, found primarily on the extensor surfaces of the lower extremities and buttocks, helps to confirm the diagnosis.

Vascular Malformations   Both syndromic and nonsyndromic forms of vascular malformations may cause GI bleeding. Capillary hemangiomas typically present with painless bleeding. Fifty percent of affected children will also have cutaneous hemangiomas. In the blue-rubber bleb syndrome there are small (<1 cm), dark, cutaneous and gastrointestinal hemangiomas. Hereditary hemorrhagic telangiectasias may present with painless UGI or LGI bleeding. These patients have telangiectasias on the lips, tongue, ears, fingertips, or nail beds.

Other Etiologies   Any cause of a severe upper GI bleed may present as lower GI bleeding. Gastroesophageal varices may cause massive UGI bleeding. The patient may have signs of chronic liver disease (splenomegaly, jaundice, caput medusae). Congenital or acquired blood dyscrasias or coagulation disorders will rarely present solely with GI bleeding. Intestinal duplication may contain ectopic gastric mucosa and mimic a Meckel's diverticulum.

Diagnosis

Determine that the red or black color in the stool is truly blood by obtaining stool for guaiac. *Beets, gelatin, artificially colored drinks,* and certain medications may turn the stools red. *Iron, Pepto-Bismol, spinach,* and *licorice* can cause stools to have a dark appearance. Occasionally *genitourinary tract bleeding* can be confused with LGI bleeding, especially in patients wearing diapers.

Bright-red blood or streaking of blood on the stool surface suggests a low rectal lesion (*fissure, polyp*). Flecks of blood admixed with mucus in a diarrheal stool is indicative of colonic inflammation (*gastroenteritis, pseudomembranous colitis, milk-protein intolerance, inflammatory bowel disease*). Blood originating from the small bowel (*polyp, gastroenteritis, intussusception, Henoch-Schönlein purpura, Meckel's diverticulum, vascular malformation*) varies from dark to bright red depending on volume and transit time. Melena in association with UGI bleeding is caused by lesions above the ligament of Treitz (*varices, ulcers, swallowed blood*) but has also been reported in bleeding Meckel's diverticuli and other sources of bleeding in the ascending colon. Consider *duodenal bleeding* as a cause of melena in older children and adolescents with peptic symptoms.

Once the presence of blood is confirmed, inquire about a history of fever, vomiting, diarrhea, or constipation. Ask about aspirin or steroid use (*ulcer, gastritis, erosion*); prior antibiotic use (*pseudomembranous colitis*); previous bleeding episodes (*Meckel's diverticulum, polyps*); weight loss or arthralgias (*inflammatory bowel disease*); and jaundice, liver disease, or a complicated neonatal course with umbilical vein catheterization (*varices*). On examination look for signs of *liver disease* (jaundice, hepatospleno-megaly, caput medusae), purpura (*Henoch-Schönlein purpura*), perioral pigmentation (*Peutz-Jeghers syndrome*), an abdominal mass (*intussusception, volvulus*), and *anal fissure* or sentinel tag. Perform a rectal examination on all patients to check for polyp, mass, intussusception, and constipation and to test the stool for blood.

If the patient is having bloody diarrhea, a *bacterial etiology* is suggested by the presence of neutrophils in the stool. Smear a small amount of stool onto a slide, add two drops of methylene blue, and cover with a coverslip. Wait several minutes, then examine the specimen for polymorphonuclear leukocytes (PMNs) under high power. An afebrile, nontoxic young infant (younger than 4 months) with small amounts of blood and mucus in the stool and negative stool cultures may have *cow's milk protein intolerance*. This can occur in breast-fed as well as bottle-fed infants.

ED Management

Stabilization of the vital signs is the priority. Check for signs of volume depletion (orthostatic vital sign changes, skin color and temperature, capillary filling, mental status). If volume depletion is present or bleeding is ongoing in the ED, insert a large-bore IV and resuscitate with isotonic fluid followed by whole blood if bleeding persists (see Shock, pp 18–22). Obtain blood for a CBC, spun hematocrit, platelet count, PT and PTT, type and cross-match, electrolytes, glucose, and liver function test and consult a radiologist and a pediatric surgeon.

If the patient has a significant unexplained LGI bleed, insert a nasogastric tube and lavage with 5 mL/kg of *room temperature* normal saline. Bright-red blood or coffee grounds on lavage is consistent with a UGI source of bleeding. However, a negative lavage does not rule out a duodenal bleeding site.

Obtain an abdominal flat-plate x-ray in any child whose LGI bleeding is associated with vomiting or abdominal pain to look for signs of intestinal obstruction (intussusception, volvulus, duplication). Brisk, painless bleeding is most often due to a Meckel's diverticulum, and a Meckel's scan is indicated. Other lesions that present with brisk, painless GI bleeding, such as vascular malformations, may require a nuclear bleeding scan or angiography to make the diagnosis. In the instance in which the bleeding source is unidentified, a diagnostic laparotomy may be indicated.

GI bleeding due to severe colitis (painful, bloody, mucoid stools) warrants both an investigation for infection and lower endoscopy to investigate the possibility of inflammatory bowel disease. Note that severe colonic bleeding that has been reported in the hemolytic-uremic syndrome may occur in the absence of stool leukocytes.

Treat an anal fissure in a well-appearing infant under 1 year of age with petrolatum to the anus at each diaper change. Also, use dietary measures (malt extract, increased fluids, prune juice) to treat coexistent constipation. If the patient has diarrhea and the stool smear evaluation reveals the presence of PMNs, collect a stool sample for culture. Also obtain a CBC and blood culture if the patient is febrile (>38.9°C; 102°F) and less than 3 months of age.

Treat suspected cow's milk protein intolerance by switching a formula-fed infant to a protein hydrolysate formula (Alimentum, Nutramigen). Advise the breast-feeding mother to discontinue cow's milk protein from her diet and begin a calcium supplement. Arrange for follow-up within 2 to 3 days.

Patients with stable vital signs who definitely have a polyp (past history, polyp seen or palpated) may be discharged with referrals to a primary care provider and pediatric gastroenterologist. If the bleeding consists of more than streaking or if anemia is suspected (history of significant blood loss, pallor, tachycardia), obtain a spun hematocrit. Suspected inflammatory bowel disease (weight loss in association with abdominal pain or arthralgias) is an indication to also obtain an ESR.

The ED management of intussusception (pp 239–240), volvulus (pp 213–215), and gastroenteritis (pp 217–222) is detailed elsewhere.

Follow-up

- Cow's milk protein intolerance: 1 to 2 days
- Polyp (with stable vital signs): pediatric gastroenterologist in 1 to 2 weeks

Indications for Admission

- Signs of intravascular volume depletion
- UGI bleeding or significant LGI bleeding
- Infants <3 months of age with fever and colitis (PMNs in stool)
- Severe abdominal pain

BIBLIOGRAPHY

Fox VL: Gastrointestinal bleeding in infancy and childhood. *Gastroenterol Clin North Am* 2000;29:37–66.
Silber G: Lower gastrointestinal bleeding. *Pediatr Rev* 1990;12:85–92.
Squires RH: Gastrointestinal bleeding. *Pediatr Rev* 1999;20:95–101.

MECKEL'S DIVERTICULUM

Meckel's diverticulum is the most common intestinal malformation, occurring in approximately 2% of the population. It is usually located within the terminal 100 cm of the ileum and may be connected by a fibrous cord to the abdominal wall. In about one-half of the cases there is ectopic mucosa, which is gastric in almost 90% of cases. In addition to ectopic gastric mucosa, ectopic pancreatic, small bowel, or colonic mucosa can also be present. Meckel's diverticulum is the most common cause of massive LGI bleeding in children.

Clinical Presentation

Most cases of Meckel's diverticulum are asymptomatic, with the diverticulum noted as an incidental surgical or postmortem finding. Signs or symptoms of hemorrhage, obstruction, or diverticulitis occur in 25 to 30% of cases. Bleeding occurs secondary to ulceration of ileal mucosa adjacent to the ectopic gastric tissue and is seen in 40 to 60% of symptomatic patients. Many children present with massive painless rectal bleeding. Alternatively, chronic blood loss or tarry stools can occur. Intestinal obstruction occurs in 20% of symptomatic patients.

Intestinal obstruction can occur secondary to intussusception with the diverticulum acting as a lead point, volvulus around the fixed tip of the diverticulum, internal herniation, or incarceration in an inguinal hernia. One-half of cases of intussusception due to Meckel's diverticulum occur in infancy, with a presentation that is identical to that of idiopathic intussusception.

Diverticulitis and perforation occasionally occur, possibly secondary to peptic ulceration. These are clinically indistinguishable from acute appendicitis, although the area of most intense pain is closer to the midline.

Diagnosis and ED Management

A history of previous episodes of LGI bleeding is important, as many patients with a bleeding Meckel's diverticulum will have had a similar episode in the past. Once it has been established that the bleeding is coming from the LGI tract, insert a large-bore IV if there is active bleeding, there are changes in orthostatic vital signs, or there is tachycardia or hypotension. Give fluid resuscitation with normal saline boluses (20 mL/kg) as needed. Obtain blood for a CBC with differential, platelet count, type and cross-match, PT, and PTT.

Order a technetium-99m sodium pertechnetate abdominal scan (Meckel's scan) for a stable patient with painless LGI bleeding. It is a simple, noninvasive method for identifying a Meckel's diverticulum with ectopic gastric mucosa, with a sensitivity of 80 to 90% and a specificity of >95%. To increase the accuracy of the scan, give oral cimetidine (20 mg/kg/day) or, for an emergency scan, subcutaneous pentagastrin (6 μg/kg). Treatment is operative after correction of anemia and/or fluid and electrolyte imbalances. Notify a surgeon when a patient presents with a possible Meckel's diverticulum, as surgery may be required on an emergent basis.

Indications for Admission

- Positive Meckel's scan
- Significant LGI blood loss with evidence of hypovolemia

BIBLIOGRAPHY

Arnold JF, Pellicane JV: Meckel's diverticulum: a ten-year experience. *Ann Surg* 1997;63:354–355.

Brown RL, Azizkhan RG: Gastrointestinal bleeding in infants and children: Meckel's diverticulum and intestinal duplication. *Semin Pediatr Surg* 1999;8: 202–209.

Faubion WA, Perrault J: Gastrointestinal bleeding, in Walker WA, Durie PR, Hamilton JR, et al (eds): *Pediatric Gastrointestinal Disease*. Philadelphia: Decker, 2000, pp 164–178.

RECTAL PROLAPSE

Rectal prolapse is usually a benign, self-limited condition that occurs predominantly in the first 2 years of life.

Clinical Presentation and Diagnosis

Rectal prolapse appears as a sausage-shaped, erythematous mass that protrudes from the anus. It occurs during defecation and recedes spontaneously. Predisposing factors include constipation, diarrhea, cystic fibrosis, parasitic infection, and neurologic or anatomic anomalies. A protruding *polyp or hemorrhoid* can easily be differentiated from a prolapsed rectum by simple inspection.

ED Management

If the prolapsed rectum does not reduce spontaneously, lubricate the prolapsed tissue and manually reduce it gently. Treat any underlying constipation or diarrhea. Perform careful physical and neurologic examinations, paying careful attention to the anus, spine, and lower extremities. Refer the patient to a primary care setting to arrange for serial stool collection for ova and parasites and a sweat chloride determination (to rule out cystic fibrosis).

Follow-up

- Primary care follow-up in 1 week

BIBLIOGRAPHY

Johnson S, Jaksic T: Perianal lesions, in Walker WA, Durie PR, Hamilton JR, et al (eds): *Pediatric Gastrointestinal Disease*. Philadelphia: Decker, 2000, pp 456–462.

Siafakas C, Vottler TP, Andersen JM: Rectal prolapse in pediatrics. *Clin Pediatr (Phila)* 1999;38:63–72.

UMBILICAL LESIONS

Most umbilical lesions are benign. The umbilical cord begins to dry shortly after birth and typically separates completely and falls off by the end of the second week. The more aseptic the care, the longer the cord may stay attached. Delayed separation, defined as occurring after 6 weeks of age, is rarely secondary to abnormal neutrophil function.

Clinical Presentation

Umbilical Hernia   An umbilical hernia presents as a bulging out of the umbilicus that is most prominent when the baby is crying or stooling. The hernia can be quite large and occurs more commonly in African Americans. It typically closes by 2 or 3 years of age as the abdominal musculature grows. Very rarely, a piece of mesentery can become incarcerated, causing local pain and tenderness.

Granuloma   The most common of all umbilical lesions is persistence of granulation tissue at the site of cord separation. A granuloma is a reddish mass protruding from the umbilicus. There may be a small amount of a blood-tinged discharge.

Omphalitis   In newborns, a small rim of erythema around the umbilicus can be normal. Omphalitis presents with a foul odor and erythematous streaking, particularly in the direction of the liver. The infant may present with fever, irritability, decreased oral intake, and lethargy.

Persistent Omphalomesenteric Duct and Urachus   After the cord separates, a persistent omphalomesenteric duct may present with fecal drainage. A persistent urachus may allow the drainage of urine from the umbilicus. Either remnant may also persist as a blind sinus with a purulent or egg-white discharge.

Diagnosis

Normally, once the umbilical cord separates, there is no erythema or tenderness of the surrounding skin, although there can be a small amount of blood-tinged discharge. If the drainage smells like feces, consider a persistent *omphalomesenteric duct.* If there is a large amount of clear watery discharge, a *persistent urachus* is possible. Purulent drainage or material resembling egg whites suggests a persistent sinus secondary to one of the two preceding conditions.

ED Management

Umbilical Hernia   The treatment is education and reassurance, since most umbilical hernias resolve without intervention. Inform the parents that home remedies are of no benefit (binders, tape, a quarter taped to the umbilicus). Surgical repair is not indicated until the child is at least 3 years old. However, instruct the parents to seek medical attention if the hernia cannot be easily reduced. If the patient presents with an incarcerated hernia, manually reduce the incarcerated mesentery and arrange for surgical repair. Urgent surgical reduction is required if bowel incarcerates (very rare).

Granuloma   The treatment is cauterization with a silver nitrate stick. Moisten the stick with tap water and apply to the granuloma until the entire surface changes from red to a grayish color. Avoid contact with normal skin. Advise the family to not bathe the baby for several days. See the infant in 1 week and repeat the cauterization if necessary. If the mass is particularly large when first seen, tie a ligature (3-0 nylon) around the base and see the patient again in 1 week. At that time, sever the granuloma at its base, then cauterize the stump.

Omphalitis   Omphalitis is potentially life-threatening. Perform a full sepsis workup, admit the infant, and treat with IV nafcillin (100 mg/kg/day divided q 6 h). Consider an anaerobic infection in the case of severe necrotizing omphalitis. The infant appears toxic, with associated cellulitis or peritonitis. Add either clindamycin (40 mg/kg/day divided q 6 h) or metronidazole (30 mg/kg/d divided q 8 h).

Persistent Omphalomesenteric Duct and Urachus   If a persistent omphalomesenteric duct or urachus is suspected, consult with a pediatric surgeon to confirm the diagnosis.

Delayed Cord Separation   Obtain a CBC with differential to look for neutropenia, and instruct the parents to keep the cord dry. Refer the infant to a primary care provider for follow-up within 1 week.

Follow-up
- Umbilical granuloma, delayed cord separation: primary care visit within 1 week

Indications for Admission
- Omphalitis
- Incarcerated or strangulated umbilical hernia
- Persistent omphalomesenteric duct or urachus

BIBLIOGRAPHY

Haddock G, Wesson D: Hernias, in Walker WA, Durie PR, Hamilton JR, et al (eds): *Pediatric Gastrointestinal Disease.* Philadelphia: Decker, 2000, pp 445–449.

O'Donnell KA, Glick PL, Caty MG: Pediatric umbilical problems. *Pediatr Clin North Am* 1998;45:791–799.

Siegel JD: Skin and soft tissue infections, in McMillan JA, DeAngelis CD, Feigin RD, Warshaw JB (eds): *Oski's Pediatrics.* Philadelphia: Lippincott Williams & Wilkins, 1999, pp 530–531.

CHAPTER 10

Emergencies Associated with Genetic Syndromes

Robert W. Marion

Congenital malformations are present in approximately 3% of newborns in the United States. Malformations may occur as isolated conditions, as in the case of a simple cleft lip or palate, or may cluster together in recognizable patterns, or syndromes, such as trisomy 13. Early diagnosis of a specific syndrome expedites the detection of associated internal anomalies and facilitates appropriate counseling of the family.

For the physician working in the emergency department (ED), recognition of a syndromic diagnosis is of special importance. Often, presenting symptoms are due to internal manifestations associated with that syndrome, and early identification of such associated problems can be lifesaving. Table 10-1 lists some commonly occurring congenital malformation syndromes and the possible conditions with which affected individuals may present to the ED.

BIBLIOGRAPHY

Buyse ML: *Birth Defects Encyclopedia.* New York: Liss, 1990.
Jones KL: *Smith's Recognizable Patterns of Human Malformation,* 5th ed. Philadelphia: Saunders, 1997.

Table 10-1   Emergencies Associated with Genetic Syndromes*

SYNDROME	EXTERNAL MANIFESTATIONS	PRESENTATION/POSSIBLE EMERGENCY
Achondroplasia (autosomal dominant)	Short stature Prominent forehead Proximal limb shortening	Apnea/SIDS: narrowed foramen magnum Vomiting, irritability: ↑ICP secondary to hydrocephalus "Sciatica": nerve root compression secondary to narrow spinal canal
Beckwith-Wiedemann syndrome (multiple etiologies)	Somatic overgrowth Omphalocele "Coarse facies," large tongue Ear creases Hemihypertrophy	Hypoglycemia: hyperinsulinism Abdominal mass, vomiting: Wilms' tumor (occurs in 5–10%)
Craniosynostosis syndromes (including Crouzon, Apert, and Pfeiffer) (most autosomal dominant)	Unusual head shape Ocular proptosis Hypertelorism Some with limb defects	Obstructive apnea: choanal stenosis Vomiting, irritability: ↑ICP secondary to premature suture closure
Down's syndrome (trisomy 21)	Hypotonia Typical face Midfacial hypoplasia Brachydactyly Developmental delay	Poor feeding, tachypnea: CHF Vomiting: intestinal obstruction secondary to duodenal atresia or annular pancreas Constipation: Hirschsprung's disease Sudden paralysis below neck: cord compression secondary to atlantoaxial instability Failure to thrive, sluggishness: hypothyroidism Anemia, bone pain, fever: leukemia
Ectodermal dysplasias (multiple) (autosomal dominant and recessive; X-linked)	Alopecia Hypodontia/adontia Hypoplastic nails	Hyperthermia, febrile seizures: lack of sweat glands

Table 10-1 *(Continued)*

SYNDROME	EXTERNAL MANIFESTATIONS	PRESENTATION/POSSIBLE EMERGENCY
Marfan's syndrome (autosomal dominant)	Tall, thin body Long fingers	Sudden chest pain: dissection of ascending aortic aneurysm Sudden decreased vision: lens dislocation or retinal detachment
Myelomeningocele (multifactorial)	Spinal defect Paraplegia Orthopedic abnormalities Hydrocephalus	Vomiting, irritability: ↑ICP secondary to hydrocephalus Stridor, apnea: Arnold-Chiari malformation (neurosurgical emergency) Fever, foul-smelling urine: UTI secondary to neurogenic bladder Fever, irritability, vomiting: ventricular shunt infection Deteriorating lower extremity strength, gait, bowel, bladder function: tethering of spinal cord Anaphylaxis: latex allergy
Neurofibromatosis I (autosomal dominant)	Café-au-lait spots Axillary freckling Neurofibromas	Gradual vision loss: optic glioma Scoliosis Headache, irritability, vomiting: ↑ICP secondary to tumor
Neurofibromatosis II (autosomal dominant)	Café-au-lait spots Neurofibromas Iris hamartomas	Hearing loss, tinnitus: acoustic neuromas Headache, irritability, vomiting: ↑ICP secondary to tumor Hypertension: pheochromocytoma, neurofibroma
Osteogenesis imperfecta type I (autosomal dominant)	Blue sclerae Bone fragility ± Dentinogenesis imperfecta	Fractures after trivial trauma: fragile bones (must consider child abuse) Gradual hearing loss: otosclerosis ± Multiple caries
Osteogenesis imperfecta type IV (autosomal dominant)	White sclerae Bone fragility ± Dentinogenesis imperfecta Bowing of some bones	Fractures after trivial trauma: fragile bones ± carious teeth Gradual hearing loss: otosclerosis ± Multiple caries
Pierre-Robin malformation sequence (often part of another syndrome)	Micrognathia U-shaped cleft palate Glossoptosis	Upper airway obstruction: glossoptosis

Table 10-1 *(Continued)*

SYNDROME	EXTERNAL MANIFESTATIONS	PRESENTATION/POSSIBLE EMERGENCY
Prader-Willi syndrome (15q11-13 deletion)	Obesity Hypotonia Developmental delay Hypoplastic genitalia	Polydipsia/uria: diabetes mellitus Upper airway obstruction
Sturge-Weber syndrome (usually sporadic; some autosomal dominant)	Port wine stain overlying dermatome supplied by deep ophthalmic branch of fifth nerve	Enlarged, hazy cornea, decreased vision: glaucoma secondary to hemangioma blocking angle Seizures: "railroad track" calcifications in cerebral cortex
Turner syndrome (monosomy X)	Female Short stature Webbed neck Puffy hands and feet Broad chest	Hypertension, decreased leg pulses: coarctation of aorta Fever, dysuria: UTI secondary to renal anomaly Poor growth, constipation, obesity: hypothyroidism Failure to enter puberty: gonadal dysgenesis
Williams syndrome (7p deletion)	"Elfin" facies Short stature Developmental delay	Constipation, irritability: hypercalcemia CHF: supravalvular aortic stenosis Hypertension: renal artery stenosis Chest pain, sudden death: MI secondary to coronary artery stenosis Syncope, weakness: CVA due to narrowing of cerebral arteries and moyamoya disease

ABBREVIATIONS: SIDS, sudden infant death syndrome; ICP, intracranial pressure; CHF, congestive heart failure; UTI, urinary tract infection; MI, myocardial infarction; CVA, cerebrovascular accident.

CHAPTER 11

Genitourinary Emergencies

Alfred Winkler and Alfred Kohan

BALANOPOSTHITIS

Balanitis is inflammation of the glans penis, which may be associated with inflammation of the preputial tissue surrounding the glans (posthitis). Balanoposthitis occurs in approximately 3% of boys, particularly if uncircumcised. Poor hygiene and accumulation of smegma lead to bacterial proliferation about the glans and prepuce. In circumcised boys without residual foreskin or glans penis adhesions, balanitis may be secondary to contact dermatitis from urine, laundry soaps, powders, or ointments. In adolescents with a retractable foreskin, poor hygiene and sexually transmitted diseases are etiologies.

Clinical Presentation and Diagnosis

Balanoposthitis presents with erythema, edema, and pain of the distal phallus, particularly the glans penis. There may be secondary meatitis with resultant dysuria and reluctance to void. The foreskin will be difficult to retract and a discharge may be present. In severe cases, the cellulitis can extend down the shaft of the penis and onto the lower abdominal wall or the scrotum. Palpable inguinal adenopathy is often present.

Recurrent episodes of posthitis can result in phimosis, whereas repeated episodes of balanitis may result in meatal stenosis, with a poor stream and dribbling of urine.

ED Management

Acute localized infections usually respond to frequent warm-water sitz baths followed by drying of the penis and topical antibiotics (bacitracin) thrice daily. If there is voluntary retention, fever, or cellulitis extending onto the penile shaft, treat with oral antibiotics for 7 days. Use 40 mg/kg/day of either cephalexin (divided qid) or cefadroxil (divided bid).

More severe infections with purulent discharge and widespread cellulitis require admission and treatment with parenteral antibiotics (nafcillin 150 mg/kg/day divided q 6 h).

Failure of posthitis to respond to warm soaks and systemic antibiotics may be due to inadequate drainage secondary to phimosis. An urgent incision of the dorsal inner foreskin is indicated if there is a poor urinary stream or dribbling.

Follow-up

- Inability to void: immediate. Otherwise primary care follow-up in 1 week.

Indications for Admission

- Severe infection
- Urinary retention

BIBLIOGRAPHY

Lundquist ST, Stack LB: Diseases of the foreskin, penis, and urethra. *Emerg Med Clin North Am* 2001;19:529–546.
Schwartz RH, Rushton HG: Acute balanoposthitis in young boys. *Pediatr Infect Dis J* 1996;15:176–177.
Waugh MA: Balanitis. *Dermatol Clin* 1998;16:757–762.

RENAL AND GENITOURINARY TRAUMA

Renal Trauma   Renal trauma occurs most frequently as a result of blunt injury (motor vehicle accidents, falls, athletic injuries); in the pediatric population penetrating trauma is less common. The pediatric kidney is particularly susceptible to injury because of the relative paucity of surrounding fat, its size in relation to surrounding organs, and an immature thoracic cage, which provides inadequate protection. Because abnormal kidneys are more easily injured, an underlying congenital anomaly is found in up to 20% of cases of traumatic hematuria, including ureteropelvic junction obstruction, primary obstructive megaureter, or ectopic or solitary kidneys. Although most renal trauma occurs as an isolated injury, other organs are injured in 25% of cases of blunt and 80% of penetrating abdominal trauma, particularly the liver.

Ureteral Trauma   Ureteral trauma is relatively uncommon; when present, it is usually associated with multiple intraabdominal injuries. Children are particularly susceptible to avulsion at the ureteropelvic junction, a relatively fixed point in the course of the ureter.

Bladder Trauma   The pediatric bladder is particularly susceptible to blunt trauma, especially from motor vehicle accidents. Patients with pelvic fractures are also at risk for associated bladder injury.

Urethral Trauma   Urethral injury is usually the result of blunt trauma to the lower abdomen or a straddle injury to the perineum. There can also be iatrogenic injury from urethral instrumentation.

Clinical Presentation

Renal Trauma   The patient will commonly present with flank pain, which may be localized or radiate to the ipsilateral groin. There may also be costovertebral tenderness, flank ecchymoses, or a palpable flank mass if there is extravasation of blood or urine into the perirenal tissues. Associated findings include ipsilateral rib fractures and fractured transverse processes of the vertebral bodies. Either gross or microscopic hematuria is nearly always present, although the degree of hematuria can be variable and does not correlate with the degree of injury.

Ureteral Trauma   The early presentation of ureteral trauma is nonspecific and may be obscured by other associated injuries that are paramount on initial presentation. Hematuria is initially present in only 70% of cases. Later, there may be fever or flank or abdominal pain. A high level of clinical suspicion is required for early diagnosis.

Bladder Trauma   Since a bladder injury most commonly occurs in association with a pelvic fracture, the signs of the bony trauma may obscure the urologic injury. A patient with a ruptured bladder presents with suprapubic and abdominal pain with tenderness on palpation, hematuria, and occasionally inability to void.

Urethral Injury   Males with posterior urethral injuries have generally suffered severe blunt trauma and have significant associated injuries. Lower abdominal and pelvic swelling, tenderness, and ecchymosis are commonly seen, with hematuria and blood at the external meatus. With complete disruption of the urethra, the patient may be unable to void.

Bulbar urethral trauma commonly accompanies a straddle injury. Perineal ecchymosis, usually in a butterfly distribution, and scrotal hematomas may be noted. Bleeding from the meatus is the hallmark of urethral injury and may be associated with an inability to void.

Penile and Scrotal Injuries

Most penile injuries in boys occur as a result of circumcision. The injuries vary from an inappropriate amount of skin removed (too little or too much) to complete transection of the penis. Penile injuries due to blunt or penetrating trauma in childhood are rare but may be associated with urethral injury. Penile and scrotal zipper injuries are common in boys and usually present with skin avulsion. Scrotal trauma can present with acute swelling, bleeding manifesting itself as ecchymosis or hematocele, and testicular injury with disruption of the tunica albuginea. In severe cases, blood and/or urine extravasates into the upper abdominal wall and into the perineum along the Colles' fascia.

Diagnosis and ED Management

On urinalysis, there is usually significant hematuria. However, there is no consistent relationship between the number of red cells and the degree of urinary tract injury, particularly with renal injuries. In fact, the absence of blood does not exclude a major injury, such as a ureteral transection or an injury to the renal vasculature. Therefore, suspect a renal injury in any victim of blunt trauma with gross or microscopic hematuria on urinalysis or with signs or symptoms suggestive of renal injury (flank pain or hematoma, lower rib fracture, shock), particularly with rapid deceleration as the mechanism of injury. Always consider the possibility of sexual abuse in a child presenting with trauma to the external genitalia.

If the blood pressure is not stable, obtain immediate surgical and urologic consultation. For the stable patient, arrange for a computed tomography (CT) scan with contrast for proper staging of injuries and identification of any other associated intraabdominal injuries.

Renal Trauma   If an isolated renal injury is likely, promptly obtain a CT scan of the abdomen and pelvis after administration of IV contrast.

The staging of renal injuries is shown in Table 11-1. Maintain the patient at bed rest with close hemodynamic monitoring and consult a urologist.

Ureteral Trauma   If a ureteral injury is suspected, obtain a CT scan of the abdomen and pelvis with contrast. Extravasation of contrast is the hall-

Table 11-1   Staging of Renal Injuries

GRADE	FINDINGS	TREATMENT
Grade 1	Contusion with microscopic or gross hematuria No intraparenchymal laceration	Bed rest Serial hematocrits
Grade 2	Subcapsular nonexpanding hematoma Perirenal nonexpanding hematoma Laceration with a parenchymal tear <1 cm No involvement of the collecting system No extravasation of urine	Bed rest Serial hematocrits
Grade 3	Laceration with parenchymal tear >1 cm No involvement of the collecting system No extravasation of urine	Bed rest Serial hematocrits
Grade 4	Laceration with extensive parenchymal injury Involvement of the collecting system Vascular damage to the hilar vessels	Ureteral stent Possible renal exploration with reconstruction or nephrectomy
Grade 5	Parenchymal destruction (shattered kidney) Hilar vascular injury with devascularization	Ureteral stent Possible renal exploration with reconstruction or nephrectomy

mark of ureteral injury. Hydronephrosis, ureteral deviation, or lack of visualization of contrast in the distal ureter may also be noted. Emergent treatment is indicated, either intraoperative repair or urinary diversion with a nephrostomy tube. A preoperative retrograde pyelogram may be necessary to delineate the degree of injury. Arrange emergent urologic consultation.

Bladder Trauma   Inability to void, a distended bladder, and gross hematuria are warning signs. Call a urologist immediately, as urethral integrity must be assured before catheterization is performed. A rectal examination may demonstrate a boggy mass palpated in the area of urethral disruption. A retrograde urethrogram is indicated in the male. After evaluation of urethral integrity, obtain a gravity cystogram for all patients. Calculate the age-adjusted bladder capacity before administering the contrast material [in mL, < 2 years: (weight in kg) $\times$ 7; > 2 years: (2 + age in years) $\times$ 30]. Bladder injuries are classified by extravasation of contrast into either the extra- or intraperitoneal space, although combined intra- and extraperitoneal injuries can also occur, particularly with penetrating trauma.

Treat a patient with extraperitoneal extravasation with either a suprapubic or urethral catheter. Intraperitoneal extravasation is an indication for intraoperative repair and suprapubic diversion of urine.

Urethral Injury   Blood at the urethral meatus indicates a urethral injury; consult a urologist to perform a retrograde urethrogram. Do not catheterize the patient before urethral integrity is fully evaluated, as catheterization may further damage a partial disruption, creating a complete one. After the level and degree of urethral injury are ascertained, suprapubic catheter placement is indicated for temporary urinary diversion pending more definitive repair on an emergent or expectant basis.

External Genital Trauma   Treat *penile hair-tourniquet trauma* with an ice bag to ease the pain and shrink the swelling. Application of soapy water to the hairs facilitates removal. Wrap any size *penile amputation* in a saline gauze, put it in a plastic bag, and place it on ice, with pressure and sterile dressings applied to the remaining shaft. Immediate reanastomosis surgery may be successful. Treat an *amputation or avulsion of scrotal skin* with sterile saline-soaked towels and consult a urologist to determine the need for surgery. If there is a *urethral foreign body*, arrange for cystoscopy and transurethral extraction after percutaneous placement of a suprapubic catheter by a urologist. If gentle attempts to remove *penile skin caught in a zipper* are unsuccessful, inject 1% lidocaine (without epinephrine) into the foreskin. Then the zipper can be closed, cut through at its base, and opened from the base, releasing the entrapped skin.

Indications for Admission

- Abnormal CT scan (renal contusion, laceration, collecting system injury, major vessel injury)
- Penile or scrotal amputation
- Bladder or urethral contusion, laceration, or rupture
- Inability to void

BIBLIOGRAPHY

Ahn JH, Morey AF, McAninch JW: Workup and management of traumatic hematuria. *Emerg Med Clin North Am* 1998;16:145–164.

Chapple CR: Urethral injury. *BJU Int* 2000;86:318–326.

Elshihabi I, Elshihabi S, Arar M: An overview of renal trauma. *Curr Opin Pediatr* 1998;10:162–166.

MEATAL STENOSIS

Meatal stenosis is a narrowing of the urethral meatus, usually secondary to recurrent episodes of subclinical meatitis. Etiologies include ammoniacal diaper irritation (circumcised boys) and recurrent balanoposthitis (uncircumcised boys). However, acquired meatal stenosis occurs very rarely in uncircumcised boys because the foreskin acts as a protective cover for the meatus. Congenital meatal stenosis is also very rare.

Clinical Presentation

Obstructive symptoms occasionally occur, including hesitancy, straining, urgency, frequency, and postvoiding dribbling. An abnormal urinary stream may be seen, with either spraying or upward deflection. However, urinary retention is rare. If there is an associated meatitis, an erythematous, swollen meatus is noted, often with a purulent discharge.

Diagnosis

When the typical findings are present, the diagnosis can be assumed to be meatal stenosis. However, observe the urinary stream, since the subjective impression (on visual inspection) of a narrowed meatus does not constitute a valid diagnosis of meatal stenosis. Radiographic studies are seldom necessary to confirm the diagnosis.

ED Management

Treat purulent meatitis with warm-water sitz baths and oral antibiotics for 7 days. Use 40 mg/kg/day of either cephalexin (divided qid) or cefadroxil (divided bid). Refer all patients to a urologist for confirmation of the diagnosis and further evaluation. Immediately consult a urologist for the rare case of acute urinary retention.

Follow-up

- Meatitis without retention: urology follow-up in 1 to 2 weeks

Indication for Admission

- Urinary retention

BIBLIOGRAPHY

Gausche M: Genitourinary surgical emergencies. *Pediatr Ann* 1996;25:458–464.

Lundquist ST, Stack LB: Diseases of the foreskin, penis, and urethra. *Emerg Med Clin North Am* 2001;19:529–546.

PARAPHIMOSIS

Paraphimosis is entrapment of a retracted foreskin behind the coronal sulcus of an uncircumcised or inadequately circumcised penis. It occurs when a tight, phimotic foreskin is retracted proximal to the glans penis without immediate reduction. This produces a tourniquet effect, with resultant venous congestion and edema of the glans.

Clinical Presentation and Diagnosis

Glans edema is proportional to the duration of the paraphimosis and the tightness of the foreskin. On examination, there is a severely painful, edematous, blue, congested glans with a tight proximal collar of swollen tissue. The glans congestion can progress to ischemia (white), with eventual gangrene. The tightness of the foreskin along with resultant edema may lead to urethral obstruction at the coronal level. The patient then complains of difficulty voiding and urinary retention. Direct erosion into the urethra rarely occurs.

ED Management

Place an ice bag on the foreskin and give anesthesia, either EMLA cream or a penile block, and/or sedate the patient (see Sedation and Analgesia, pp 626–633). Reduce the edema by applying manual circumferential compression for several minutes. Then, grasp the penile shaft with the index and third fingers of each hand with the thumbs on the glans. Firm downward pressure on the glans against counterpressure on the shaft usually advances the foreskin back over the glans. Alternatively, following the application of EMLA cream with an occlusive dressing (30 min to 1 h), inject 1 mL of hyaluronidase (150 U/mL) into one or more sites in the edematous prepuce. Resolution of the edema is almost immediate, and the foreskin can then be gently retracted over the glans. It is critical to attempt to advance the most distal foreskin ring (the foreskin closest to the coronal margin). If this tight ring can be reduced, the remainder of the foreskin will follow. Occasionally, there is tearing of the skin with bleeding, which can be controlled by compression. Instruct the patient to avoid retracting his foreskin for several days. Refer the patient to a urologist for follow-up and evaluation of the need for an elective circumcision.

If the paraphimosis cannot be reduced, consult a urologist immediately to perform a dorsal slit to release the constricting ring of tissue.

Follow-up

- Reducible paraphimosis: urology follow-up in 1 to 2 weeks

BIBLIOGRAPHY

DeVries CR, Miller AK, Packer MG: Reduction of paraphimosis with hyaluronidase. *Urology* 1996;48:464–465.
Gausche M: Genitourinary surgical emergencies. *Pediatr Ann* 1996;25:458–464.
Hartmann RW Jr, Tunnessen WW Jr: Picture of the month. Paraphimosis. *Arch Pediatr Adolesc Med* 1997;151:315–316.

PHIMOSIS

Phimosis is the inability to retract the foreskin over the glans penis. In 50% of uncircumcised boys, the foreskin is retractable at 1 year of age, and 90% are retractable by 4 years. The remaining 10% may not become retractable until puberty. If associated infections (local or more proximally in the urinary tract) or voiding difficulties occur, correction may be indicated.

Clinical Presentation and Diagnosis

Acquired phimosis is a result of poor hygiene with inflammation of the glans. Accumulated smegma may form aggregates that appear as whitish, globular masses under the nonretractile foreskin. Associated inflammatory conditions may coexist, including balanoposthitis (pp 257–258), and meatitis (p 262). With severe phimosis, the foreskin may balloon during voiding as the urine collects under it and then dribbles out from the tight opening. The adolescent may complain of pain on erection, secondary to tension on the foreskin from the glandular adhesions.

ED Management

Treat accumulated smegma without any associated infection with gentle retraction of the foreskin (as far as it can go) during bathing. Depending on the patient's age, if there is no infection, refer him to a urologist for consideration of elective circumcision. If there is ballooning of the foreskin with a dribbling urinary stream or an associated urinary tract infection (UTI), consult a urologist. Gentle dilation may be necessary, after which an elective circumcision or preputialplasty (surgical widening of the phimotic ring) is indicated.

Follow-up

- Phimosis without associated difficulty voiding: urology follow-up in 1 to 2 weeks

BIBLIOGRAPHY

Gausche M: Genitourinary surgical emergencies. *Pediatr Ann* 1996;25:458–464.
Lundquist ST, Stack LB: Diseases of the foreskin, penis, and urethra. *Emerg Med Clin North Am* 2001;19:529–546.
Shankar KR, Rickwood AM: The incidence of phimosis in boys. *BJU Int* 1999; 84:101–102.

PRIAPISM

Priapism is a persistent and often painful erection. It most frequently occurs in association with sickle cell disease (pp 319–323) but may also result from spinal cord injury, leukemic infiltration, or trauma.

Clinical Presentation and Diagnosis

Priapism presents with a persistent painful and tender erection. Urinary retention may result, with a palpably distended bladder noted on examination. Persistence of the priapism can lead to corporal fibrosis, with resultant erectile dysfunction. In boys with sickle cell disease, other manifestations of the crisis may be present.

ED Management

The cornerstones of management irrespective of the etiology are analgesia, sedation, hydration, and oxygenation. If the patient has sickle cell disease, determine the percent of hemoglobin S (HgbS). Specific therapy for the sickle cell patient is aimed at reducing the HgbS to 30 to 35% by exchange transfusion. Institute HgbS-reduction therapy promptly; the goal is to achieve a therapeutic reduction within the first 24 h. If the priapism persists in spite of adequate reduction of HgbS, consult a urologist to perform aspiration of blood from the corpora cavernosa, followed by irrigation with a dilute epinephrine solution. Most commonly, however, reduction of HgbS is sufficient to effect resolution of the priapism. On occasion, acute bladder drainage with a Foley catheter may be necessary.

Indication for Admission

- Priapism

BIBLIOGRAPHY

Harmon WJ, Nehra A: Priapism: diagnosis and management. *Mayo Clin Proc* 1997;72:350–355.

Mantadakis E, Ewalt DH, Cavender JD, et al: Outpatient penile aspiration and epinephrine irrigation for young patients with sickle cell anemia and prolonged priapism. *Blood* 2000;95:78–82.

Pitetti RD, Nangia A, Bhende MS: Idiopathic priapism. *Pediatr Emerg Care* 1999; 15:404–406.

SCROTAL SWELLINGS

A number of conditions can produce an acutely erythematous and tender hemiscrotum. However, expedient diagnosis of testicular torsion is always the priority in managing any case of painful scrotal swelling.

Clinical Presentation

Testicular Torsion Testicular torsion is a true surgical emergency. It is caused by twisting of the spermatic cord, leading to venous, lymphatic, and eventual arterial occlusion. Although testicular torsion is possible at any age, the peak is 14 years (range 12–18 years). About 60% of patients experience the sudden onset of severe testicular pain, which may radiate to the groin or lower abdomen. Other symptoms include nausea, vomiting, and a wide-based gait. Younger patients may complain only of abdominal or inguinal pain.

On physical examination, there is hemiscrotal swelling and erythema. The involved testis may lie higher in the scrotum, with a horizontal (rather than vertical) orientation. The hemiscrotal swelling does not transilluminate, and elevation of the testicle does not diminish the pain. Most commonly the ipsilateral cremasteric reflex is absent. There is no fever or dysuria, and in about half of the cases there is a history of subacute bouts of scrotal pain (previous intermittent torsion).

Torsion of the Testicular Appendage   The appendix testis is a remnant of the müllerian duct at the upper pole of the testicle. Torsion of the testicular appendage on its vascular pedicle can mimic testicular torsion, most often in adolescent boys. There is the acute onset of pain and tenderness localized to the superior pole of the testis. At times a characteristic bluish nodule can be seen through the thin scrotal skin (blue dot sign). More often, however, the bluish dot is not evident until several days after the surrounding scrotal edema and erythema have resolved. The swelling does not transilluminate, although there may be an associated reactive hydrocele that does. Elevation of the testis does not relieve the pain, there is no fever, and there are no urinary symptoms. Previous subacute episodes are uncommon.

Epididymoorchitis   Epididymoorchitis is caused by the spread of an infection from the bladder or urethra to the epididymal and testicular ducts and tubules. It may be confused with a testicular torsion, although it is uncommon in boys under 14 years of age. Etiologies in preadolescents include mumps, infectious mononucleosis, varicella, and coxsackievirus. When epididymitis occurs in boys who are not sexually active, there may be a history of a urinary tract anomaly (ectopic ureter, vesicoureteral reflux), recent urethral instrumentation, or an associated urinary tract infection. In postpubertal adolescents, the etiology of epididymitis is usually a sexually transmitted organism such as *Gonococcus, Chlamydia,* or *Ureaplasma* (pp 286–293).

Symptoms include the gradual onset of localized testicular and possibly abdominal pain, nausea, vomiting, fever, and dysuria. On examination, there may be localized testicular or epididymal tenderness, nontransilluminating scrotal swelling, and a thickened epididymis. Manual scrotal elevation often relieves the pain in epididymoorchitis (Prehn's sign) but not in testicular and appendiceal torsions. However, this sign is unreliable in prepubertal boys.

Inguinal Hernia   Inguinal hernias are most common in the first year of life, especially if the infant was premature. They are predominantly indirect, secondary to a patent processus vaginalis. Males are affected 10 times more often than females, and hernias are more common on the right side. Typically, recurrent episodes of painless, nonerythematous scrotal and inguinal swelling occur, often when the baby is crying or irritable. Bowel sounds may be heard in the scrotum, and transillumination is variable. In females, an ovary may be palpated in the hernial sac. Incarceration within the inguinal ring can occur and present with acute tenderness, erythema, and induration. Over the course of a few hours, strangulation and bowel obstruction ensue, with vomiting, decreased bowel sounds, abdominal distention, and possible fluid and electrolyte imbalances.

Hydrocele   Hydroceles are most common during the first year of life, especially on the right side. The mass transilluminates, and the testicle is usually palpable posteriorly in the scrotum. The swelling generally does not extend into the inguinal canal. Hydroceles are categorized according to whether the processus vaginalis is patent (communicating) or obliterated (noncommunicating).

Communicating hydroceles typically present with recurrent episodes of painless, nonerythematous scrotal swellings that vary in size. It may be possible to completely reduce the hydrocele fluid by gentle pressure. Noncommunicating hydroceles are usually present at birth, are stable in size without waxing and waning, and are not reducible with gentle pressure.

Varicocele   A varicocele is a collection of dilated spermatic cord veins. They are most commonly found on the left side, usually not before puberty. The patient may complain of a sensation of heaviness or dull ache in the scrotum. However, most are detected as an asymptomatic swelling. Examination in the upright position reveals a nontender, nonerythematous scrotum with a "bag of worms" inside. This may be accentuated by having the patient perform a Valsalva maneuver.

Idiopathic Scrotal Edema   Idiopathic scrotal edema is an inflammatory condition of unknown etiology causing an erythematous discoloration and swelling of the scrotal wall with a normal underlying testis.

Hematocele   A hematocele can occur after scrotal trauma or in association with a bleeding diathesis. A painful bluish scrotal swelling is seen. When examination of the ipsilateral testis is difficult, scrotal ultrasound can assess the integrity of the involved testicle.

Testicular Tumor   Testicular tumors are rare, and most occur in patients under 3 years of age. There is diffuse or localized testicular enlargement that is firm or rock-hard and painless. There can be an associated reactive hydrocele that confuses the picture.

Diagnosis

The diagnosis in patients with acute hemiscrotal pain and swelling is *testicular torsion until proved otherwise*. An appendicular torsion and epididymoorchitis may closely resemble a testicular torsion. If there is any suspicion of torsion, *immediately* obtain urologic consultation. When there is any doubt, confirm the diagnosis at surgery. However, imaging studies, if available within 1 h of the patient's presentation, may help differentiate among the causes of an acute hemiscrotum. These include color Doppler ultrasound (decreased blood flow in testicular torsion, increased with appendicular torsion and epididymoorchitis) and radioisotope scrotal scanning (cold in testicular torsion, normal or hot in appendicular torsion, hot with epididymoorchitis).

With *appendicular torsion*, pain and swelling may be localized to the superior testicular pole and a blue dot may be seen through the thin scrotal skin. Dysuria with pyuria and possible bacteriuria may occur in *epididymoorchitis*, along with fever and an elevated white blood cell count.

Inguinal hernias, hydroceles, hematoceles, and varicoceles can usually be distinguished by the clinical findings. If a strangulated inguinal hernia cannot be ruled out, obtain immediate surgical consultation. If time allows, obtain a KUB. Dilated intestinal loops with air-fluid levels may be seen along with a loop of bowel in the scrotum.

ED Management

Testicular Torsion   All suspected cases must be evaluated immediately by a urologist, as testicular survival depends on the duration and degree of ischemia. The testicular salvage rate approaches 100% if the patient is explored within 6 h of the onset of symptoms, but it drops to 20% after 12 h. However, duration of symptoms for more than 24 h is not a reason to defer surgery, as the testis may twist and untwist, and variable degrees of torsion may occur. The intermittent nature of the torsion increases the chance of survival in spite of the long duration. In preparation for surgery, make the child NPO and obtain a complete blood count (CBC), type and cross-match, and a urinalysis.

In extreme circumstances, when a surgeon or operating room is unavailable or if the child has recently eaten, manual detorsion may be tried. Sedate the child, then rotate the left testis 180 to 360 degrees clockwise, or the right testis counterclockwise ("when in doubt, turn it out") until the torsion is relieved as documented by relief of pain or increased blood flow by Doppler. Surgery is still necessary, as retorsion often occurs acutely.

Torsion of Appendix Testis   Surgery is indicated when testicular torsion cannot be clinically excluded, or if unremitting swelling or pain continues for several days. Otherwise, treat with analgesics.

Epididymoorchitis   Treat the prepubertal male with antibiotics [trimethoprim-sulfamethoxazole (8 mg/kg/day of TMP divided bid, or amoxicillin 40 mg/kg/day divided tid) for 10 days, analgesics, bed rest, and scrotal support. The treatment of sexually transmitted epididymitis is detailed elsewhere (p 291).

Inguinal Hernia   An easily reducible hernia requires no acute treatment. Refer the patient to a surgeon so that elective repair can be arranged. The vast majority of incarcerated inguinal hernias can be reduced manually. Manual reduction and elective repair are less hazardous than operating on an incarcerated hernia in an infant or child. If the contents of the hernial sac cannot be easily pushed back into the abdomen, sedate the patient (pp 619–626) and place him in the Trendelenburg position with an ice bag on the hernia. After 30 min, attempt to push the hernia back into the abdomen by bimanual reduction. Apply pressure to the internal inguinal ring with one hand while milking the entrapped gas and fluid of the incarcerated bowel into the intraabdominal intestines with the other. This will usually facilitate reduction of the entire bowel. If reduction is successful, refer the patient for prompt elective repair. If reduction is not successful, admit the patient for correction of any fluid and electrolyte imbalances prior to emergency herniorrhaphy.

Hydrocele   Almost all noncommunicating hydroceles resolve spontaneously prior to 12 months of age. Thereafter, refer the patient to a urologist for possible correction. Refer patients with communicating hydroceles for elective surgical repair and caution the parents about the possible presence of an associated inguinal hernia.

Varicocele   Refer the patient to a urologist for evaluation. There is a 20% risk of subsequent subfertility due to the effect of the varicocele on spermatogenesis. Prompt surgery is indicated in cases of loss of testicular volume.

Idiopathic Scrotal Edema   No treatment is required other than rest, analgesia, and antihistamines (diphenhydramine 5 mg/kg/day divided qid).

Hematocele   Obtain an ultrasound to rule out rupture of the tunica albuginea, which is an indication for surgical exploration. Otherwise, treat with rest and analgesia. If the patient has a bleeding diathesis, employ appropriate measures (pp 302–306) and consult with a urologist.

Testicular Tumor   If there is any suspicion of a testicular tumor, obtain a scrotal ultrasound. If a mass is detected, obtain serum for beta human chorionic gonadotropin (beta-HCG), alpha-fetoprotein, and lactate dehydrogenase (LDH) and immediately consult with a urologist.

Follow-up
- Appendiceal torsion: 2 to 3 days if the pain persists
- Epididymoorchitis, unincarcerated inguinal hernia, idiopathic scrotal edema: primary care follow-up in 7 to 10 days
- Hematocele: 3 to 5 days

Indications for Admission
- Suspected testicular torsion
- Incarcerated inguinal hernia

BIBLIOGRAPHY

Frush DP, Sheldon CA: Diagnostic imaging for pediatric scrotal disorders. *Radiographics* 1998;18:969–985.
Kapur P, Caty MG, Glick PL: Pediatric hernias and hydroceles. *Pediatr Clin North Am* 1998;45:773–789.
Kass EJ, Lundak B: The acute scrotum. *Pediatr Clin North Am* 1997;44:1251–1266.

UNDESCENDED TESTIS

The prevalence of undescended testis is 4% at birth (full-term) and 0.8% at 1 year of age, after which spontaneous descent of an undescended testicle is unlikely. Histologic deterioration begins during the second year of life, and this has been correlated with infertility even in unilateral cases. Therefore medical or surgical descent should be accomplished after the first birthday. An undescended testis is at higher risk for torsion, trauma, and, possibly, malignant degeneration.

Clinical Presentation and Diagnosis

Eighty percent of undescended testes are *palpable* in the groin (in the inguinal canal or the superficial inguinal pouch) or in an ectopic location. There may be an associated inguinal hernia. Some of these testes are actually *retractile* and will reenter the scrotum during a warm bath or can be milked into the scrotum easily without a tendency to spring back up to the groin when released.

Most *impalpable* testes are ultimately found within the abdomen or on occasion in the groin if they are atrophic or dysplastic. In the remaining cases there is unilateral or bilateral *testicular absence*, most commonly vanishing testis syndrome.

ED Management

No acute treatment is necessary. Refer infants under 1 year of age to a primary care provider and instruct the parent to examine the scrotum while the child is in a warm bath. At 1 year of age, refer patients to a urologist. If an inguinal hernia is present, arrange for early surgical correction of the cryptorchidism and the hernia, regardless of the patient's age.

BIBLIOGRAPHY

Fonkalsrud EW: Current management of the undescended testis. *Semin Pediatr Surg* 1996;5:2–7.
Gill B, Kogan S: Cryptorchidism. Current concepts. *Pediatr Clin North Am* 1997; 44:1211–1227.
Pillai SB, Besner GE: Pediatric testicular problems. *Pediatr Clin North Am* 1998; 45:813–830.

URINARY RETENTION

Ninety percent of all newborns void within the first 24 h of life, and 99% do so by 48 h. Thereafter, urinary retention is defined as failure to urinate for more than 12 h.

In the male infant, posterior urethral valves are the most common congenital cause of retention. Other etiologies include a urethral polyp, urethral stricture, urethral diverticulum, meatal stenosis, and fecal impaction. In the female infant, retention is most often secondary to a prolapsing ureterocele, urethral prolapse, or foreign body.

Infections (cystitis, urethritis, meatitis), iatrogenic or self-instrumentation, spinal cord lesions, medications (antihistamines, decongestants, bronchodilators, tricyclic anticholinergics, propantheline), and psychogenic retention are other causes of urinary retention. Also, urinary retention and dysfunctional voiding may be the presenting symptom of sexual abuse.

Clinical Presentation and Diagnosis

Urinary retention in a newborn male presents as dribbling or a poor stream. In the female, a bulging introital mass may be seen, representing a ureterocele. In either sex, the bladder may be persistently palpable.

In older patients, urinary retention may be associated with urgency, hesitancy, frequency, dribbling, a poor stream, recurrent urinary tract infections, and a distended, palpable bladder. Dysuria (*cystitis* or *urethritis*), a urethral discharge (*urethritis*), or an inflamed, swollen urethral meatus (*meatitis*) may be present. Confirm that uncircumcised males do not have *balanoposthitis* or *phimosis*.

Patients with *spinal cord abnormalities* usually have a visible deformity of the back (sacral dimple, tuft of hair, sinus). On neurologic examination, there may be altered lower extremity reflexes, decreased anal sphincter tone, a sensory level, or differential responses to sensory testing in the lower extremities compared with the upper extremities.

Psychosomatic retention usually occurs in females with no previous history of voiding abnormalities. The initiating stress factor is often unrecognized by the patient and parents, and no other congenital or acquired etiology can be found.

Consider the possibility of *sexual abuse* if the history and physical examination are not consistent with any other etiologies for urinary retention.

ED Management

Obtain blood for blood urea nitrogen (BUN) and creatinine and urine for urinalysis; immediately refer all infants with dribbling, poor stream, or failure to void within 48 h of birth to a urologist.

The management of cystitis (pp 613–616), urethritis (pp 286–293), and meatitis (p 262) is discussed elsewhere.

Treat retention secondary to urinary tract instrumentation with sitz baths thrice daily and phenazopyridine hydrochloride (Pyridium, 12 mg/kg/day divided tid, max 300 mg/dose, for 1–2 days), but warn the family that the urine will turn orange. Discontinue any medication that may be causing retention.

If a spinal cord lesion is suspected, consult with a neurologist. However, intermittent catheterization or an indwelling catheter may be required as a temporizing measure.

If psychosomatic retention is suspected, immediately refer the patient to a psychiatrist. Once again, temporary intermittent catheterization or an indwelling catheter may be required. The management of possible sexual abuse is discussed elsewhere (pp 541–550).

In cases of urinary retention secondary to fecal impaction, rapid treatment of the impaction (see Constipation, pp 236–238) leads to resolution of the urinary retention.

Indication for Admission

- Urinary retention that cannot be relieved in the ED

BIBLIOGRAPHY

Choong S, Emberton M: Acute urinary retention. *BJU Int* 2000;85:186–201.
Jayanthi VR, Khoury AE, McLorie GA: The nonneurogenic neurogenic bladder of early infancy. *J Urol* 1997;158:1281–1285.

URETHRITIS

Urethritis is an inflammation of the urethral mucosa caused by local irritation (chemical, infection, foreign-body insertion). While infectious causes of urethritis are rare in prepubertal children, sexually transmitted infection is the most common etiology in sexually active adolescents.

Clinical Presentation and Diagnosis

Irritation   Bubble bath or chlorine may cause a chemical irritation of the distal urethral and penile meatus. The patient presents with meatal pain, itching, and dysuria. The urine culture is negative.

Anatomic Abnormalities   A *prolapsed urethra* most commonly occurs in young African-American females. The prolapsed mucosa is visible and becomes irritated and congested, then hemorrhagic.

Other abnormalities, such as *urethral diverticulum, urethral polyp*, and *valve of Guérin,* are uncommon. They usually present with difficulty voiding, gross hematuria, voiding pain at the dorsal glans penis, and blood spotting on the underpants.

Foreign Body   A urethral foreign body causes a bloody urethritis. There may be a history of insertion, the object may be palpable in the urethra, or it may be radiopaque.

Posterior Urethritis   This is a nonspecific urethral inflammation in boys 5 to 15 years old. It presents with urethral discharge, urethral bleeding, or terminal hematuria. The physical examination is normal, and routine cultures of the discharge and the urine are sterile.

Sexually Transmitted Urethritis   In males, *Neisseria gonorrhoeae, Chlamdia,* or *Ureaplasma* cause dysuria, urethral discharge, and occasionally epididymitis or prostatitis. In females, *Chlamydia* commonly causes the acute urethral syndrome (dysuria, urgency, suprapubic tenderness, pyuria) or pelvic inflammatory disease (pp 286–293).

Obtain a urinalysis and routine urine culture and perform a Gram's stain and culture (gonococci, chlamydia) of the urethral discharge.

ED Management

Irritation   Discontinue the chemical irritant if known; if the symptoms are severe, give phenazopyridine hydrochloride (Pyridium 12 mg/kg/day, 300 mg maximum dose, divided tid) for 1 or 2 days only.

Anatomic Abnormalities   Treat a prolapsed urethra with sitz baths three times a day. Consult a urologist if marked edema causes voiding difficulty. Refer patients with gross hematuria associated with penile voiding pain to a urologist.

Foreign Body   Immediately consult a urologist.

Posterior Urethritis   Treat with antibiotics for 10 days (<8 years: amoxicillin 40 mg/kg/day divided tid; >8 years: trimethoprim-sulfamethoxazole (8 mg/kg/day of TMP divided bid). There is a high rate of recurrence, and bulbar urethral stricture can result. Therefore refer the patient to a urologist.

Sexually Transmitted Urethritis   Treat with a single dose of ceftriaxone 125 mg IM, followed by a 7-day course of either PO doxycycline 100 mg bid (over 8 years of age) or erythromycin 40 mg/kg/day divided qid (under 8 years of age). Ofloxacin 300 mg PO bid for 7 days is an alternative, although it is contraindicated in prepubertal patients.

Follow-up
- Urethritis: primary care follow-up in 7 to 10 days

Indications for Admission
- Inability to void
- Urethral foreign body

BIBLIOGRAPHY

Docimo SG, Silver RI, Gonzalez R, et al: Idiopathic anterior urethritis in prepubertal and pubertal boys: pathology and clues to etiology. *Urology* 1998;51:99–102.
Farhat W, McLorie G: Urethral syndromes in children. *Pediatr Rev* 2001;22:17–21.

CHAPTER 12

Gynecologic Emergencies

Anthony J. Ciorciari and Jodi J. Sutton

BREAST DISORDERS

Common breast disorders are neonatal hypertrophy, premature thelarche in prepubertal girls, breast abscesses in newborns and pubertal girls, and gynecomastia in adolescent boys.

Clinical Presentation

Neonatal Breast Hypertrophy Neonatal breast hypertrophy occurs in up to two-thirds of normal newborns of both sexes. It presents as palpable breast tissue, present from birth, in an otherwise healthy infant. Occasionally, in female infants, there is also galactorrhea (sometimes known as "witch's milk"), clitoral hypertrophy, and a bloody vaginal discharge. Most cases resolve within 4 weeks, but the condition can persist for several months, particularly in breast-fed infants.

Premature Thelarche Premature thelarche is defined as breast enlargement in the absence of other signs of puberty. It usually occurs in girls 1 to 5 years old and either regresses or does not progress. There is no associated nipple change, growth spurt, axillary or pubic hair, clitoral enlargement, acne, or nipple discharge. In the presence of any of the above conditions, consider pathologic causes including true precocious puberty, central nervous system (CNS) disorders, ovarian tumors, and exogenous estrogens.

Breast Abscesses Breast abscesses can occur in newborns as well as adolescent females. *Staphylococcus aureus* is the most common pathogen. The abscess presents as a warm, erythematous, tender mass that may be fluctuant.

Gynecomastia Gynecomastia, or enlargement of the male breast, is seen in 40% of teenage boys but is rare in preadolescents. It occurs at 12 to 15 years of age in healthy, often obese boys who are experiencing normal male pubertal development. The enlargement is usually bilateral but may be unilateral, and tenderness is not uncommon. It is most noticeable in boys who are virilizing rapidly. The enlargement regresses spontaneously. Gynecomastia has been associated with Klinefelter's syndrome (XXY karyotype and small testes), hypo- or hyperthyroidism, and medication use [tricyclic antidepressants, phenothiazines, benzodiazepines, theophylline, angiotensin converting enzyme (ACE) inhibitors, calcium channel blockers] and substance abuse (marijuana, anabolic steroids, heroin). Prepubertal gynecomastia is rare and is always considered to be pathologic.

Diagnosis

Premature Thelarche   Perform a thorough physical examination, looking for other secondary sexual characteristics, café au lait spots (*neurofibromatosis, McCune-Albright syndrome*) or ash-leaf macules (*tuberous sclerosis*), an abdominal or ovarian mass (perform a rectal examination), and visual field disturbances.

Breast Abscess   The diagnosis is usually evident on inspection. In addition, there may be an associated cellulitis or purulent discharge.

Gynecomastia   First, assess whether the breast enlargement is secondary to adipose tissue (*pseudogynecomastia*) or consists of true breast tissue. Insert an index finger directly into the nipple. With adipose tissue, it feels like the hole of a doughnut, whereas breast tissue is firm. If there is true gynecomastia, palpate the abdomen for hepatomegaly, and examine the testicles to evaluate their size and rule out a mass. Look for findings suggestive of *hypo-* or *hyperthyroidism*.

ED Management

Neonatal Breast Hypertrophy   Reassurance, cool compresses, and avoidance of breast massaging are all that is necessary. Refer the infant to a primary care provider.

Premature Thelarche   If there are no other signs of puberty, refer the patient to a primary care physician for routine follow-up. However, if other signs of puberty are present, so that a pathologic etiology cannot be ruled out in the ED, refer the patient to a pediatric endocrinologist for a prompt evaluation.

Breast Abscesses   Treat neonates with 40 mg/kg/day of oral cephalexin (divided qid) or cefadroxil (divided bid) and warm soaks. If the baby has a fever higher than 100.6°F (38.1°C) or looks "toxic," perform a complete sepsis workup (including lumbar puncture) and treat with IV nafcillin (150 mg/kg/day divided q 6 h).

Treat an afebrile adolescent female with a small abscess with 40 mg/kg/day (maximum 2 g) of oral cephalexin (divided qid) or cefadroxil (divided bid) for 3 to 4 weeks. Follow up in 24 h; if the mass enlarges or becomes fluctuant or the patient develops fever, admit her for intravenous antibiotics and drainage *by an experienced surgeon.* Extensive breast abscesses may not appear fluctuant and ready for drainage until a large amount of breast tissue has been destroyed. Therefore these infections must be followed carefully.

Gynecomastia   Reassure healthy pubertal males with normal growth and arrange for primary care follow-up. Refer prepubertal boys to a pediatric endocrinologist for prompt evaluation.

Follow-up
- Premature thelarche associated with other secondary sexual characteristics: endocrinologist within 1 week
- Breast abscess: 24 h
- Prepubertal male with gynecomastia: endocrinologist within 1 week

Indications for Admission
- Breast abscess in a febrile or toxic neonate or febrile adolescent
- Enlarging breast abscess, despite oral antibiotics, in an adolescent female

BIBLIOGRAPHY

Neinstein LS: Breast disease in adolescents and young women. *Pediatr Clin North Am* 1999;46:607–629.
Sher ES, Migeon CJ, Berkovitz GD: Evaluation of boys with marked breast development at puberty. *Clin Pediatr (Phila)* 1998;37:367–371.
Sloand E: Pediatric and adolescent breast health. *Lippincotts Prim Care Pract* 1998;2:170–175.

DYSFUNCTIONAL UTERINE BLEEDING

Normal menstrual bleeding does not occur more often than every 21 days; the flow lasts no more than 8 days; and no more than 6 well-soaked pads or 10 well-soaked tampons are used in 24 h.

Dysfunctional uterine bleeding (DUB) is irregular, painless bleeding of endometrial origin. Most cases are secondary to anovulation, which is common during the first 2 years after menarche. Pathologic causes of anovulation include stress, recent weight gain or loss, chronic illness, drug abuse, ovarian cyst, and birth control pills. In addition, however, abnormal vaginal bleeding may be associated with local or systemic disease and therefore must be evaluated carefully.

Clinical Presentation

A typical pattern of DUB is prolonged or excessive flow alternating with periods of amenorrhea. Pain, fever, chills, and vaginal discharge are absent.

Mild DUB   With mild DUB, the menses may be somewhat prolonged or the cycle shortened for 2 to 3 months. The hemoglobin and hematocrit are normal, >12 g/dL and >36 to 38%, respectively.

Moderate DUB   Moderate DUB is characterized by prolonged periods and an increased flow severe enough to cause a decrease in hemoglobin and hematocrit to 10 to 12 g/dL and 28 to 35%, respectively.

Severe DUB   Severe DUB results in significant decreases in the hemoglobin and hematocrit, to <10 g/dL and <28%, respectively. There are clinical signs of acute blood loss (tachycardia, orthostatic vital sign changes, delayed capillary refill).

Diagnosis

DUB is a diagnosis of exclusion. By definition, it is painless. The most frequent causes of painful vaginal bleeding are complications of *pregnancy* and *uterine infections*. See Table 12-1 for the differential diagnosis of abnormal vaginal bleeding.

Inquire about the age of menarche, date of last normal menstrual period, frequency and regularity of menses, length of flow, and the number of pads or tampons used. Ask about other bleeding manifestations, sexual activity (including *genital trauma*), *foreign bodies*, medication use (particularly *oral contraceptives*), *endocrine disorders*, *exposure to diethylstilbestrol (DES)* in utero, *emotional stress*, and *chronic illnesses.*

Table 12-1   Differential Diagnosis of Dysfunctional Uterine Bleeding

Complications of pregnancy	*Genital trauma*
Abortion	First intercourse
Ectopic	Rape
Gynecologic infection	*Foreign body*
Cervicitis	Diaphragm
Pelvic inflammatory disease	Tampon
Bleeding disorder	*Anatomic abnormality*
Von Willebrand disease	Ovarian cyst
	Fibroids
Endocrine disorders	DES exposure in utero (rare)
Hypo- or hyperthyroidism	
Adrenal disorders	*Chronic illness*
Diabetes mellitus	Inflammatory bowel disease
Polycystic ovary syndrome	Chronic renal disease
	Liver disease
Medication use	
Warfarin	*Malignancy*
Birth control pills	*Stress*

Obtain a family history of *abnormal bleeding* (epistaxis, easy bruising, bleeding gums).

On physical examination, the priorities are the vital signs, manifestations of a bleeding diathesis, and the gynecologic examination. Check for orthostatic hypotension, bradycardia (*hypothyroidism*), tachycardia (*hyperthyroidism, significant blood loss*), delayed capillary refill, petechiae or ecchymoses (*bleeding diathesis*), or evidence of a chronic illness. Examine the breasts for signs of *pregnancy* (fullness, tenderness, enlarged and darkened areola, galactorrhea) and the abdomen for an enlarged uterus, mass, or tenderness (suggesting *pelvic inflammatory disease*).

A gynecologic examination is indicated for any teenager with moderate or severe DUB. Inspect the external genitalia for signs of *trauma* or bleeding sources. Next, perform a speculum examination looking for evidence of trauma, *exposure to DES* (vaginal adenosis, cockscomb cervix), *pregnancy* (bluish color to the cervix), *abortion* (opening of the internal os), or *infection* (cervical discharge). Upon bimanual (or rectoabdominal) examination, check the cervix for softness (pregnancy) and tenderness on motion (salpingitis), palpate the uterus to determine size and tenderness, and examine the adnexae for masses and tenderness.

Pregnancy (pp 282–286) is suggested by a history of fatigue, nausea, vomiting, and urinary frequency; a positive serum hCG confirms the diagnosis. Breast tenderness and an enlarged uterus may be noted. *Salpingitis* (pp 286–293) may present with a vaginal discharge, lower abdominal pain, fever, chills, and cervical motion tenderness. With a *bleeding disorder* (pp 302–306), there may be other bleeding manifestations, such as petechiae, ecchymoses, epistaxis, bleeding gums, hematuria, and, rarely, hematochezia.

ED Management

For all patients, obtain a complete blood count (CBC) with platelet count, thyroid function tests, and a urinalysis. If the patient is sexually active, obtain a Pap smear, cultures for *Neisseria gonorrhoeae* and *Chlamydia trachomatis,* VDRL (Venereal Disease Research Laboratory) test, and pregnancy test. Clotting studies [prothrombin time (PT), partial thromboplastin time (PTT)], bleeding time, serial hematocrits, and type and crossmatch are indicated for moderate, severe, or prolonged bleeding or if there is excessive bleeding at menarche. If a pelvic mass is appreciated, obtain an ultrasound.

Mild DUB   Observation and reassurance are all that is needed. Advise the patient to keep a menstrual calendar. Iron supplementation (300 mg/day of ferrous sulfate) may be necessary, but the majority of these patients convert spontaneously to normal menstrual cycles within several months.

Moderate DUB   Treat with oral contraceptives [1 mg progesterone, 35 mg estrogen (e.g., Ortho-Novum 1:35)]: Give four pills per day for 4 days, then three pills per day for 4 days, then two pills per day for 13 to 19 days. Withdrawal bleeding for 7 days will follow. On the Sunday after the withdrawal bleeding stops, resume the 1:35 oral contraceptive or a triphasic preparation (e.g., Ortho-Tricyclen) and continue for 3 months.

Severe DUB   The priority is restoration of adequate perfusion (see Shock, pp 18–22) with 20-mL/kg boluses of isotonic crystalloid (normal saline or Ringer's lactate). A transfusion of packed red cells (10 mL/kg) is indicated if the patient remains orthostatic or symptomatic at rest (tachycardia, dizziness) after two 20-mL/kg boluses of crystalloid. Admit the patient for treatment and observation. If the bleeding is severe enough to warrant a transfusion, treat with a conjugated estrogen (25 mg IV over 20 min q 4–6 h) until the bleeding stops. An antiemetic may be needed [prochlorperazine maleate (Compazine) 10 mg PO q 6 h or 25 mg PO bid]. If a transfusion is not needed, treat with a 1:35 oral contraceptive, as for moderate DUB. Continued bleeding beyond 24 h is rare. It may signal an anatomic abnormality and is an indication for gynecologic consultation to consider examination under general anesthesia with possible dilation and curettage. Iron therapy and ongoing hormonal therapy are also indicated, as for patients with moderate DUB. After the withdrawal bleeding, use a 1:50 oral contraceptive (Ortho-Novum 1:50) for the next 3 months.

Follow-up

- Mild DUB: routine primary care follow-up.
- Moderate DUB: 1 to 2 days; refer to a gynecologist if the bleeding does not stop within 2–3 days.

Indication for Admission

- Severe DUB (hematocrit <28%, orthostatic changes, transfusion needed)

BIBLIOGRAPHY

Bravender T, Emans SJ: Menstrual disorders. Dysfunctional uterine bleeding. *Pediatr Clin North Am* 1999;46:545–553.
Chen BH, Giudice LC: Dysfunctional uterine bleeding. *West J Med* 1998;169: 280–284.
Lavin C: Dysfunctional uterine bleeding in adolescents. *Curr Opin Pediatr* 1996;8: 328–332.

DYSMENORRHEA

Dysmenorrhea (painful menstruation) is very common in teenagers and may be a response to elevated levels of prostaglandin. Dysmenorrhea may be classified as primary or secondary. The majority of cases are primary, presenting within 2 years of menarche and not associated with significant pelvic pathology. In secondary dysmenorrhea, there is pelvic pathology, most often salpingitis, endometriosis, or genital tract obstruction.

Clinical Presentation

Primary Dysmenorrhea   Primary dysmenorrhea usually presents within 6 to 12 months of menarche. Typically, colicky suprapubic pain begins several hours before or after the start of a period. The pain may radiate to the back or down the thighs. In 50% of patients there may be nausea, vomiting, diarrhea, and headache. The symptoms usually last from a few hours to several days.

Secondary Dysmenorrhea   Secondary dysmenorrhea generally presents years after menarche. As in primary dysmenorrhea, the pain occurs during menstruation. There may be a history of pelvic inflammatory disease, menorrhagia, endometriosis, or use of an intrauterine device (IUD) for contraception.

Diagnosis

Document the age at menarche and the frequency and severity of the pain and its relation to the periods. Ask about a history of vaginal discharge, sexual activity, and IUD use. If the patient is sexually active, perform a pelvic examination looking for causes of secondary dysmenorrhea.

The pain of *salpingitis* may be exacerbated during periods. On examination, there may be fever, a vaginal discharge, cervical motion tenderness, and adnexal enlargement. The pain of *endometriosis* typically starts before the period and persists after the bleeding has stopped. The uterus or ovaries may be tender or enlarged, and the uterus may be nodular and sensitive to motion. *Genital tract obstruction* presents with cyclic lower abdominal pain in an amenorrheic patient. On examination, the uterus is enlarged.

In addition, consider nongynecologic causes of pelvic pain, such as *chronic constipation, inflammatory bowel disease*, and *psychogenic disorders*.

ED Management

Primary Dysmenorrhea   Oral prostaglandin synthetase inhibitors are effective in 70 to 100% of patients. If menstrual cramps do not interfere with a teenager's normal activity, use ibuprofen 400 mg qid. However, if the pain is more substantial, use mefenamic acid (500 mg to start, then 250 mg q 6 h) or naproxen sodium (550 mg to start, then 275 mg q 6–8 h). Advise the patient to start the medication at the onset of each period. If one drug is ineffective, try an alternative. Side effects include nausea, dizziness, dyspepsia, and gastric irritation. These medications are contraindicated in patients with ulcers or aspirin allergy; use with caution in patients taking anticoagulants or those with liver or kidney disease.

Suppression of ovulation by oral contraceptives is effective, but reserve this therapy for the primary care setting, where appropriate follow-up can be arranged.

Secondary Dysmenorrhea   Refer the patient to a gynecologist to treat the underlying cause. The management of salpingitis is discussed on pp 286–293. Prostaglandin synthetase inhibitors may be helpful, particularly if the patient has an IUD. If endometriosis is suspected, refer the patient to a gynecologist to arrange for laparoscopic confirmation of the diagnosis, followed by hormone therapy.

Follow-up

- Primary dysmenorrhea: primary care follow-up before the next period
- Secondary dysmenorrhea: gynecologic follow-up before the next period

BIBLIOGRAPHY

Davis AR, Westhoff C: Primary dysmenorrhea in adolescent girls and treatment with oral contraceptives. *J Pediatr Adolesc Gynecol* 2001;14:3–8.

O'Connell BJ: The pediatrician and the sexually active adolescent. Treatment of common menstrual disorders. *Pediatr Clin North Am* 1997;44:1391–1404.

Schroeder B, Sanfilippo JS: Dysmenorrhea and pelvic pain in adolescents. *Pediatr Clin North Am* 1999;46:555–571.

PREGNANCY AND COMPLICATIONS

It is estimated that 1 of 10 teenage girls becomes pregnant each year. Spontaneous abortions complicate 10 to 15% of pregnancies. Ectopic pregnancies occur in approximately 2% of pregnancies in North America and are more common among nonwhite ethnic groups.

Clinical Presentation

Knowledge of whether a patient is pregnant is essential in evaluating her complaints and determining management. The first step is to interview the teenager privately and assure her that the discussion is confidential. Often the pregnant patient presents with vague complaints of "abdominal pain" or "not feeling right" because she does not want her family to suspect the possible pregnancy. The patient may not realize or deny that she is pregnant. Also, she may not volunteer the information that she has missed a period or had unprotected intercourse.

During early pregnancy, a teenager may report "missing" her period or that it was "different" (longer or shorter than usual). Fatigue, dizziness, syncope, nausea, and vomiting (especially in the morning), urinary frequency, and weight gain may be noted by 2 weeks. Nipple discharge (colostrum) can occur at 6 weeks.

On examination, the breasts have darkened areolae and enlarged nipples. Often, there is protrusion of Montgomery's glands. Findings on pelvic examination depend on the time elapsed since the last normal period. At 5 weeks, the examination may be normal; at 6 weeks, there may be softening of the upper cervix (Hegar's sign); at 8 weeks, the cervix and vaginal mucosa may have a bluish tinge (Chadwick's sign) and the uterus may be soft and slightly enlarged; and by 10 to 12 weeks. the fetal heart may be heard with Doppler ultrasound. At 12 weeks, the globular uterus can be palpated at the level of the pubic symphysis; at 16 weeks, at the midpoint between the symphysis and umbilicus; and at 20 weeks, at the level of the umbilicus.

Threatened and Imminent Abortion   With a threatened abortion, the history is compatible with early pregnancy. There is vaginal bleeding with or without cramps, and the internal cervical os is closed. With an imminent abortion, the cervix becomes shortened and dilated.

Inevitable and Complete Abortion   An inevitable abortion resembles an imminent abortion except that tissue is seen protruding from the dilated, effaced cervix. The embryo and placenta are completely expelled in a complete abortion.

Incomplete Abortion   With an incomplete abortion, fragments of placenta remain in the uterus; there are persistent cramps as well as bleeding and cervical dilation.

Missed Abortion   A missed abortion is a fetal death in utero before the 20th week, but with the pregnancy retained. The patient is amenorrheic, with or without uterine growth.

Ectopic Pregnancy   An ectopic pregnancy occurs when the blastocyst implants in a location other than the uterus; the vast majority of such implantations are in the fallopian tubes. Predisposing factors include pelvic inflammatory disease and a previous ectopic pregnancy. The classic presentation is amenorrhea with symptoms of early pregnancy, followed by abdominal pain and mild to moderate vaginal bleeding. Amenorrhea (late or missed period) occurs in 75% of patients, followed by vaginal spotting or bleeding. Brisk or heavy bleeding is uncommon. Initially the pain is unilateral and crampy. After several hours (to days), there is the sudden onset of sharp pain secondary to tubal rupture and bleeding into the peritoneum. Later, the pain becomes generalized. As blood accumulates under the diaphragm, the pain can be referred to the shoulder and increase when the patient lies supine or inhales. Syncope and hypovolemic shock are less common presentations.

Physical examination findings include abdominal, pelvic, and cervical motion tenderness. An adnexal mass, typically 5 to 7 cm in diameter, can be identified in 50% of patients. Most importantly, there is often a discrepancy between the palpated uterine size and what is expected based on the date of the last menstrual period. Although only 15% of patients have the classic ectopic presentation, approximately 90% complain of mild pelvic discomfort and 80% have abnormal vaginal bleeding, often mild and intermittent. However, the history and physical examination can be normal. The patient is usually afebrile with a normal to slightly elevated white blood cell count.

Diagnosis

Pregnancy tests detect the presence of hCG in the blood or urine. The standard urine pregnancy test is 99% sensitive and specific, detecting 5 to 25 mIU/mL of hCG. In normal pregnancies, it may be positive as early as 3 to 4 days after implantation and virtually always by the expected date of the missed period. The serum hCG by radioimmunoassay can be positive within 7 days of conception (before a period has been missed). With an intrauterine pregnancy, the hCG rises by at least 60% every 2 days, up to a titer of 50,000 IU/mL. With an ectopic pregnancy, the hCG is lower and does not rise as fast. However, a single hCG measurement is of limited value, since the exact gestational age is not often known and there is some overlap in the range of hCG levels found in the two conditions. Therefore, obtain serial hCG determinations 2 days apart. Doubling of the hCG within 48 h suggests an intrauterine pregnancy. A slower doubling time, or a rise of less than 66% over 2 days, suggests *but does not confirm* an ectopic pregnancy.

The serum progesterone is useful for diagnosing an ectopic pregnancy. In a normal pregnancy, the level is >25 ng/mL, while a level <5 ng/mL is strongly associated with an ectopic pregnancy. Values between 5 and 25 ng/mL are indeterminate.

It is not always safe to wait 2 days to confirm the diagnosis. Using transabdominal ultrasound, a normal intrauterine pregnancy can be detected with an hCG >6500 mIU/mL. However, transvaginal ultrasound is far more sensitive (90–95%). A gestational sac can be confirmed at an hCG of 1000 to 1500 mIU/mL, or within 1 week of the first missed period (before tubal rupture is common). The diagnostic and therapeutic approach to ectopic pregnancy is summarized in Fig. 12-1.

The differential diagnosis of an ectopic pregnancy includes a normal pregnancy with another cause for the abdominal or pelvic pain. Among the gynecologic conditions that may complicate pregnancy and can be evaluated by ultrasound are an *ovarian cyst, ovarian* or *tubal torsion, ruptured corpus luteum,* and *stretched ligaments.* Alternatively, the pathology may be nongynecologic, such as an *appendicitis* (anorexia prominent, no vaginal bleeding) or a *renal stone* (renal colic, vomiting common, hematuria, no vaginal bleeding). Other conditions can be ruled out during the pelvic examination, including a *spontaneous abortion* (more active bleeding) and *pelvic inflammatory disease* (fever, bilateral pain).

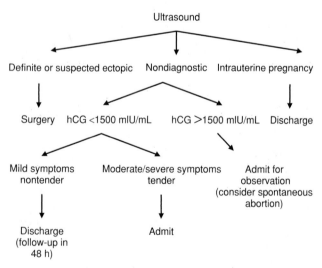

Figure 12-1   Management of suspected ectopic pregnancy.

ED Management

The priority is *expedient diagnosis and management of an ectopic pregnancy*. Suspect an ectopic pregnancy in any pubertal female with moderate vaginal bleeding and/or lower abdominal pain, especially if her period is late. Perform a pelvic examination; cervical motion tenderness and an adnexal mass suggest the possibility of an ectopic pregnancy. Immediately arrange for gynecologic consultation, obtain blood for hCG, CBC, type and cross-match; insert a large-bore IV and monitor the patient carefully, with frequent checking of vital signs and serial hematocrits.

If a *ruptured ectopic pregnancy is likely* (rebound tenderness, changes in orthostatic vital signs, or falling hematocrit associated with a positive hCG), *immediate surgical exploration is indicated.*

If a ruptured ectopic pregnancy is not likely and the patient is not in shock, obtain an ultrasound and hCG and follow the management plan outlined in Fig. 12-1. If the ultrasound is nondiagnostic, the hCG is less than 1500 mIU/mL, and the symptoms (abdominal pain, cervical tenderness) are moderate or severe, admit the patient. If the patient has no abdominal tenderness, she may be discharged for outpatient serial hCG measurements every 48 h *provided that reliable follow-up is guaranteed.* A normal increase suggests an intrauterine pregnancy, which must be confirmed by transvaginal ultrasound. An abnormal hCG rise or no intrauterine pregnancy on ultrasound are indications for surgery.

If the hCG is greater than 1500 mIU/mL and the ultrasound is nondiagnostic, admit the patient for observation (possible spontaneous abortion) and gynecologic consultation. If the ultrasound is not immediately available, admit the patient for close observation, serial hCG measurements, and possible laparoscopy. Culdocentesis is now indicated only if transvaginal ultrasound is not available. It is very specific: nonclotting blood in the cul-de-sac mandates surgical exploration. However, sensitivity is poor, as "dry taps" can occur and straw-colored fluid excludes only a ruptured ectopic.

If the gestation is less than 4 cm and there is no evidence of rupture or leakage, consult a gynecologist to attempt medical management of a confirmed ectopic pregnancy. Up to 95% of cases will resolve after one dose of methotrexate (50 mg/m^2). Reliable, close follow-up is absolutely necessary.

Manage *threatened abortions* expectantly, with complete bed rest and no intercourse. If bleeding continues, hospitalize the patient and obtain a type and cross-match in case a transfusion becomes necessary (hematocrit <18%; symptoms of hypovolemia not relieved by crystalloid fluid resuscitation).

Admit patients with *imminent, inevitable*, and *incomplete abortions* and consult with a gynecologist for dilation and curettage. In the ED, insert a large-bore IV and obtain a CBC, spun hematocrit, and a type and hold.

If the patient shows symptoms of acute blood loss, order a type and cross-match and begin fluid resuscitation with isotonic crystalloid (pp 18–22).

The patient with a *complete abortion* can be sent home unless there are signs of serious blood loss, in which case insert a large-bore IV and obtain a CBC and type and cross-match.

Check the Rh status for any patient with a threatened, imminent, inevitable, complete, incomplete, or missed abortion or an ectopic pregnancy. If she is Rh-negative, IM RhoGAM is required. Give a minidose (50 µg) during the first trimester; use 300 µg beyond the first trimester.

If a *normal intrauterine pregnancy* is diagnosed, make an appointment for the teenager (and her boyfriend) to be seen within a few days in an adolescent gynecology or family planning clinic for appropriate counseling and management. Social work referral may also be indicated.

Follow-up

- Possible ectopic pregnancy without abdominal tenderness: at once for dizziness or abdominal or shoulder pain. Otherwise, follow up in 48 h.

Indications for Admission

- Ectopic pregnancy (confirmed or probable)
- Ectopic pregnancy unlikely (nondiagnostic ultrasound, hCG <1500 mIU/mL), but follow-up not guaranteed
- Ultrasound nondiagnostic and hCG <1500 mIU/mL, but patient has moderate or severe abdominal pain or cervical motion tenderness
- Ultrasound nondiagnostic and hCG >1500 mIU/mL
- Imminent, incomplete, or inevitable abortion
- Severe acute blood loss

BIBLIOGRAPHY

Lehner R, Kucera E, Jirecek S, et al: Ectopic pregnancy. *Arch Gynecol Obstet* 2000;263:87–92.
Polaneczky M, O'Connor K: Pregnancy in the adolescent patient: screening, diagnosis, and initial management. *Pediatr Clin North Am* 1999;46:649–670.
Tenore JL: Ectopic pregnancy. *Am Fam Physician* 2000;61:1080–1088.

SEXUALLY TRANSMITTED DISEASES

One of four teenagers will have a sexually transmitted disease (STD) before graduating from high school. Pelvic inflammatory disease, or salpingitis, is the most serious and affects over 200,000 teenagers per year. *N. gonorrhoeae* and *C. trachomatis* are responsible for most cases of salpingitis, while *Chlamydia* and *Ureaplasma urealyticum* cause at least 70% of the cases of nongonococcal urethritis. *Treponema pallidum*, the agent responsible for syphilis, can cause severe systemic disease, and *human papillomavirus* (HPV) has been associated with cervical cancer. There are no cures for any of the sexually transmitted viruses (including herpes and HIV).

Clinical Presentation

Salpingitis   Salpingitis can be acute, subacute, chronic, or subclinical, and none of the causative organisms produces a distinctive clinical picture. Classic acute salpingitis presents within 1 week of the onset of a menstrual period, although the disease can occur at any time in the cycle. Symptoms include vaginal discharge, high fever, shaking chills, and severe unilateral or, more commonly, bilateral lower abdominal pain. On abdominal examination, there is marked lower abdominal tenderness, guarding, and rebound tenderness. On pelvic examination, a purulent cervical discharge, cervical motion tenderness (especially side to side), tender adnexae, and a normal-size uterus are noted. The white blood count (WBC) is usually greater than 10,000 to 15,000/mm³ and the erythrocyte sedimentation rate (ESR) is elevated (>50 mm/h).

Just as often, the presentation is subacute, with lower abdominal pain in the absence of fever, with or without vaginal discharge, and without elevation of the WBC and/or ESR. The *FitzHugh–Curtis syndrome* (perihepatitis in association with salpingitis) presents with right-upper-quadrant pain, occasionally accompanied by right-sided pleuritic chest and shoulder pain.

Urethritis   Urethritis is the most common manifestation of STD in males. Dysuria and a urethral discharge occur, occasionally in association with epididymitis. In females, *Chlamydia* commonly causes the *acute urethral syndrome,* with dysuria, urgency, suprapubic tenderness, pyuria without hematuria, and a negative routine urine culture.

Cervicitis and Proctitis   Cervicitis and proctitis can be seen with *N. gonorrhoeae* and/or *Chlamydia*. Both are associated with purulent discharge.

Syphilis   The hallmark of primary syphilis is the chancre, which develops 3 to 4 weeks after exposure. It appears as a painless ulcer with a smooth clean base, raised indurated borders, and scanty yellow discharge. In males the chancre is most frequently seen on the penis, scrotum, or anus or in the mouth. In females, it occurs on the vulva, vagina, cervix, or urethra or in the mouth. Fifty percent of patients have more than one chancre, and enlarged, firm regional lymph nodes are seen in 60 to 80% of patients. Untreated, the chancre resolves in 3 to 6 weeks; it may be followed in 6 to 8 weeks by the signs of secondary syphilis.

Several skin (and mucous membrane) eruptions are typical of secondary syphilis. Commonly, there are nonpruritic, well-demarcated, brownish red macules and papules symmetrically distributed on the trunk and extremities. These are often also found on the palms and soles. Condylomata lata are highly contagious, flat, moist, pink papules that occur in warm, moist intertriginous areas. When the maculopapules involve the mucous membranes of the mouth, they appear as shallow gray ulcers called mucous patches. Other signs of secondary syphilis include "moth-eaten" alopecia and nontender, firm, or rubbery lymphadenopathy. Constitutional symptoms—including low-grade fever, headache, fatigue, sore throat, weight loss, arthralgias, and myalgias—occasionally accompany the above findings.

Chancroid (Haemophilus Ducreyi)   Chancroid causes genital ulcers. It typically presents as multiple purulent ulcers, often with ragged edges and tender inguinal nodes.

Lymphogranuloma Venereum   LGV is also associated with ulcers and is caused by three serotypes of *C. trachomatis*. It is rare and more often seen in males. The ulcer is usually transient, and the patient typically seeks medical attention for late sequelae, such as large inguinal nodes or rectal strictures.

Genital Herpes   Genital herpes is usually due to type 2 herpes simplex virus, but 5 to 15% can be secondary to type 1 infections. In primary infections, vesicles appear on the anogenital area, then rupture within several days and become small painful ulcers. The patient may complain of dysuria in addition to local burning. Inguinal nodes enlarge, and the patient may complain of a headache, fever, myalgias, and malaise. Symptoms may last up to 3 weeks. Recurrent herpes infections are less marked and shorter in duration (3–5 days). Often a 24-h prodrome of neuralgia is noted prior to the development of lesions.

Anogenital Warts   Condylomata acuminata are skin-colored growths with a cauliflower-like surface. Varying in size, most are asymptomatic, but they can cause itching, burning, and pain, and they can bleed. They are caused by the human papillomavirus (HPV) and are primarily transmitted by sexual contact. Suspect sexual abuse if they are noted in a child beyond infancy.

Lice   Pediculosis pubis (pp 106–108) causes itching in the pubic region.

Diagnosis

Salpingitis   The priorities are to identify salpingitis and rule out an ectopic pregnancy. Have the parent leave the room and ask about intercourse (including anal), number of partners, oral-genital contact, contraceptive use, and a history of salpingitis or other STDs. The risk of salpingitis increases with nonuse of barrier contraception, multiple partners, and a history of previous episodes. Ask when menarche began, and note the regularity and duration of menses and the dates of the previous period as well as the one before. Symptoms beginning within 1 to 2 weeks of the last period suggest salpingitis.

On physical examination, look for evidence of *pregnancy*, surgical scars on the abdomen, and signs of respiratory distress (tachypnea, retractions), since *pneumonia* can present with severe lower abdominal pain. Examine the abdomen carefully for tenderness, rebound, guarding, and the presence and quality of bowel sounds.

Perform a pelvic examination if a postmenarchal female complains of vaginal discharge, abdominal pain, or menstrual abnormalities or if she has physical signs of pregnancy. On speculum examination, use a Dacron swab to obtain endocervical cultures for *N. gonorrhoeae* (modified Thayer-Martin-Jembec Transgrow or Thayer-Martin medium) and *Chlamydia*. Prepare a slide for Gram's stain and perform a Pap smear as well. Although *Neisseria* species are normally found in the female genital tract, the presence of gram-negative intracellular diplococci on the Gram's stain of a purulent endocervical discharge is highly suggestive of gonococcal infection. After the speculum examination, perform a bimanual examination, attempting to elicit side-to-side cervical motion tenderness suggestive of tubular pathology. Examine the adnexae for the presence of a mass or bogginess (ovarian mass, tuboovarian abscess). Also obtain urine for culture (two separate clean-catch specimens or a catheter specimen if a vaginal discharge is present) and a urinalysis. Obtain anal and pharyngeal cultures from patients with extragenital contact, since some of the treatment regimens may be ineffective for infection in these sites. Obtain blood for CBC, ESR, blood culture and a serum hCG, and a type and cross-match if an *ectopic pregnancy* cannot be ruled out with certainty. Obtain liver function tests if *FitzHugh–Curtis syndrome* is suspected.

In the differential diagnosis of salpingitis, consider *gastroenteritis* (diarrhea), *inflammatory bowel disease* (weight loss, bloody stools, change in bowel pattern), *acute appendicitis* (periumbilical pain localizing to the right lower quadrant), *urinary tract infection* (suprapubic or flank pain, dysuria, bacteriuria in association with pyuria), *right- lower-lobe pneumonia* (cough, tachypnea, rales, right-upper-quadrant pain), and, rarely, *cholecystitis* (right-upper-quadrant pain, intolerance of fatty foods). In all these, the pelvic examination is normal. Always consider an *ectopic pregnancy* when there has been amenorrhea or abnormal menses preceding the episode. There may be pregnancy symptoms and a positive serum pregnancy test (pp 282–286), but fever and marked leukocytosis are absent. In many females, the diagnosis is not certain from the history and physical examination. Consult a gynecologist, who may recommend abdominal ultrasound, culdocentesis, or laparoscopy. Insert a large-bore IV if a patient who might have an ectopic pregnancy must leave the ED for diagnostic tests.

Urethritis   Obtain a urinalysis and urine culture if there are symptoms of urethritis. Ask sexually active males to try to express any discharge, which must be cultured for *N. gonorrhoeae* and *Chlamydia*. If the patient has noticed a discharge previously but none is present at the time of examination, insert a Caligswab 2.5 cm into the urethra to obtain specimens for culture and Gram's stain. Assume that an asymptomatic male has urethritis if there are >4 WBCs per high-power field (oil) on Gram's stain of an intraurethral smear. If gram-negative intracellular diplococci are seen on the Gram's stain of the discharge in a male, the diagnosis is *gonococcal urethritis*.

Syphilis   Suspect all genital lesions of being syphilitic. Chancres can be confused with *chancroid* (multiple soft, tender ulcers; very tender contiguous adenopathy), *granuloma inguinale* (soft, smooth, granulating painless lesion), *lymphogranuloma venereum* (transient vesicular ulceration with very enlarged tender nodes), or *lichen planus* (annular flat-topped papules). Also, rule out *herpes* (multiple superficial, painful lesions), a *pyogenic granuloma* (a single painful, erythematous lesion, history of trauma or surgery), *molluscum contagiosum* (grouped, umbilicated, flesh-colored papules, similar lesions elsewhere on body), and *condyloma acuminatum* (dry, single or clustered warty lesions). The maculopapular eruption of *pityriasis rosea* is not present on the palms and soles, although it can otherwise resemble the rash of secondary syphilis. The scaly plaques of *psoriasis* can be on the penis and elsewhere on the body.

Send wet smears from lesions for dark-field microscopy, and obtain a VDRL or other nontreponemal serologic test for syphilis (STS). A newly positive test or a fourfold rise in titer of the STS from the previous level is diagnostic. These tests are reactive within 3 to 4 weeks of the appearance of the chancre. If the VDRL is positive, the fluorescent treponemal antibody absorption (FTA) test should also be positive. False-positive VDRLs (usually low titer) occur with hepatitis, mononucleosis, collagen vascular disease, tuberculosis, viral pneumonia, malaria, varicella, measles, and narcotics abuse.

Chancroid and LGV   The diagnosis of chancroid is made by excluding syphilis and herpes; it is extremely difficult to culture *Haemophilus ducreyi.* LGV is diagnosed by titer.

Herpes   The diagnosis of herpes is confirmed by culture but may also be made by seeing multinucleated giant cells and inclusions on a Tzanck smear (Wright's stain of a scraping).

Lice   The diagnosis of lice is made by inspection; small, moving particles resembling dandruff flakes or nits firmly attached to hair shafts are seen.

Warts   Warts are diagnosed by inspection (pp 119–120).

ED Management

Antibiotic treatment is summarized in Table 12-2. Obtain a VDRL if the patient is sexually active and might have an STD. Remind the patient that the sexual partner(s) must be examined and treated, and arrange a follow-up visit with a primary care provider for a test-of-cure evaluation.

Obtain a CBC, ESR, and liver function tests and secure an IV if there are signs or symptoms of *acute salpingitis.* Because of the tremendous risk of subsequent infertility, ectopic pregnancy, and chronic pelvic pain, admit an adolescent suspected of having salpingitis for IV therapy.

Treat an afebrile patient with *cervicitis* (cervical discharge and friability but no cervical motion tenderness) or *proctitis* on an outpatient basis with oral medications. Schedule a follow-up office visit within a week of completing therapy; emphasize both the avoidance of intercourse until the patient's partner is cultured and treated and the use of condoms to prevent both future infections and pregnancy. Oral contraception may be started in the ED if the patient is within a week of the end of the last period.

Treat a male with presumptive or definite *urethritis* and schedule a revisit within 48 to 72 h to evaluate progress and another within a week of completing the medication for repeat cultures. Until the patient's sexual partner is cultured and treated, intercourse must be avoided.

Treat a female with *acute urethral syndrome* for chlamydial urethritis and schedule a follow-up office visit within a week.

Treat a patient with primary or secondary *syphilis,* and arrange for follow-up serologic testing 3, 6, 12, and 24 months after treatment. Evalu-

Table 12-2   Treatment of Sexually Transmitted Diseases

CHLAMYDIA TRACHOMATIS

Chlamydial urethritis, cervicitis, conjunctivitis, and proctitis or nongono-
coccal nonchlamydial urethritis and cervicitis:

a. Doxycycline* 100 mg PO bid × 7 days *or*
b. Azithromycin 1 g PO as one dose *or*
c. Ofloxacin[†] 300 mg PO bid × 7 days *or*
d. Erythromycin 500 mg PO qid × 7 days

GONORRHEA[‡]

Urethral, cervical, rectal, or pharyngeal:
   One dose of one of the following: ceftriaxone[§] 125 mg IM *or* cefixime
   400 mg (8 mg/kg) *or* ciprofloxacin[†] 500 mg PO *or* ofloxacin[†] 400 mg PO
   or levofloxacin 250 mg PO

EPIDIDYMITIS

Ofloxacin[†] 300 mg bid × 10 days *or* ceftriaxone[§] 250 mg IM once, *followed*
by doxycycline* 100 mg PO bid × 10 days

PELVIC INFLAMMATORY DISEASE

Inpatient. Give one of the following regimens:

a. Cefotetan 2 g IV q 12 h *or* cefoxitin 2 g IV q 6 h *plus* doxycycline* 100 mg
   PO bid or IV q 12 h, until improved
b. Clindamycin 900 mg IV q 8 h *plus* gentamicin 2 mg/kg IV once, *followed*
   by gentamicin 1.5 mg/kg IV q 8 h, until improved
c. Ofloxacin[†] 400 mg IV q 12 h *plus* metronidazole 500 mg IV q 8 h until
   improved
d. Ampicillin/sulbactam 3 g IV q 6 h *plus* doxycycline* 100 mg PO bid or
   IV q 12 h until improved
e. Ciprofloxacin 200 mg IV q 12 h *plus* doxycycline* 100 mg PO or IV bid
   q 12 h *plus* metronidazole 500 mg IV q 8 h, until improved

Once improved, give doxycycline* 100 mg PO bid to complete a 14-day course

Outpatient. Give one of the following regimens:

a. Ofloxacin[†] 400 mg PO bid × 14 days *plus* metronidazole 500 mg PO bid
   × 14 days
b. Ceftriaxone[§] 250 mg IM once, *followed by* doxycycline* 100 mg PO bid
   × 14 days
c. Cefoxitin 2 g IM once *plus* probenecid 1 g PO once, *followed by* doxycycline* 100 mg PO bid × 14 days

---

SYPHILIS

Primary, secondary, early latent (<1 year)	a. Benzathine penicillin G 2.4 million units IM as a single dose
	b. Doxycycline* 100 mg PO bid × 14 days

Table 12-2   Treatment of Sexually Transmitted Diseases (*continued*)

SYPHILIS (*continued*)

Late (duration >1 year, late-latent)	a. Benzathine penicillin G 2.4 million units IM weekly × 3 weeks b. Doxycycline* 100 mg PO bid × 14 days

CHANCROID

a. Azithromycin 1 g PO once *or*
b. Ceftriaxone§ 250 mg IM once *or*
c. Ciprofloxacin† 500 mg PO bid × 3 days *or*
d. Erythromycin 500 mg PO tid × 7 days

HERPES SIMPLEX

First episode	a. Acyclovir 400 mg PO tid × 7–10 days or 200 mg PO 5 times/day × 7–10 days *or* b. Famciclovir 250 mg PO tid × 7–10 days *or* c. Valacyclovir 1 g PO bid × 7–10 days
Recurrent	a. Acyclovir 400 mg PO tid × 5 days *or* b. Famciclovir 125 mg PO bid × 5 days *or* c. Valacyclovir 500 mg PO bid × 3–5 days
Daily suppressive therapy	a. Acyclovir 400 mg PO bid *or* b. Famciclovir 250 mg PO bid *or* c. Valacyclovir 500 mg–1 g PO qd

PEDICULOSIS

Apply a pyrethrin-based product (A200, Rid), leave in pubic area for 10 min, then wash out. Comb through hair and wash affected clothes and sheets.
Use lindane shampoo if the infestation persists.

GENITAL WARTS (HPV)

No treatment eradicates the virus, and no single therapy is uniformly effective at removing the warts and preventing recurrences.
Refer the patient to a dermatologist or gynecologist.

LYMPHOGRANULOMA VENEREUM (LGV)

Doxycycline* 100 mg PO bid × 21 days
Erythromycin 500 mg PO qid × 21 days

* Use only if >8 years old and not pregnant.
† Safety not established in patients <15 years of age or during pregnancy.
‡ Also give a course of treatment effective against *Chlamydia*.
§ Preferred where penicillinase-producing *N. gonorrhoeae* is prevalent. Also effective for pharyngeal and rectal gonorrhea.

Adapted from Abramowicz M (ed): Drugs for sexually transmitted diseases. *Med Lett Drugs Ther* 1999;41:85–90, and

Workowski KA, Levine WC: Sexually transmitted diseases treatment guidelines 2002. *MMWR Morb Mortal Wkly Rep* 2002;51:1–78 ate and treat sexual partners, and remind the patient to avoid sexual activity until that time.

Clinical response to the treatment of *chancroid* can be seen within 7 days. Examine and treat any individuals with whom the patient had sexual contact within 10 days preceding the onset of symptoms.

Treatment of primary *herpes* (pp 100–104) will shorten the duration of symptoms and the amount of viral shedding. It will also prevent the formation of new lesions. It is not curative, nor does it prevent later recurrences. The treatment of pubic lice (pp 106–108) is detailed elsewhere. Refer a patient with *genital warts* to a gynecologist or dermatologist for treatment, which may include cryotherapy, podophyllin, trichloroacetic acid, or bichloroacetic acid.

Follow-up

- Cervicitis, proctitis, female with acute urethral syndrome, chancroid, primary or recurrent herpes, pubic lice: primary care follow-up in 1 week
- Male with urethritis: 48 to 72 h
- Primary or secondary syphilis: 1 month
- Genital warts: gynecology or dermatology follow-up within 1 to 2 weeks

Indications for Admission

- Acute salpingitis
- Pregnant female with secondary syphilis (risk of a Herxheimer reaction)

BIBLIOGRAPHY

Abramowicz M (ed): Drugs for sexually transmitted diseases. *Med Lett Drugs Ther* 1999;41:85–90.

Gevelber MA, Biro FM: Adolescents and sexually transmitted diseases. *Pediatr Clin North Am* 1999;46:747–766.

Pletcher JR, Slap GB: Pelvic inflammatory disease. *Pediatr Rev* 1998;19:363–367.

VULVOVAGINITIS

The prepubertal vagina is a good culture medium due to the thinness of its epithelium and labia, neutral to alkaline pH, and lack of estrogenic stimulation. Also, younger girls are more likely to manipulate themselves with dirty hands or to insert foreign objects. In pubertal girls, sexual activity is the major etiologic factor of vulvovaginitis.

Clinical Presentation

Prepubertal Girls

Nonspecific Vaginitis   Eighty percent of prepubertal vaginitis is nonspecific. That is, routine bacterial and fungal cultures are negative and there is no obvious etiology. Included in this group are girls who use bubble bath, wear tight synthetic underpants, or have poor perineal hygiene.

The inflammation is generally low-grade yet persistent and may be associated with dysuria and pruritus.

Gonorrhea and Chlamydia   In this age group, gonorrhea and *Chlamydia* cause vaginal (not cervical) infections. These infections present with a copious, yellowish, purulent discharge with labial swelling, dysuria, and genital pruritus. The vagina can be very inflamed and excoriated. Often there is no definite history of sexual contact; however, nonsexual acquisition of these organisms is exceedingly rare. Suspect child abuse and alert the child protective services whenever a sexually transmitted disease is diagnosed in a prepubertal child.

Other Bacterial Infections   An overgrowth of normal vaginal coliform bacteria can occur secondary to poor hygiene; other bacteria (*S. aureus, Pneumococcus, Proteus*) can be transferred to the vagina. A low-grade, foul-smelling discharge results.

Some 7 to 10 days after an upper respiratory illness, infection by group A beta-hemolytic streptococci can cause hyperemia and irritation of the vulva and vagina. Symptoms include dysuria, pruritus, and discomfort when walking. *Shigella* can cause a bloody discharge in a girl who has recently had gastroenteritis.

Foreign Body   A vaginal foreign body produces a foul-smelling discharge that can be bloody. Toilet paper remnants are the most common objects found.

Pubertal Girls
Vaginitis   In addition to a discharge, dysuria is very common, often in association with pyuria.

Candida Albicans (Monilia)   *Candida albicans* is a common cause of vaginitis in diabetics and girls taking antibiotics or oral contraceptives. A thick, white, cheesy discharge is noted, with extreme pruritus and inflammation.

Trichomonas Vaginalis   This infection is usually acquired by sexual contact. A gray, bubbly, malodorous discharge occurs, often associated with pruritus or dyspareunia.

Gardnerella Vaginalis   This organism, in synergy with various anaerobes, is thought to be responsible for bacterial vaginosis. Infections usually present with a grayish, malodorous discharge.

Gonorrhea and Chlamydia   Adolescents may complain of a vaginal discharge, although the infection is actually higher in the genital tract (pp 286–293).

Foreign Body   The most common objects are forgotten tampons or remnants of masturbation aids (candle, vegetable). A purulent, brownish, malodorous discharge occurs.

Contact Reaction   A contact vaginitis may be caused by soap, bubble bath, douche, deodorant, or contraceptive foam or jelly.

Physiologic Leukorrhea   Adolescents may sometimes complain of a clear or mucoid discharge, either prior to menses or at midcycle. The discharge is nonpathologic, composed of epithelial cells and endocervical mucus.

Psychosocial Etiologies   When the patient's complaints are not consistent with the objective findings, consider psychosomatic illness, sexual molestation, and school phobia.

Diagnosis

Perform a brief physical examination, focusing on the breasts (Tanner stage, signs of pregnancy), abdomen (pregnancy, mass, tenderness), and inguinal area (lymphadenopathy). Next, inspect the introitus for Tanner stage, inflammation, and signs of trauma.

The vaginal examination of the prepubertal child is easily performed with the patient lying prone, in a knee-chest position, with the buttocks in the air and the knees 6 to 8 inches apart. Instruct the patient to relax and let her belly sag downward, then gently spread the labia to view the vagina. It is helpful to have the patient's mother in the room, possibly assisting by spreading the labia. Specimens can then be obtained with a sterile medicine dropper or a cotton swab moistened with saline. Perform a Gram's stain, looking for gram-negative intracellular diplococci (*gonorrhea*), and culture for routine bacteria, *N. gonorrhoeae*, and *Chlamydia*. If the discharge is bloody or particularly foul-smelling, inspect the vagina for a foreign body. Solid objects can often be palpated on rectal examination.

Perform a wet prep on a sample of every vaginal discharge. After the specimen is obtained with a cotton swab, place it in a test tube containing a small amount of saline. Place several drops of this solution on a slide and observe under high power. Budding yeast are seen with *candidal* infection; pseudohyphae can be seen after 10% potassium hydroxide (KOH) is added and the slide is gently heated. *Trichomonads* appear as live, flagellated, motile organisms. With *Gardnerella*, the wet prep has clue cells (epithelial cells stippled with dark granules); the odor becomes fishy with the addition of KOH.

Do not assume that an adolescent with dysuria and/or pyuria has a urinary tract infection (UTI). If a sexually active female has dysuria associated with a vaginal discharge, pruritus, or foul odor, perform a pelvic examination. Obtain endocervical cultures for gonorrhea and *Chlamydia* and evaluate the discharge via wet prep. If a UTI is a consideration in a girl with a vaginal discharge, the urine must be obtained by catheter.

ED Management

Prepubertal Girls

Nonspecific Vaginitis   Treat with plain-water sitz baths three times a day. Teach the parents proper hygiene techniques, and have the patient avoid tight-fitting pants (cotton underpants preferred). If symptoms persist after 2 to 3 weeks, prescribe an oral antibiotic (amoxicillin 40 mg/kg/day divided tid) for 10 days.

Gonorrhea and Chlamydia   In this age group, a positive Gram's stain or culture is indicative of sexual abuse (pp 547–550). Treat the child with ceftriaxone 125 mg IM or spectinomycin 40 mg/kg IM for gonorrhea; add erythromycin (<8 years of age: 50 mg/kg/day divided qid) or doxy-cycline (>8 years of age: 100 mg bid) for 7 to 10 days for *Chlamydia*. Report the case to the child protection services.

Other Bacterial Etiologies   If the culture is positive, treat with a culture-specific antibiotic for 7 to 10 days. Amoxicillin (40 mg/kg/day divided tid) for coliforms; penicillin VK (50,000 U/kg/day divided qid) for group A *Streptococcus* and *Pneumococcus*; and trimethoprim-sulfamethoxazole (8 mg/kg/day of TMP divided bid) for *Shigella*.

Foreign Bodies   Usually, removal can be accomplished with a forceps. On occasion, sedation or general anesthesia is required.

Pubertal Girls

Candida Albicans   Treat with an imidazole derivative (miconazole, clotrimazole) cream or suppository at bedtime for 1 week or double-strength cream at bedtime for 3 days. An alternative is one oral dose of fluconazole (150 mg), although there may be nausea, vomiting, or diar-rhea in 10% of patients. Advise the patient to avoid pantyhose and tight clothing. Treatment can be continued during menses. It is not necessary to treat sexual partner(s) unless the patient quickly becomes reinfected.

Trichomonas Vaginalis   Treat the patient and her partner(s) with one oral dose of metronidazole (2 g). Advise the patient to avoid alcohol on the day of treatment and for 2 days afterward. Determine whether the patient might be pregnant; avoid metronidazole during the first trimester.

Gardnerella Vaginalis   Treat with metronidazole, either orally (500 mg bid for 7 days or 2 g in a single dose) or as a vaginal gel [Metrogel, one applicator, (5 g) intravaginally bid for 5 days]. It is not necessary to treat sexual partner(s) unless the patient quickly becomes reinfected.

Foreign Bodies   These can usually be removed with a forceps or via warm saline irrigation.

Contact Reaction   Avoidance of the offending agent is usually all that is required. Treat severe pruritus with hydroxyzine (2 mg/kg/day divided tid). A medium-potency topical corticosteroid cream (0.1% triamcinolone tid) for 2 to 3 days may also help.

Physiologic Leukorrhea   No treatment is necessary, although panty liners may be helpful.

Psychosocial Etiologies   Have an experienced interviewer speak with the patient. Attempt to ascertain whether sexual molestation has occurred. Refer all patients without a definite etiology to a primary care provider.

Follow-up

- Prepubertal girl with nonspecific vaginitis or culture-proven bacterial vaginitis: primary care follow-up in 7 to 10 days
- Pubertal girl with vaginitis: primary care follow-up in 1 week

Indications for Admission

- Suspected sexual abuse if the patient's family is unable to provide the necessary support
- Severe vulvovaginitis with urinary retention or systemic signs (fever, toxicity)

BIBLIOGRAPHY

Abramowicz M (ed): Drugs for sexually transmitted diseases. *Med Lett Drugs Ther* 1999;41:85–90.
Nyirjesy P: Vaginitis in the adolescent patient. *Pediatr Clin North Am* 1999;46: 733–735.
Sobel JD: Vaginitis. *N Engl J Med* 1997;337:1896–1903.

CHAPTER 13

Hematologic Emergencies

Mark Weinblatt

ANEMIA

The criteria for anemia vary with age (Table 13-1); the lower limits of a normal hemoglobin level range from 9.5 g/dL at 3 months of age to 11 g/dL in the teenager. Anemia is never an isolated diagnosis but a sign of some underlying condition that can vary from a minor lab curiosity to a serious or even life-threatening disorder. As such, it requires an appropriate investigation to determine the cause.

Table 13-1 Hemoglobin, Hematocrit, and Determinations of Mean Corpuscular Volume (Mean, and Lower Limits of Normal)

Age (years)	Hemoglobin g/dL		Hematocrit %		MCV fL	
	Mean	Lower Limit	Mean	Lower Limit	Mean	Lower Limit
Birth	16.5	13.5	51	42	108	98
2 months	11.5	9.0	35	28	96	77
3–6 months	11.5	9.5	35	29	91	74
0.5–1.9	12.5	11.0	37	33	77	70
2–4	12.5	11.0	38	34	79	73
5–7	13.0	11.5	39	35	81	75
8–11	13.5	12.0	40	36	83	76
12–14						
Female	13.5	12.0	41	36	85	78
Male	14.0	12.5	43	37	84	77
15–17						
Female	14.0	12.0	41	36	87	79
Male	15.0	13.0	46	38	86	78
>18						
Female	14.0	12.0	42	37	90	80
Male	16.0	14.0	47	40	90	80

Adapted from Dallman PR, Siimes M: Percentile curves for hemoglobin and red cell volume in infancy and childhood. *J Pediatr* 1979;94:26–31.

Clinical Presentation

The signs and symptoms of anemia result from the decreased oxygen-carrying capacity of the blood and depend on the degree and rapidity of onset. Exercise intolerance, pallor, tachycardia, fatigue, and systolic murmurs may occur with moderate anemia. Severe or rapidly developing anemia causes nonexertional dyspnea, dizziness, changes in orthostatic vital signs, cardiac gallop, syncope, hypotension, and heart failure.

Diagnosis

A thorough history will often yield significant clues as the etiology of anemia. A complete dietary history is important when there is suspicion of a nutritional cause of anemia (such as *iron deficiency* caused by the intake of large amounts of cow's milk in infants, or, in older children, certain strict vegetarian diets containing no reliable source of iron). Unusual cravings, such as pagophagia and pica, are occasionally seen in patients with iron deficiency and may further complicate the picture (as with lead-containing paint chips). A history of recent infection may suggest hemolysis induced by *Epstein-Barr virus* (EBV) or *Mycoplasma pneumoniae* or suppression of the bone marrow (particularly in patients with chronic hemolytic disorders) due to *parvovirus*. Inquire about *blood loss*, such as irregular menstrual bleeding, hematuria, or gastrointestinal bleeding. A history of unexplained or prolonged bleeding may, in fact, uncover a *hemostatic disorder* that is contributing to anemia. Ask about chronic medical problems and inflammatory disorders, such as *juvenile rheumatoid arthritis* or *inflammatory bowel disease*. Recurrent bouts of jaundice suggest hemolytic disorders such as *G-6-PD deficiency*, *hemoglobinopathies*, and *spherocytosis*. A patient with a hemolytic disorder may have a positive family history of anemia, cholecystectomy, or splenectomy (*hereditary spherocytosis, sickle cell disease*, and some enzyme deficiencies). Ask about medication use, since many medications can suppress erythropoiesis (e.g., sulfa drugs and anticonvulsants) or trigger hemolysis in patients with G-6-PD deficiency.

On examination, a healthy, vigorous child is more likely to have mild *iron deficiency anemia, thalassemia trait*, or a mild *chronic hemolytic anemia*; a patient with a *malignancy, severe malnutrition, severe chronic disease*, or *bone marrow infiltration* usually appears ill. Jaundice, often accompanied by abdominal pain, splenomegaly, and dark urine, is frequently seen in *hemolytic processes*. Untreated or undiagnosed *thalassemia major* is associated with frontal bossing, malar prominence, hepatosplenomegaly, and dental malocclusion. Generalized lymphadenopathy and hepatosplenomegaly are frequent features of *myeloproliferative disorders* and *malignancies* (especially *leukemia* and *lymphoma*). Petechiae, purpura, and multiple ecchymoses can be expected in *hemostatic disorders*. Orthopedic anomalies may suggest *Fanconi's anemia* (abnormal radii or thumbs) or *Diamond-Blackfan syndrome* (triphalangeal or bifid thumbs).

In the emergency department (ED), anemia is often discovered when a complete blood count (CBC) is obtained during the evaluation of some other clinical problem. Despite the many diverse etiologies of anemia, a CBC with red-cell indices, a reticulocyte count, and examination of the peripheral smear will help narrow the differential diagnosis and guide further laboratory examinations (see The Abnormal CBC, pp 307–309).

Iron Deficiency   Iron deficiency is the most likely diagnosis in an otherwise well child with mild-to-moderate microcytic, hypochromic anemia. While inadequate dietary intake of iron (particularly in a patient who ingests large amounts of cow's milk) is the most common cause in a young child, blood loss is the more likely one in an older child or adolescent. Administering a diagnostic and therapeutic trial of oral iron supplementation prior to any further laboratory workup is reasonable. A rising hemoglobin and hematocrit and reticulocytosis after 1 week usually confirms the diagnosis of iron deficiency. If the mean corpuscular volume (MCV) is available, the Menser index [MCV in fL divided by the red blood cells (RBC) in millions: MCV/RBC] is one formula that can help differentiate the microcytic anemias. If the ratio is less than 11:1, then *thalassemia minor* is likely, while ratios greater than 14:1 suggest *iron deficiency, lead intoxication,* or the *anemia of chronic disease.*

ED Management

Iron Deficiency   Treat with oral ferrous sulfate, 6mg/kg/day of elemental iron divided twice daily between meals. Give with juice (vitamin C enhances iron absorption) but not with milk (impairs iron absorption). If there is difficulty with administration, the entire daily dose can be given as once daily. A rise in hemoglobin and reticulocyte count 1 week later confirms both the diagnosis and adherence to the regimen. Lack of response suggests a wrong diagnosis, ongoing blood loss, incorrect dose, malabsorption, or noncompliance with medication. Warn the patient or parents that gastrointestinal complaints, particularly constipation and darkening of the stools, may result from iron therapy. For occasional epigastric discomfort, divide the doses into smaller volumes at more frequent intervals or give the iron with food (not milk).

Blood Loss   Acute blood loss may require treatment with the transfusion of packed red blood cells, particularly if the patient is symptomatic (tachycardia, orthostatic hypotension, syncope). Do not rely solely on the level of the hematocrit to decide whether a transfusion is necessary, since children often tolerate extremely low red cell counts without exhibiting any symptoms, especially when given sufficient time for the body to adjust and compensate. Consider associated clinical findings, such as resting heart rate and respiratory rate, as well as the likelihood of a further imminent decrease in the hematocrit. In addition to overt or occult blood loss, other conditions that might warrant a transfusion include disorders associated with decreased erythrocyte production, as seen in bone marrow failure (aplastic anemia, transient erythroblastopenia of childhood, nutritional anemias, and drug-induced marrow suppression) or marrow replacement (leukemia, neuroblastoma, storage disorders). Consult a pediatric hematologist before giving blood to these patients (see Transfusion Therapy, pp 306–307).

Autoimmune Hemolytic Anemia   Initially treat with prednisone (2 mg/kg/day) after consultation with a pediatric hematologist. A red-cell transfusion might be required, but these conditions are frequently associated with a high risk of transfusion reactions.

Institute specific therapy for any underlying conditions. However, therapy of most primary hematologic etiologies of anemia other than iron deficiency, lead intoxification, and bleeding requires consultation with a pediatric hematologist.

Follow-up

- Iron deficiency anemia: 1 week, for a hemoglobin and reticulocyte count

Indications for Admission

- Significant cardiovascular or cerebral symptomatology (fainting, tachycardia, heart failure)
- Acute blood loss requiring transfusion
- Pancytopenia or suspicion of a malignancy
- Acute Coombs-positive or extrinsic hemolytic anemia with hemoglobin <8 g/dL
- Chronic hemolytic disease with acute reticulocytopenia and significant fall in hematocrit (aplastic crisis seen in sickle cell disease and spherocytosis)
- Severe deficiency of glucose-6-phosphate dehydrogenase (G-6-PD) with exposure to oxidant stress (e.g., infections, mothballs, sulfonamides, antimalarials)
- Hemoglobin <6 g/dL

BIBLIOGRAPHY

Glader BE: Hemolytic anemia in children. *Clin Lab Med* 1999;19:87–111.
Miller DR: Anemias—general considerations, in Miller DR, Baehner RL (eds): *Blood Disorders of Infancy and Childhood.* Philadelphia: Mosby, 1995, pp 111–139.
Oski FA, Brugnara C, Nathan DG. A diagnostic approach to the anemic patient, in Nathan DG, Oski FA (eds): *Hematology of Infancy and Childhood,* 5th ed. Philadelphia: Saunders, 1998, pp 375–384.

HEMOSTATIC DISORDERS

Hemostasis is dependent on a complex interaction among circulating platelets, coagulation proteins, and vascular endothelium. Any of these components may be dysfunctional and lead to abnormal bleeding. There is also a delicate balance between the competing coagulation and fibrinolytic systems, with often profound consequences if one dominates the other.

Thrombocyte disorders most commonly involve a decrease in the number of circulating platelets secondary to underproduction, as in marrow failure (aplasia, infections, or drugs) or marrow replacement (leukemia, storage disorders, histiocytosis); increased peripheral destruction [immune thrombocytopenic purpura (ITP), hypersplenism, infections, hemangiomas]; ineffective production (myelodysplasia); or microangiopathic processes [hemolytic-uremic syndrome, disseminated intravascular coagulation (DIC)].

In addition to thrombocytopenia, symptoms related to platelet dysfunction can also cause bleeding manifestations. These disorders of platelet function can be acquired (uremia, ingestion of aspirin or other non-steroidal anti-inflammatory medications) or inherited (von Willebrand disease, storage pool disorder).

The reverse situation, thrombocytosis, can occur with a variety of disorders, because the platelet count often behaves as an acute-phase reactant. Thrombocytosis may be seen in children with recent infections or major stress or as a "rebound" phenomenon after a period of bone marrow suppression. Underlying disorders associated with thrombocytosis include malignancies (chronic myelogenous leukemia, neuroblastoma), Kawasaki syndrome, sarcoid, chronic inflammatory disorders (inflammatory bowel disease), chronic hemolytic disorders, and iron deficiency.

Coagulation factors are necessary for the formation of fibrin strands at bleeding sites. Hemorrhage can occur when any of these proteins are either decreased in amount or dysfunctional. Factor activity is decreased in inherited deficiencies (von Willebrand disease), vitamin K deficiency [normal newborns, sodium warfarin (Coumadin) therapy, prolonged oral antibiotic therapy], liver failure, and DIC. Abnormal proteins with markedly diminished or absent function, as in hemophilia and dysfibrinogenemia, are less common.

The endothelium is responsible for the production of factor VIII and prostacyclin (a platelet inhibitor) and the insulation of coagulation factors and platelets from exposure to underlying collagen. Dysfunction of the endothelial system is observed in vasculitis (lupus erythematosus, Henoch-Schönlein purpura) and infections (meningococcemia, rickettsemia).

Clinical Presentation

The presenting complaint of hemostatic disorders may vary greatly, depending on the location, rapidity, and severity of bleeding. Platelet abnormalities are commonly associated with petechial or mucosal bleeding that occurs immediately after the trauma and usually responds to local pressure. With ITP, skin and mucosal bleeding often follows a benign viral illness or measles vaccination. Patients with coagulation factor abnormalities, particularly the hemophilias, may have delayed, posttraumatic deep tissue hemorrhages into muscles and joints. In the first few weeks of life, a coagulopathy may present with delayed, persistent bleeding from the circumcision site or the umbilical stump. Abrasions and tooth extractions respond poorly to local pressure and can continue to ooze and bleed for days. Bleeding secondary to vasculitis (such as Henoch-Schönlein purpura) usually presents as palpable purpura.

Diagnosis

Suspect a bleeding disorder in a child who presents with a history of bruising or bleeding out of proportion to the level of trauma, bleeding in unusual locations, spontaneous hemorrhage, and prolonged or recurrent bleeding. Ask about a family history of any inherited hemorrhagic disorders, such as hemophilia A and B (X-linked), factor XI deficiency (autosomal recessive), and von Willebrand disease (autosomal dominant), or unexplained significant bleeding, particularly if a blood transfusion was necessary. A seriously ill child may have leukemia (pallor, fever, fatigue, hepatomegaly, lymphadenopathy), hemolytic-uremic syndrome (lethargy, diarrhea, oliguria), liver disease (vomiting, jaundice, hepatomegaly, dark urine, acholic stools), or DIC.

The final identification of the underlying disease can be facilitated by a few simple screening tests: platelet count (normal: 150,000–300,000/mm^3); either the prothrombin time (PT) (normal: within 2 s of control or <14 s) or International Normalized Ratio (INR) (normal: <1.2), both of which test the extrinsic clotting system (factors I, II, V, VII, X); partial thromboplastin time (PTT), which tests the intrinsic system (factors I, II, V, VII, IX, X, XI, XII; (normal: within 5 s of control or <35–40 s); and bleeding time, which assesses the platelet-endothelium interaction (normal: <8 min). As shown in Table 13-2, the results of these tests suggest the most likely diagnosis.

Abnormal clot formation with thrombosis is uncommon in children. Ask about any indwelling catheters, particularly in the neonatal period or in patients treated with PICC lines or central venous catheters. Dehydration and prolonged periods of immobilization can lead to localized stasis and thrombosis. Other risk factors include pregnancy, use of oral contraceptive pills, and smoking. Signs and symptoms include painful swelling of an extremity or sudden respiratory distress from an embolus migrating to the lungs. On physical examination, there may be tender swelling of an extremity or decreased breath sounds.

ED Management

For the patient with vitamin K deficiency who is actively bleeding, give 5 to 10 mg of vitamin K by slow IV infusion. Correction of the coagulation factor levels begins within hours, with marked improvement by 24 h. However, treat severe bleeding with an infusion of fresh frozen plasma to correct the deficiencies rapidly. If there is a history of warfarin ingestion, a repeat administration of vitamin K might be necessary.

Treat thrombocytopenic conditions with local pressure to superficial bleeding sites. If this is unsuccessful or the platelet count is <50,000/mm^3, obtain a type and cross-match and consult a pediatric hematologist. Treat a patient with documented ITP and serious, life-threatening bleeding with high-dose intravenous gamma globulin (0.25–0.5 g/kg over 4–5 h) or high-dose corticosteroids (methylprednisolone 20–40 mg/kg over 1 h) while awaiting consultation with a hematologist. A patient who is Rh-positive can also be treated with WinRho at a dose of 50 μg/kg. For patients with

Table 13-2   Differential Diagnosis of Bleeding

Platelet Count	Prothrombin Time	Partial Thromboplastin Time	Diagnoses
Normal	Prolonged	Normal	Moderate liver disease Warfarin ingestion Factor VII deficiency
Normal	Normal	Prolonged	von Willebrand disease Heparin effect Factor VIII, IX, XI, or XII deficiency
Decreased	Prolonged	Prolonged	Disseminated intra-vascular coagulation Giant hemangioma Congenital heart disease
Decreased	Normal	Normal	Thrombocytopenia
Normal	Prolonged	Prolonged	Severe liver disease Vitamin K deficiency High-dose heparin or warfarin therapy Factor II, V, or X deficiency Dysfibrinogenemia
Normal	Normal	Normal (obtain bleeding time)	von Willebrand disease Platelet dysfunction Factor XIII deficiency Henoch-Schönlein purpura Connective tissue disease

thrombocytopenia caused by decreased production (leukemia, other marrow failure syndromes), transfuse single-donor apheresis platelets (see Transfusion Therapy, pp 306–307).

Obtain a computed tomography (CT) scan of the head for a patient with a hemostatic disorder who has a moderate or severe headache or any neurologic symptoms (irritability, lethargy, vomiting, ataxia, loss of consciousness) after head trauma.

As a general rule, 1 U/kg of factor VIII will raise a patient's factor level by 2%. However, consult with a hematologist before treating a coagulopathy patient with factor replacement, as the selection and dose of the factor product varies greatly. Avoid giving aspirin and other medications that can inhibit proper platelet function to any patient with a bleeding diathesis.

Follow-up

- Patient with ITP: repeat platelet count in 1 to 2 days, if initial platelet count <100,000/mm^3.
- Patient treated with factor VIII: next day

Indications for Admission

- Massive bleeding that causes hypovolemic symptomatology or requires transfusion of packed RBCs
- Suspected or proven intracranial hemorrhage
- Hemophiliac or patient with other severe hemostatic disorder who sustains significant head trauma (e.g., lethargy, skull fracture, abnormal neurologic finding, or loss of consciousness)
- Significant hematemesis, hematochezia, or hematuria
- Newly diagnosed thrombocytopenia (platelet count <50,000/mm^3)
- Severe inherited coagulopathy with gross hematuria, large laceration, or severe abdominal pain
- Clinical features suspicious for marrow replacement, DIC, hemolytic-uremic syndrome, or hepatic failure
- Generalized petechial or purpuric eruption in an acutely ill febrile child (to rule out sepsis)
- Suspicion of venous thrombosis or pulmonary embolus

BIBLIOGRAPHY

Blanchette V, Carcao M: Approach to the investigation and management of immune thrombocytopenic purpura in children. *Semin Hematol* 2000;37:299–314.

Grabowski EF, Corrigan JJ: Hemostasis: general considerations, in Miller DR, Baehner RL, Miller LP (eds): *Blood Diseases of Infancy and Childhood,* 7th ed. Philadelphia: Mosby, 1995, pp 849–865.

Schneppenheim R, Thomas KB, Sutor AH: Von Willebrand disease in childhood. *Semin Thromb Hemost* 1995;21:261–275.

TRANSFUSION THERAPY

The primary purposes of red cell transfusions are to rapidly ameliorate hypovolemia, particularly in situations of acute blood loss, and to increase oxygen carrying capacity. Criteria for transfusions vary depending on the patient, the underlying illness or situation, the desired effect, and the risks of transfusion versus the anticipated benefits.

If the patient has a slowly evolving anemia, appropriate compensatory mechanisms, and a normal blood pressure, transfuse a maximum volume of 10 to 15 mL/kg of packed red cells slowly, over 2 to 3 h. Each 1 mL/kg of blood raises the hematocrit approximately 0.7%. For very severe, chronic, or well-compensated anemias, administer the blood in smaller aliquots of 5 mL/kg, with several hours between transfusions to allow for the removal of excess fluid from the vascular compartment. A diuretic, such as furosemide (0.5 mg/kg IV), may be required between transfusions to prevent volume overload and heart failure. In treating acute or ongoing blood loss, particularly if there is hypovolemia or hypotension, administer the blood rapidly. This includes splenic sequestration crises in patients with sickle cell disease who require rapid blood transfusion to correct severe anemia and hypovolemia.

The patient's history dictates what RBC processing is indicated prior to transfusion. For patients who have received several transfusions in the past, or those who have experienced prior febrile, nonhemolytic transfusion reactions, use leukocyte depleted RBCs to decrease the likelihood of transfusion reactions.

Request irradiated RBCs for any immunodeficient patient, including neonates, patients with malignancies or immunodeficiency diseases, bone marrow transplant candidates, and patients on immunosuppressive therapy. Irradiation destroys white cells that might cause serious graft-versus-host disease in the recipient.

As a rule, it is usually beneficial to administer premedication to decrease the risk of febrile nonhemolytic transfusion reactions. At a minimum, give acetaminophen (15 mg/kg) prior to the transfusion. For a patient with a history of frequent reactions, particularly if urticarial, give diphenhydramine (1 mg/kg PO or 0.5 mg/kg IV); and if there is a history of more significant prior allergic reactions, give corticosteroids (hydrocortisone 1 mg/kg PO or IV).

A patient with an autoimmune hemolytic anemia who requires transfusions poses additional difficulties. It may be impossible to find a completely compatible donor unit, so the least reactive unit is often the only alternative. If a cold antibody is present, infuse the RBCs through a warmer (usually a warm winter bath immersing the IV tubing) to decrease the amount of hemolysis. Because of the very high risk of reactions, given high-dose steroids (hydrocortisone 1–1.5 mg/kg IV) prior to the transfusion and every 3 h during it.

Platelet transfusions can help stop bleeding in a thrombocytopenic patient who is not producing platelets (leukemia, aplastic anemia). Platelet transfusions are of little value in patients with ITP unless severe internal bleeding develops. Generally, use single-donor apheresis platelets. Once again, administer premedications, as reactions with platelets are more common than with transfused RBCs.

BIBLIOGRAPHY

Kevy SV, Gorlin JB: Red cell transfusion, in Nathan DG, Oski FA (eds): *Hematology of Infancy and Childhood*, 5th ed. Philadelphia: Saunders, 1998, pp 1784–1801.

Kulkarni R, Gera R: Pediatric transfusion therapy: practical considerations. *Indian J Pediatr* 1999;66:307–317.

Nugent DJ: Platelet transfusion, in Nathan DG, Oski FA (eds): *Hematology of Infancy and Childhood,* 5th ed. Philadelphia: Saunders, 1998, pp 1802–1817.

THE ABNORMAL CBC

RBC Abnormalities

After determining that a patient is anemic for age, the most expeditious way of establishing a diagnosis is by using an algorithm based on the red cell size (see Table 13-1). Microcytic anemias are due to delayed or abnormal hemoglobin formation, with disorders of the iron, globin chain, or porphyrin ring components. These conditions include *iron deficiency*, the *thalassemias, sideroblastic anemias* (including *lead poisoning*), *porphyrias*, and the *anemia of chronic inflammation*. These disorders typically have decreased MCV, with a peripheral blood smear revealing hypochromic red cells exhibiting enlarged central pallor and small size. To further establish a diagnosis, consider additional testing such as iron and ferritin levels, hemoglobin electrophoresis, and a lead level.

The less common macrocytic anemias, with MCV >100 outside of the newborn period, result from delayed nuclear maturation or elevated fetal hemoglobin content. These include the megaloblastic anemias (*vitamin B_{12} and folic acid deficiencies*), *liver disease, hypothyroidism,* and *inherited aplastic anemia or pure red cell hypoplasia* with elevated fetal hemoglobin.

The normocytic anemias comprise the largest differential, with disorders that include *marrow failure or replacement, immune and extrinsic hemolysis, hemoglobinopathies, membrane disorders,* and *enzyme deficiencies.*

In differentiating among these disorders, some features of the red cells other than size can help establish the diagnosis. These features include the following:

Red Cell Shape   Sickle cells (both crescent and "box-car" shapes); target cells, often seen in hemoglobinopathies (especially *Hgb C disease* and the microcytic *thalassemia syndromes*) and liver disease; burr cells (renal disease, hemolysis); spherocytes (*spherocytosis, ABO immune hemolysis*); schistocytes (*hemolysis*).

Color   Polychromasia occurs with increased RBC production in association with decreased life span or marrow recovery. This is usually indicative of an elevated reticulocyte count

Inclusions   Howell-Jolly bodies (decreased splenic function); basophilic stippling (thalassemia, lead poisoning, some enzyme deficiencies); parasites (malaria, babesiosis).

Platelet Abnormalities

In contrast to RBCs, the platelet count can be quickly and reliably estimated from examining the peripheral blood smear. In any high-power field, each platelet seen represents a total of 10,000 to 15,000/mm³ so a normal smear has 10 to 35 platelets per high-power field. (see p 308 for thrombocytopenia).

In addition to platelet number, platelet size can give important information. Enlarged platelets are seen in disorders of increased peripheral destruction (especially *immune thrombocytopenic purpura*) and some inherited thrombocytopenias (*Bernard Soulier syndrome, May-Hegglin anomaly*). Small platelets are typically seen in *Wiskott-Aldrich syndrome* and frequently in *leukemias*.

Finally, platelet color can yield important clues in the diagnosis of bleeding disorders. Normally, Wright-stained platelets appear gray with purple granulation. The absence of granules is characteristic of *storage pool disorder*, a lifelong bleeding disorder resulting from abnormal platelet aggregation.

Leukocyte Disorders

While the automated Coulter counter can give much information regarding the white cell count and differential, additional information can be gleaned from examination of the peripheral blood smear. The presence of increased numbers of eosinophils may suggest a *parasitic infection* or *allergic disorders*. Basophilia most commonly is seen in *chronic myelogenous leukemia*. Elevated numbers of mature granulocyte are the hallmark of *infections, inflammation,* and *stress reactions*. Large numbers of immature cells with decreased numbers of mature leukocytes usually indicate a *leukemic process*. Serious infections are often associated with inclusions (Döhle bodies) and toxic granulation. Inclusions can also be diagnostic of inherited granulocyte disorders (*May-Hegglin anomaly*). Leukopenia may be the result of *viral infections, overwhelming bacterial infections,* and *marrow failure* or *marrow replacement*. The presence of large numbers of atypical lymphocytes, particularly if accompanied by monocytosis, is most commonly a result of viral infections, including but not limited to *Epstein-Barr virus (EBV)* and *cytomegalovirus (CMV)*.

BIBLIOGRAPHY

Miller DR: Normal blood values from birth through adolescence, in Miller DR, Baehner RL (eds): *Blood Diseases of Infancy and Childhood.* Philadelphia: Mosby, 1995, pp 30–53.

INFECTION AND THE IMMUNOCOMPROMISED HOST

After the first few months of life, most infants have the ability to resist serious infections. The hallmark of an immunocompromised patient, however, is an increased susceptibility to infection, including increased frequency, duration, and severity, as well as infection caused by unusual pathogens.

Clinical Presentation

Although symptoms will vary with the organism and site of infection, the patient may have recurrent respiratory infections and repeated severe bacterial illnesses (sepsis, pneumonia, meningitis). Persistent lymphadenopathy and hepatosplenomegaly are common findings in many of these disorders. The patient may have chronic diarrhea with some form of malabsorption and failure to thrive (IgA deficiency, exocrine pancreatic insufficiency). A variety of skin lesions may be seen, including eczema (Wiskott-Aldrich syndrome), pyoderma (cyclic neutropenia, Kostmann's syndrome, Job syndrome), and diffuse dermatitis (chronic granulomatous disease).

Human immunodeficiency virus (HIV) infection may present in a variety of ways: lymphadenopathy, hepatosplenomegaly, and failure to thrive in an infant with maternal risk factors; a hemophiliac or multiply transfused child with interstitial pneumonitis; or a child with poorly responsive immune thrombocytopenic purpura.

Although most children with sickle cell disease are identified early in life by newborn hemoglobinopathy screening, a Caucasian child of Mediterranean background may present with frequent bouts of bone pain, leukocytosis, and a chronic hemolytic anemia.

Lymphoma in an adolescent can present with cervical adenopathy, fever, weight loss, splenomegaly, and herpes zoster or prolonged varicella infection.

Diagnosis

Prior to proceeding with an extensive immunologic evaluation, try to distinguish the immunodeficient child from the one with frequent colds and normal immunologic function. Many children have up to 8 or 10 respiratory infections in any given year, but these are usually mild, self-limited, occasionally accompanied by fever, with complete recovery between bouts. Allergy is more likely in children with repeated or persistent infections limited to the upper respiratory tract. Likewise, infections limited to a particular organ suggest specific disease entities: recurrent pneumonias in *cystic fibrosis, foreign body, collagen vascular diseases, bronchiectasis*, or *cow's milk sensitivity, celiac disease*, and *inflammatory bowel disease* with chronic diarrhea and failure to thrive. Many chronic diseases predispose patients to frequent infections (*rheumatic disorders, chronic renal disease, sickle cell disease, diabetes, nutritional deficiencies*, and *malignancies*). Finally, a history in the patient or parent of blood product administration, intravenous drug abuse, or high-risk sexual activity suggests the possibility of *HIV infection*.

ED Management

If the child has had either two or more serious infections (pneumonia, meningitis, sepsis, osteomyelitis) in a short period of time or an infection with an unusual pathogen, obtain a CBC with differential and platelet count, erythrocyte sedimentation rate (ESR), and quantitative immunoglobulins. In addition, evaluate cell-mediated immunity by measuring T-cell subsets and consider skin testing [*Candida*, streptokinase-streptodornase, mumps, and purified protein derivative (PPD)]. Assume that any patient with a history of treatment with chemotherapeutic drugs for malignancy or autoimmune disorders or with immunosuppressive medications (including corticosteroids for conditions like asthma) is at high risk for infections. Consult a pediatric hematologist or immunologist for further evaluation with specific definitive tests.

Treatment of a patient with a chronic immunodeficiency or granulocyte disorder is usually supervised by a pediatric hematologist or immunologist. However, these children are often seen in an ED. When a patient with a known immunodeficiency or neutrophil disorder presents with a fever (>38.6°C, 101.5°F), a very conservative approach is mandatory. Obtain a CBC and cultures of the blood, urine, and any wound prior to initiating treatment. If there are central nervous system (CNS) symptoms, perform a lumbar puncture with additional fluid evaluated for unusual organisms (mycobacteria, India ink stain for *Cryptococcus*), in addition to the standard cultures and Gram's stain.

Treat a neutropenic patient with combination IV antibiotic therapy: an aminoglycoside such as tobramycin or gentamicin (6 mg/kg/day divided q 8–12 h) and either a semisynthetic penicillin (piperacillin/tazobactam 250 mg/kg/day divided q 6 h) or ceftazidime (100 mg/kg/day divided q 8 h) for adequate *Pseudomonas* coverage. Treat a child with defective cell-mediated immunity who has fever and respiratory symptoms with trimethoprim-sulfamethoxazole (20 mg/kg/day of TMP divided q 6 h) along with broad-spectrum antibiotics (as above). Treat a patient with splenic dysfunction with ceftriaxone or cefuroxime (100 mg/kg/day). If the patient has a very high fever or appears toxic, add vancomycin (40 mg/kg/day divided q 6 h) because of the increasing incidence of resistant *Pneumococcus*. Consult a hematologist for a patient with a neutrophil disorder who has a serious infection, as granulocyte transfusions or granulocyte colony stimulating factor (G-CSF), 5 mg/kg/day, may be indicated.

Follow-up

- Immunocompromised patient with low-grade fever not treated with antibiotics: next day

Indications for Admission

- Fever (>38.5°C, 101.5°F) in a patient with a granulocyte count <1000/mm^3, a documented phagocytic defect, or other immunodeficiency
- Immunocompromised patient with pneumonia, an abscess, or localized infection (e.g., otitis, cellulitis) not responding to initial antibiotic therapy
- Patient with sickle cell disease with fever > 39.4°–40°C (103°–104°F)
- Suspected malignancy
- Immunocompromised patient with a toxic appearance, regardless of the temperature
- Varicella or herpes zoster infection in a child with defective cell-mediated immunity

BIBLIOGRAPHY

Freifeld AG, Walsh TJ, Pizzo PA: Infectious complications in the pediatric cancer patient, in Pizzo PA, Poplack DG (eds): *Principles and Practice of Pediatric Oncology,* 3rd ed. Philadelphia: Lippincott-Raven, 1997, pp 1069–1114.
Patrick CC, Slobod KS. Opportunistic infections in the compromised host, in Feigin RD, Cherry JD (eds): *Textbook of Pediatric Infectious Disease,* 4th ed. Philadelphia: Saunders, 1998, pp 980–994.

LEUKEMIA AND LYMPHOMA

The most common pediatric malignancy is acute lymphoblastic leukemia (ALL), and lymphomas are second only to brain tumors in frequency of solid tumors. While these are relatively infrequent diseases in childhood, parental fear often prompts a medical evaluation in a child with persistent nonspecific symptoms. Early recognition of these diseases is imperative so that effective therapy can be instituted as soon as possible.

Clinical Presentation

Leukemia   The presenting symptoms of ALL usually result from the absence of normal hematopoietic elements, along with the proliferation and accumulation of abnormal cells. Clinical findings are related to the degree of anemia (pallor, fatigue, light-headedness, palpitations), thrombocytopenia (petechiae, purpura, epistaxis), and neutropenia (infections).

Other signs and symptoms include joint or bone pain, hepatosplenomegaly, lymphadenopathy, skin nodules, and gingival hypertrophy. CNS involvement can be asymptomatic; alternatively, there can be symptoms related to elevated intracranial pressure (headache, vomiting, irritability, visual disturbances) or unusual constellations of findings such as an isolated cranial nerve paresis or the "hypothalamic syndrome" (marked hyperphagia with weight gain, personality changes). Leukemic infiltration in organs such as the testes, kidneys, and ovaries can lead to firm, painless enlargement.

Hodgkin's Disease   Hodgkin's disease most commonly presents with either firm, nontender, asymptomatic lymphadenopathy (particularly the cervical, supraclavicular, mediastinal, and paraaortic nodes) or constitutional symptoms (fever, night sweats, cough, weight loss). Pruritus rarely occurs in children, and complications such as jaundice and superior vena cava obstruction are uncommon. Prolonged varicella or a history of herpes zoster is often reported.

Non-Hodgkin's Lymphomas   The non-Hodgkin's lymphomas may also present with isolated, nontender, firm lymphadenopathy, but children more frequently have widespread disease. A primary mediastinal mass may cause dyspnea, cough, pleural effusion, and superior vena cava obstruction (respiratory distress; distended neck and arms). Children can have primary tumors in Waldeyer's ring, presenting with tonsillar involvement misdiagnosed as a peritonsillar abscess. Primary gastrointestinal lymphomas (Peyer's patches of the distal ileum) can cause asymptomatic abdominal distention, vomiting and diarrhea, intussusception, or intestinal obstruction. Burkitt's lymphoma can present with retroperitoneal or mesenteric tumors and occasionally with involvement of the maxillary sinus, but jaw masses are uncommon in the United States.

Diagnosis

In addition to cytopenia, the hallmark of leukemia is the presence of large numbers of primitive leukocytes (blasts) in the blood and bone marrow. While metastatic neuroblastoma may also replace the bone marrow with malignant cells, these cells do not appear in the peripheral blood.

Most often confused with leukemia and lymphomas are *infectious mononucleosis* and *mono-like syndromes* (CMV, toxoplasmosis), which can present with fever, lymphadenopathy, hepatosplenomegaly, cytopenias, and immature leukocytes on blood smear. However, these cells can usually be distinguished from leukemic blasts. *Pertussis* can induce a profound leukocytosis (on occasion >100,000/mm^3) and neutropenia, but the cells are mature and anemia is not usually present. Children with *ITP* do not appear chronically ill, the platelets are usually large, and other cytopenias are absent. Storage disorders (*Gaucher's disease*) may present with hepatosplenomegaly and pancytopenia, necessitating enzyme assays, a bone marrow examination, or liver biopsy for confirmation.

A lymphoma-like picture can be seen with *sinus histiocytosis, diphenylhydantoin therapy*, and, rarely, in *Kawasaki syndrome*. A node biopsy is indicated if there is weight loss or supraclavicular lymphadenopathy or the node is nontender, firm, and progressively enlarging.

ED Management

If leukemia or lymphoma is suspected, obtain a CBC with differential, platelet count, reticulocyte count, heterophile antibody or Monospot test, elecrolytes, liver function tests, lactic dehydrogenase, a blood culture, and chest x-ray. Consult with a pediatric hematologist-oncologist and admit patients with blasts on peripheral smear, pancytopenia, or lymphadenopathy that meets the criteria for biopsy.

Follow-up

- Asymptomatic patient with lymphadenopathy: 7 to 10 days

Indications for Admission

- Newly diagnosed or suspected malignancy
- Pancytopenia
- Suspicion of mass pressure on a vital structure

BIBLIOGRAPHY

Miller DR: Hematologic malignancies—leukemia and lymphoma, in Miller DR, Baehner RL (eds): *Blood Diseases of Infancy and Childhood*, 7th ed. Philadelphia: Mosby, 1995, pp 660–762.

Pui CH, Childhood leukemias. *N Engl J Med* 1995;332;1618–3160.

Thomas DA, Kantarjian HM: Lymphoblastic lymphoma. *Hematol Clin North Am* 2001;15:51–95.

LYMPHADENOPATHY

Palpable lymph nodes may be a normal finding or a sign of disease, either minor or life-threatening. Lymph nodes are not usually palpable in infants under a few months of age. Afterward there is a steady increase in the body's normal lymphoid tissue, so that by puberty nearly 100% of children will have at least some palpable nodes, most commonly in the cervical and inguinal areas. Although the presence of lymph node enlargement is an alarming finding to parents concerned about the possibility of malignant disease, a variety of factors must be considered in deciding whether to pursue a workup for enlarged nodes.

Clinical Presentation

Generalized Lymphadenopathy

Generalized lymphadenopathy is defined as enlargement in at least three noncontiguous lymph node regions. It is always abnormal, and usually nonlymphoid features of the primary disease process are evident (fever, rash, pharyngitis, arthritis, arthralgia, bruising, pallor, hepatosplenomegaly, etc.). The most common etiology is infection, particularly viral disease like infectious mononucleosis or mono-like illnesses (CMV, toxoplasmosis). Other infectious etiologies include the exanthematous viral infections of childhood (measles, rubella, varicella), enteroviruses (echo, coxsackie), tuberculosis, hepatitis B, syphilis, malaria, and HIV. Noninfectious causes include rheumatoid diseases (juvenile rheumatoid arthritis, systemic lupus erythematosus), serum sickness, drug reactions (diphenylhydantoin), sarcoidosis, storage diseases, and eczema. Malignancies to consider include leukemia, lymphoma, and histiocytosis.

Localized Lymphadenopathy
Reactive Adenopathy   Localized lymphadenopathy is most often a response to a regional infection (reactive lymphadenopathy). The location often suggests the underlying infection. For example, occipital lymphadenopathy occurs in response to scalp conditions such as seborrhea, tinea capitis, and pediculosis; preauricular enlargement is secondary to conjunctivitis; and submandibular and submental nodes may enlarge with infection of the gingiva, teeth, buccal mucosa, and tongue. Axillary lymphadenopathy can be caused by cat-scratch fever, rat-bite fever, or a recent immunization, while inguinal involvement occurs with venereal diseases (syphilis, gonorrhea, lymphogranuloma venereum, chancroid) and lower extremity infections. However, since the supraclavicular nodes drain from the lungs and mediastinum, enlargement here is always a concern. Etiologies include infections (tuberculosis, histoplasmosis, coccidioidomycosis), neoplasms (lymphomas), and sarcoidosis. For any node site, a proximal cellulitis, dermatitis, or local pyogenic infection will cause reactive enlargement.

Adenitis   A second category of local lymphadenopathy is primary infection of the node, or adenitis, Most often this is bacterial in origin. The most common organisms are *Staphylococcus aureus* and group A *Streptococcus*, although anaerobes, *Mycobacterium tuberculosis*, atypical mycobacteria, and HIV are other etiologies to consider.

Diagnosis

A complete history and physical examination are necessary to locate a primary infection, document a local adenitis, or diagnose a disease causing generalized lymphadenopathy. Note any fever, weight loss, rash, jaundice, arthritis, arthralgias, bruising, pallor, pharyngitis or upper respiratory symptoms, hepatosplenomegaly, contact with contagious diseases, history of a cat scratch or rat bite, and sexual activity. In examining the involved node(s), there are six features to consider:

1. *Location*: Significant generalized lymphadenopathy always warrants further investigation, as does supraclavicular adenopathy. Isolated cervical, inguinal, and occipital nodes are less likely to be caused by a serious disease.

2. *Size*: Generally, consider nodes larger than 1 cm in diameter to be abnormal. However, in the cervical area, a node may be 2 to 3 cm in the absence of serious disease.

3. *Rate of Enlargement*: Rapid enlargement is most commonly caused by an infection, either an adenitis or a reactive hyperplasia. Slow growth suggests a malignancy or a systemic disease.

4. *Mobility*: A node fixed to adjacent structures or matted to other nodes suggests an infiltrative disease that demands further evaluation. A freely mobile node is generally benign.

5. *Consistency*: Soft, shotty nodes are usually normal or represent reactive enlargement. Adenitis causes fluctuance, while malignancy is associated with hard, rubbery nodes.

6. *Overlying Skin*: Bacterial adenitis causes erythema and warmth of the overlying skin. Adherence of the skin to the node occurs in cat-scratch fever and atypical mycobacterial infection. A reactive node does not affect the overlying skin.

While abnormality of any one of these characteristics might not be worrisome, if multiple features are abnormal (e.g., a firm, fixed, supraclavicular node), suspect an underlying serious disorder, particularly a malignant disease, and expedite further investigation.

ED Management

Generalized Lymphadenopathy

If infectious mononucleosis is suggested by the clinical findings (fever, fatigue, pharyngitis, hepatosplenomegaly), obtain a CBC with differential (to look for atypical lymphocytosis or monocytosis) and a Monospot or heterophile antibody test to confirm the diagnosis. However, since the heterophile is likely to be negative in a child <6 years old with active mononucleosis, obtain EBV serology, including IgM. Treatment is supportive (bed rest, acetaminophen as needed). Instruct the patient to avoid contact sports because of the risk of splenic rupture. Admission and steroid therapy (prednisone 2 mg/kg/day divided bid) are indicated for neurologic symptoms, respiratory distress, massively enlarged tonsils, or cytopenias.

For other situations, the clinical picture guides the evaluation, although in general a CBC with differential, ESR, liver function tests, VDRL (Venereal Disease Research Laboratory) test, hepatitis B antigen, heterophile antibody, PPD, and chest x-ray are often indicated. If any risk factors are present, obtain HIV serology.

Localized Lymphadenopathy

Reactive Adenopathy In most cases a contiguous infection will be found and reactive adenopathy diagnosed. Treat the primary infection appropriately. The reactive node(s) will shrink as the infection resolves.

Adenitis Treat an adenitis with 40 mg/kg/day of cefadroxil (divided bid), cephalexin (divided qid), or erythromycin (divided qid). Alternatives include cefprozil (20 mg/kg/day divided bid), clarithromycin (15 mg/kg/day divided bid), or azithromycin (12 mg/kg/day for 5 days). Warm compresses applied for 15 to 30 min every 3 to 4 h are an important adjunct. Reevaluate the patient in 48 to 72 h. If there has been a response, continue the antibiotic for a full 10-day course (5 days for azithromycin). If there has been no change in the node in an otherwise asymptomatic child, change the antibiotic to clindamycin (20 mg/kg/day divided qid) or amoxicillin-clavulanate (45 mg/kg/day of amoxicillin divided bid) and follow up in 2 days. However, if there is no improvement and the patient appears ill, or if the node continues to enlarge, obtain a CBC and blood culture and admit the patient for further evaluation (including surgical consultation) and parenteral antibiotics [100 mg/kg/day of either nafcillin (divided q 6 h) or ceftriaxone (divided q 12 h)]. If malignancy is suspected at any time because of a change in the nature of the node, unresponsiveness to treatment, or associated physical or laboratory findings, request an immediate oncology consultation for node biopsy and/or other definitive diagnostic procedures.

Follow-up

- Adenitis treated with oral antibiotics: 2 days

Indications for Admission

- Systemic toxicity
- Suspicion of a malignancy or AIDS, to facilitate the workup and management
- Adenitis unresponsive to oral antibiotics

BIBLIOGRAPHY

Morland B. Lymphadenopathy. *Arch Dis Child* 1995;73:476–479.
Peters TR, Edwards KM. Cervical lymphadenopathy and adenitis. *Pediatr Rev* 2000;21:399–405.
Steuber CP, Nesbit ME: Clinical assessment and differential diagnosis of the child with suspected cancer, in Pizzo PA, Poplack DG (eds): *Principles and Practice of Pediatric Oncology*, 3rd ed. Philadelphia: Lippincott-Raven, 1997, pp 130–132.

ONCOLOGIC EMERGENCIES

A patient with a malignancy, under the care of an oncologist, may be brought to the ED if the family notices an acute change in the child's condition. The most common serious problems are fever, acute neurologic symptomatology, superior vena cava obstruction, respiratory distress, metabolic derangements, and intestinal perforation.

Clinical Presentation

Since malignant diseases and their treatments are associated with immunodeficiency and neutropenia, patients are particularly susceptible to infectious complications, typically manifest by fever (>38.6°C, 101.5°F).

The immunodeficient patient with pneumonia is at risk for opportunistic infections (*Pneumocystis, Aspergillus, Candida, Legionella pneumophilia*). An absolute neutrophil count <500/mm^3 places the patient at risk for gram-negative and fungal infections. Indwelling central venous catheters increase the risk of staphylococcal and streptococcal infections.

Acute neurologic symptomatology may result from spinal cord or nerve root compression and from intracranial involvement. Spinal cord or nerve root compression can cause back pain, lower extremity weakness and sensory loss, and bladder and bowel dysfunction. Headache, vomiting, and isolated cranial nerve paresis can occur with intracranial involvement.

A patient with lymphoma or leukemia who presents with a mediastinal mass can have superior vena cava obstruction causing dyspnea, edema of the head and neck, and prominence of the superficial veins on the upper body. Mediastinal masses may also compress the tracheobronchial tree and cause respiratory distress.

A patient who develops mucositis, particularly in combination with prolonged neutropenia, is at risk for intestinal perforation. The possibility increases with superimposed diarrhea. Because of the decreased inflammatory response and neutropenia, a perforation may present without the classic physical findings of peritoneal irritation, although there may be abdominal pain, fever, and distention.

A patient with a large tumor burden and rapidly proliferating disease is at risk for significant metabolic derangements, including hyperuricemia (oliguria), hyperkalemia (muscle weakness, and peaked T waves, PR prolongation, and QRS widening on the electrocardiogram), and hypocalcemia (tetany, laryngospasm, carpopedal spasm, seizures).

Diagnosis and ED Management

For all febrile [>38.6°C (101.5°F)] oncology patients, obtain a CBC with differential, urinalysis, chest x-ray (if there are respiratory symptoms), and cultures of the throat, blood, urine, and wound (if any). If there is granulocytopenia (<1000/mm^3), consult the oncologist and admit the patient for IV antibiotics pending culture results. The ultimate choice of antibiotic is best determined after checking the sensitivities of the local hospital flora. Give combination IV antibiotic therapy with an aminoglycoside such as tobramycin or gentamicin (6 mg/kg/day divided q 8–12 h) and either a semisynthetic penicillin (piperacillin/tazobactam 250 mg/kg/day divided q 6 h) or ceftazidime (100 mg/kg/day divided q 8 h). If an interstitial pneumonia is found, add trimethoprim-sulfamethoxazole (20 mg/kg/day of TMP divided q 6 h). If the patient has a central venous catheter with erythema surrounding any part of the catheter or port, consider adding vancomycin (40 mg/kg/day divided q 6 h).

The treatment of varicella exposure in a patient with a negative history (and negative varicella titers) is zoster-immune globulin (VZIG), 1 vial per 10 kg (5 vials maximum) given within 4 days of exposure; there is no benefit of VZIG if the patient is seen 4 days or more after the exposure. Regardless of VZIG treatment, if clinical varicella develops, admit the patient and treat with IV acyclovir (10 mg/kg IV q 8 h).

If spinal cord compression is suspected, obtain plain films of the spine and consult the oncologist and neurologist immediately. Definitive diagnosis often requires a magnetic resonance imaging (MRI) scan or myelogram. A patient with signs of intracranial involvement requires emergency CT or MRI. If a mass lesion is found, immediately consult with a neurosurgeon and an oncologist. Treatment often entails emergency radiation therapy and high-dose dexamethasone, and, on some occasions, surgical intervention.

The diagnosis of superior vena cava obstruction is confirmed by finding an anterior mediastinal mass on chest x-ray or chest CT. Obtain a CBC with differential, platelet count, and reticulocyte count while awaiting consultation with an oncologist. Secure IV access in a lower extremity to avoid aggravating the condition with IV fluids directed toward the superior vena cava. The treatment is radiation or chemotherapy.

Treat elevation of the uric acid (>10 mg/dL) with hydration (twice maintenance), allopurinol (10 mg/kg/day PO divided bid-qid), and alkalinization of the urine with sodium bicarbonate (1 to 2 mEq/kg). Treat hyperkalemia >6 mEq/L with kayexalate enemas (1 g/kg). If the hyperkalemia is associated with ECG changes (peaked T waves), give insulin (0.1 U/kg IV) and glucose (0.5 g/kg IV). If there is an associated QRS widening or PR lengthening, also give calcium chloride (20 mg/kg IV over 3–5 min). Dialysis is indicated for a serum potassium >7.5. Treat hypocalcemia (pp 164–165) <7.5 mEq/L with 75 mg/kg/day of elemental oral calcium, divided q 6 h, and aluminum hydroxide gel (Amphojel) 500 mg PO to lower the phosphorus.

If intestinal perforation is suspected, obtain an upright abdominal x-ray or right and left lateral decubitus films of the abdomen looking for free air. A CT scan often confirms the diagnosis. Immediately treat with broad-spectrum antibiotics (as for febrile patient, see above), including additional anaerobic coverage (metronidazole 30 mg/kg/day, divided q 6 h). Carefully monitor the blood pressure, since these patients can rapidly develop both hypovolemia and septic shock. Treat hypotension (pp 18–22) expeditiously with isotonic fluid and packed red cell transfusions, along with vasopressors. Consult a surgeon to arrange for laparotomy.

Indications for Admission

- (>38.5°C, 101.5°F) and granulocytopenia (<1000/mm^3), pneumonia, or evidence of any serious infection
- Clinical varicella
- Spinal cord compression, CNS leukemia, superior vena cava obstruction, airway obstruction
- Significant complication of therapy or serious metabolic derangement (uric acid >10 mg/dL; potassium >6 mEq/L; calcium <7.5 mEq/L)
- Suspected intestinal perforation

BIBLIOGRAPHY

Kelly KM, Lange B: Oncologic emergencies. *Pediatr Clin North Am* 1997;44: 809–830.

Lange B, O'Neill JA, Goldwein JW, et al: Oncologic emergencies, in Pizzo PA, Poplack DG (eds): *Principles and Practice of Pediatric Oncology*. 3rd ed. Philadelphia: Lippincott-Raven, 1997, pp 1025–1050.

SICKLE CELL DISEASE

The sickle cell syndromes are inherited disorders characterized by a chronic hemolytic anemia of variable severity as well as recurrent obstruction of the microvasculature.

Clinical Presentation

Crisis
Children with sickle cell disease (SCD) may present with a constellation of signs and symptoms, termed *crises*.

Vasoocclusive Crisis   The most common type is the vasoocclusive crisis, which is secondary to stasis of sickled RBCs in capillaries and small veins. Multiple organ systems are frequently involved, with severe pain, fever, and symptoms that can mimic many infections and inflammatory disorders. A common finding is bone pain in multiple sites, particularly the extremities and back. Other presentations may include priapism, pneumonia, limp, hematuria, acute hemiplegia (stroke), acute visual impairment caused by retinal vein occlusion or proliferative retinopathy, and leg ulcers. Right-upper-quadrant pain and jaundice occur in an older patient secondary to cholelithiasis from chronic hemolysis. In a child under 2 years of age, vasoocclusive crises often take the form of dactylitis, or the "hand-foot" syndrome, with pain and swelling in the hands, feet, fingers, and toes.

Aplastic Crisis   In addition to the vasoocclusive events, several other crises are seen in children with SCD. Aplastic crises are manifest by worsening anemia and reticulocytopenia. These crises, lasting 7 to 10 days, usually follow viral infections (particularly parvovirus B19) that transiently suppress the bone marrow. Patients present with fatigue, light-headedness, tachycardia, and palpitations. With parvovirus B19 infection, the patient may have a prodrome of fever, malaise, and myalgias, but the characteristic rash is usually absent.

Sequestration Crisis   Splenic sequestration crises, with pooling of RBCs in a rapidly enlarging spleen, are most often seen in young patients doubly heterozygous for HbS and another abnormal hemoglobin, such as β-thalassemia (S-Thal) or hemoglobin C (S-C disease). The patient may present with cold, clammy skin, marked tachycardia, extreme pallor, and profound hypotension as well as a large left-sided abdominal mass (spleen). If unrecognized, deterioration can be rapid, with a fatal outcome.

Hyperhemolytic Crisis   A hyperhemolytic crisis with a falling hematocrit, increasing jaundice, and markedly elevated reticulocyte counts (>20%) is rare and may in reality be the resolving phase of an aplastic crisis. Increased hemolysis with a rise in bilirubin can also be seen in a patient with concurrent G-6-PD deficiency.

Megaloblastic Crisis   A megaloblastic crisis, due to folate depletion, is rare and may be diagnosed by finding hypersegmented polymorpho-nuclear leukocytes (PMNs) and pancytopenia.

Infection
Infections account for many of the serious problems in patients with SCD. Hyposplenism (initially functional, then anatomic) in conjunction with decreased antibody production, decreased serum-opsonizing activity, vasoocclusion, and defective neutrophil function places these children at risk for fulminant overwhelming sepsis, particularly with encapsulated organisms such as *Streptococcus pneumoniae*. They are also at increased risk for *meningitis, pneumonia, pyelonephritis,* and *osteomyelitis* (particu-larly due to *Salmonella*). Until recently, the polyvalent pneumococcal vaccine did not reliably prevent serious pneumococcal infections in chil-dren under 2 years of age. The newer Prevnar conjugate vaccine is very effective in young infants and may help to further decrease the incidence of life-threatening pneumococcal disease.

Diagnosis

Test all undiagnosed children who present with any of the classic sickle cell symptoms noted above for SCD. Confirm the sickle prep with hemo-globin electrophoresis to determine the particular form of the disease (S-S, S-C, S-Thal). Suspect the diagnosis in an asymptomatic patient whose peripheral blood picture reveals anemia, sickle cells, and reticulocytosis (>5%). In addition, the smear will often reveal target cells, "helmet" cells, polychromasia, and Howell-Jolly bodies.

A major diagnostic problem in children with SCD lies in determining the cause of certain symptomatology, in particular, differentiating between infection and infarction. A vasoocclusive crisis is always a diagnosis of exclusion. Leukocytosis (>18,000–20,000/mm^3) is typical in SCD, and fever is not helpful in distinguishing the different entities. Particular diffi-culties are seen with the symptoms described below.

Bone Pain   Differentiating between bone infarcts and osteomyelitis can be very difficult, particularly when only one site is involved. X-rays and bone scans are often unreliable, necessitating needle aspiration to obtain a specimen for culture. An elevated ESR and an increased number of bands (>10% of the total white blood cells) on peripheral smear may indicate an infection, but a normal ESR does not rule out infection. Aseptic necrosis of the head of the femur or humerus presents with bone pain and, in most cases, abnormal radiographs of the affected limb. An MRI scan is often necessary to detect early osteonecrosis.

Right Upper Quadrant Abdominal Pain   Consider hepatitis (especially for patients on chronic transfusion therapy), hepatic infarction, and cholelithiasis, all of which can cause severe pain and fever and elevated bilirubin. With hepatic infarcts, abnormal liver chemistries return to base-line in a much shorter time (days) than with hepatitis, while an abdominal sonogram often detects biliary stones. However, right-lower-lobe pneu-monia, rib infarcts, intestinal wall infarcts, and renal disorders (pyelo-nephritis and papillary necrosis) can all cause pain in a similar location, although other physical and laboratory findings, including urinalysis and x-rays, help to differentiate among these conditions.

Chest Pain and Respiratory Distress   The major differential is between vasoocclusion (pulmonary infarct) and infection (pneumonia). Fever, leukocytosis, and similar radiographic and auscultatory findings occur with both diseases. In addition, either illness can lead to the other, so it is prudent to treat for both entities. A ventilation/perfusion scan may differ-entiate between the two, although therapy will generally not be any different, as infection and infarction are treated simultaneously. Finally, chest pain can be secondary to rib infarcts and abdominal disorders.

ED Management

Crises

Vasoocclusive Crisis   Hydroxyurea is currently in use for selected pa-tients to increase the fetal hemoglobin level and thus prevent sickling. However, since no safe, effective antisickling agent to abort acute crises is available for young children, therapy consists of treating the triggering event and potentiating factors as well as supportive care, including the following:

1. *Vigorous Hydration:* The patient often presents with decreased plasma volume secondary to fever, vomiting, and chronic hyposthenuria. In addition to ad lib oral intake, administer several hours of intravenous hydration at a $1\frac{1}{2} \times$ maintenance rate except for a patient with a pul-monary infarct (give maintenance fluids, since these patients can rapidly develop pleural effusions and worsening respiratory status). The type of fluid is controversial, but $D_5\frac{1}{2}NS$ is satisfactory.
2. *Sodium Bicarbonate:* Reserve sodium bicarbonate (1 mEq/kg) only for marked acidosis (pH <7.20).
3. *Analgesics:* For mild vasoocclusive crises, give aspirin (15 mg/kg), ibuprofen (10 mg/kg), or acetaminophen (15 mg/kg) with codeine (0.5 mg/kg). For a teenager, 5 mg oxycodone plus 325 mg acetamino-phen (Percocet) q 3 to 4 h is an alternative. Occasionally, a single injection of hydromorphone (Dilaudid) or morphine, in conjunction with a few hours of vigorous hydration, can prevent hospital admis-sion. Another alternative is 0.5 mg/kg q 6 h of ketorolac, a potent non-narcotic analgesic that is less likely to cause respiratory depression.
4. *Antipyretics:* Fever leads to further dehydration and sickling, so treat with aspirin (15 mg/kg q 4 h), ibuprofen (10 mg/kg q 6 h), or aceta-minophen (15 mg/kg q 4 h).
5. *Bed Rest:* Muscular activity can produce lactate and worsen the acidosis.

6. *X-ray:* If the patient is limping, a radiograph of the hip must be obtained to rule out asceptic necrosis of the femoral head. If positive, immediately institute bed rest and consult with an orthopedist.

7. *Oxygen:* Oxygen therapy has not been shown to be of benefit for the management of most painful crises, and in fact may be detrimental, since there can be a "rebound" crisis with an outpouring of sickle cells from the bone marrow after therapy is stopped. Indications for supplementary oxygen include severe anemia, pneumonia or pulmonary infarction (particularly if there is documented hypoxia), and shock from infection or splenic sequestration.

Aplastic Crisis   If the patient has not yet begun to recover, as manifest by a brisk reticulocytosis, follow the hemoglobin closely; these patients often have little reserve. A transfusion is usually necessary if the hematocrit is <15% with a reticulocyte count <1%.

Sequestration Crisis   If the patient is hypotensive, immediately infuse Plasmanate (10–20 mL/kg), followed by a transfusion of packed red cells (5–10 mL/kg) if the hematocrit is <15%. This is one instance where rapid red cell transfusion can be lifesaving.

Megaloblastic Crisis   If the hematocrit is >20%, the absolute granulocyte count >1000/mm^3, and the platelet count >50,000/mm^3, administer 1 mg/day of folic acid. Repeat the blood count in 4 to 7 days.

Fever

For a patient above age 2 in no distress with a temperature <39.4°C (103°F) and no obvious source for the fever, obtain a blood culture, CBC, and, for girls, a urinalysis and urine culture. If there is no marked left shift and the absolute band count is <3000/mm^3, the non-ill-appearing patient may be sent home. Give one dose of ceftriaxone (50 mg/kg IM) and observe for 1 to 2 hours before discharge from the ED. Arrange for follow-up in 24 h, or sooner if the temperature goes higher.

Admit the patient with a temperature ≥ 39.4°C (103°F). Also admit a toxic-appearing patient and a child younger than 2 years with a temperature >38.3°C (101°F). Treat with IV ceftriaxone (100 mg/kg/day divided q 12 h). For a patient taking hydroxyurea (which can cause neutropenia), broad-spectrum antibiotic coverage is indicated (p 311) if the absolute neutrophil count is <500/mm^3.

In addition to the basic fever workup, if there are any respiratory symptoms, obtain a chest x-ray, regardless of the auscultatory findings. Admit and treat any SCD patient with a pulmonary density as having a pneumonia. Give ceftriaxone (100 mg/kg/day divided q 12 h), oxygen, and a red cell transfusion; if the patient is over 5 years of age, add azithromycin (10 mg/kg, once on day 1, followed by 5 mg/kg/qd on days 2 to 5) for possible mycoplasmal infection. If there is any suspicion of an osteomyelitis (fever, swelling, point tenderness of a single bone), consult an orthopedist and arrange for a needle aspiration for Gram's stain, cell count, and culture. Indications for a lumbar puncture include a febrile, irritable infant under 2 years of age and a lethargic older patient with a temperature >39.2°C (103°F) and no fever source.

Follow-up

- Vasoocclusive crisis: next day
- Megaloblastic crisis: 4 to 7 days
- Patient >2 years old with temperature <39.4°–40°C (103°–104°F): 24 h or sooner if the temperature goes higher

Indications for Admission

- Serious symptoms, including acute hemiplegia, gross hematuria, acute visual disturbance, severe right upper quadrant pain, or respiratory distress, priapism
- Splenic sequestration or aplastic crisis with hematocrit <15%
- Patient with temperature ≥ 39.4°C (103°F) with or without an identifiable source
- Severe or prolonged vasoocclusive crisis with pain unresponsive to usual therapeutic measures
- Irritable infant with hand-foot syndrome
- Clinical pneumonia or any newly discovered pulmonary density on chest x-ray
- Severe megaloblastic crisis (hematocrit <20%, platelet count <50,000/mm^3, or granulocyte count <1000/mm^3

BIBLIOGRAPHY

Overturf GD: Infections and immunizations of children with sickle cell disease. *Adv Pediatr Infect Dis* 1999;14:191–218.

Quinn CT, Buchanan GR: The acute chest syndrome of sickle cell disease. *J Pediatr* 1999;135:416–422.

Wethers DL: Sickle cell disease in childhood: Part II. Diagnosis and treatment of major complications and recent advances in treatment. *Am Fam Physician* 2000;62:1309–1314.

Yaster M, Kost-Byerly S, Maxwell LG: The management of pain in sickle cell disease. *Pediatr Clin North Am* 2000;47:699–710.

SPLENOMEGALY

A palpable spleen tip that is slightly below the costal margin is a frequent finding on routine physical examination in normal infants up to 1 year of age, as well as in patients with fevers or colds. However, a spleen that extends 2 cm below the costal margin or persists for more than 2 months warrants further investigation. Most often, a viral infection (EBV, adenovirus, CMV) is implicated, but a more serious, nonmalignant or malignant condition may be the etiology (Table 13-3).

Table 13-3   Etiologies of Splenomegaly

Infections
  Viral: Epstein-Barr, adenovirus, cytomegalovirus, HIV
  Bacterial: syphilis, tuberculosis, SBE
  Fungal: histoplasmosis
  Rickettsial: Rocky Mountain spotted fever
  Parasitic: malaria, Leishmania
Neoplasms: leukemia, lymphomas
Outflow obstruction: cirrhosis, cystic fibrosis, Budd-Chiari syndrome,
  portal vein thrombosis
Storage diseases: sarcoid, histiocytosis, Hurler's syndrome, Gaucher's disease
Inflammatory/autoimmune disorders: SLE, serum sickness, JRA
Benign cyst
Trauma: splenic hematoma
Extramedullary hematopoiesis: thalassemia, myelofibrosis
Hemolysis: sickle cell disease, autoimmune hemolytic anemia, hereditary
  spherocytosis

KEY: SBE, subacute bacterial endocarditis; SLE, systemic lupus erythematosus;
JRA, juvenile rheumatoid arthritis

Clinical Presentation

Associated clinical findings depend on the primary disease. Regardless of
etiology, massive splenomegaly can cause anemia (pallor, tachycardia,
weakness), leukopenia, and thrombocytopenia (petechiae, purpura, frank
bleeding).

Diagnosis

Inquire about risk factors for HIV infection in the patient or parents,
recent travel to endemic areas of disease (*Plasmodium, Leishmania,
Histoplasma*), and a family history of inherited disorders (*thalassemia,
sickle hemoglobinopathies, Gaucher's disease, Hurler's syndrome*), or
splenectomy *(thalassemia, hereditary spherocytosis).* Ask about fevers
(infection, inflammation, malignancy), easy bruising or bleeding *(leukemia, lymphoma, marrow replacement),* hematemesis *(cirrhosis),* and
transfusions *(hemoglobinopathy).*

On physical examination, look for evidence of infection (adenopathy,
exanthem, pharyngitis), storage disorders (asymptomatic organ enlargement), malignancy (weight loss, bruising, bleeding, adenopathy, hepatomegaly, fever), or connective tissue disorders (arthritis).

Although generalized adenopathy and hepatomegaly might be significant findings, they are associated with splenomegaly of many etiologies,
and therefore are usually not helpful in making the diagnosis. One of the
most common constellations is fatigue, fever, pharyngitis, generalized
adenopathy, and hepatosplenomegaly consistent with *infectious mononucleosis, a mono-like syndrome (CMV),* and, rarely, more serious illnesses *(leukemia).*

ED Management

Laboratory examination is usually not immediately necessary for an infant or child who appears well and has a palpable spleen tip. Arrange for follow-up to repeat the abdominal examination. Undertake further evaluation if the spleen remains palpable for more than 2 months, enlarges to >2 cm below the costal margin, or becomes associated with other signs or symptoms.

If the patient presents with fatigue, upper respiratory congestion, and pharyngitis, obtain a CBC and a Monospot test, or, in a younger child, EBV titers, to confirm the diagnosis of infectious mononucleosis.

A more thorough laboratory evaluation is indicated for the child who has a history of weight loss or persistent splenomegaly or exhibits any serious signs and symptoms, such as pallor, ecchymoses, arthritis, or a toxic appearance. Admit the patient and obtain a CBC with differential, platelet and reticulocyte counts, an ESR, blood chemistries, and a chest x-ray, and place a 5 TU PPD. If the clinical picture is suggestive of an infection, obtain a blood culture. Obtain a sonogram or CT scan to determine the consistency and size of the spleen.

Isolated splenomegaly usually does not cause significant problems except for cytopenias and rupture following trauma. The patient may attend school (if otherwise well) but caution against participating in contact sports and other activities that increase the risk for abdominal injury. Otherwise, management depends on the underlying etiology.

Follow-up

- Well child with palpable spleen tip: primary care follow-up in 2 to 4 weeks

Indications for Admission

- Suspected malignancy
- Splenomegaly and neutropenia (<1000/mm^3) with associated fever, thrombocytopenia (<40,000/mm^3), or hematemesis
- Massive, unexplained splenomegaly for evaluation
- Splenomegaly with anemia and abdominal pain, particularly with a history of abdominal trauma

BIBLIOGRAPHY

Miller D and Ladisch S. Disorders of the spleen and monocyte-macrophage system, in Miller DR, Baehner RL (eds): *Blood Diseases of Infancy and Childhood.* Philadelphia: Mosby, 1995, pp 805–816.

Pearson HA: The spleen and disturbances of splenic function, in Nathan DG, Oski FA: *Hematology of Infancy and Childhood,* 5th ed. Philadelphia: Saunders, 1998, pp 1051–1068.

ADVERSE EFFECTS OF CANCER THERAPY

Aggressive chemotherapy has dramatically increased the response and cure rates for malignancies, but often at a cost of significant adverse effects. While these complex treatment regimens are usually administered by pediatric oncologists, patients often present to the ED with significant complications. It is crucial for the ED staff to recognize potential and existing problems related to the cancer therapy.

Chemotherapeutic agents share many common side effects—including myelosuppression, nausea, and alopecia—but each drug has the potential for specific toxicities (Table 13-4). Consult a pediatric oncologist during the evaluation of a patient receiving treatment for a malignancy who presents to the ED with possible side effects.

Table 13-4   Side Effects of Chemotherapy

DRUG	POTENTIAL ADVERSE EFFECTS
Asparaginase	Allergic reactions, anaphylaxis, pancreatitis, fever, coagulopathy, hepatotoxicity
Bleomycin	Fever, chills, allergic reactions, nausea and vomiting, pulmonary fibrosis, mucositis
Busulfan	Myelosuppression, pulmonary fibrosis, glossitis, skin darkening
Carboplatin	Myelosuppression, nausea and vomiting, ototoxicity, fatigue, nephrotoxicity
Carmustine (BCNU)	Myelosuppression, nausea and vomiting, nephrotoxicity, mucositis, fever, pulmonary fibrosis, phlebitis
Chlorambucil	Myelosuppression, nausea and vomiting, diarrhea, pulmonary fibrosis, skin rash
Cisplatin	Nausea and vomiting, nephrotoxicity, neurotoxicity, hypomagnesemia, ototoxicity, hepatotoxicity
Cladribine	Myelosuppression, fever, cough, nausea and vomiting
Cyclophosphamide	Myelosuppression, nausea and vomiting, SIADH,* hemorrhagic cystitis, immunosuppression, cardiotoxicity, skin darkening
Cytosine arabinoside	Myelosuppression, nausea and vomiting, hepatotoxicity, mucositis, conjunctivitis, fever, neurotoxicity
Dacarbazine	Myelosuppression, nausea and vomiting, hepatotoxicity, blistering
Dactinomycin	Myelosuppression, nausea and vomiting, hepatotoxicity, mucositis, blistering
Daunorubicin	Myelosuppression, cardiotoxicity, blistering, mucositis, diarrhea
Dexamethasone	Weight gain, hypertension, diabetes, moodiness
Doxorubicin	Myelosuppression, nausea and vomiting, cardiotoxicity, blistering, mucositis, diarrhea
Etoposide	Myelosuppression, nausea and vomiting, hypotension, hepatotoxicity
Fludarabine	Myelosuppression, nausea and vomiting, blurred vision, mucositis, fatigue, diarrhea
5-Fluorouracil	Myelosuppression, nausea and vomiting, diarrhea, mucositis, headache, dermatitis
Gemtuzumab	Nausea and vomiting, chills, fever, mucositis, headache, hepatotoxicity, hypotension
Hydroxyurea	Myelosuppression, nausea and vomiting, mucositis, diarrhea

Table 13-4   Side Effects of Chemotherapy (*continued*)

DRUG	POTENTIAL ADVERSE EFFECTS
Idarubicin	Myelosuppression, nausea and vomiting, cardio-toxicity, blistering, diarrhea
Ifosfamide	Myelosuppression, nausea and vomiting, nephro-toxicity, neurotoxicity, hemorrhagic cystitis
Lomustine (CCNU)	Myelosuppression, nausea and vomiting, hepato-toxicity, nephrotoxicity, anorexia
Mechlorethamine	Myelosuppression, nausea and vomiting, blistering, phlebitis, diarrhea, mucositis
Melphalan	Nausea and vomiting, mucositis, pulmonary fibrosis
6-Mercaptopurine	Myelosuppression, nausea and vomiting, hepatotoxicity
Methotrexate	Myelosuppression, nausea and vomiting, hepatotoxicity, neurotoxicity, nephrotoxicity, mucositis
Mitoxantrone	Myelosuppression, cough, gastrointestinal bleeding, mucositis, diarrhea, headache
Prednisone	Weight gain, hypertension, diabetes, moodiness
Procarbazine	Myelosuppression, nausea and vomiting, neurotoxicity, fever, mucositis, diarrhea, myalgias, fatigue
Teniposide (VM-26)	Myelosuppression, nausea and vomiting, mucositis, allergic reactions, diarrhea
6-Thioguanine	Myelosuppression, nausea and vomiting, hepato-toxicity, mucositis
Thiotepa	Myelosuppression, mucositis, neurotoxicity
Topotecan	Myelosuppression, nausea and vomiting, abdominal pain
Tretinoin	Abdominal pain, muscle pain, constipation, anorexia
Vinblastine	Myelosuppression, nausea and vomiting, blistering
Vincristine	Peripheral neuropathy, SIADH, constipation, seizures
Vinorelbine	Myelosuppression, neuropathy, anorexia, constipation

*Syndrome of inappropriate antidiuretic hormone.

BIBLIOGRAPHY

Balis FM, Holcenberg JS, Poplack: General principles of chemotherapy, in Pizzo PA, Poplack DG (eds): *Principles and Practice of Pediatric Oncology*, 3rd ed. Philadelphia: Lippincott-Raven, 1997, pp 215–272.

Gootenberg JE, Pizzo PA: Optimal management of acute toxicities of therapy. *Pediatr Clin North Am* 1991;38:269–298.

MacKenzie JR: Complications of treatment of paediatric malignancies. *Eur J Radiol* 2001;37:109–119.

CHAPTER 14

Infectious Disease Emergencies

David M. Jaffe and Gregg Rusczyk
- Michael Rosenberg (contributor—HIV-Related Emergencies)
- Steven R. Levine (contributor—Lyme Disease)

BOTULISM

Botulism is a paralyzing disease caused by a neurotoxin elaborated by *Clostridium botulinum*, a gram-positive spore-forming obligate anaerobe whose natural habitat is the soil. Botulinum toxin is tasteless, odorless, and extremely toxic. It acts by irreversibly blocking the release of acetylcholine in peripheral somatic and autonomic synapses as well as at the motor end plates. Raw, home canned, or inadequately prepared foods may be contaminated with the toxin, which is heat-labile. Heating food to the boiling point destroys the toxin, but the bacterial spores are resistant to heat and may survive the home canning process. Canned fish, vegetables, and potatoes have been implicated in outbreaks of botulism.

In children, botulism usually occurs after the ingestion of preformed botulinum toxin in spoiled food. Since infants lack the *Clostridium*-inhibiting bile acids and protective bacterial flora found in the normal adult intestinal tract, ingested botulinum spores can germinate in the intestinal tract. There are approximately 100 cases of infant botulism annually in the United States, with a peak incidence between 2 and 4 months of age; honey consumption is a significant risk factor. Botulism has been implicated in some cases of sudden infant death syndrome.

In wound botulism, *C. botulinum* grows in the injured tissue and produces toxin. Most cases in the United States occur in intravenous drug users or patients with compound fractures of an extremity.

Clinical Presentation

Symptoms of food-borne botulism begin within 12 to 36 h of ingestion of contaminated food. The patient develops blurred vision, diplopia, ptosis, ophthalmoplegia, dysarthria, and dysphagia. Autonomic signs include constipation, dry mouth, postural hypotension, urinary retention, and pupillary dilatation with a sluggish or absent light reflex. Nausea and vomiting may also occur in one-third of patients. A descending weakness follows, which, in severe cases, may involve the respiratory muscles. Weakness is usually bilateral but may be asymmetric. The sensory nerves and mentation are notably spared.

Infantile botulism begins gradually, 2 to 4 weeks after ingestion of the spores. Breast-fed infants are infected later than formula-fed infants, and breast feeding may moderate the severity of the illness. Constipation is often the first symptom, followed by weak cry, weak suck, drooling, difficulty feeding, dysphagia, loss of head control, signs of a descending cranial nerve palsy, and hypotonia. Progressive paralysis can lead to respiratory failure.

After a 4- to 14-day incubation period, the presentation of wound botulism is similar to that of food-borne botulism. There may be fever but not nausea and vomiting. The wound may exhibit no signs of infection.

Diagnosis

Consider other causes of paralysis, including *Guillain-Barré syndrome* (ascending paralysis with an elevated CSF protein), *poliomyelitis* (asymmetric involvement, fever, CSF pleocytosis), *myasthenia gravis* (muscle fatigability, reversal of ptosis with Tensilon), *spinal muscular atrophy* (severe weakness, absent DTRs, tongue fasciculations), and *tick paralysis* (rapidly progressive generalized paralysis, absent DTRs, normal CSF protein, possible dysesthesias). In a febrile infant who is lethargic and feeding poorly, consider *bacterial sepsis* or *meningitis*. Metabolic causes of acute weak-ness include *hypokalemia, hypo-* and *hypercalcemia,* and *hypo-* and *hyperthyroidism.* The diagnosis can be confirmed by analyzing suspected food, serum, gastrointestinal contents, or wound exudates for evidence of toxin or organisms.

ED Management

Admit the patient to an ICU for monitoring, as respiratory arrest can occur at any time. Antitoxin is available from the Centers for Disease Control and Prevention for older children but is not recommended for infants because it is of equine origin and is associated with hypersensitivity reactions. Antibiotics are not necessary to eradicate the bowel colonization of infants. If sepsis cannot be excluded, obtain a CBC, blood culture, and lumbar puncture and start age-appropriate antibiotics (see pp 337–338). Aminoglycosides are contraindicated because they may potentiate the effects of the toxin. In infants and children, recovery takes about 4 weeks and is generally complete.

Indication for Admission

- Suspected botulism

BIBLIOGRAPHY

Cherington M: Clinical Spectrum of Botulism. *Muscle Nerve* 1998;21:701–710.
Committee on Infectious Disease: *2000 Red Book: Report of the Committee on Infectious Disease,* 25th ed. Elk Grove Village, IL: American Academy of Pediatrics, 2000, pp 212–214.
Muensterer OJ: Infant botulism. *Pediatr Rev* 2000;21:427.

CAT-SCRATCH DISEASE

Cat-scratch disease (CSD) is caused by *Bartonella henselae*, a gram-negative bacillus whose reservoir is the cat flea. The disease is associated with scratches or bites by cats. Although there is no evidence that fleas transmit the disease directly to humans, the precise mechanism of cat-to-human transmission is unclear. Approximately 22,000 cases are reported each year, with most occurring in the southern states, Hawaii, and California. The disease occurs more often in the fall and winter months, and clusters occur in families with new pets. Sixty percent of cases are noted in children.

Clinical Presentation

During a 7- to 12-day incubation period, one or more erythematous papules may erupt at the site of inoculation and persist from 1 to 7 weeks (median 12 days), after which proximal lymphadenopathy develops. In 50% of cases, only a single node is affected. In other cases, several nodes draining the site of inoculation become involved, including the axillary, cervical, submandibular, preauricular, epitrochlear, femoral, and inguinal lymph nodes. The infected node is usually tender and swollen, and the overlying skin may become erythematous, warm, and indurated. Lymph nodes remain enlarged for 2 to 4 months and may be associated with fever (38–39°C, 100.4–102.2°F), malaise, anorexia, fatigue, and headache in 30% of patients. An evanescent, polymorphic maculopapular rash may occur early in the course of the disease. If the primary inoculation site is near the eye, Parinaud oculoglandular syndrome may ensue, with mild to moderate conjunctivitis and preauricular lymph node involvement.

Rarely, within 6 weeks of the onset of lymphadenopathy, CSD can cause encephalitis, with high fever and convulsions. Other uncommon complications include osteolytic bone lesions, granulomatous hepatitis, mesenteric lymphadenitis, pneumonia, arthralgia, subacute iritis, chorioretinitis, optic neuritis, urethritis, lymphedema, and thyroiditis.

Diagnosis

Suspect CSD if a patient with persistent regional lymphadenitis (>3 weeks) has a history of contact with a cat and an identifiable inoculation site. Indirect immunofluorescence and enzyme immunoassay serologic tests for *B. henselae* are available. The differential diagnosis of CSD includes most causes of lymphadenopathy (see pp 313–316).

ED Management

To date, no data demonstrate that CSD responds to antibiotics. Therefore, reserve antibiotic therapy [trimethoprim-sulfamethoxazole (TMP-SMX), 8 mg/kg/day of TMP divided bid; azithromycin, 12 mg/kg qd; erythromycin 40 mg/kg/day divided tid or qid] for a patient with severe systemic symptoms, hepatomegaly, large, painful adenopathy, or immunocompromise. Surgical excision of affected nodes is unnecessary, although needle aspiration of painful, suppurative nodes may relieve symptoms. The systemic symptoms usually resolve in 2 weeks, and neurologic complications are rare.

Indication for Admission

- CSD with encephalitis, seizures, severe liver disease.

BIBLIOGRAPHY

Bass JW, Vincent JM, Person SA: The expanding spectrum of *Bartonella* infections: II. Cat-scratch disease. *Pediatr Infect Dis J* 1997;16:163–179.
Conrad DA: Treatment of cat-scratch disease. *Curr Opin Pediatr* 2001;13:56–59.
Margileth AM: Recent advances in diagnosis and treatment of cat scratch disease. *Curr Infect Dis Rep* 2000;2:141–146.

ENCEPHALITIS

Encephalitis is characterized by inflammation of the brain. Approximately 20,000 cases of encephalitis occur in the United States each year, most of which are mild. The two endemic causes of encephalitis in the United States are the herpes simplex viruses (HSV 1 and 2) and the rabies virus. Other viral etiologies include arthropod-borne viruses (St. Louis encephalitis, California encephalitis, eastern, western, Venezuelan equine encephalitis, West Nile virus), other herpesviruses (varicella zoster, Epstein-Barr, cytomegalovirus), and enteroviruses (enterovirus, echovirus, coxsackievirus). Bacterial causes include *Haemophilus influenzae*, *Neisseria meningitides*, *Streptococcus pneumoniae*, and *Mycobacterium tuberculosis*, although these organisms more often cause meningitis (see pp 366–369). Spirochetal infections include *Treponema pallidum*, *Leptospira* species, and *Borrelia burgdorferi* (Lyme disease). Other nonviral causes of encephalitis include *Chlamydia psittaci* and *Chlamydia pneumoniae*, rickettsial infections, mycoplasmal infections (*Mycoplasma pneumoniae* and *Mycoplasma hominis*), and fungal infections (*Coccidioides immitis*, *Cryptococcus neoformans*). Additionally, *Toxoplasma gondii* and *Listeria monocytogenes* can cause encephalitis in an immunocompromised patient.

Parainfectious encephalitis is thought to be due to an autoimmune phenomenon initiated by a viral pathogen, most often influenza, varicella, or measles. Characteristically, there is a latent phase between the acute illness and the onset of neurologic symptoms.

Clinical Presentation

Encephalitis most commonly begins as an acute systemic illness with fever and headache. Most patients have diffuse disease with behavioral or personality changes, altered level of consciousness, or generalized seizures. The patient may have localized findings, such as ataxia, cranial nerve defects, hemiparesis, or focal seizures. Alternatively, there may be high fever, convulsions with bizarre movements, and hallucinations alternating with periods of clarity. Nuchal rigidity, if present, is less pronounced than with meningitis.

Herpesviruses   Herpes can affect newborns as well as older children and adults. Both HSV-1 and HSV-2 cause CNS infection in about 50% of newborns with herpes infection. Morbidity and mortality depend on whether the infant has isolated CNS involvement or disseminated disease. However, the mortality rate, even with antiviral therapy, is 60%, while approximately 40% of survivors have neurologic impairment. In an older child or adolescent, encephalitis is usually secondary to HSV-1. Fever, focal or generalized seizures, focal neurologic signs, and altered level of consciousness can occur. Although therapy improves survival, more than 50% of patients progress to significant neurologic impairment or death. *Epstein-Barr virus (EBV) encephalitis* causes a focal encephalopathic disease in conjunction with fever, pharyngitis, lymphadenopathy, atypical lymphocytosis, and a positive heterophile test. Recovery is usually complete. *Varicella encephalitis* follows the distinctive exanthem and may lead to nystagmus, dysarthria, and cerebellar ataxia.

Arthropod-Borne   The responsible agents are transmitted by mosquitoes and ticks, and outbreaks occur primarily during the summer and fall seasons. Recently, the West Nile virus that previously caused sporadic cases and outbreaks in Europe has been documented in the northeastern United States. Mosquitoes that prey on birds and humans are the principal vectors. After an incubation period of 3 to 6 days, there is the abrupt onset of a febrile, flu-like illness with headache, sore throat, myalgias, and fatigue. In addition, there may be conjunctivitis, retrobulbar pain, and a maculopapular rash that spreads from the trunk to the extremities and head. Anorexia, nausea, abdominal pain, diarrhea, respiratory symptoms, nuchal rigidity, confusion, somnolence or altered consciousness, abnormal reflexes, and seizures may occur. The patient may develop hepatitis, pancreatitis, myocarditis, and hepatosplenomegaly. Recovery is usually complete in children.

Enteroviral   Enteroviral infection usually occurs in the summer. Following a prodrome of fever and upper respiratory tract symptoms, the patient develops acute neurologic findings such as confusion, altered level of consciousness, or irritability. Neurologic manifestations are usually global rather than focal. Other possible manifestations include photophobia and a macular or petechial rash.

Rabies   Rabies has an average incubation period of 4 to 6 weeks (range from 5 days to 6 years). Rabies infection is transmitted by the bite of an infected animal and is invariably fatal. Clinically, there is anxiety, dysphagia, and hydrophobia (see Rabies, pp 670–672).

Parainfectious   A patient with measles parainfectious encephalitis presents with the abrupt onset of fever, neurologic symptoms, and altered mental status while recovering from the acute infection. Neurologic sequelae occur in most survivors and may include intellectual, motor, psychiatric, epileptic, visual, or auditory deficits. Approximately 50% of patients have seizures.

Diagnosis

Obtain a detailed history, including whether there has been any exposure to ill contacts (human or animal), mosquitoes, ticks, or animals. Inquire about recent travel or injections and the possibility of accidental exposure to heavy metals or pesticides. Perform a thorough physical examination, looking for focal neurologic abnormalities, cerebellar signs, and evidence of increased intracranial pressure (including funduscopy).

Consider metabolic diseases such as *hypoglycemia, uremic* or *hepatic encephalopathy*, and *inborn errors of metabolism* (disorders of glucose or ammonia metabolism), toxic disorders (*drug ingestion, Reye's syndrome*), and *mass lesions* (tumor or abscess). Also consider subarachnoid hemorrhage from an *arteriovenous malformation* or *aneurysm* and embolic lesions from *bacterial endocarditis*. Acute demyelinating disorders, including *multiple sclerosis, acute hemorrhagic leukoencephalitis*, and *status epilepticus* are also possible diagnoses. Postinfectious disease including *Guillain-Barré syndrome* and *Miller-Fisher syndrome, brainstem encephalitis*, and *acute cerebellar ataxia* are also in the differential diagnosis of encephalitis.

ED Management

Perform an immediate lumbar puncture to exclude bacterial meningitis unless focal neurologic signs are found or there is evidence of increased intracranial pressure. In such a case, give IV ceftriaxone (50 mg/kg) immediately and arrange for a CT scan of the head prior to performing the lumbar puncture. Send the CSF for Gram's stain, cell count, protein, glucose, culture, rapid antigen identification test, viral culture, and, if tuberculosis is a possibility, acid-fast stain or culture for *Mycobacterium.* The CSF in viral encephalitis is usually clear, and the leukocyte count can range from none to several thousand, with a polymorphonuclear predominance early in the course. The protein is normal to moderately elevated, and the glucose is initially normal.

Obtain a CBC, platelet count, electrolytes, BUN, creatinine, glucose, blood culture, and urin-alysis. If specific viral etiologies are being considered, send urine, stool, CSF, and throat swabs for viral diagnostic tests and sera for viral titers (repeat the titer in 2–4 weeks). In particular, if herpes simplex virus (HSV) is a possibility, send CSF for HSV polymerase chain reaction analysis.

Admit patients with encephalitis for close monitoring of vital signs and fluid status. Give antibiotics directed at organisms causing bacterial meningitis (pp 366–369) and be prepared to treat complications including seizures, cerebral edema, hyperpyrexia, respiratory insufficiency, fluid and electrolyte abnormalities, aspiration, gastrointestinal bleeding, cardiac decompensation, DIC, and cardiopulmonary arrest.

If *herpes* is a possibility, treat with acyclovir for 14 to 21 days (60 mg/kg/day divided q 8 h). Isolate the patient until a specific agent is identified. If *rabies* is suspected, immediately initiate passive and active immunization for personnel whose mucous membranes or open wounds have contacted the patient's saliva, CSF, or brain tissue.

During *enteroviral* epidemics in the summer and fall, a patient >6 years of age who develops encephalitis without meningitis (mild to moderate headache that responds to acetaminophen or ibuprofen, nontoxic appearance, CSF with a monocytic pleocytosis and normal chemistries) may be sent home for bed rest, fluids, and antipyretic therapy. Admit any patient with nuchal rigidity, moderate to severe headache, unresponsive to acetaminophen or ibuprofen, or lethargy.

Follow-up

• Nontoxic patient with probable enteroviral infection: daily

Indication for Admission

• Encephalitis or meningoencephalitis except for mild enteroviral infection

BIBLIOGRAPHY

Hinson VK, Tyor WR: Update on viral encephalitis. *Curr Opin Neurol* 2001;14: 369–374.
Kimberlin D, Lin C, Jacobs R, et al: Safety and efficacy of high-dose intravenous acyclovir in the management of neonatal herpes simplex virus infections. *Pediatrics* 2001;108:230–238.
Marfin AA, Gubler DJ: West Nile encephalitis: an emerging disease in the United States. *Clin Infect Dis* 2001;33:1713–1719.
Whitley RJ, Kimberlin DW: Viral encephalitis. *Pediatr Rev* 1999;20:192–198.

EVALUATION OF THE FEBRILE CHILD

Fever is one of the most common causes for a visit to the ED It is defined here as a rectal temperature greater than 38°C (100.4°F). It may be the presenting sign of a viral illness, a minor bacterial infection, or a life-threatening bacterial process. While fever most typically indicates the presence of an infection, on rare occasions it may be the presenting sign of poisoning (aspirin, phenothiazines), collagen vascular disease, or malignancy. Although a patient can have sepsis without fever, it is more likely that a seriously ill child has some elevation in temperature.

Clinical Presentation

Clinical impression is a component of every strategy for evaluating febrile infants and young children. The best known tool is the Yale Observation Scale (YOS), an objective scoring system based on the child's alertness, playfulness, interaction with the environment, color, state of hydration, quality of cry, and ability to be consoled. The older the patient, the more reliable the clinical impression becomes as a predictor of serious underlying illness. In addition, an older child is more likely to have specific localizing signs of illness.

A young infant (<8 weeks) may have bacterial sepsis without many clinical findings. The YOS has been shown to be neither sensitive nor specific for identifying which young febrile infant is at risk for serious bacterial infection.

There may be a history of excessive crying, irritability, lethargy, or decreased feeding. Unfortunately, an infant is at highest risk for sepsis in the first few days of life, when there has been little time for behavior patterns to develop. Therefore, the history is often not helpful. However, a history of a cyanotic episode or a seizure in an infant with fever is extremely worrisome and mandates a full evaluation for sepsis.

On physical examination, the young infant may be pale or mottled, tachypneic, tachycardic, with weak cry and grunting respirations. Alternatively, the infant may simply be sleeping and difficult to arouse. Focal infections typically do not present with localized findings. Meningeal signs may be absent despite the presence of meningitis, and there may be no ear tugging with otitis media. The infant with a UTI may have only a fever, perhaps accompanied by vomiting or diarrhea.

Beyond 8 weeks of age, clinical impression becomes more accurate, at least when applied to young, febrile children with serious bacterial infections such as pneumonia or meningitis. The child with sepsis does not smile and is rarely interested in its surroundings. The parent often reports that there is a definite change in the child's behavior. Moreover, localized infections are often associated with focal complaints. The older child (toddler age) with meningitis usually has nuchal rigidity and positive Kernig's and/or Brudzinski's signs.

The evaluation of nontoxic-appearing febrile young children from 3 months to 3 years for "occult" bacteremia (OB) has been the subject of considerable study and debate. The introduction of the conjugated pneumococcal vaccine is likely to render obsolete prior findings on the epidemiology of OB and therefore invalidate previously published management guidelines. The risk for OB is extremely low in children with temperatures less than 38.9°C (102°F) and increases as the temperature rises above 39°C (102.2°F). The patient may have symptoms of an upper respiratory infection or pharyngitis but no other detectable etiology for the fever. Despite efforts to develop reliable methods of diagnosis, these children may be clinically indistinguishable from children with self-limited viral diseases, and they may have no localizing signs whatsoever.

A temperature greater than 41.1°C (106°F) is unusual. However, these children have the same risk of serious infection as children with temperatures between 38.5 and 41.1°C (101.3 and 106°F).

Diagnosis and ED Management

The priority is the identification of the child with a serious bacterial infection (SBI). Clinical impression and physical examination are the mainstays of diagnosis. Certain laboratory tests may help predict the risk of serious infection when the results of the clinical evaluation are equivocal. A white blood cell count (WBC) >15,000/mm^3, band to neutrophil ratio >0.2 (in infants 0–2 months of age), and an ESR >30 mm/h have been shown to correlate with SBI or a risk of OB. However, because of the low prevalence of bacteremia, the positive predictive value of any single test remains low.

The management of febrile infants and children is summarized below. These guidelines may have to be modified if unusual pathogens are suspected (immunocompromised host, CSF shunt, recent course of antibiotics).

Below 8 Weeks of Age
Since clinical impression is difficult to apply to young infants, perform a full evaluation for sepsis, including CBC with differential count, blood and urine cultures, urinalysis, and lumbar puncture for cell count, glucose, protein, Gram's stain, and culture. Obtain urine by catheter insertion or suprapubic aspiration (not clean-catch bag). A chest radiograph is indicated only if there are respiratory signs or symptoms. The following criteria have been used to identify infants at low risk for sepsis:

1. Well appearance
2. No identifiable source of infection on physical examination
3. No known immunodeficiency
4. Urinalysis with ≤10 WBCs per high-power field and no bacteria on Gram's stain
5. CSF with <8 WBC/mm³ and no bacteria on Gram's stain
6. WBC <15,000/mm³
7. ESR <30 mm/h or a band:neutrophil ratio <0.2
8. If the infant has diarrhea, the stool is heme-negative, and there are ≤5 WBCs per high-power field
9. Normal chest radiograph

Below 4 Weeks of Age   Admit the infant and treat with ampicillin (<1 week of age: 100 mg/kg/day, divided q 12 h; >1 week of age: 200 mg/kg/day, divided q 6 h) *and* cefotaxime (<1 week, 100 mg/kg/day, divided q 12 h; 1–4 weeks; 150 mg/kg/day, divided q 8 h). If meningitis is suspected, increase the cefotaxime dose to 200 mg/kg/day divided q 6 h.

4 to 8 Weeks of Age   There is a growing consensus that an infant in this age group who meets the criteria for low risk for SBI may be managed as an outpatient, without expectant antibiotic therapy. However, admit an infant who appears clinically ill or has evidence of SBI and treat with ceftriaxone (100 mg/kg/day divided q 12 h). Obtain all cultures, including a lumbar puncture, before starting antibiotics unless the infant is in shock or has evidence of respiratory distress.

8 Weeks to 6 Months of Age
Clinical impression is more reliable in this age group. Try to observe the infant carefully at its best. If no fever source can be found, examine and culture the urine. Also obtain a chest radiograph if there are any respiratory signs, including tachypnea. Administer appropriate therapy for focal infections such as otitis media, suspected UTI, and pneumonia, and admit an infant <3 months of age with presumed bacterial pneumonia (pp 591–595) or UTI (pp 613–616).

The most important aspects of care are careful and frequent follow-up and parental vigilance for clinical deterioration. One of the true arts of pediatrics is the ability to distinguish irritability associated with otitis media or nonspecific viral febrile illness from that associated with meningitis or sepsis. Give a dose of acetaminophen (15 mg/kg) or ibuprofen (10 mg/kg) to a patient who seems irritable but has normal vital signs and is not lethargic and reevaluate in 30 min. Admit a patient who appears toxic (lethargic, inconsolable, poor perfusion, grunting), but discharge the patient who is consolable and feeds well in the ED. Arrange for a follow-up examination the next day.

6 Months to 36 Months of Age
Some of the guidelines for evaluating younger children still pertain, but this is an area of intense debate. With the widespread use of pneumococcal vaccine, the risk of OB is under 1 to 2% in a child with a temperature >39.5°C (103°F).

Above 36 Months of Age
Localizing findings are generally reliable. Look for meningeal signs, evidence of focal infection, or petechiae.

All Infants and Children with Fever without a Source
When there is no identified source of the fever, management includes the following:

1. Perform a lumbar puncture if there is any suspicion of sepsis or meningitis. Admit and treat any toxic-appearing child.
2. Obtain a urinalysis and urine culture in boys <1 year of age and girls <2 years of age. Infants and young children still in diapers are unable to give a midstream sample; obtain urine by suprapubic aspiration or catheter insertion. Approximately 8% of uncircumcised boys <1 year of age and up to 16% of girls ≤2 years of age with fever without a source will have a UTI. The Gram's stain is 99% sensitive for UTI, although only a culture can prove or exclude an infection.
3. The chest radiograph is usually negative in a child without signs or symptoms of respiratory illness, although a patient beyond the newborn period can have "occult pneumonia." Usually the child will have persistent fever, dehydration, chest pain or discomfort, or decreased breath sounds. A chest radiograph is indicated in any child with tachypnea unresponsive to antipyretic therapy and/or with persistent cough or rhonchi. Pneumonia may be diagnosed clinically in the febrile child with rales.
4. Send a stool culture if the patient has bloody diarrhea or >5 WBCs per high-power field in a stool smear. Obtain a blood culture and begin antibiotic therapy in a febrile infant with a stool culture positive for *Salmonella* (see Diarrhea, pp 217–222). An older child with *Salmonella* enteritis rarely needs specific antimicrobial therapy.

In evaluating (at a follow-up visit) a patient with documented *S. pneumoniae* bacteremia, obtain a repeat blood culture if the child is still febrile or afebrile for <24 h. Admit the child, complete the workup for sepsis, and treat with IV penicillin G (100,000 U/kg/day divided q 6 h). Because of emerging patterns of resistant *S. pneumoniae,* check local antibiotic sensitivities and use a third-generation cephalosporin plus vancomycin (10–15 mg/kg q 8 h) if resistance is a concern. If a patient with *S. pneumoniae* bacteremia has been afebrile for >24 h and is well-appearing, treat as an outpatient with oral penicillin (50 mg/kg/day divided qid) for 7 days. Give the parents specific guidelines for temperature control (15 mg/kg of acetaminophen q 4 h) and for assessing the child at home (increased irritability or lethargy, decreased PO intake) and provide for a follow-up visit within 24 to 48 h, or sooner if the patient seems worse to the parents.

Follow-up

- 4 to 8 weeks: daily, until cultures are negative
- 8 weeks to 6 months: daily, until afebrile
- 6 to 36 months: 24 to 48 h
- >36 months: 2 to 3 days, if still febrile

Indications for Admission

- All infants <4 weeks of age with a temperature greater than 38.1°C (100.6°F) or the temperature cutoff in your hospital
- Most infants <3 months of age with focal bacterial infection other than otitis media
- Toxic appearance regardless of age or degree of fever
- Patient recalled for *S. pneumoniae* or *Salmonella* in the blood who is ill appearing, febrile, or afebrile for <24 h
- Patient recalled for any other gram-negative organism in the blood

BIBLIOGRAPHY

Alpern ER, Alessandrini EA, Bell LM, et al: Occult bacteremia from a pediatric emergency department: current prevalence, time to detection, and outcome. *Pediatrics* 2000;106:505–511.

Baker MD: Evaluation and management of infants with fever. *Pediatr Clin North Am* 1999;46:1061–1072.

Baraff LJ: Management of fever without source in infants and children. *Ann Emerg Med* 2000;36:602–614.

Kuppermann N: Occult bacteremia in young febrile children. *Pediatr Clin North Am* 1999;46:1073-1109.

Kuppermann N, Fleisher GR, Jaffe DM: Predictors of occult pneumococcal bacteremia in young febrile children. *Ann Emerg Med* 1998;31:679–687.

Shaw KN, Gorelick M, McGowan KL, et al: Prevalence of urinary tract infection in febrile young children in the emergency department. *Pediatrics* 1998;102:e16.

HIV-RELATED EMERGENCIES

Human immunodeficiency virus (HIV) is transmitted horizontally, via sexual contact or exposure to contaminated blood or blood products (e.g., transfusions, used needles), and vertically from mother to fetus. Zidovudine (AZT) prophylaxis and improved medical and obstetric management of HIV-infected pregnant women have reduced vertical transmission rates to an estimated 1 to 4% nationwide. In addition, potent combination antiretroviral therapy (ART) has been shown to slow disease progression and reduce the risk of opportunistic infections, so that in some children, immune reconstitution has occurred. At this time, perinatally infected infants and children constitute the largest group of pediatric AIDS patients and, as the HIV epidemic "matures," there will be more infected adolescents with severe immunodeficiency and its attendant complications. Victims of rape or sexual abuse and teenagers engaging in unprotected sex also present to the ED for HIV counseling, testing, and postexposure chemoprophylaxis.

Clinical Presentation and Diagnosis

Children and adolescents with HIV can experience the same spectrum of acute illnesses as uninfected patients. However, because of HIV-induced immunodeficiency, the presentation, clinical course, and response to therapy may differ.

Acute Fever   HIV-infected children with fever may have otitis media, a viral infection, or a serious bacterial or opportunistic infection. They develop bacteremia with the same organisms that affect other children, such as *pneumococci, meningococci*, and gram-negative bacilli *(Salmonella, Pseudomonas)*. In addition, patients with indwelling catheters or soft tissue infections are prone to bacteremia from *S. aureus,* or other, coagulase-negative staphylococci. Prolonged courses of antibiotics predispose patients to infections by multiple drug resistant bacteria (e.g., penicillin resistant pneumococci, gram-negative bacilli) and fungi, especially *Candida* species.

The sexually active teenager with signs and symptoms suggestive of a mononucleosis-like illness—including fever, malaise, headache, pharyngitis, rash, and generalized lymphadenopathy—may have the acute retroviral syndrome, which can result in clinical syndromes indistinguishable from classic EBV-related mononucleosis.

Chronic Fever   Fever lasting more than 2 weeks may be due to undiagnosed or untreated HIV infection or may be secondary to an occult abscess, opportunistic infection, or malignancy. Disseminated *Mycobacterium avium-intracellulare* (MAI) infection may cause chronic fevers. It is often associated with anemia due to bone marrow infiltration. In contast, tuberculosis is far more common among HIV-positive adults than among HIV-infected children.

Skin and Soft Tissue Infections   HIV-infected children with common cutaneous disorders such as impetigo or cellulitis may have a more extensive and rapid spread of infection. Also, scabies may present with a generalized papulosquamous eruption or with diffuse areas of crusting and scale, indicating severe infestation.

Exanthematous Diseases   Viral exanthems are common. In some cases of chickenpox, the lesions do not resolve or take much longer to resolve than in immunocompetent children. Complications include dehydration secondary to poor fluid intake from severe mucous membrane involvement and visceral dissemination to the lung, liver, pancreas, or brain. Herpes zoster presents with characteristic lesions in a dermatomal distribution usually involving the trunk. Secondary dissemination involving multiple dermatomes and viscera can occur.

Head, Ear, Eye, Nose, and Throat Infections   Acute otitis media, chronic suppurative otitis media with perforation, conjunctivitis, sinusitis, and pharyngitis are common. Bacterial sinusitis is the second most frequent clinically diagnosed infection after pneumonia. Oropharyngeal candidiasis, mucosal ulcerations, and esophagitis can develop in patients with advanced immunosuppression. HIV-infected children are more prone to gingivitis and periodontitis, and, in cases of poor dental hygiene, dental abscesses. Parotid infiltration or adenopathy increases the risk of bacterial superinfection. Lymphadenitis and parotitis can then present with erythema, warmth, tenderness, and induration.

Pulmonary   Respiratory problems are a common cause of morbidity and mortality. Reactive airway disease and community-acquired pneumonia are the most prevalent conditions treated in the ED. *Pneumocystis carinii* pneumonia (PCP) is the most common opportunistic infection. It usually occurs in children under 18 months of age and is associated with rapid onset of respiratory distress, with tachypnea, fever, and dry cough. In older children, it can present in an insidious fashion with wheezing, mild cough, and progressive dyspnea. The pulmonary examination reveals wheezing, diminished breath sounds, and occasionally rales. Hypoxia ($Po_2 < 70$ mmHg) is common, with an A-a O_2 gradient > 30 mmHg. The typical radiologic finding is a diffuse interstitial process; occasionally there is a pattern of adult respiratory distress syndrome (ARDS), with complete opacification of the lung fields. Rarely, the chest radiograph may show clear lungs, slight hyperinflation, or cystic changes. Serum LDH levels are often markedly elevated (> 500 IU/L). A normal LDH level is strong evidence against PCP.

The etiology and presentation of bacterial pneumonia (pp 591–595) is the same as for immunocompetent patients. In addition, pneumonia due to *Moraxella, Legionella,* and *Nocardia* can occur. Patients receiving antibiotics or who have recently been hospitalized are at risk for antibiotic-resistant gram-positive and gram-negative pneumonias.

Cardiac   Wheezing unresponsive to bronchodilators can be due to heart failure secondary to HIV cardiomyopathy. Heart failure usually presents in older children with tachypnea, rales, decreased activity, or wheezing. Hepatomegaly is often found, though it is not specific. Radiographic examination shows an enlarged cardiac silhouette, but definitive diagnosis may require an echocardiogram. Consider infective endocarditis (pp 55–57) in a patient who presents with fever, toxicity, and a new cardiac murmur.

Gastrointestinal   Nausea, vomiting, and diarrhea (acute and chronic) are common complaints in HIV-infected children. In addition to the usual viral causes of acute gastroenteritis, these children are susceptible to unusual gastrointestinal pathogens. *Cryptosporidium*, a protozoan, can cause intractable watery diarrhea associated with abdominal pain and vomiting. The diagnosis is made by staining the stool with a modified acid-fast stain. *Isospora belli* may cause a similar syndrome. Diagnosis is made by identification of oocytes in the stool. MAI can cause multisystem disease characterized by wasting, recurrent fevers, night sweats, abdominal pain, and diarrhea. MAI can be isolated from the blood, liver biopsy, lymph node, bone marrow, or the GI tract of infected patients. Cytomegalovirus (CMV) colitis can also present with bloody diarrhea; diagnosis of this disorder usually requires histologic verification.

Salmonella gastroenteritis causes fever, vomiting, and malaise in addition to watery or bloody diarrhea. It is a common cause of bacteremia and can lead to sepsis, septic arthritis, and meningitis. These complications can develop weeks to months after recovery from the acute enteritis.

Medications are often responsible for causing GI symptoms. Protease inhibitors such as ritonavir, amprenavir, and lopinavir can cause nausea and vomiting, while nelfinavir can cause loose stools. Use of didanosine has been associated with pancreatitis, but this complication is uncommon in children.

Hematologic   Hematologic complications are common. Medications, infections, nutritional deficiencies, and HIV itself can cause bone marrow dysfunction and result in a spectrum of mild to severe cytopenias. Undiagnosed HIV infection occasionally presents with asymptomatic thrombocytopenia. Bleeding is rare in these circumstances, but the risk of potentially catastrophic intracranial hemorrhage increases as the platelet count falls below $10,000/mm^3$.

Genitourinary/Renal   The incidence and clinical manifestations of UTIs are not influenced by the presence of HIV infection. African-American children with advanced disease are at higher risk of developing HIV nephropathy, a condition characterized by nephrotic-range proteinuria and eventual progression to renal failure. The protease inhibitor indinavir can cause nephrolithiasis, which may be asymptomatic or present with flank pain, hematuria, and crystalluria.

Neurologic   Bacterial meningitis and most aseptic meningitis syndromes are not more common or virulent in asymptomatic HIV-infected children than in seronegative controls. In addition to HIV-related encephalopathy, children with low T-cell counts ($<50–100/mm^3$) are susceptible to opportunistic CNS infections such as cryptococcal meningitis, progressive multifocal leukoencephalopathy (PML), and cerebral toxoplasmosis. CNS lymphoma can also occur, but is rare.

ED Management

Fever   Occult bacteremia is a concern in HIV patients, although the period of susceptibility is beyond 3 years of age. Take a history and perform a careful examination, focusing on any possible localized infection.

Well-Appearing   If the patient appears well but has a fever over 39°C (102.2°F), obtain a CBC and blood culture; and if the child is still in diapers, obtain a urinalysis. If the urinalysis is abnormal or if the child is irritable, has CVA tenderness and/or any urinary complaints, obtain a urine culture. If there are any respiratory findings, including isolated tachypnea or cough or an elevated WBC count with a left shift, obtain a chest radiograph. Baseline CBCs are helpful in evaluating these children, since many of them are leukopenic. If such values are not available, use a WBC >15,000/mm^3 as abnormal. If no obvious focus of infection is found, treat with ceftriaxone (50 mg/kg/day IM) pending culture results. Alternatively, prescribe a beta-lactamase–stable antibiotic such as amoxicillin-clavulanic acid (875/125 formulation, 45 mg/kg/day divided bid) or an oral second-generation cephalosporin such as cefuroxime(30 mg/kg/day divided bid). Schedule a follow-up visit for the next day, but advise the family to return if symptoms worsen or if the patient becomes lethargic.

Ill-Appearing   Obtain cultures of the blood, urine, and, stool if indicated. If there is meningismus, altered mental status, or an underlying abnormal mental status that makes evaluation unreliable, perform a lumbar puncture (unless the child is unstable). Start an IV and give ceftriaxone (one 75 mg/kg dose followed by 100 mg/kg/day q 12 h). Add vancomycin (60 mg/kg/day divided q 6 h) for suspected bacterial meningitis.

If the patient has recently been taking antibiotics or has an indwelling catheter, administer broad-spectrum IV antibiotics such as ticarcillin-clavulanic acid (200–300 mg/kg/day divided q 6 h) or nafcillin (150 mg/kg/day divided q 6 h) *and* ceftazidime (150 mg/kg/day divided q 8 h).

Chronic Fever   The goal of the ED evaluation is to rule out possible bacterial infection. Obtain a CBC, ESR or C-reactive protein, urinalysis, chest and sinus x-rays, and blood, urine, and stool cultures. Also obtain a blood culture for MAI; use culture bottles that are specific for the isolation of mycobacteria (Bactec 13A system). If there is no obvious source of infection and the laboratory evaluation is negative, admit the patient to begin a diagnostic workup for fever of unknown origin.

Skin, Soft Tissue, and HEENT Infections   Obtain a CBC, blood culture, and wound culture. Treat a well-appearing child with a well-circumscribed infection as an outpatient. For parotitis, prescribe an antibiotic active against *S. aureus* and oral streptococci, such as amoxicillin-clavulanic acid (875/125 formulation, 45 mg/kg/day divided bid), clindamycin (20 mg/kg/day divided tid), or a cephalosporin (cefadroxil 40 mg/kg/day divided bid; cefuroxime (30 mg/kg/day divided bid). Frequent warm-water rinses are a useful adjunctive measure. Treat cellulitis due to a break in the skin with amoxicillin-clavulanic acid or a first-generation cephalosporin. Treat a dental abscess with clindamycin (20 mg/kg/day divided tid). Reevaluate the child within 48 h; if there is no improvement, admit for parenteral antibiotics. Also admit any child who appears toxic, has a large area involved, or whose infection impinges on important structures (i.e., the airway) for parenteral antibiotic therapy.

Varicella Zoster Virus (VZV) Infection   Carefully evaluate the child's hydration, mental, and respiratory status and order a chest x-ray if the patient is tachypneic. Admit a patient with a low CD4+ cell count (<500) and primary VZV infection for IV acyclovir (1500 mg/m^2/24 h divided q 8 h). Give oral acyclovir (80 mg/kg/day divided qid) for the treatment of a mild infection in a patient with good immune function. Newer antiviral agents such as famciclovir and valacyclovir are approved for the treatment of zoster in adults and may be useful in older children and adolescents who can swallow pills. Instruct the caretaker to bring the child back if the rash starts to disseminate. Reevaluate the patient within 48 h, and if there is no improvement, admit for IV acyclovir. For an unimmunized child who has not had chickenpox or shingles and reports an exposure to varicella, administer IM varicella zoster immune globulin (VZIG; 1 vial/ 10 kg, 5 vials max) within 4 days of exposure. If another exposure occurs more than 3 weeks after the initial administration of VZIG in a recipient who did not develop varicella, give another dose of VZIG. Patients receiving monthly infusions of IV immune globulin (IVIG) or who have had chickenpox or varicella vaccine in the past do not require VZIG for later exposure.

Pneumonia   If pneumonia is suspected, obtain a CBC, blood culture, chest radiograph, and either an arterial blood gas or oxygen saturation (pulse oximetry). Obtain a serum LDH to help differentiate PCP from a bacterial process. If the child is over 1 year of age, not in respiratory distress, taking fluids well, and has an arterial oxygen saturation >95% and an x-ray consistent with bacterial pneumonia, treat as an outpatient with cefuroxime (30 mg/kg/day divided bid) for children <5 years old; for a patient >5 years of age, use azithromycin (12 mg/kg/day for 5 days). Schedule a follow-up visit within 24 h, and instruct the guardian to bring the child back to the ED if the condition worsens at any time. If PCP is suspected start TMP-SMX (20 mg/kg/day of TMP divided q 6 h) and prednisone (2–4 mg/kg/day divided q 6 h).

Admit a child with pneumonia who appears ill, is hypoxic, or is under 1 year of age. Treat suspected bacterial pneumonia with IV cefuroxime (100 mg/kg/day divided q 8 h) or ceftriaxone (100 mg/kg/day divided q 12 h). Suspect PCP if the chest x-ray shows a diffuse interstitial pattern or ARDS, the LDH is >500 IU/L, or if the child has an A-a gradient of >30 mmHg. Admit for IV TMP-SMX (20 mg/kg/day of TMP divided q 6 h). Treat patients with profound hypoxia (PO$_2$ <70 mmHg) with steroids. Use prednisone (2 mg/kg/day) or the IV equivalent. Do not delay antibiotic therapy until definitive diagnosis can be made by bronchoalveolar lavage. PCP does not resolve rapidly; clinical improvement within 24 to 48 h suggests a bacterial etiology for the pneumonia.

Consider an atypical organism (*Mycoplasma, Chlamydia, Legionella*) if there is an interstitial pneumonitis without a significant increase in the LDH. Treat with azithromycin (12 mg/kg/day for 5 days).

If an older patient with a history of bronchiectasis presents with an exacerbation of the underlying lung disease (worsening cough and sputum production, fever, persistent rales), give an antipseudomonal antibiotic such as ciprofloxacin (20–30 mg/kg/day divided bid) or levofloxacin (250–500 mg qd for 5–7 days).

Wheezing The treatment of wheezing is the same as for HIV-negative children (see pp 569–575). Discharge a patient who responds well to bronchodilator therapy, has a respiratory rate <40/min, an oxygen saturation >95%, and is taking fluids well. Prescribe the usual medications for asthma, including a short course of prednisone, if it would otherwise be indicated for an immunocompetent child with reactive airway disease. Obtain a chest x-ray if the patient has a temperature greater than 39°C (102.2°F) to help determine whether a pneumonia is present.

A young child less than 1 year of age who presents with wheezing for the first time most likely has bronchiolitis, which can be treated in the usual manner (pp 575–578). However, PCP can present with wheezing, so the patient must have a normal oxygen saturation (>95%) in room air prior to discharge home. Otherwise, obtain a chest x-ray and serum LDH and admit the patient. If PCP is suspected, give TMP-SMX (as above) in addition to bronchodilator therapy, consult a pulmonologist, and arrange for bronchoalveolar lavage to confirm the diagnosis.

Heart Failure Prior to admission, obtain a chest x-ray to assess cardiac size, an ABG or pulse oximetry, electrolytes, and liver function tests (LFTs). Therapy is the same as for an immunocompetent patient (see Congestive Heart Failure, pp 48–50).

Diarrhea The ED treatment of diarrhea is similar to that for immunocompetent patients. Focus on the history of possible exposures, recent infections, the duration and severity of symptoms, and fluid intake. Note the patient's state of hydration, and perform a careful physical examination. Test the stool for blood; also order a stool smear for PMNs, a stool culture, and a test for parasites.

A patient who appears well hydrated and has no blood or PMNs in the stool can be treated symptomatically with dietary management and close follow-up visits. If the child appears well but examination of the stool shows either blood or >5 PMNs per high-power field, treat with oral TMP-SMX (10 mg/kg/day of TMP divided bid) for possible *Salmonella* infection. Treat suspected *Campylobacter* enteritis with a macrolide antibiotic such as erythromycin (40 mg/kg/day divided qid) or clarithromycin (15 mg/kg/day divided bid). If the child attends day care, instruct the caretaker to keep the child at home until the illness resolves and the culture is negative. Arrange for follow-up with the patient's primary care provider. Admit the child with diarrhea who appears ill or dehydrated for IV hydration and antibiotics.

If diarrhea with negative bacterial cultures is unresponsive to dietary therapy, order an examination of the stool for ova and parasites and send a stool sample (not a swab) to test for *Clostridium difficile* toxin. Treat

C. difficile infection with metronidazole (15–35 mg/kg/day divided tid). Do not use oral vancomycin for *C. difficile* owing to the increasing prevalence of vancomycin-resistant enterococci.

Bleeding   If a child presents with evidence of bleeding (e.g., petechiae, bruising, mucosal bleeding), obtain a medication history, perform a careful physical examination, and draw blood for a CBC and prothromin time/partial thromboplastin time (PT/PTT). In patients with HIV-related thrombocytopenia and platelet counts >50,000/mm^3, no intervention is required. When severe bleeding episodes such as intracranial or internal hemorrhage occur, admit the patient for urgent platelet transfusions and supportive therapy. In milder cases of immune thrombocytopenia (platelet count 20,000–50,000/mm^3), treat with IVIG (1–2 g/kg) and consult with an HIV specialist and a pediatric hematologist.

Seizures, Meningismus, Altered Mental Status   Knowledge of the patient's past medical history, current immune function, and medications (especially those for opportunistic infection prophylaxis) may be helpful in excluding certain CNS disorders associated primarily with advanced immunodeficiency (e.g., cryptococcal meningitis, toxoplasmosis, lymphoma, progressive multifocal leukoencephalopathy (PML), and cerebral vasculitis syndromes). Computed tomography or magnetic resonance imaging of the neuraxis may be necessary to demonstrate bleeding, edema, infarction, space-occupying lesions, or other pathology. Although extremely rare in children, if cryptococcal meningitis is suspected, send serum and CSF for cryptococcal antigen determination and ask the lab to perform a CSF India ink test to confirm the diagnosis. In unusual cases or those associated with fastidious or nonculturable pathogens (e.g., JC virus of PML, CMV encephalitis, VZV-associated vasculitis), collect and refrigerate an extra tube of CSF. In these situations the saved CSF can later be analyzed using sophisticated molecular tests such as PCR to aid in making a definitive diagnosis and guiding treatment.

Indications for Admission

- Ill appearance, with or without fever
- Soft tissue infection involving a large area, not well circumscribed, impinging on important structures, or unresponsive to oral antibiotics
- Suspected PCP
- Pneumonia in a child less than 1 year old
- Persistent respiratory distress despite appropriate ED management (tachypnea, oxygen saturation <95% or 5% below patient's baseline, retractions, or flaring)
- Inadequate oral intake
- Varicella or disseminating zoster
- Uncontrolled or excessive bleeding, CNS hemorrhage
- New-onset seizures
- Altered mental status

Universal Precautions

Human immunodeficiency virus has been isolated from all body fluids: blood, semen, and cervical secretions are most often associated with viral transmission. Transmission has not been shown to occur through tears, saliva, urine, stool, sweat, or via casual contact. The risk to health care workers, therefore, comes largely from contact with blood, either from needle-stick injuries or onto abraded skin or mucous membranes. The risk of seroconversion following needle-stick injuries involving blood of infected patients is approximately 1 in 300.

Compliance with the CDC's "universal precautions," which follow, will help prevent transmission of HIV to health care workers in the ED setting:

1. Wear gloves for all procedures that involve touching blood or body fluids, mucous membranes, or nonintact skin.
2. Wash hands immediately after removing gloves or if contaminated by blood or body fluids.
3. Do not recap needles. Dispose of them in puncture-resistant containers, which should be located near all work areas.
4. Minimize the need for mouth-to-mouth resuscitation by keeping ventilation devices available in areas where they are likely to be needed.
5. Wear glasses or goggles and a mask when performing procedures that may cause blood or bodily fluids to splash (e.g., irrigating a wound).

Guidelines for Managing Exposures to Blood and Body Fluids

General Considerations   The efficacy of HIV postexposure prophylaxis (HIV PEP) following sexual assault/abuse, accidental needle-stick injuries, and human bites in nonoccupational settings is unknown and has led to a lack of consensus among public health authorities. Therefore, emergency consultation with a pediatric infectious disease or HIV specialist or an immunologist may be required. In contrast, the management of occupational exposures is clear: after notification of the employee health department, immediate treatment is indicated.

The per-episode risk of infection following sexual exposure is difficult to define, although it is highest with unprotected receptive anal intercourse (0.8–3.2%), followed by receptive vaginal intercourse (0.05–1.5%), and insertive vaginal intercourse (0.03–0.09%). Although no per-contact estimates of risk with insertive anal intercourse or with oral sex have been published, seroconversion as a result of such an exposure has been documented. In comparison, the estimated risk following a percutaneous occupational exposure is 0.32%, and that following sharing of a needle is 0.67%. Therefore accidental needle-stick injuries following exposure to discarded needles, as in parks or alleyways, is likely to carry a small risk for HIV exposure. Other types of exposure among children that carry an unknown but probably minimal risk are bites and sports-related injuries resulting in exposure to blood or blood-tinged secretions.

**Table 14-1   HIV Postexposure Prophylaxis (PEP):
General Considerations**

CONSIDERATION	COMMENTS
Assessment of HIV risk	See Tables 14-2 and 14-3
Timing of HIV PEP	Initiate as soon as possible after exposure; limited efficacy if started past 72 h.
Choice of antiretroviral drugs	Offer a dual-drug regimen comprising zidovudine and lamivudine, or, in certain cases, stavudine and didanosine. Consult with an HIV expert for addition of a protease inhibitor for high-risk exposures. See Table 14-4 for age-specific drug dosages. Duration of PEP: 4 weeks.
Evaluation for HIV PEP toxicity	See Table 14-4 for drug-related side effects/toxicities.
Baseline laboratory testing	HIV serologies, liver function tests, CBC, and pregnancy testing (if indicated).
Psychosocial counseling	Medical social worker or psychiatric nurse familiar with crisis intervention.
Involvements of parents/ legal guardian	The parent or legal guardian must sign informed consent to allow HIV testing of the child (unless the patient is an emancipated minor).
Established follow-up arrangement	Initial follow-up: 24-72 h, in person or by telephone, with a physician comfortable with the use of antiretroviral drugs in children. Assess medication compliance, side effects, and financial barriers. Follow-up visit with physician: within 1 week.
Other considerations	Forensic evidence collection, hepatitis B and C evaluation, PEP for other sexually transmitted diseases, emergency contraception, wound care, assessment of tetanus immunization status.

Adapted from Babl FE, Cooper ER, Damon B, et al: HIV postexposure prophylaxis for children and adolescents. *Am J Emerg Med* 2000;18:282–287.

Recommendations   General considerations and specific elements necessary for a rational and consistent approach to HIV PEP after potential HIV exposure in children and adolescents are outlined in Tables 14-1 through 14-4. The various HIV diagnostic tests are summarized in Table 14-5. In a case involving no to low-risk exposures, reassure the caregiver that the child will not contract HIV infection and that PEP is not necessary. For an individual presenting to the ED 72 h or more after an exposure has occurred, chemoprophylaxis is not indicated except for high-risk exposures. Consult an HIV expert, especially with regard to the selection

Table 14-2 Risk Assessment for Providing Sexual PEP

PEP recommended
1. The HIV exposure is high-risk, specifically:
   a. Unprotected receptive anal or vaginal intercourse.
   b. Unprotected insertive anal or vaginal intercourse.
   c. Unprotected receptive fellatio with ejaculation.
2. The patient's partner is known to be either HIV-infected or in an HIV risk group (homosexual or bisexual male, IV drug user, prostitute).
3. The exposure is isolated or the patient has made a commitment to safer sex in the future. If the unsafe practices are expected to continue, PEP is not indicated.
4. The exposure occurred no more than 72 h earlier.

PEP not recommended
1. After other sexual exposures, including:
   a. Cunnilingus*
   b. Receptive fellatio without ejaculation*

*Except when there are factors that increase the chance of transmission (such as exposure to menstrual blood).

Adapted from Katz MH, Gerberding JL: Care of persons with recent sexual exposure to HIV. *Ann Intern Med* 1998;128:306–312.

of alternative prophylactic drug regimens. If local expertise is not available, advice may be obtained 24 h/day from PEPLine (1-888-HIV-491). These guidelines are subject to modification based upon the epidemiology of HIV in your community, resource availability, and the continued advancement of knowledge in this complex area.

Table 14-3 Risk Assessment for Providing HIV PEP following Accidental Needle-Stick Injuries and Human Bites

Needle-stick injuries
Characteristics of injury
   Penetrates the skin (more than a scratch)
   Large hollow-bore needle
   Visible blood on needle
   Needle placed directly in vein/artery of source

Other factors
   Source patient with known HIV risk factors
   Prevalence of HIV infection among local IV drug users

Human bites
Bite recipient
   Break in the skin
   Presence of bleeding gums or other lesions facilitating admixture of blood and saliva
   Known HIV risk factors in bite inflictor

Bite inflictor
   Exposure to blood of bite wound victim with known HIV risk factors
   Presence of oral/mucosal lesions

Table 14-4   Management Guideline for HIV PEP: Drug Regimens and Pediatric Dosing Directions

AGE/DRUGS	DOSE	FREQ	FORMULATION	INSTRUCTIONS	MAJOR TOXICITIES
<12 years					
Zidovudine (ZDV)	160 mg/m2 (300 mg max)	tid	10-mg/mL syrup 100 mg caps	Take with or without food	Anemia, headaches
Lamivudine (3TC)	4 mg/kg (150 mg max)	bid	10-mg/mL syrup 150 mg tabs	Take with or without food	Headache, rash, abdominal pain, pancreatitis
Nelfinavir (NFV)	40-50 mg/kg	bid	50-mg/scoop powder 250 mg tabs	Take with food	Watery diarrhea
>12 years					
Zidovudine	300 mg	bid	100-mg caps	As above	As above
Lamivudine	150 mg	bid	150-mg tabs	As above	As above
Combivir	One tab	bid	300 mg ZDV + 150 mg Lamivudine	As for ZDV and 3TC (above)	As for ZDV and 3TC (above)
Nelfinavir	1250 mg	bid	250-mg tabs	Take with food	As above

Babl FE, Cooper ER, Damon B, et al: HIV postexposure prophylaxis for children and adolescents. *Am J Emerg Med* 2000;18:282–287.

Table 14-5 Spectrum of Tests for the Diagnosis and Monitoring of HIV-1 Infection

ASSAY	OTHER NAMES	COMMENTS
Routine serology	HIV antibody test HIV serologies HIV enzyme Immunoassay (EIA) Western blot (WB)	Gold-standard for diagnosis of HIV infection Readily available and inexpensive Informed consent required If EIA is positive, must confirm with WB Seroconversion detectable 6–12 weeks following infection 95% of infected patients seropositive by 6 months Serology not useful in HIV-exposed infant <18 months old
OraSure Test System	Salivary test Saliva HIV test HIV spit test	Salivary collection device to collect IgG for EIA and WB Sensitivity/specificity comparable to standard blood tests
Calypte 1	Urine HIV test Urine test	EIA test to detect HIV antibodies in urine Must be administered by physician Positive result must be verified by serology
DNA PCR	DNA PCR test Virus DNA test Virus test	Used to detect cell-associated proviral DNA Requires confirmation Test of choice for diagnosis of neonatal HIV infection Usually positive by 2–4 weeks of age
Quantitative HIV-RNA	Viral load HIV RNA-PCR (Roche) bDNA assay (Chiron) NASBA (Organon)	Quantification of plasma viral RNA using reverse transcription and amplification by PCR Results reported as copies per milliliter Dynamic range varies according to assay used Can measure between 20–10,000,000 copies per milliliter Used to monitor response to antiretroviral therapy Not FDA-approved for diagnosis of established HIV infection Acute HIV infection associated with high viral loads and lack of HIV antibodies (window period) Consider this test in settings of recent, high-risk HIV exposure, especially in adolescents presenting with mononucleosis-like syndrome
CD4 cell count	T-cell count T-cell subsets T helper-cell count CD4+ T-cell count	Number of CD4+ T lymphocytes circulating in blood These cells are depleted during course of HIV infection Marker of host's current immune status Presented as percentage or absolute number of CD4+ cells: >25% considered normal in children; <15% indicates profound immunosuppression

REFERENCES

Abrams EJ: Opportunistic infection and other clinical manifestations of HIV disease in children. *Pediatr Clin North Am* 2000;47:79–108.

Babl FE, Cooper ER, Damon B, et al: HIV postexposure prophylaxis for children and adolescents *Am J Emerg Med* 2000;18:282–287.

Bartlett JG, Gallant JG: *Medical Management of HIV Infection.* Baltimore: Port City Press, 2000.

Katz MH, Gerberding JL: Care of persons with recent sexual exposure to HIV. *Ann Intern Med* 1998;128:306–312.

Laufer M, Scott GB: Medical management of HIV disease in children. *Pediatr Clin North Am* 2000;47:127–153.

INFECTIOUS MONONUCLEOSIS

Infectious mononucleosis (IM) is a clinical syndrome consisting of prolonged fever, pharyngitis, and lymphadenopathy. EBV causes most (80–90%) cases of IM. Other conditions and infections that produce a mononucleosis-like syndrome include CMV, human herpesvirus 6, HIV, adenovirus, *Toxoplasma gondii*, *Corynebacterium diphtheriae*, hepatitis A, influenzae A and B, rubella, *Coxiella burnetii*, malignancies (lymphoma, leukemia), and medications (phenytoin, sulfa).

EBV is a ubiquitous herpesvirus that replicates in epithelial cells and B lymphocytes. It infects children and young adults primarily. By adulthood, 90% of people worldwide have serologic evidence of prior EBV infection. The incidence is 30 times higher in whites than in African Americans, with no known gender differences. There is no obvious seasonal pattern of EBV infection.

Transmission occurs primarily through exposure to oropharyngeal secretions, although transmission via blood products has also been reported. Although the virus has been found in cervical mucosa and semen, sexual transmission has not been demonstrated. The virus infects the oral epithelial cells and spreads to B lymphocytes, triggering a massive, self-limited immunologic response. The infection stimulates the production of antibodies against EBV antigens as well as unrelated antigens (heterophile antibodies). EBV remains in the body for life.

Clinical Presentation

Clinical manifestations of IM are influenced by age. After an incubation period that can range from 30 to 50 days, a young child (<4 years old) is usually asymptomatic or has mild, nonspecific symptoms, such as a URI, tonsillopharyngitis (without exudate), or a prolonged febrile illness with or without lymphadenopathy. This age group has a higher frequency of organomegaly. An older child is more likely to develop the classic triad of fever, sore throat, and lymphadenopathy. The patient may have a prodromal illness consisting of 1 to 2 days of malaise, anorexia, fatigue, headache, and high fever (40°C, 104°F). In contrast, there may be the abrupt onset of focal symptoms. Pharyngitis is often most severe in the first 3 to 5 days, and 30% of patients have exudative pharyngitis. There may also be palatal petechiae.

An enlarged spleen is palpated in 17% of patients, but splenomegaly has been noted on ultrasound in 100% of patients. Bilateral, nontender, posterior and anterior cervical lymphadenopathy often occurs. Less common clinical features include upper airway compromise, abdominal pain, hepatomegaly, jaundice, and periorbital edema.

Rash occurs in 5% and may be macular, petechial, scarlatiniform, urticarial, or similar to erythema multiforme. In 90 to 100% of patients, a nonallergic pruritic rash develops after receiving ampicillin, 7 to 10 days after the first dose.

The duration of illness is variable. Symptoms peak at 7 days after onset and dissipate over the next 1 to 3 weeks. The fever can last 1 to 2 weeks; splenomegaly usually resolves within 4 weeks of the onset of symptoms, but the fatigue often persists.

Complications include thrombocytopenia (25–50%), upper airway obstruction (<5%), hemolytic anemia (3%), and splenic rupture (<0.5%). Neurologic complications occur in 1 to 5% of cases, including meningoencephalitis, Guillain-Barré syndrome, transverse myelitis, encephalitis, and cranial nerve palsies. An "Alice in Wonderland" syndrome, characterized by metamorphopsia (distortion of sizes, shapes, and spatial relations of objects), has been reported.

Diagnosis

Although the diagnosis of IM is clinical, laboratory testing is useful for confirming the diagnosis, especially when the presentation is atypical. Specifically, the diagnosis is proven if there is a lymphocytosis (≥50%) with 10% or more atypical forms or a positive heterophile titer or Monospot test. The percentage of patients with acute EBV infection who have heterophile antibodies increases relative to the time since onset of symptoms but may be negative in up to 50% of patients <4 years old. EBV titers are indicated for a patient with an atypical presentation or negative heterophile antibody test or who is severely ill or immunocompromised. In such a case, obtain serum for viral capsid antigen (VCA) IgG and IgM and for EBV nuclear antigen (EBNA) IgG.

Other laboratory abnormalities associated with IM include a two- to threefold increase in transaminase levels (90% of cases) and abnormalities on urinalysis, including proteinuria, pyuria, and microscopic hematuria.

ED Management

Treatment for IM is supportive. Obtain a throat culture to rule out *Streptococcus* and treat, if positive (pp 143–146). Encourage rest and fluids and recommend acetaminophen (15 mg/kg q 4 h) or ibuprofen (10 mg/kg q 6 h), for symptomatic relief from sore throat or headache.

Admit a patient with significant upper airway obstruction (stridor). Continuously monitor the oxygen saturation and treat with elevation of the head of the bed, IV hydration, humidified air, and systemic corticosteroids (prednisone 2 mg/kg/day divided bid, 60 mg/day maximum). However, steroids have not been proven to provide significant or reproducible benefit for lymphadenopathy or hepatosplenic involvement. More than half of all splenic ruptures occur in patients without a palpable spleen. Therefore advise the patient not to participate in contact sports or strenuous activities for approximately 4 weeks.

Follow-up

- Primary care follow-up in 2 to 4 weeks. Instruct the family to return immediately for stridor or inability to swallow (persistent drooling).

Indications for Admission

- Upper airway obstruction
- Inability to take adequate oral fluids
- Neurologic complication

BIBLIOGRAPHY

Hickey SM, Strasburger VC: What every pediatrician should know about infectious mononucleosis in adolescents. *Pediatr Clin North Am* 1997;44:1541–1556.
Jenson HB: Acute complications of Epstein-Barr virus infectious mononucleosis. *Curr Opin Pediatr* 2000;12: 263–288.
Peter J, Ray G: Infectious mononucleosis. *Pediatr Rev* 1998;19:276–279.

INFECTIOUS DISEASE ASSOCIATED WITH EXANTHEMS

Illnesses with cutaneous manifestations are caused by a variety of agents, including viruses, *chlamydiae, rickettsiae, mycoplasma,* bacteria, fungi, and protozoa. Today, enteroviruses are the leading cause of exanthematous diseases. Although most exanthematous illnesses are benign, the differential diagnosis is important because the early signs of potentially fatal bacterial and rickettsial diseases frequently involve the skin.

Clinical Manifestations

Nonspecific Viral Exanthems   The most common etiologies of nonspecific viral exanthems are enteroviruses (coxsackieviruses, echovirus, enterovirus) and respiratory viruses (adenovirus, rhinovirus, parainfluenza virus, respiratory syncytial virus, influenza virus). Most summertime exanthems are due to enteroviruses, while the respiratory viruses predominate during the colder months. The typical nonspecific viral exanthem presents as blanching, erythematous macules and papules distributed diffusely on the trunk and extremities, with occasional facial involvement. Associated symptoms can include fever, headache, upper respiratory tract or GI symptoms, myalgias, and fatigue.

Coxsackie A4 virus causes fever and herpangina (1- to 5-mm vesicles and ulcers of the posterior pharynx). An erythematous maculopapular exanthem can develop after the patient defervesces. In some patients, the lesions become vesicular, spread to the extremities, and regress to a brownish discoloration in 1 to 2 weeks. Fever and an erythematous rash that starts on the face and neck, then spreads to the trunk and extremities, characterize *Coxsackie A9* virus infection. There may be an associated aseptic meningitis. *Coxsackie A16* virus causes hand-foot-mouth syndrome, which presents with a mild fever, anorexia, malaise, and a sore mouth, followed by a vesicular eruption on the hands and/or feet associated with herpangina-like intraoral lesions. The rash associated with *coxsackie B5* virus is usually maculopapular, but it can be petechial at times. Rarely, there may be concomitant aseptic meningitis or myocarditis.

Echovirus 9 and *enterovirus 71* cause a nonspecific febrile illness, which can be associated with aseptic meningitis. The rash of echovirus 9 is usually rubelliform or petechial, whereas the rash associated with enterovirus 71 varies from erythematous maculopapular to vesicular.

Measles (Rubeola)   Although vaccination has greatly reduced the incidence of measles in the United States, outbreaks continue to occur, primarily during the winter and spring. Measles is spread by direct contact with infectious droplets or by airborne spread, with a subsequent incubation period of 8 to 12 days. Measles classically presents with the "three C's": cough, coryza, and conjunctivitis, usually associated with a high fever (up to 40°C, 104°F). During the prodrome, pathognomonic Koplik's spots appear. They are small (1-2 mm) white spots with a red background on the buccal mucosa. Koplik's spots usually disappear within 48 h of the onset of exanthem, which typically appears on the fourth day of the illness. Nonpruritic erythematous macules and papules appear first on the face and spread to the trunk and extremities. The rash fades in the same order as it appeared. Complications include pneumonia, otitis, bronchitis, encephalitis, and myocarditis.

Two other types of measles are now recognized, modified measles and atypical measles. Modified measles occurs in a partially immunized patient, presenting with a shorter prodrome, a less severe rash, and the possible absence of Koplik's spots. Atypical measles has been reported rarely among patients who received the live attenuated vaccine. Atypical measles presents with abrupt onset of high fever, myalgias, and cough. In contrast to typical measles, the rash begins on the extremities 2 to 5 days later and spreads centrally. Lobar pneumonia is frequently present.

Erythema Infectiosum   Also known as fifth disease, this viremia is caused by parvovirus B19. It is most common in the spring, primarily affecting 4- to 10-year-olds. Transmission is by respiratory droplets, followed by an incubation period of 6 to 14 days. Some patients have a mild prodrome of headache, low-grade fever, malaise, pharyngitis, joint pain, and GI symptoms before the onset of the rash. The eruption begins with the sudden appearance of "slapped cheeks" (erythematous patches on the cheeks). It then progresses to the trunk and extremities, where it appears as erythematous macules and papules, before developing into a lacy reticular pattern. Arthralgia and arthritis can be present in 10% of patients. Parvovirus can suppress the bone marrow, so that patients with shortened red blood cell life spans (sickle cell disease, thalassemia, hereditary spherocytosis, pyruvate kinase deficiency) are at risk for a transient aplastic crisis. Parvovirus infection during pregnancy can cause fetal hydrops and death.

Roseola Infantum   Roseola, thought to be caused by human herpesvirus-6, is transmitted by respiratory droplets. It affects children between 6 months and 2 years of age, with a peak incidence at 6 to 7 months. It is generally a self-limited, benign illness characterized by 3 to 5 days of high fever (39–40.5°C, 102.2–104.9°F), which peaks in the evening. Other symptoms are rare but can include mild respiratory symptoms, irritability, and malaise. The fever ends abruptly, followed by the rash within

24 to 48 h. The eruption is characterized by pink, blanching, discrete macules and papules over the trunk. The rash is rarely pruritic and usually fades over 1 to 2 days.

Rubella   Prior to the rubella vaccine, the peak incidence of infection was in children 5 to 14 years of age, but the disease is now seen in nonimmune older children and adults. After a 14- to 21-day incubation period, rubella presents with an upper respiratory infection. The rash of rubella is variable, beginning on the face and then spreading to other areas. It starts as maculopapules, which may become pinpoint papules, similar to those seen in scarlet fever. Mild pruritus may be present and resolution usually occurs within 72 h. Rose-colored macules may develop on the soft palate immediately preceding the rash, and the patient may have tender retroauricular, posterior cervical, and occipital lymphadenopathy. The patient will shed virus for 7 days prior to and after the rash. Rubella can cause a severe fetal infection if a susceptible pregnant woman is exposed.

Varicella (Chickenpox)   Once an exceedingly common childhood disease, varicella is now seen much less frequently as a result of the vaccination. It is a highly contagious disease with an incubation period of 11 to 21 days. The patient presents with fever, malaise, headache, anorexia, and abdominal pain. After 24 to 48 h, an intensely pruritic rash appears on the face, scalp, or trunk and spreads peripherally. It begins as erythematous macules, which evolve into papules and then vesicles containing serous fluid ("dew drop on a rose petal"). The vesicles spontaneously rupture and develop into crusts before resolving. Subsequent crops of lesions develop over 4 to 6 days, so that the presence of lesions in different stages is characteristic of varicella. The patient is infectious from the beginning of the prodromal illness (about 2 days before the rash erupts) until each pox has a crust, about 7 to 10 days. Complications include bacterial superinfection of the skin (which may rarely progress to necrotizing fasciitis), pneumonia, thrombocytopenia, arthritis, hepatitis, cerebellar ataxia, encephalitis, meningitis, and glomerulonephritis. The virus establishes latency in the dorsal root ganglia during primary infection, and reactivation results in herpes zoster (shingles).

Herpes Zoster   Herpes zoster is caused by reactivation of the varicella virus. Pain and tenderness along a dermatome precede the eruption of classic chickenpox lesions clustered within one to three continuous dermatomes. The pain, tenderness, as well as localized lymphadenopathy persist as long as the skin lesions are present (1–2 weeks).

Herpes Simplex   Primary HSV gingivostomatitis (pp 72–76) causes fever, irritability, and lesions involving the gingival and mucous membranes of the mouth. Genital herpes, characterized by vesicular lesions, is most common in adolescents. Consider sexual abuse if genital herpes is seen in a prepubertal child. Reactivation of the latent virus causes "cold sores," single or grouped vesicles in the perioral region but not inside the mouth, or as lesions on the external genitalia. Neonatal HSV can present as a focal or systemic infection (p 104), appearing at any time from the day of birth until 4 to 6 weeks of life.

Meningococcemia (Neisseria meningitides)   is a gram-negative diplococcus that is carried in the upper respiratory tract in up to 25% of adolescents. Disease occurs more commonly in the winter and early spring, and the majority of cases are seen in children <2 years of age. The disease can progress extremely rapidly, presenting with a range of severity from self-resolving bacteremia to meningitis to septic shock and coma. The rash usually presents with nonblanching petechiae and purpura, classically described as asymmetric gunmetal gray palpable purpura of the extremities. However, maculopapular, bullous, and pustular lesions can also occur.

Scarlet Fever   Scarlet fever is caused by group A beta-hemolytic streptococci. After an incubation period of 1 to 7 days, the illness presents with fever, vomiting, headache, and pharyngitis. The tonsils are hyperemic and edematous and may be covered with exudates; there may be palatal petechiae; and the tongue may have a strawberry appearance. The rash is usually erythematous, punctate, or finely papular, with the texture of sandpaper. It appears in the axillae, groin, and neck first and generalizes within 24 h. Accentuation in the flexion creases (Pastia's lines) and circumoral pallor are common. Desquamation begins on the face at the end of the first week and proceeds over the trunk and then to the hands and feet.

Diagnosis

Determination of exposure, season, and knowledge of incubation period are important in diagnosing patients with a rash. Inquire about exposure to a similar illness as well as immunization and medication histories. The appearance, progression, and distribution of the rash can be very helpful, as can the time elapsed between the exposure and the current illness.

The age of the child and season of the year can provide useful clues in determining the diagnosis. Certain diseases occur more commonly in particular age groups. Roseola infantum occurs primarily in 6 to 36 month-olds, erythema infectiosum in 2- to 12-year-olds, and scarlet fever in school-age children. Some diseases have seasonal predilection, such as scarlet fever, which tends to be seen in the late winter and early spring, and enteroviruses, which appear most often during the summer and fall.

The time elapsed between the onset of fever and the appearance of the rash provides an important clue to the diagnosis. The rash in rubella occurs simultaneously with the fever. A patient with scarlet fever is generally febrile for 12 to 24 h prior to the onset of the rash, while a patient with roseola has 3 to 5 days of fever and then defervesces prior to the onset of the rash. While these relationships are not absolute, they represent the norm and are therefore valuable adjuncts in determining the diagnosis.

The appearance, progression, and distribution of the rash can also be very helpful in determining the diagnosis. Maculopapular rashes are the most common and are usually associated with enteroviral infections. Vesicular exanthems present either as single or localized lesions (herpes simplex, herpes zoster), generalized lesions (varicella), or in a peripheral distribution (hand-foot-mouth disease).

Pertinent physical findings include the patient's appearance and the presence of regional or generalized lymphadenopathy, conjunctivitis, hepatomegaly, or GI involvement. Children who are very ill-appearing may have meningococcemia, Rocky Mountain spotted fever, Kawasaki disease, or measles.

Adenopathy is particularly important in considering the diagnosis of rubella (postauricular and suboccipital adenopathy) and infectious mononucleosis (generalized with hepatosplenomegaly). Koplik's spots on the buccal mucosa can confirm measles prior to the appearance of the exanthem in a febrile child.

The differential diagnosis of these diseases includes many of the infectious illnesses with fever and rash. The first phase of erythema infectiosum resembles scarlet fever, but the patient appears well and there is no evidence of streptococcal infection. Infection may be confirmed, if necessary, by serum B19–specific antibody. A roseola-like illness has been ascribed to an enterovirus. Many children with the prodromal fever of roseola are given antibiotics, so the rash is occasionally diagnosed as a *drug allergy* or *amoxicillin rash*.

Measles can be confused with scarlet fever (cough and coryza absent), Kawasaki disease (stomatitis, rash does not spread down the body), and rubella (shorter prodrome and rash duration, patient appears much less sick). In none of these are Koplik's spots seen. The diagnosis can be confirmed by viral isolation from nasopharyngeal secretions, conjunctiva, blood, and urine during the febrile phase or by comparing paired acute and convalescent sera. Some laboratories can detect measles-specific IgM antibody with a single serum sample. The diagnosis of rubella can be confirmed by IgM-specific antibody or virus isolated from nasal secretions, throat swab, blood, urine, or CSF.

Varicella has a typical appearance. However, mild eruptions can be confused with *bullous impetigo* and *insect bites*, although these lesions do not erupt in crops or go through a series of stages. Zoster may resemble a *contact dermatitis* in which pruritus is more common than pain.

The rash of meningococcemia can be confused with that of other causes of *bacterial sepsis, viral infections, idiopathic thrombocytopenic purpura*, and *Rocky Mountain spotted fever*. Unroofing a skin lesion and Gram's staining the contents may reveal the pathognomonic gram-negative intracellular diplococci. The diagnosis is confirmed by a positive blood culture.

If diagnostic confirmation of an enterovirus is needed, the organism can be isolated from the throat and rectum. PCR may be available for the identification of virus in serum.

ED Management

There is no specific treatment for many of these diseases. Therapy consists largely of reassurance and supportive care. Treat fever with acetaminophen (15 mg/kg q 4 h) or ibuprophen (10 mg/kg q 6 h). Assess the hydration status and give intravenous fluids when appropriate. Generally, blood tests and cultures are not necessary unless the patient appears seriously ill.

Measles   Treatment is supportive. Admit a patient with pneumonia (for antibiotic therapy), and perform a lumbar puncture if the child presents with lethargy, excessive irritability, or nuchal rigidity. Notify public health officials of any suspected case of measles so that appropriate community measures can be instituted. Vitamin A decreases the morbidity and mortality of measles in children with vitamin A deficiency; give vitamin A (50,000 U/day) to children 6 months to 2 years of age who are hospitalized with complications of measles.

Rubella   Treatment is supportive. If rubella is suspected, refer pregnant contacts to their obstetricians immediately for titers.

Varicella   Treat pruritus with antihistamines (diphenhydramine 5 mg/kg/day divided qid or hydroxyzine 2 mg/kg/day divided tid) and oatmeal baths. Do not use aspirin because it is associated with an increased risk of Reye's syndrome. Oral acyclovir is not routinely recommended in otherwise healthy children with varicella. Possible indications include an exposed patient >12 years of age who does not have a history of varicella, a child with chronic cutaneous or pulmonary disorders, a patient receiving long-term salicylate therapy, and a patient receiving glucocorticoids, including short, intermittent, or aerosolized courses. Give 80 mg/kg/day divided qid for 5 days (3200 mg/day maximum).

Give postexposure immunization to a susceptible patient within 72 h and possibly up to 120 h after varicella exposure. A newborn whose mother develops varicella within 5 days before delivery or up to 48 h after delivery, a patient with varicella pneumonia, or an immunocompromised patient with zoster has a serious risk of overwhelming infection. Admit these patients and consult with an infectious disease specialist regarding antiviral therapy.

VZIG is recommended if significant exposure (5 to 60 min of face-to-face play, residing in the same household) occurs in an immunocompromised patient who does not have a history of chickenpox, susceptible pregnant women, and newborns whose mothers develop chickenpox within 5 days before to 48 h after delivery. Give VZIG, 1 vial (125 U) IM for each 10 kg of body weight (5 vials maximum, 1 vial minimum) within 96 h of exposure (preferably within 48 h).

If a patient with varicella is hospitalized, implement airborne and contact precautions for a minimum of 5 days after the onset of the rash and as long as the rash remains vesicular.

Herpes Zoster   Treatment is supportive and includes analgesia for these painful lesions [ibuprofen, 10 mg/kg per dose or acetaminophen with codeine, (1 mg/kg per dose)]. Consult with a pediatric infectious disease specialist to determine the need for therapy.

Herpes Simplex   The treatment of primary and recurrent herpes is summarized on pp 72–73. Consult an ophthalmologist if there is ocular involvement (p 496). Treat suspected neonatal HSV infection with IV acyclovir (60 mg/kg/day divided tid for 21 days).

Meningococcemia   If meningococcemia is suspected, immediately obtain a blood culture and initiate antibiotic therapy with IV cefotaxime (200 mg/kg/day divided q 6 h) or ceftriaxone (100 mg/kg/day divided q 12 h). Perform a lumbar puncture if there are meningeal signs or consciousness is altered (see Meningitis, pp 366–369). If meningococcemia is confirmed, treat with IV penicillin (250,000 U/kg/day in 6 divided doses) or cefotaxime. Give prophylactic rifampin (10 mg/kg bid, 600 mg maximum, for 2 days), IM ceftriaxone (<12 years: 125 mg; >12 years: 250 mg), or ciprofloxacin (500 mg once) to household, day care, and nursery school contacts, persons having direct contact with the patient's secretions (kissing, shared toothbrush, eating utensils), and any medical provider who has had close contact with the patient's secretions (unprotected mouth-to-mouth resuscitation, intubation, suctioning).

Scarlet Fever   The treatment is the same as for streptococcal pharyngitis (p 145).

Follow-up

- Possibly susceptible pregnant patient in the third trimester exposed to varicella: obstetrical follow-up immediately
- Possibly susceptible pregnant patient in the first trimester exposed to rubella or parvovirus: obstetrical follow-up within 2 to 3 days
- Herpes zoster: 2 to 3 days

Indications for Admission

- Measles pneumonia or encephalitis
- Varicella or suspected HSV in immunocompromised patients and newborns
- Suspected meningococcemia
- Dehydration requiring IV fluid therapy
- Respiratory distress

BIBLIOGRAPHY

Cherry JD: Cutaneous manifestations of systemic infections, in Feigin RD, Cherry JD (eds): *Textbook of Pediatric Infectious Diseases,* 4th ed. Philadelphia: Saunders, 1998, pp 713–735.

Committee on Infectious Disease: *2000 Red Book: Report of the Committee on Infectious Disease,* 25th ed. Elk Grove Village, IL: American Academy of Pediatrics, 2000.

Gable EK, Liu G, Morrell DS: Pediatric exanthems. *Primary Care* 2000;27:353–369.

Mancini AJ: Exanthems in childhood: an update. *Pediatr Ann* 1998;27:163–170.

KAWASAKI SYNDROME

Kawasaki syndrome (KS) is an acute, self-limited, multiorgan vasculitis. It predominately affects young children, with a peak incidence between 6 and 12 months of age. More than 50% of patients are younger than 2 years and 80% are younger than 4 years; KS rarely occurs in children older than 8 years or younger than 3 months. In the United States an estimated 3000 children are hospitalized each year with KS. The etiology of KS is unknown, but it is believed to be due to an infectious agent, with immune system activation playing a role in its pathogenesis. Epidemics may last from 2 to 5 months.

Clinical Presentation

There are three distinct stages of the illness. The acute stage (days 1 to 10) is characterized by an abrupt onset of high fever, typically over 40°C (104°F), without prodrome, for at least 5 days. The fever persists for a mean of 12 days if untreated. Within 2 to 5 days of the onset of fever, the patient develops other characteristic features of the illness including at least four of the following five:

- Conjunctival injection without exudate
- Erythema of the mouth and pharynx, a strawberry tongue, and cracked, red lips
- Erythematous rash of almost any pattern
- Induration of the hands and feet with erythematous palms and soles
- Isolated, unilateral cervical lymphadenopathy (>1.5 cm), typically seen on the first day of fever

Cardiac manifestations in the first stage may include tachycardia (60%), myocarditis with associated pericardial effusion (30%), and electrocardiographic (ECG) changes such as prolongation of the PR interval (first-degree heart block).

In the subacute stage (days 11 to 24), the fever, rash, and lymphadenopathy resolve. Periungual and perineal desquamation occur during the second to third weeks of the illness. Patients may remain irritable and anoretic after defervescence. Cardiac complications, including coronary artery aneurysms, coronary obstruction and thrombosis, and myocardial and endocardial inflammation occur in as many as 20 to 25% of untreated patients. Males and infants are at highest risk.

In the final stage (after day 24) there is resolution of the external findings. The cardiovascular complications either improve or progress to myocardial infarction or chronic myocardial ischemia.

Other clinical features of KS include arthralgias and arthritis, involving the small joints during the acute phase and later the large, weight-bearing joints. Myringitis, urethritis with sterile pyuria, aseptic meningitis, uveitis and, rarely, hydrops of the gallbladder may be present. Other features include diarrhea, vomiting, abdominal pain, cranial nerve palsies, and thrombosis.

Atypical presentations of KS occur, especially among young infants. Patients may have fever and fewer than four of the principal diagnostic features. Detection of coronary artery abnormalities by echocardiography is diagnostic.

Cardiac sequelae are not uncommon in KS, especially in males under 6 months of age. Myocardial infarction and subsequent heart failure are the most likely clinical sequelae from previous KS. Young children with an MI present with shock, vomiting, and excessive or "hard" crying, rather than chest pain.

Laboratory abnormalities, which persist for 6 to 10 weeks, include leukocytosis with a predominance of neutrophils, anemia, thrombocytosis, elevated liver transaminases, and increased bilirubin and alkaline phosphatase. Additionally there may be elevated levels of acute-phase reactants such as ESR, C-reactive protein (CRP), and serum alpha$_1$ antitrypsin.

Diagnosis

KS is diagnosed if a patient has fever for >5 days in association with four of the five other major manifestations. Consider KS likely if the patient has fever and three of these features. Obtain a CBC with differential, platelet count, ESR or CRP, blood culture, urinalysis, throat culture, chest radiograph, and ECG.

The differential diagnosis of KS includes staphylococcal or streptococcal *toxic shock syndrome* (hypotension, renal involvement with elevated BUN and creatinine), *rheumatic fever, scarlet fever* (pharyngitis, Pastia's lines, no conjunctivitis), *staphylococcal scalded skin syndrome* (desquamation early with positive Nikolsky's sign), *Rocky Mountain spotted fever* (petechial and purpuric rash, no enanthem), and *leptospirosis* (icterus, proteinuria). It also includes *viral illnesses* (less sick-appearing, no or dissimilar extremity involvement) such as *measles* (Koplik's spots, different progression of exanthem), *influenza,* and *EBV* and *adenovirus* infections. Noninfectious diseases include *Stevens-Johnson syndrome, erythema multiforme, adverse drug reactions* (use of presumptive agent), and *juvenile rheumatoid arthritis.*

ED Management

Management in the acute phase is aimed at reducing inflammation in the myocardium and coronary artery wall and at preventing thrombosis. Give aspirin (80–100 mg/kg/day divided qid) plus high-dose IV immunoglobulin (2 g/kg IVSS over 10–12 h). Admit the patient because of the high rate of cardiac complications during the subacute stage and consult a pediatric cardiologist.

Indication for Admission

- Suspected Kawasaki syndrome

BIBLIOGRAPHY

Leung DY, Meissner HC: The many faces of Kawasaki syndrome. *Hosp Pract (Off Ed)* 2000;35:77-81, 85–86, 91–94.

Rowley AH: Controversies in Kawasaki syndrome. *Adv Pediatr Infect Dis* 1998; 13:127–141.

Rowley AH, Shulman ST: Kawasaki syndrome. *Pediatr Clin North Am* 1999;46: 321–329.

LYME DISEASE

Lyme disease, caused by the spirochete *Borrelia burgdorferi,* is the most common vector-borne illness in the United States. The *Ixodes* (deer) tick is the most important vector. The 2-year life cycle of the tick includes larval, nymph, and adult forms. The tiny nymphs are most prevalent in the spring and summer and feed on white-footed mice, while white-tailed deer are the preferred hosts of mature ticks, which feed throughout the fall, winter, and early spring. Both nymphs and mature ticks may attach to humans and transmit the spirochete.

Although cases have been reported from all parts of the country, the Northeast, mid-Atlantic states, northern Midwest, and Pacific Northwest are endemic areas. In the East and Midwest, the majority of infections are acquired between May and August; in the West, between January and May. However, infection may occur from early spring to late fall in endemic areas.

Clinical Presentation

The disease is categorized into two stages: early and late infection (see Table 14-6). Early Lyme disease is further subdivided into localized or disseminated disease. Early localized infection is characterized by erythema migrans (EM), which is found in over 90% of cases of pediatric Lyme disease. It is a distinctive skin lesion that usually appears between 2 and 32 days after a tick bite as an erythematous macule at the site of the bite that enlarges to >5 cm over several days to weeks. Most often, as the lesion evolves, there is central clearing, so that it resembles a ring or target. EM is usually asymptomatic, although pruritus, tenderness, or warmth can occur. If left untreated, it will resolve spontaneously over

Table 14-6 Signs and Symptoms of Lyme Disease

	EARLY LOCALIZED	EARLY DISSEMINATED	LATE
Skin	Erythema migrans (1 lesion)	±Multiple erythema migrans lesions	Acrodermatitis chronica atrophicans
Lymph-adenopathy		Regional or generalized adenopathy	
Musculo-skeletal	±Arthralgias, ±Myalgias	Arthralgias Oligo-/polyarthritis Migratory polyarthritis	Chronic/ recurrent arthritis
Neurologic		Meningitis Seventh nerve palsy Radiculopathy Peripheral neuropathy	Chronic encephalo-myelitis Peripheral neuropathy
Cardiac		Myo- or pericarditis AV block	
Constitutional symptoms	±Fever, ±Malaise	Fever, malaise, fatigue	Chronic fatigue

several weeks. However it is not a transient rash that will disappear within hours or a few days.

The onset of early disseminated infection is several weeks to months after the tick bite. Manifestations include multiple lesions of EM, fever, headache, myalgias, arthralgias, arthritis, meningitis, cranial nerve palsy, or acute radiculopathy. GI and respiratory symptoms are rare. Acute arthritis is usually monarticular, most often involving large joints, especially the knee. The typical "Lyme knee" is swollen and tender, but erythema and warmth are notably absent. Migratory arthritis and polyarthritis may also occur. Twenty percent of patients have neurologic involvement, including meningoencephalitis, seventh nerve palsy, and peripheral radiculoneuropathy. Cardiac manifestations, such as AV block, myocarditis, and pericarditis, are seen in up to 10% of patients. Conjunctivitis, hepatitis, nonexudative pharyngitis, microscopic hematuria, and proteinuria can also occur.

Late Lyme disease, characterized by persistent or relapsing symptoms, is relatively uncommon in children. Chronic and recurrent episodes of arthritis and chronic encephalomyelitis occur most frequently. The cutaneous manifestation, acrodermatitis chronica atrophicans, is seen far more commonly in Europe than in North America. It is a progressive lesion, presenting with hyperpigmentation and swelling, followed by hypopigmentation and atrophy of the skin on an extremity. In addition, during the late Lyme period, many patients will complain for months, even after treatment, about recurrent arthralgias, headaches, and malaise. However, these symptoms do not reflect active disease but rather a self-limited immune response. Prolonged or repeated antibiotic courses are not necessary to treat these symptoms.

Diagnosis

A history of a tick bite or travel to an endemic area is helpful, but absence of this information does not eliminate the possibility of Lyme disease.

EM can resemble an *insect bite reaction, nummular eczema, tinea corporis, cellulitis,* and, rarely, *erythema marginatum* or *erythema multiforme.* However, EM is typically asymptomatic and macular without scaling, and it enlarges over days or weeks into a ringlike lesion (see Table 5-4, Differential Diagnosis of Annular Lesions).

The generalized systemic symptoms may also occur in *influenza* and *enteroviral* infections, and *acute* and *chronic EBV* infection. *Viral syndromes* are far more likely to cause vomiting, diarrhea, and hepatosplenomegaly. In endemic areas, consider Lyme disease for all patients with flu-like illnesses occurring outside flu season.

Septic arthritis, trauma, transient synovitis, and rheumatologic diseases *(ARF, JRA, SLE, Crohn's disease)* can all resemble Lyme disease. Acute joint swelling with fever always raises the concern of septic arthritis, which presents with a hot, red, tender joint. With Lyme arthritis, however, although the joint may be swollen and tender, warmth and erythema are absent.

Ehrlichiosis (pp 377–380) is a relatively uncommon tick-borne illness caused by an organism that can also be transmitted by *Ixodes* ticks. It presents with an abrupt flu-like syndrome (fever, headache, myalgias), similar to early Lyme disease. In addition, there may be anorexia, nausea, abdominal pain, vomiting, and acute weight loss. About 1 week into the illness, a maculopapular or petechial rash develops on the extremities, but the palms and soles are usually spared. Thrombocytopenia, along with leukopenia and elevation of liver transaminases, is often present. Coinfection with *B. burgdorferi* may occur.

Also consider Lyme disease in the differential diagnosis of *Bell's palsy* (pp 453–455). CSF changes in Lyme meningitis are similar to the findings in *viral meningitis* (pleocytosis with normal glucose and mild protein elevation), though the pleocytosis found with Lyme is less marked (CSF WBCs <100/mm^3).

The diagnosis can be confirmed with positive antibody titers in the serum, CSF, or joint fluid. Current recommendations for serologic testing involve the use of a sensitive enzyme immunoassay (EIA) or immunofluorescent assay (IFA) in association with a Western immunoblot. When a patient is being tested early in the disease (less than 4 weeks duration of symptoms), obtain IgM and IgG tests. False-negative test results can occur if the specimen is obtained too early in the course of the disease or if the antibody rise has been blunted by antibiotic therapy. If initial testing is negative but early Lyme disease is strongly suspected, repeat the testing in 2 to 4 weeks. Confirm all positive or borderline results of EIA and IFA testing by Western immunoblot. Consider IgM Western immunoblot positive if two of the following three bands are present: 24, 39, and 41 KD; IgG Western blot is positive if 5 of the following 10 bands are present: 18, 21, 28, 30, 39, 41, 45, 58, 66, and 93 KD. False-positive tests can be seen with viral illnesses including EBV and CMV, as well as with syphilis and connective tissue disease.

ED Management

If Lyme disease is suspected but typical EM is not present, obtain blood for a Lyme titer, CBC, and ESR. If the patient has a flu-like illness, obtain EBV titers or a heterophile antibody test; obtain radiographs of any arthritic joints (see Arthritis, pp 501–505). If the patient has meningeal signs or a change in mental status, perform a lumbar puncture and send the CSF for Lyme serology. An ECG is indicated if the patient has disseminated disease. Do not withhold antibiotic therapy while awaiting the confirmatory titer results in patients with suspected early disseminated or late disease.

Ticks attach themselves by secreting a chemical, as well as screwing themselves into the skin in a clockwise direction. To remove an attached tick intact, rub a cotton ball or gauze soaked in a warm soapy water solution directly over the tick, in a counterclockwise circular motion, to dissolve the chemical attachment and "unscrew" the tick from the skin.

Amoxicillin (50 mg/kg/day divided tid, 3 g/day maximum, for 21 days) is the treatment for early disease in a child under 8 years of age. Give an older child doxycycline (100 mg bid) or amoxicillin. Cefuroxime (30 mg/kg/day divided bid, 500 mg bid maximum) is an acceptable alternative. Macrolides, including erythromycin and azithromycin, are not as effective and are indicated only for patients who are allergic to amoxicillin, doxycycline, and cefuroxime. Once antibiotic therapy is initiated, symptoms usually resolve within the first few days or week.

Treat Lyme meningitis, carditis, and polyarthritis with systemic toxicity with IV ceftriaxone, 100 mg/kg/day divided q 12 h (2 g/day maximum). Bell's palsy without meningitis and monarticular arthritis may be successfully treated with oral antibiotics for 28 days. Use the IV regimen for patients who have not responded to oral therapy.

Ticks must be attached for at least 24 h to transmit the disease. In addition, not all deer ticks are infected. Even in endemic areas, only 1 to 4% of deer tick bites result in transmission of infection. Although recent evidence suggests that two doses of doxycycline (200 mg) given 12 h apart following removal of an engorged deer tick may be effective in preventing Lyme disease, prophylactic administration of antibiotics following tick bites is not currently recommended for children.

Follow-up

- Early disease: 3 to 5 days

Indications for Admission

- Meningitis
- Third-degree AV block
- Arthritis with systemic toxicity

BIBLIOGRAPHY

Characterization of Lyme meningitis and comparison with viral meningitis in children. *Pediatrics* 1999;103:957–960.

Committee on Infectious Disease, American Academy of Pediatrics: *Report on Committee on Infectious Diseases,* 25th ed. Elk Grove Village, IL: American Academy of Pediatrics 2000, pp 374–379.

Seltzer EG, Gerber MA, Cartter ML, et al: Long-term outcomes of persons with Lyme disease. *JAMA* 2000;283:609–619.

Wormser GP, Nadelman RB, et al: Practice Guidelines for the Treatment of Lyme Disease. *J Clin Infect Dis* 2000;31:1–14.

MENINGITIS

Meningitis is an inflammation of the membranes surrounding the brain and spinal cord. It is caused by a wide variety of agents, most commonly bacteria and viruses. Fungi and parasites can be etiologies in immunosuppressed patients. Widespread use of the *Haemophilus influenzae* type B vaccine in the United States has changed the mean age of patients with meningitis from 15 months in 1986 to 25 years in 1995. However, the morbidity and mortality have not changed substantially in the last 15 years. Up to 20% of neonates and 5 to 10% of infants and children die from meningitis and sequelae occur in 25 to 50% of survivors. The etiology of meningitis varies by age and immunologic status.

Neonates　The most common bacterial agents are group B *Streptococcus, Escherichia coli,* and *Listeria monocytogenes.* Viral etiologies include herpes simplex virus, enteroviruses, and, rarely, cytomegalovirus.

1 to 3 months　The most common bacterial agents in this age group are *S. pneumoniae* and *N. meningitides.* Group B *Streptococcus* and *E. coli* can still be pathogens up to 3 months of age. Viral pathogens are the same for neonates.

3 months to 3 years   The principle bacterial causes of meningitis in this age group are *S. pneumoniae* and *N. meningitides*. *H. influenzae* type B used to be one of the principal causes of meningitis in this age group; however, the use of the HIB vaccine in the United States has dramatically decreased its incidence, although it continues to be prevalent in other parts of the world where the vaccine is not routinely used. Viral pathogens include the enteroviruses, arboviruses, and herpesviruses.

3 to 21 years   Viral meningitis caused by enteroviruses, arboviruses, and herpesviruses (see Encephalitis, pp 332–335) accounts for most of the cases of meningitis in this age group. Common bacterial causes are *S. pneumoniae* and *N. meningitides*. Other agents include EBV, human herpesvirus 6, and influenza A and B viruses. Immunocompromised patients are also susceptible to meningitis caused by *Cryptococcus*, *Toxoplasma gondii*, tuberculosis, and fungi.

Clinical Manifestations

Meningitis presents with fever, headache, neck pain and stiffness, nausea, vomiting, photophobia, and irritability. Young infants may exhibit irritability, somnolence, bulging fontanelle, and low-grade fever. Nuchal rigidity in older children may be elicited by a positive Kernig's sign (while the hip and knee are flexed 90 degrees, passive knee extension produces spasm and/or pain) and Brudzinski's sign (passive neck flexion causes hip flexion). Seizures occur in 20 to 30% of patients, and the syndrome of inappropriate antidiuretic hormone (SIADH) occurs in 30 to 60%.

Diagnosis

In *bacterial meningitis*, the CSF has a pleocytosis with a PMN predominance, decreased glucose, and elevated protein (Table 14-7). Latex agglutination and immunoelectrophoresis may help identify the etiologic agent, particularly if the patient has already received antibiotics. Gram's stain

Table 14-7   Typical Cerebrospinal Fluid Findings

	WBC/mm^3	%PMN	PROTEIN, mg/dL	GLUCOSE, mg/dL	RBC/mm^3
Normal infant <2 weeks	0–30	<60	<170	30–115	0–2
Normal child	0–6	0	20–30	40–80	0–2
Bacterial meningitis	>1000	>50	>100	<30	0–10
Viral meningitis	100–500	<40	50–100	>30	0–2
Herpes meningitis	10–1000	<50	>75	>30	10–500
Tuberculous meningitis	100–500	<30	50–80	<40	—

and culture of the CSF remain the standard for establishing the etiologic diagnosis of bacterial meningitis.

Viral meningitis can mimic bacterial meningitis. During the enterovirus epidemics of summer, older children with viral meningitis can have fever, headache, photophobia, myalgias, meningeal signs, and an exanthem that occasionally can be petechial. Herpes simplex virus can cause meningitis or encephalitis (pp 332–335), particularly in newborns, frequently without skin lesions. Suspect HSV infection in a neonate (birth to 4 weeks of age) with irritability and seizures. Meningitis with milder, self-limited findings usually associated with HSV-2 occurs in older infants and children. There may be an associated Bell's palsy, atypical pain syndromes, or trigeminal neuralgia. In viral meningitis, the spinal fluid has a normal glucose, slightly elevated protein, and a mononuclear predominance, although early in the course there can be a predominance of PMNs.

ED Management

Maintain a high index of suspicion in a patient with any of the presenting signs and symptoms. One of the most important signs of meningitis is a subtle change in the patient's affect or state of alertness, which may be noted only by the parent. In an infant, check for a bulging fontanelle; in any febrile child, check for meningeal signs, irritability, or lethargy. If meningitis is suspected, perform a lumbar puncture as quickly as possible. The only contraindications are increased intracranial pressure, impending respiratory failure, or extreme toxicity with inability to tolerate the procedure. Obtain a CT scan prior to lumbar puncture if these is papilledema, focal neurologic signs, or lethargy, but give antibiotics (Table 14-8) before obtaining the CT scan.

**Table 14-8   Empiric Antibiotic Therapy
for Suspected Bacterial Meningitis**

AGE	ANTIBIOTICS
Neonates	
0–1 weeks	
<2 kg	Ampicillin 100 mg/kg/day divided q 12 h *plus* cefotaxime 100 mg/kg/day divided q 12 h
>2 kg	Ampicillin 150 mg/kg/day divided q 8 h *plus* cefotaxime 150 mg/kg/day divided q 8 h
1–4 weeks	Ampicillin 200 mg/kg/day divided q 6 h *plus* cefotaxime 150 mg/kg/day divided q 6 h
*Older patients**	
4–8 weeks	Ampicillin 200 mg/kg/day divided q 6 *plus:* *either* ceftriaxone 100 mg/kg/day divided q 12 h *or* cefotaxime 200 mg/kg/day divided q 6 h
>8 weeks*	*either* ceftriaxone 100 mg/kg/day divided q 12 *or* cefotaxime 200 mg/kg/day divided q 6 h

*Add vancomycin (60 mg/kg/day divided q 6 h, 1 g/day maximum) if S. *pneumoniae* infection likely.

CSF analysis must include protein, glucose, cell count with differential, and culture. Gram's stain of a CSF smear is essential and can be performed quickly. Other important diagnostic tests include blood cultures, urinalysis and urine culture, CBC, platelet count, electrolytes, and liver enzymes. If viral meningitis is suspected, send CSF as well as throat and fecal swabs for viral culture. Also obtain serum and CSF for viral PCR, if available.

Monitor the patient for SIADH, which is characterized by hyponatremia, low serum osmolality, and high urine specific gravity. If the patient is not in shock or dehydrated, restrict IV fluids to two-thirds maintenance. However, give sufficient IV fluids to maintain a normal systolic blood pressure and preserve cerebral perfusion pressure. The normal autoregulatory mechanisms that maintain cerebral perfusion may be ablated in meningitis.

If pneumococcal meningitis is suspected, add vancomycin (60 mg/kg/day divided q 6 h) to the initial antibiotic regimen. If the Gram's stain suggests HIB meningitis, give dexamethasone (0.6 mg/kg/day divided q 6 h, 2 g/day maximum) 20 min before the first antibiotic dose. See p 334 for the treatment of herpes.

Indications for Admission

- Severely ill patient with meningitis of any etiology
- Suspected bacterial meningitis

BIBLIOGRAPHY

Booy R, Kroll JS: Bacterial meningitis and meningococcal infection. *Curr Opin Pediatr* 1998;10:13–18.

Feigin RD, Pearlman E: Bacterial meningitis beyond the neonatal period, in Feigin RD, Cherry JD (ed): *Textbook of Pediatric Infectious Diseases,* 4th ed. Philadelphia: Saunders, 1998, pp 400–424.

Wubbel L, McCracken GH Jr: Management of bacterial meningitis: 1998. *Pediatr Rev* 1998;19:78–84.

PARASITIC INFECTIONS

As many as 20% of Americans are infected with nematodes, and outbreaks of other parasitic infections are frequently reported. Immigrants from regions where parasites are endemic have high rates of infection, and travelers to endemic areas can become infested with a number of organisms.

Clinical Presentation

Pinworms   Pinworm (*Enterobius vermicularis*) is the most common parasite in North America. Pinworms are acquired from ingestion of eggs, which hatch in the duodenum and migrate to the cecum. Adult females lay eggs on the perianal skin, and the larvae return through the rectum. Although pinworms can be asymptomatic, anal pruritus is the most common complaint. Cystitis, with microscopic hematuria, can occur in young girls if worms enter the urethra, and vaginal discharge and vulvar itching can rarely occur if a worm has migrated into the vagina. There is no tissue migration of the larvae and no eosinophilia.

Roundworms   Roundworm (*Ascaris lumbricoides*) infection, or ascariasis, is usually asymptomatic while the worm inhabits the intestine. Roundworms enter the body through ingestion of eggs, which hatch in the small intestine and migrate by lymphatics or venules into the portal circulation and then travel to the liver, right side of the heart, and lungs. The larvae penetrate the capillaries, enter the airways, travel over the glottis to the esophagus, and mature in the small intestine. Larval migration through the lungs can cause fever, cough, malaise, and eosinophilia. Other less common complications are intestinal obstruction, blockage of the bile or pancreatic ducts, appendicitis, intussusception, and volvulus. Ascariasis can also affect the nutritional status of an infected child by causing malabsorption of fats, proteins, and carbohydrates.

Hookworms   Hookworm (*Necator americanus* and *Ancylostoma duodenale*) disease is most commonly found in the southern United States. The infection is acquired through exposure of skin to moist soil infested with larvae. Penetration of the soles of the feet by the larvae causes pruritus (ground itch). The worms migrate to the intestines and attach themselves to the mucosa, where they suck blood. The subsequent blood loss leads to a hypochromic, microcytic anemia that can be accompanied by hypoalbuminemia. In heavy infections, the acute intestinal phase is characterized by abdominal pain, diarrhea, nausea, and anorexia. Fever, headache, nausea, dyspnea, and cough can result from pulmonary migration. Eosinophilia is common.

Threadworm   The life cycle of the threadworm (*Strongyloides stercoralis*) is similar to that of the hookworm, with infection acquired by penetration of the skin by larvae in the soil. Although the majority of patients are asymptomatic, those with moderate or heavy infections have intense diarrhea with watery, mucous stools. Repeated exposure of the perirectal skin in immunocompetent individuals results in larva currens, a progressing linear urticarial trail extending from the anal area down the upper thighs. In massive strongyloidiasis, there may be invasion by larvae of all tissues, including the CNS. Overwhelming infection can occur in the immunocompromised host, with fever, severe abdominal pain, gram-negative sepsis, and shock.

Whipworm   Whipworm (*Trichuris trichuria*) infections are usually asymptomatic, although heavy infections can cause nausea, vomiting, diarrhea, abdominal distention and tenderness, rectal prolapse, and occasionally intestinal bleeding.

Giardia Lamblia   This organism is usually transmitted by contaminated water, although epidemics can occur in day care centers. Many infections are asymptomatic; however, usually within 3 weeks of ingestion of the cysts, there is the onset of diarrhea with watery, foul-smelling, steatorrheic stools. Nausea, anorexia, flatulence, abdominal distention, and epigastric pain and tenderness are common. Eosinophilia does not occur, and symptoms usually persist for days but can linger for months. Fever is uncommon, although a syndrome of chronic malabsorption can occur, with weight loss, protuberance of the abdomen, and anemia. Peripheral or generalized edema and pallor may also occur. Untreated, this illness may last for months or years.

Entamoeba Histolytica   Although infection with this organism is usually asymptomatic, there can be a spectrum of disease from mild intermittent episodes of loose, foul-smelling stools to fulminant and fatal dysentery. Less than half of children with amoebic dysentery present with fever, but almost all have abdominal pain, with bloody, mucous diarrhea. Abdominal discomfort, dull sacral pain, tenesmus, and flatulence are common. Peritonitis, perforation, and hemorrhages are complications associated with dysentery. Amoebas can also cause liver abscesses. Spread to the lungs, pleura, and skin can then occur by direct extension.

Malaria   Malaria is caused by members of the *Plasmodium* genus, *P. falciparum, P. vivax, P. ovale,* and *P. malariae. P. falciparum* is the most commonly seen malarial infection in the United States. The infection is transmitted by an infected female mosquito, with an incubation period ranging from 6 to 30 days, depending on the *Plasmodium* species. Unless properly treated, *P. vivax* and *P. ovale* persist in a dormant stage that can cause periodic relapses for as long as 4 years after initial infection. Untreated *P. malariae* infection can also persist subclinically for more than 30 years, with periodic recrudescence.

Typical attacks last 10 h, beginning with cycles of chills, tachycardia, nausea, vomiting, frequent micturition, and a fever to 40 to 41.1°C (104 to 106°F) within an hour. Severe headache with continued nausea and vomiting occur, followed by profuse diaphoresis for 2 to 3 h as the fever breaks. The cycles repeat themselves every 2 or 3 days, depending on the infecting species. Other symptoms include arthralgia and abdominal and back pain. Fever and chills are more typical of *P. vivax* and *P. ovale* infections. Severe infections caused by *P. falciparum* can result in coagulopathy, renal and hepatic failure, shock, encephalopathy, coma, and death. Jaundice and pallor are seen with hemolysis; blackwater fever is a hemolytic anemia due to *P. falciparum.* It is characterized by massive intravascular hemolysis, hemoglobinuria, acute renal failure, and a high mortality rate.

Diagnosis

The diagnosis of most parasitic infections can be made only if the possibility is considered. Recent travel to or emigration from endemic areas makes infestation likely. A history of chronic or bloody diarrhea, dysentery, weight loss, or cutaneous eruptions suggests the possibility of a parasitic infection. Eosinophilia suggests *roundworms, hookworms, threadworms,* and *whipworms.* Occasionally the patient or parent will report seeing a worm in the stool, vomitus, or sputum or in the perianal region. Often the physical examination is not helpful in determining the diagnosis.

Pinworm infestation is most easily confirmed by early morning application of transparent adhesive tape to the perianal region. The eggs adhere to the tape and can then be visualized under the microscope.

The diagnosis of other parasitic infections can be confirmed by microscopic examination of a fresh stool specimen (stool for ova and parasites). Ninety percent of infections will be detected by the collection of samples on *three* successive mornings. Refrigerate stool that cannot be examined within 1 h. *Ascaris, Strongyloides, Trichuris,* and *hookworm* are diagnosed by finding eggs in the stool. Stool identification requires patience and experience and is best performed by trained laboratory personnel.

Stool examination is negative in up to 50% of *Giardia* infections. If *Giardia* is suspected after three negative stool examinations by a parasitology laboratory, refer the patient to a gastroenterologist for presumptive therapy or a string test (Enterotest).

Entamoeba is diagnosed by finding amoebic cysts or trophozoites in the stool. A proctoscopic examination may be helpful by revealing amoebic colitis with mucosal ulcerations in the rectum. Extraintestinal amoebic infections can be accurately diagnosed with indirect hemagglutination, indirect immunofluorescence, or enzyme-linked immunosorbent assay (ELISA) antibody techniques. CT and MRI can also demonstrate extraintestinal amebiasis.

The diagnosis of *malaria* is made by the demonstration of *Plasmodium* on peripheral blood smear. Thick smears are more sensitive in detecting organisms, while thin smears may help to determine the species.

ED Management

Although a pinworm infection may be treated on the presumptive evidence of rectal itching in the absence of local pathology, treat other parasitic infections only if positive identification is available. Otherwise, arrange for the collection of specimens and refer the patient for primary care follow-up.

Parasitic infections can now be treated with safe, effective broad-spectrum medications (Table 14-9). Appropriate follow-up includes repeated stool cultures 1 to 2 weeks after the completion of therapy.

Mebendazole is possibly the most effective medication against nematodes except for *Strongyloides*. It is safe, effective treatment for *Trichuris* and only rarely causes side effects (abdominal pain, diarrhea). However, it has been shown to be teratogenic in animals; do not use it during pregnancy. A newer drug, albendazole, is less effective for *Trichuris* but has higher cure rates for *Necator* and *Ancylostoma* than mebendazole.

Pyrantel treats *Enterobius, Necator, Ancylostoma*, and *Ascaris* and is considered an alternative to mebendazole. Occasional side effects include GI disturbances, headache, dizziness, rash, and fever.

Thiabendazole is the drug of choice for *Strongyloides* (including disseminated disease), but its usefulness is limited by frequent side effects (nausea, vomiting, vertigo) and relapses. Leukopenia, rash, hallucinations, olfactory disturbances, erythema multiforme, and Stevens-Johnson syndrome occasionally occur with this drug.

Eighty percent of *Giardia* infections will be eradicated by quinacrine or metronidazole. If there is a therapeutic failure, a second course of the same medication may be successful. Quinacrine frequently causes dizziness, headache, vomiting, and diarrhea, and it has been associated with yellow discoloration of the skin, toxic psychosis, insomnia, blood dys-

Table 14-9   Treatment of Parasitic Infections

PARASITE	DRUG	DOSE
Entamoeba histolytica		
Asymptomatic	Iodoquinol	30–40 mg/kg/day divided tid × 20 days
Intestinal or	Metronidazole,	35–50 mg/kg/day divided tid × 10 days
extraintestinal	followed by	
disease	iodoquinol	30–40 mg/kg/day divided tid × 20 days
Ascaris lumbricoides		
Drug of choice	Mebendazole	100 mg bid × 3 days or 500 mg once
Alternatives	Pyrantel pamoate	11 mg/kg once (1 g maximum)
	Albendazole	400 mg once
Enterobius vermicularis		
Drug of choice	Pyrantel pamoate	11 mg/kg once (1 g maximum); repeat in 2 weeks
Alternative	Mebendazole	100 mg once; repeat in 2 weeks
Giardia lamblia		
Drug of choice	Metronidazole	15 mg/kg/day divided tid × 5 days
Alternatives	Quinacrine	2 mg/kg tid × 5 days (300 mg/day maximum)
	Furazolidone	6 mg/kg/day divided qid × 7–10 days
Ancyclostoma duodenale and *Necator americanus*		
Drug of choice	Mebendazole	100 mg bid × 3 days or 500 mg once
Alternatives	Pyrantel pamoate	11 mg/kg (1 g max) × 3 days
	Albendazole	400 mg once
Strongyloides stercoralis		
Drug of choice	Ivermectin	200 µg/kg/day × 1–2 days
Alternative	Thiabendazole	50 mg/kg/day divided bid (3 g/day max) × 2 days
Trichuris trichuria	Mebendazole	100 mg bid × 3 days or 500 mg once

Adapted from Committee on Infectious Disease: *2000 Red Book: Report of the Committee on Infectious Disease*, 25th ed. Elk Grove Village, IL: American Academy of Pediatrics, 2000, pp 693–717.

crasias, and urticaria. Side effects of metronidazole include nausea, headache, dry mouth, and metallic taste and occasionally vomiting, diarrhea, insomnia, weakness, stomatitis, vertigo, and paresthesias. Advise the patient to avoid alcohol and alcohol-containing medications during treatment with metronidazole because the mixture of the two can cause intense nausea and vomiting [disulfiram (Antabuse) effect]. Furazolidone, an alternative, is available in liquid form.

The therapy of amoebiasis depends on the location and severity of the disease. Treat intraluminal infestation and asymptomatic cyst carriers with iodoquinol, although prolonged use can result in optic atrophy. Metronidazole is effective for colitis and hepatic infections. For severe extraintestinal disease, use both.

The treatment of malaria is outlined in Table 14-10.

Table 14-10　Treatment of Malaria

DRUG	DOSE
I. All Plasmodium *species except chloroquine-resistant* P. falciparum *and* P. vivax	
A. Oral drug of choice	
Chloroquine phosphate	10 mg base/kg (600 mg maximum), then 5 mg base/kg at 6, 24, and 48 h after the initial dose
B. Parenteral drugs of choice	
Quinidine gluconate	10 mg/kg loading dose (600 mg maximum) in NS slowly over 1-2 hours, followed by a continuous infusion of 0.02 mg/kg/min, until oral therapy can be started
Quinine dihydrochloride	20 mg/kg salt loading dose in 10 ml/kg D_5W over 4 h, followed by 10 mg/kg salt over 2–4 h q 8 h (1800 mg/day maximum) until oral therapy can be started
II. Chloroquine-resistant P. falciparum	
A. Oral drugs of choice	
Quinine sulfate	25 mg/kg/day divided tid × 3–7 days (2 g/day maximum)
plus either	
1. Pyrimethamine-sulfadoxine	<1 year: single dose of ¼ tablet
(give on last day of quinine)	1–3 years: single dose of ½ tablet 4–8 years: single dose of 1 tablet 9–14 years: single dose of 2 tablets >14 years: single dose of 3 tablets
or	
2. Doxycycline (≥ 8 years)	2 mg/kg/day × 7 days (100 mg/day maximum)
or	
3. Tetracycline (≥ 8 years)	6.25 mg/kg qid × 7 days (1 g/day maximum)
B. Alternative oral drug	
Mefloquine	< 45 kg: 15 mg/kg once followed by 10 mg/kg 8–12 hours later > 45 kg: 750 mg followed by 500 mg 12 h later
C. Parenteral drugs of choice (give with 1 of oral option)	
Quinidine gluconate	Same as above
Quinine dihydrochloride	Same as above
III. Prevention of relapses: chloroquine-sensitive areas	
A. Oral drug of choice	
Chloroquine phosphate	5 mg/kg base once per week (300 mg maximum)
IV. Prevention of relapses: chloroquine-resistant areas	
A. Oral drug of choice	
Mefloquine*	<15 kg: 5 mg/kg once per week 15–19 kg: 1/4 tablet once per week 20–30 kg: 1/2 tablet once per week 31–45 kg: 3/4 tablet once per week

*Start 2 weeks prior to travel to endemic area and continue for 4 weeks after leaving area.

Adapted from Committee on Infectious Disease: *2000 Red Book: Report of the Committee on Infectious Disease*, 25th ed. Elk Grove Village, IL: American Academy of Pediatrics, 2000, pp 705–710.

Follow-up

- Primary care follow-up at the completion of therapy

Indications for Admission

- Dehydration, severe weight loss, or ill-appearence
- Extraintestinal amoebiasis
- Strongyloidiasis in immunocompromised patients
- Malaria with infection of greater than 3% of blood cells or any systemic complication

BIBLIOGRAPHY

Committee on Infectious Disease: Red Book 2000: *Report on Committee on Infectious Diseases*, 25th ed. Elk Grove Village, IL: American Academy of Pediatrics, 2000.

Drugs for parasitic infections. *Med Lett Drugs Ther* 1998;40:1–12.

Feigin RD, Cherry JD (eds): *Textbook of Pediatric Infectious Diseases*, 4th ed. Philadelphia:WB Saunders, 1998.

Noyer CM, Brandt LJ: Parasitic infections of the gastrointestinal tract. *Curr Gastroenterol Rep* 1999;1:282–291.

PERTUSSIS

Pertussis (whooping cough) is a highly communicable disease of the respiratory tract caused by *Bordetella pertussis*, for which humans are the only known host. The disease occurs worldwide and affects all age groups, but is recognized primarily in children and is most serious in young infants. The majority of deaths due to pertussis occur in unimmunized infants <6 months of age. Transmission occurs by droplets from a coughing patient and is most likely early in the illness. Pertussis is most common in the summer and fall, and epidemics occur in 2- to 5-year intervals, suggesting that immunization does not prevent transmission of the organism. Unrecognized disease in adults is an important source of infection in unimmunized or partially immunized children; attack rates in susceptible household contacts range from 70 to 100%.

Clinical Presentation

The clinical presentation of pertussis varies by age. After an incubation period of 7 to 10 days, the classic illness occurs in children 1 to 10 years of age and consists of three stages: catarrhal, paroxysmal, and convalescent. The catarrhal stage lasts 2 weeks and resembles an upper respiratory infection with rhinorrhea, conjunctival injection, low-grade or no fever, and a mild cough that gradually worsens. In the paroxysmal stage, the coughs increase in severity and number over a 2- to 4-week period. Repetitive, forceful coughs in a series of 5 to 10 occur during a single exhalation. These paroxysms are followed by a massive inspiratory effort, producing the characteristic whoop as air is inhaled forcefully through a narrowed glottis. Posttussive emesis, cyanosis, and apnea may occur. The paroxysms are exhausting and the patient may appear dazed and apathetic. The convalescent stage is characterized by less frequent coughing spells and a decrease in the severity of episodes over a 1- to 2-week period. Most young infants are unable to generate sufficient respiratory effort to whoop, so they are mistakenly diagnosed with a respiratory virus. Older children, adolescents, and adults typically have milder symptoms, and in them the diagnosis of pertussis is often not entertained.

Common complications associated with pertussis include pneumonia and otitis media. Other complications include seizures, activation of latent tuberculosis, epistaxis, melena, subconjunctival hemorrhages, subdural hematomas, rectal prolapse, dehydration, SIADH, and apnea. The most important but rare systemic complication of pertussis is encephalopathy, whose cause is not known.

Diagnosis

Whooping does not occur in all children, especially infants <6 months of age. Suspect pertussis in any patient with coughing spasms and vomiting (especially posttussive), especially if the primary DTaP vaccination series has not been completed. Obtain a CBC, looking for a leukocytosis with a lymphocytosis. The chest radiograph is usually normal, but it may have some perihilar, lobar, and diffuse or patchy infiltrates. Definitive diagnosis is made by nasal culture or specific antibody studies. Alert the laboratory that you will be sending a nasal culture for pertussis, as they have to prepare the Bordet-Gengou medium and plate the specimen promptly. Obtain the specimen using a Dacron or calcium alginate swab.

A pertussoid illness can be caused by *adenovirus* and *Bordetella parapertussis*, but confirming an etiologic diagnosis is not crucial to proper management. *Chlamydia pneumoniae* presents with a staccato cough in an afebrile, tachypneic infant younger than 12 weeks of age (p 592). Rhinorrhea is usually absent, but eosinophilia and bilateral infiltrates on chest x-ray are characteristic. Also consider *bronchiolitis* (pp 575–578), *bacterial pneumonia* (pp 591–596), *cystic fibrosis, tuberculosis* (pp 383–387), and an *airway foreign body.*

ED Management

Treatment consists of supportive therapy, avoidance of stimuli that trigger coughing attacks, maintenance of hydration and nutritional needs, and antibiotics. Erythromycin (40–50 mg/kg/day divided q 6 h for 14 days) reduces infectivity and, if started during the catarrhal stage, may reduce the severity of the illness. Azithromycin (10 mg/kg day 1; 5 mg/kg qd days 2–5) may also be effective. If erythromycin is given, inform parents about the risks of developing pyloric stenosis and watch for projectile vomiting. Treat close contacts for 14 days as well, regardless of immunization status. If the contact is unimmunized or has had fewer than four doses of pertussis vaccine, begin or continue immunization according to the standard schedule. Also give a vaccine dose to a patient who received a third dose 6 months or more before exposure. If a patient <7 years of age has had four doses of pertussis vaccine, give a booster dose of DTaP unless a dose has been given within the last 3 years. Admit a patient who is under 6 months of age, or if these is cyanosis or respiratory distress. Isolate hospitalized patients with droplet precautions for 5 days after initiation of treatment.

Follow-up

- Patient >6 months of age: immediately for cyanosis, otherwise every other day until the disease is no longer progressing

Indications for Admission

- Cyanosis, respiratory distress, or feeding difficulties
- Suspected pertussis in an infant less than 6 months old

BIBLIOGRAPHY

Black S: Epidemiology of pertussis. *Pediatr Infect Dis J* 1997;16:S85–S89.

Cherry JD, Heininger U: Pertussis and other *Bordetella* infections, in Feigin RD, Cherry JD (eds): *Textbook of Pediatric Infectious Diseases,* 4th ed. Philadelphia: Saunders, 1998, pp 1423–1435.

Edwards KM: Pertussis in older children and adults. *Adv Pediatr Infect Dis* 1997;13:49–77.

RICKETTSIAL DISEASES

The rickettsial diseases, Rocky Mountain spotted fever (RMSF), ehrlichiosis, Q fever, and the typhus fevers, are a group of infectious diseases diseases that occur worldwide and throughout the United States. Signs and symptoms of rickettsial diseases are variable; therefore a high index of suspicion is needed to diagnose and manage patients appropriately.

Clinical Presentation

Rocky Mountain Spotted Fever   RMSF is the most prevalent rickettsial disease in the United States. The principal vectors are the wood tick in the western United States, the dog tick in the East, and the Lone Star tick in the Southwest. About 600 cases are reported annually, most between April and September. Two-thirds of patients are below 15 years of age. Although antibiotic therapy is effective treatment, the overall case fatality rate is 3.9%.

RMSF infection causes a systemic, small vessel vasculitis characterized by a rash, severe headache, confusion, and myalgias. The disease usually occurs 2 to 8 days after an infected tick bite, and the onset may be either gradual or abrupt. Fever tends to be high (40–40.6°C, 104–105°F) and may oscillate. The rash appears on the second or third day of the illness, as small blanching, erythematous macules that progress to become maculopapular and petechial and, in untreated patients, may become hemorrhagic and confluent. The rash appears peripherally first and then spreads to the trunk, with involvement of the palms and soles being characteristic. Rarely, the rash may be absent. The patient may appear restless, irritable, and apprehensive and may become confused or comatose. Other neurologic symptoms include nuchal rigidity, photophobia, seizures, ataxia, spastic paralysis, sixth nerve palsy, and deafness. Congestive heart failure and arrhythmias are common. Ocular manifestations include blindness, retinal edema, papilledema, retinal hemorrhages, and cotton wool spots. Other signs include edema of the hands and face and GI symptoms, including nausea, vomiting, diarrhea, and abdominal pain.

Ehrlichiosis   Human monocytic ehrlichiosis (HME) is caused by *Ehrlichia chaffeensis* and human granulocytic ehrlichiosis (HGE) is caused by an unnamed *Ehrlichia* species closely related to *E. phagocytophila* and *E. equi.* These diseases are most prevalent in the southeastern and south central areas of the United States, although they have been reported in the Northeast. The Lone Star tick is the principal vector for HME; the deer tick and dog tick are the vectors for HGE. Illness occurs primarily between March and October, presenting about 7 to 14 days after a tick bite.

HME, HGE, and RMSF have similar signs and symptoms, including acute fever, headache, anorexia, and myalgias. Rash occurs more commonly in HME and is variable in location. It may be macular, maculopapular, or petechial. Complications include pulmonary infiltrates, bone marrow hypoplasia, respiratory failure, encephalopathy, meningitis, DIC, and renal failure. Characteristic cytoplasmic inclusion bodies (morulae) can sometimes be seen in the leukocytes.

Q Fever   This disease, caused by *Coxiella burnettii,* primarily infects animals. Close contact with infected animals and consumption of raw milk are risk factors, while epidemics occur when infected animals are slaughtered. The disease has been diagnosed in an increasing number of children below 3 years of age, usually beginning abruptly with chills, high fever, malaise, myalgias, and intractable headache, 9 to 20 days after exposure to the organism. Pneumonia, with cough and chest pain, occurs in 50% of cases. Hepatosplenomegaly is common and gastroenteritis may also be present, but there is no rash. Complications include endocarditis and hepatitis.

Typhus Fevers   Three rare diseases make up this group, louse-borne typhus, Brill-Zinsser disease, and murine flea-borne typhus. The first two are transmitted by the louse and the third by the rat flea. Symptoms of louse-borne typhus occur 1 to 2 weeks after a bite by an infected louse. High fever, headache, and a rash occur, the rash appearing on the trunk and spreading peripherally. Complications are uncommon but include myocardial and renal failure, gangrene, parotitis, pleural effusion, and pneumonia. Brill-Zinsser disease is a relapse of louse-borne typhus occurring years after the initial episode. Murine typhus is a disease of rats that is accidentally transmitted to humans by a bite of the rat flea. The symptoms are similar to those of louse-borne typhus but are usually milder.

Diagnosis

RMSF   Consider RMSF if the patient has "flu" in the summertime. The diagnosis can be confirmed by a fourfold change in titer between paired acute and convalescent serum specimens (indirect IFA, enzyme immunoassay, complement fixation, latex agglutination, indirect hemagglutination, or microagglutination tests). These tests are seldom diagnostic before the seventh day of the illness. Other nonspecific laboratory findings that can suggest the diagnosis earlier include a normal or low WBC, thrombocytopenia, and hyponatremia. Anemia and elevated liver enzymes and BUN may also be present. Definitive diagnosis can also be made by fluorescent or peroxidase–tagged antibody testing of a skin biopsy of the rash.

Consider *measles* (characteristic rash, conjunctivitis, cough, coryza) and *meningococcemia* (central petechial rash), *typhoid fever* (headache, malaise, anorexia, abdominal pain, hepatosplenomegaly, rose spots), *leptospirosis* (fever, chills, myalgias, conjunctival suffusion, contact with infected mammals), *rubella* (characteristic rash), *scarlet fever* (sandpaper rash, Pastia's lines, circumoral sparing, fever, pharyngitis), *disseminated gonococcal disease* (migratory arthritis, maculopapular rash), *infectious mononucleosis* (fever, exudative pharyngitis, lymphadenopathy, hepatosplenomegaly, atypical lymphocytosis), *secondary syphilis* (maculopapular rash including the palms and soles, condyloma, lymphadenopathy, fever, splenomegaly, headache, arthralgias), *rheumatic fever, enteroviral infections, ITP, immune complex vasculitis*, and *hypersensitivity reactions*.

Ehrlichiosis   As with RMSF, consider ehrlichiosis if the patient has "flu" in the summertime. The diagnosis can then be documented by a fourfold increase in antibody titer by indirect IFA between paired acute and convalescent serum samples, PCR, detection of morula seen on peripheral smear, or a single high serum antibody titer in a patient with a consistent history. Nonspecific laboratory abnormalities include mild leukopenia, anemia, thrombocytopenia, hyponatremia, and elevated liver enzymes.

Q Fever   Diagnosis of Q fever is made by IFA, enzyme immunoassay, complement fixation, and immune adherence hemagglutination antibody tests using paired serum samples.

Typhus   The typhus fevers can be diagnosed by a fourfold change in antibody titer between paired serum specimens obtained during the acute and convalescent phases. PCR, if available, may also be useful.

ED Management
Because RMSF and ehrlichiosis are potentially fatal, if one of these infections is suspected, *immediately treat the patient, regardless of age*, with doxycycline (3.5 mg/kg/day divided bid, 100 mg bid maximum, for 7–10 days). Patient outcome is best if therapy is started before day 5 of illness (before paired antibody titer results are available). Restrict fluids to two-thirds maintenance if hyponatremia develops. Also use doxycycline for Q fever (may relapse and require repeated courses) and the typhus fevers. Treat louse-borne typhus until the patient is afebrile for 72 h (usually 7–10 days) and flea-borne typhus with a single dose of doxycycline.

Follow-up
- Tick borne disease: 2 to 3 days

Indications for Admission
- Suspected RMSF
- Severely ill patient with ehrlichiosis, Q fever, or one of the typhus fevers

BIBLIOGRAPHY

Abramson JS, Givner LB: Rocky Mountain spotted fever. *Pediatr Infect Dis J* 1999;18:539–540.

Committee on Infectious Disease: *2000 Red Book: Report of the Committee on Infectious Disease,* 25th ed. Elk Grove Village, IL: American Academy of Pediatrics, 2000, pp 234–236, 473–475, 491–493, 620–622.

Edwards MS, Feigin RD: Rickettsial diseases, in Feigin RD, Cherry JD (eds): *Textbook of Pediatric Infectious Diseases.* Philadelphia: Saunders, 1998, pp 2239–2255.

TOXIC SHOCK SYNDROME

Toxic shock syndrome (TSS) is an acute febrile illness caused by a toxin produced by *Staphylococcus aureus* and, less frequently, by invasive group A *streptococci.* TSS was initially seen with tampon use during menses. Afterwards, nonmenstrual TSS was described, most commonly associated with cutaneous and subcutaneous infections (23%), childbirth or abortion (11%), and postoperatively (18%). Other less common causes of TSS are non-menstrual-associated vaginal infections and vaginal contraceptive sponge ·or diaphragm use. Streptococcal TSS is a syndrome similar to *S. aureus* TSS and is usually caused by infections of the skin or mucous membranes.

Clinical Presentation

The onset of the illness is usually abrupt. Initial symptoms can include headache, fever, chills, malaise, conjunctival hyperemia, sore throat, myalgias, muscle tenderness, fatigue, vomiting, diarrhea, abdominal pain, orthostatic dizziness, syncope, and rash. Progression to multiple organ involvement and shock can occur. In the first 1 to 2 days, diffuse erythroderma, severe watery diarrhea, decreased urine output, and cyanosis and edema of the extremities may be present. Somnolence, confusion, irritability, agitation, and hallucinations may occur as a result of cerebral ischemia or edema or toxin-mediated CNS effects.

Within 1 to 2 weeks, desquamation occurs, especially on the fingers, palms of the hands, toes, and soles of the feet. In menstrual TSS, edema and erythema of the inner thighs and perineum may be seen. In postoperative TSS, which occurs within 12 to 48 h following surgery, there is little or no inflammation of the surgical wound.

Mild episodes of TSS may occur, particularly in menstruating women who are using tampons. These women may develop fever, headache, sore throat, diarrhea, vomiting, orthostatic dizziness, syncope, and myalgias. There can be recurrences, which are associated with either inadequate treatment or an inadequate or delayed antibody response.

While the clinical characteristics of streptococcal TSS (profound hypotension, shock, and multiorgan system failure) are similar to those found with staphylococcal TSS, the two differ in several ways. The onset of streptococcal TSS often spans several days and there is no vomiting or diarrhea. Skin involvement is variable and presents as an extremely painful sandpaper-like rash rather than erythroderma. Preexisting varicella infections have been noted in 40 to 50% of pediatric case reports, and the mortality is 40 to 50%.

Diagnosis

The diagnosis of both staphylococcal and streptococcal TSS is made on the basis of clinical criteria and presentation. The case definition of *S. aureus* TSS is based on the following major diagnostic criteria (from the CDC):

1. Fever >38.9°C (102°F)
2. Rash: Diffuse macular erythroderma
3. Desquamation: 1 to 2 weeks after onset of illness, particularly of palms, soles, fingers, and toes
4. Hypotension: systolic BP <90 mmHg for adults; <5th percentile by age for children <16 years old; orthostatic drop in diastolic BP ≥15 mmHg from lying to sitting; orthostatic syncope or dizziness
5. Involvement of three or more of the following organ systems:
   a. Gastrointestinal: vomiting or diarrhea at onset of illness
   b. Muscular: severe myalgias or CPK level > twice the upper limit of normal
   c. Mucous membranes: vaginal, oropharyngeal, or conjunctival hyperemia
   d. Renal: BUN or serum creatinine greater than twice the upper limit of normal or >5 WBCs per high-power field in the absence of a urinary tract infection
   e. Hepatic: total bilirubin, AST or ALT greater than twice the upper limit of normal
   f. Hematologic: platelets <100,000/mm^3
   g. Central nervous system: disorientation or alteration in consciousness, without focal neurologic signs, when fever and hypotension are absent
6. Negative results on the following tests: blood, throat, or CSF cultures (although blood cultures may be positive for *S. aureus*) and, if obtained, serologic tests for RMSF, leptospirosis, or measles

A probable case of *S. aureus* TSS is defined by having five of the six clinical findings described above. A confirmed case is defined by having all six clinical findings unless the patient dies before desquamation can occur.

Laboratory abnormalities include a CBC differential with >90% neutrophils, thrombocytopenia, anemia, prolongation of the PT and PTT, sterile pyuria, elevated BUN and creatinine, elevated AST or ALT, profound hypocalcemia, hypoproteinemia, and an elevated CPK. The majority of these tests will return to normal within 7 to 10 days of disease onset.

More than 80% of patients with menstrual TSS will have *S. aureus* cultured from the cervix or vagina. The same proportion of patients with nonmenstrual TSS will have *S. aureus* cultured from the focus of infection. Since 10 to 20% of healthy individuals may have *S. aureus* isolated from the anterior nares or vagina and approximately 10% of such strains can produce TSS toxin 1, the identification of toxin-producing *S. aureus* is only presumptive evidence of infection.

The differential diagnosis of TSS includes clinical entities in which a rapid onset of fever, rash, hypotension, and multisystem involvement occurs. *Septic shock*, particularly *meningococcemia*, is often associated with a petechial or purpuric rash. Consider *streptococcal* and *staphylococcal scarlatiniform eruptions* (normotensive, sandpaper-like rash), *leptospirosis* (conjunctival suffusion), *RMSF* (purpuric rash), *measles* (cough, coryza, conjunctivitis), *acute rheumatic fever* (polyarthritis, mitral regurgitation, no erythroderma), *acute pyelonephritis* (normotensive, bacteriuria), *Legionnaires' disease* (pulmonary disease predominates), *pelvic inflammatory disease* (normotensive, cervical motion tenderness), *hemolytic uremic syndrome* (acute anemia), *acute viral syndrome*, *systemic lupus erythematosus* (normotensive, butterfly rash), *gastroenteritis* (lacks multisystem involvement), and *Kawasaki syndrome* (normotensive, no erythroderma, conjunctivitis).

ED Management

If TSS is suspected, provide oxygen, assist with ventilation as needed, and establish IV access with a large-bore cannula. Begin volume replacement and vasopressors if necessary. Give 20 mL/kg of NS or lactated Ringer's solution immediately, and repeat the fluid bolus as needed until the vital signs return to normal (see Shock, pp 18–22). The patient may require large amounts of fluid replacement. Continue close monitoring of vital signs and fluid status in the ICU for moderately or severely ill patients.

Obtain blood for CBC, platelets, electrolytes, BUN, creatinine, liver transaminases, PT and PTT, CPK, and blood cultures. Order a urinalysis and obtain cultures of the throat, stool, and urine. If there is an alteration in the level of consciousness, perform a lumbar puncture (if the patient can tolerate the procedure).

Treat with a penicillinase-resistant antistaphylococcal antibiotic to eradicate the focus of toxin-producing *S. aureus* and reduce the risk of a recurrent episode. Use nafcillin (150 mg/day divided q 6 h) unless the patient is allergic to penicillin, in which case clindamycin (40 mg/kg/day divided q 6 h) is the drug of choice. This regimen is also effective for streptococcal TSS.

Remove any vaginal tampons or wound packing. Explore and drain infected wounds, even if there are no obvious signs of inflammation. Obtain cultures of the cervix, vagina, or incisional wounds.

Indication for Admission

• Suspected TSS

BIBLIOGRAPHY

Ahem S, Ayoub EM: Severe invasive group A streptococcal disease and toxic shock. *Pediatr Ann* 1998; 27:287–292.

Chesney PJ, Davis JP: Toxic shock syndrome, in Feigin RD, Cherry JD (eds): *Textbook of Pediatric Infectious Diseases,* 4th ed. Philadelphia: Saunders, 1998, pp 830–847.

Hajjeh RA, Reingold A, Weil A, et al: Toxic shock syndrome in the United States: surveillance update, 1979–1996. *Emerg Infect Dis* 1999;5:807–810.

TUBERCULOSIS

Tuberculosis (TB) is caused by *Mycobacterium tuberculosis,* an acid-fast microorganism with the ability to infect humans and then persist in a dormant state for many years. It can also cause active disease within a few months of infection. Although 20 to 45% of the world's population is infected with TB, only 4 to 6% of the population of the United States (15 million people) is infected. Risk factors include immigration from high-risk countries, lower socioeconomic status, HIV infection, drug use, homelessness, travel to high-risk areas, history of incarceration, and employment in health care facilities. Children exposed to adults in any of the high-risk groups are at increased risk of infection.

The major route of transmission of TB is respiratory, although short, casual contact is usually not sufficient for infection. For children, household contacts are the most likely source, with infection rates around 20%. Children >12 years old are generally not contagious, despite having active disease, because they have low numbers of organisms and lack the adult tussive force to expel infectious droplets.

With *TB infection*, tubercle bacilli are established in the body, usually the lung, but there is no clinical or radiologic evidence of disease despite a positive purified protein derivative (PPD) test. These individuals are not contagious. *Tuberculosis disease*, when infection produces clinical symptoms and/or radiologic findings, develops in only 5 to 10% of infected individuals. Pulmonary disease accounts for 75% of cases in children, while extrapulmonary disease may occur in any part of the body, most often (70%) in a lymph node.

Clinical Presentation

Primary Tuberculosis   Most childhood TB is primary. The hallmark is the Ghon complex, consisting of a primary pulmonary focus (site of initial seeding), lymphangitis, and regional (hilar or paratracheal) lymphadenopathy. There is no typical clinical presentation of primary TB, which is most often subtle despite significant radiographic changes. When symptoms do occur, there may be low-grade fever, cough, anorexia, weight loss, irritability, malaise, or fatigue. The cough in childhood TB is typically mild and nonproductive. Infrequently, primary TB may mimic bacterial pneumonia, with sudden onset of high fever, cough, and respiratory distress, with or without pleural effusions. Infants may have wheezing and respiratory distress from bronchial obstruction secondary to enlarged hilar nodes.

Chronic Pulmonary Tuberculosis   Reactivation disease is the most common form of TB in adults, and it also occurs in some adolescents. It results from activation of latent TB organisms in a previously infected patient who was not treated. The patient develops a cough that becomes productive, with blood streaked sputum, fever, weight loss, night sweats, and malaise.

Lymphadenitis   Tuberculous lymphadenitis presents with discrete, painless, usually bilateral cervical lymph node enlargement that is indistinguishable from other causes of lymphadenitis. The nodes may become matted, develop a sinus tract, or become fluctuant. In contrast to suppurative adenitis, the nodes are usually not warm.

Meningitis   Most cases of TB meningitis occur within 6 months of the onset of pulmonary disease, particularly in children 4 months to 6 years of age. Unlike bacterial meningitis, the initial course is indolent, with nonspecific symptoms such as headache, poor feeding, low-grade fever, and apathy. The CSF has a mononuclear predominance with an elevated protein and low glucose. If untreated, signs of increased intracranial pressure develop later in the course. The chest radiograph is positive in 50% of cases.

Miliary Tuberculosis   The patient is febrile initially and may appear toxic, although there may be no localizing signs. Later, diffuse lymphadenopathy and hepatosplenomegaly develop. The chest radiograph, which may initially be negative, displays mottling within 1 to 3 weeks of presentation.

Congenital Tuberculosis   Congenital disease occurs rarely and only in infants whose mothers have disseminated tuberculosis (e.g., miliary TB or meningitis). The infant develops failure to thrive, jaundice, anemia, hepatosplenomegaly, cough, or respiratory distress during the first few weeks of life.

Other Infections   Infections can also occur in bones, eyes, ears, skin, kidneys, adrenals, or the genitourinary or gastrointestinal tracts.

Diagnosis

The Mantoux skin test, containing 5 tuberculin units (TU) of PPD, administered intradermally, is the only practical tool for diagnosing tuberculosis infection in asymptomatic patients. If a patient has pneumonia, hemoptysis, persistent cough, pleural effusion, failure to thrive, or persistent fever or cervical lymphadenitis for more than 2 weeks, place a 5 TU PPD (intermediate strength, 0.1 mL) intradermally, to raise a wheal, on a nonhairy surface of the forearm. An anergy panel (*Candida*, mumps) is necessary if the patient has one of the host factors (young age, poor nutrition, immunosuppression, HIV or other chronic viral infection) that may decrease reactivity. Also place a PPD on recent contacts of an individual with active TB. Arrange for a health professional to read the PPD in 48 to 72 h. Note in millimeters the amount of induration, not erythema, that develops.

Greater than 5 mm: Consider positive if the patient is immunocompromised, had recent contact with an active case of TB, or has a chest x-ray consistent with TB.

Greater than 10 mm: Consider positive in children <4 years of age; immigrants from high-risk countries in Asia, Africa, and Latin America; and residents or employees of nursing homes, correctional facilities, and homeless shelters. Also consider positive in IV drug abusers, health care workers, and patients with Hodgkin's disease, lymphoma, diabetes, renal failure, malnutrition, or steroid-dependent asthma.

Greater than 15 mm: Consider positive in children >4 years without any risk factors.

False-negative reactions may occur. Measles vaccination causes suppression of the skin test reaction 48 to 72 h after vaccination, but the vaccine may be given at the same time as the skin test. Also, up to 10% of children with culture-proven TB will not react to the skin test, or the patient may be anergic. Therefore, a negative skin test does not exclude TB. False-positives for TB may occur in patients sensitized to nontuberculous mycobacteria and in those previously vaccinated with bacille Calmette-Guérin (BCG). These reactions tend to be smaller, usually <10 mm, and suggest atypical mycobacterial infection. A true-positive skin test remains positive for life and is an indication to avoid repeat skin testing.

Order a chest x-ray for all patients with a positive PPD test. Carriers have no findings. A patient with active disease often has hilar or paratracheal adenopathy, perihilar hazy densities, and pleural thickening. Alveolar densities, atelectasis, and effusion may be seen. Cavitation is rare, but both cavitation and apical lesions may be seen in chronic TB.

In children old enough to produce sputum, collect three samples for culture on consecutive mornings to identify *M. tuberculosis* and to determine drug susceptibility. The acid fast bacilli (AFB) smear is rarely positive in children with TB disease, and laboratory findings are nonspecific (elevated ESR, anemia, and a high percentage of monocytes). In infants and young children unable to give a sputum sample, arrange for gastric washings early in the morning, to prevent the swallowing of large amounts of saliva and tears, which may dilute the sample.

Thoracocentesis may be indicated, particularly if a pleural effusion is large enough to cause dyspnea, tachypnea, or hypoxia. Also, smaller effusions may be drained as an aid in establishing the diagnosis. Tuberculosis is characterized by a high protein and LDH and several hundred WBC/mm^3 (lymphocyte predominance).

A *suppurative adenitis* is usually warm and tender, as compared with tuberculous adenitis, which is firm and nontender. With nontuberculous mycobacteria (NTB) adenitis, the induration of the PPD test is usually less than 10 mm and a chest x-ray is negative. However, differentiation between TB and NTM requires biopsy and culture, since therapy differs.

ED Management

Therapy for TB is modified by knowledge of local susceptibility patterns or suspicion of resistance in the index case or patient. Suspect resistance if the patient or index case is an urban resident; an Asian, African, or Hispanic immigrant; homeless; HIV-positive; or has a history of prior antituberculosis chemotherapy. When isoniazid (INH) is used, supplement with pyridoxine if the patient is poorly nourished, pregnant, or a breast-fed infant. Routine LFTs are unnecessary unless there is concurrent hepatic disease, liver tenderness, jaundice, an INH dosage >10 mg/kg/day is used in combination with rifampin, or there is disseminated disease (miliary or meningeal).

Since most children with primary TB are not infectious, respiratory precautions and hospital isolation are unnecessary. However, AFB precautions (i.e., a single room and use of a mask until the sputum is negative and the cough abates) are indicated if the patient (particularly adolescent) is sputum-positive or has a productive cough. Also ask adult household members who accompany the patient to wear a mask, and isolate them if they are symptomatic. Refer all close contacts of a PPD-positive patient for evaluation for TB.

Positive PPD, Negative Chest Radiograph   Treat with INH (10 mg/kg/day, 300 mg maximum) for 9 months. If resistance is known, give rifampin (10–20 mg/kg/day, 600 mg maximum). Give pyridoxine supplementation (25–50 mg/day) to breast-fed infants, pregnant adolescents, symptomatic HIV-positive children, and children on meat- and milk-deficient diets.

Positive Chest Radiograph   Admit the patient and arrange for drainage of any symptomatic effusions. Signs of CNS involvement mandate a head CT and lumbar puncture. Begin treatment with INH and rifampin. If resistance is suspected, add ethambutol (15–25 mg/kg/day) or streptomycin (20–40 mg/kg/day) until susceptibilities of the patient or index case are known. Alternatively, INH, rifampin, and pyrazinamide [(PZA) 20–40 mg/kg/day, 2 g maximum] for the first 2 months, followed by 4 months of INH and rifampin, is effective. For bone and joint disease, miliary TB, and TB meningitis, give 12 months of therapy with INH, rifampin, PZA, and either ethambutol or streptomycin.

Lymphadenitis with a Positive PPD   Obtain a chest radiograph and initiate therapy as for pulmonary TB, along with antibiotics for staphylococcal coverage, because superinfection is common with TB adenitis. Biopsy and culture are frequently necessary.

Recent Contacts of a Known Case   Place a PPD, obtain a chest radiograph, and begin prophylactic therapy (as for positive PPD, negative chest radiograph) at the initial visit. Continue therapy despite a negative skin test, and repeat the PPD 10 weeks after discontinuation of contact with index case. If it is again negative, discontinue therapy. If the PPD is positive, treatment depends on the result of the chest radiograph and index case susceptibilities.

Pediatric Dosing   Avoid INH suspension because of gastrointestinal side effects; crushed pills given with semisolid food are better tolerated. Rifampin is available in capsules that a pharmacist can make into a suspension, but do not give with food.

Follow-up
- TB infection without disease: primary care follow-up in 1 to 2 weeks

Indication for Admission
- Suspected active TB disease

BIBLIOGRAPHY

Donald PR: Childhood tuberculosis. *Curr Opin Pulm Med* 2000;6:187–192.
Smith KC: Tuberculosis in children. *Curr Probl Pediatr* 2001;31:1–30.
Starke JR, Smith MHD: Tuberculosis, in Feigin RD, Cherry JD (eds): *Textbook of Pediatric Infectious Diseases,* 4th ed. Philadelphia: Saunders, 1998, pp 1196–1230.

CHAPTER 15

Ingestions

Richard Hamilton and Robert Hendrickson
  • **Katherine J. Chou (contributor—Carbon Monoxide)**

EVALUATION OF
THE POISONED PATIENT

Among toddlers, most poisonings are accidental and usually involve household products or single drugs. Adolescent ingestions, on the other hand, may involve multiple substances (usually drugs), often in the context of suicide attempts or gestures.

Clinical Presentation

Toddlers often present to the emergency department without symptoms, so it is important to differentiate exposures (e.g., child found in an area with pills available) from ingestions. Ingestions in this age group are generally of single medications or household products. Toddlers often will taste objects that they are attracted to, including brightly colored medications, and even share them with a younger companion. Many medications are remarkably similar in color, size, and shape to candy.

Adolescent ingestions are more like adult ingestions and are generally purposeful. The intent may be suicidal and can be the impulsive actions of a patient with a mood or adjustment disorder. As a result, these ingestions often involve multiple medications, illicit drugs, and alcohol and frequently result in a symptomatic patient. In addition, the adolescent may hide the ingestion from physicians for fear of punishment from authorities or parents. It is also important to consider that the patient may be despondent over an unwanted pregnancy or attempting to self-induce an abortion. The patient rarely shares this information, so it is important to obtain a pregnancy test in all female overdoses.

If the toxin is known, the physician must assess the likelihood of toxicity. Most household products (Table 15-1A) and plants (Table 15-1B) are nontoxic. However, some common plants are toxic (Table 15-1C), and several medications can be fatal in a dose of only one pill or teaspoon

(text continues on p. 392)

Table 15-1A   Readily Available Products with Limited Toxicity

Abrasives	Hand lotions and creams
Adhesives	Hydrogen peroxide (medicinal 3%)
Air fresheners	Incense
Aluminum foil	Indelible markers
Antacids	Ink (without aniline dyes)
Antibiotics (few exceptions)	Lip balm
Antiperspirants	Lipstick
Ash, fireplace	Lubricating oils
Baby skin care products	Mineral oil
Ballpoint pen inks	Motor oil
Bath oil (castor oil and perfume)	Newspaper
Bath oils	Paraffin
Bathtub floating toys	Pencil (lead-graphite, coloring)
Battery (dry cell)	Perfumes
Bleach (≤5% sodium hypochlorite)	Petroleum jelly (Vaseline)
Bubble bath soaps (detergents)	Phenolphthalein laxatives (Ex-Lax)
Calamine lotion	Photographs
Candle (beeswax or paraffin)	Plaster
Caps (toy pistols)	Plastic
Chalk (calcium carbonate)	Play-Doh
Charcoal briquettes	Porous-tip ink marking pens
Cigarette or cigar ashes	Putty (<60 g)
Clay (modeling)	Rubber cement
Cosmetics	Saccharin
Crayons (marked AP or CP)	Shampoos
Dehumidifying packets (silica or	Shaving creams and lotions
charcoal)	Sheetrock
Deodorants	Shoe polish (most do not
Deodorizers (spray and refrigerator)	contain aniline dyes)
Detergents (phosphate type, anionic)	Silly putty (99% silicone)
Elmer's glue	Soap (hand soap only)
Erasers	Soil
Etch-A-Sketch	Spackles
Fabric softeners	Styrofoam
Fertilizer	Sunscreen preparations
Fish food	Sweetening agents (saccharin,
Glowsticks	cyclamate, aspartamine)
Glues and pastes	Teething rings
Golf balls (core may cause	Thyroid hormone
mechanical injury)	Toothpaste (without fluoride)
Greases	Watercolor paints
Gum	Wax
Gypsum	Zinc oxide ointment

Table 15-1B   Household Plants with Limited Toxicity

African violet (*Saintpaulia ionantha*)
Aluminum plant (*Pilea*)
Aralia, False (*Dizygotheca elegantissima*)
Baby's tears
Begonia (botanical name)
Bloodleaf plant (*Iresine*)
Boston fern (*Nephrolepsis exata*)
Bridal veil
Cattail (*Acalypha hispida*)
Chinese evergreen
Christmas cactus (*Zygocactus truncatus*)
Coleus (botanical name)
Corn plant (*Draecaena*)
Creeping Charlie (*Pilea nummularifolia* or *Plectranthus australis*)
Crocus (spring blooming) (*Crocus*)
Dandelion (*Taraxacum officinale*)
Devil's walking stick (*Aralia*)
Donkey tail (*Sedium morganianum*)
Dracaena spp. (corn plant)
Dusty miller (*Cineraria*)
Dwarf cactus—*Epiphylum* Hybrid—*Elegantissimum*
Dwarf palm (*Chamaedorea elegans*)
Emerald ripple
Gardenia
Geranium (*Pelargonium*)
Grape hyacinth
Hawaiian Ti (*Cordyline terminalis*)
Hens and chicks (*Echeveria* or *Sempervivum tectorus*)
Hibiscus
Honeysuckle (*Lonicera*)
Impatiens
Inch plant (*Tradescantia*)
Jade plant (*Crassula argentea*)
Kalanchoe (pregnant plant)
Lady's slipper
Lilac (*Syringa*)

Lipstick plant (*Aeschynanthus lobbianus*)
Magnolia bush
Monkey plant (*Ruellia makoyana*)
Moses-in-a-boat (*Rhoea spathacea*)
Palm
Parlor palm (*Chamaedorea elegans*)
Patient Lucy
Peacock plant (*Calathea makoyana*)
Peperomia (botanical name)
Piggy-back plant (*Tolmiea menziestii*)
Pilea (botanical name)
Pink polka dot plant (*Hypoestes sanguinolenta*)
Plectranthus (botanical name)
Prayer plant (*Maranta leuconeura kerchoveana*)
Primula
Rattlesnake plant (*Calathea insignis*)
Rose (Rosa species)
Rose begonia (*Begonia semperflorens*)
Rose of Sharon
Rubber plant (*Ficus elastica*)
Scheffelera (umbrella plant)
Sensitive plant (*Mimosa pudica*)
Snake plant (*Sanservieria*)
Snapdragon (*Antirrhinum*)
Spider plant (*Anthericum* or *Chlorophytum cosmosum*)
String of hearts (*Creopegia woodii*)
Swedish ivy (*Plectranthus australis*)
Umbrella plant (*Cyperus altermfolus*)
Violets (*Saintpaulia ionantha*)
Wandering Jew (*Zebrina pendula*)
Wax plant (*Hoya*)
Weeping fig (*Ficus benjamina*)
Zebra plant (*Aphelandra squarrosa*)

Table 15-1C   Common Poisonous Plants

PLANT	POISONOUS PART
Indoor plants	
Aroids (*Dieffenbachia, Monstera*)	Leaves
Philodendron, Spathiphyllum)	Leaves, stems
Mistletoe (*Phoradendron serotinum*)	Berries
Poinsettia (*Euphorbia pulcherrima*)	Milky sap
Outdoor Plants	
Trees	
Black cherry (*Prunus serotina*)	All, except ripe fruit flesh
Black locust (*Robinia pseudoacacia*)	Seeds, leaves, inner bark
Mulberry (*Morus* spp.)	Unripe fruits and milky sap
Shrubs and bedding plants	
Azalea (*Rhododendron* spp.)	All parts
Boxwood (*Buxus* spp.)	Leaves
Caladium (*Caladium* spp.)	All parts
Cardinal flower (*Lobelia cardinalis*)	All parts
Castor bean (*Ricinus communis*)	Seeds
Heavenly bamboo (*Nandina domestica*)	Berries (potentially)
Holly (*Ilex* spp.)	Berries (eaten in quantity)
Hydrangea (*Hydrangea* spp.)	Bark, leaves, flower buds
Jimsonweed (*Datura stramonium*)	All parts
Lantana (*Lantana camara*)	Unripe fruits
Lobelia (*Lobelia* spp.)	All parts
Madagascar periwinkle (*Catharanthus roseus*)	All parts
Mountain-laurel (*Kalmia latifolia*)	All parts
Oleander (*Nerium oleander*)	All parts
Pokeweed (*Phytolacca americana*)	All mature parts
Rhododendron (*Rhododendron* spp.)	All parts

Courtesy of Krings A, Department of Botany, North Carolina State University, Raleigh, NC.

(Table 15-2). In addition, several specific medications may cause delayed toxicity (Table 15-3).

Toxicity may develop from substances that are ingested, inhaled, or absorbed through the skin. This is especially important in evaluating neonates or infants. Their relatively large ratio of body surface area to mass is such that toxicity from dermal absorption of solvents and alcohols can cause toxicity.

Diagnosis

In most instances, diagnosis is not difficult because the ingestion is the chief complaint. In adolescents and occasionally in toddlers, the parent or patient may hide the diagnosis or the ingestion may not be known. In these cases, the diagnosis requires a high index of suspicion. Consider a poisoning in any previously well child with change in mental status, lethargy, hallucinations, delirium, seizures, or coma.

Table 15-2 One Pill Can Kill: Highly Toxic Drugs and Poisons

DRUG/POISON	POTENTIALLY FATAL DOSE	TOXIC DOSE FOR A 10 KG CHILD	TOXICITY
Benzocaine	20 mg/kg	2 mL of 10% gel	Methemoglobinemia, seizures
Calcium antagonists (Verapamil)	40 mg/kg	1–2 tabs	Bradycardia, hypotension, seizures, hypoglycemia
Camphor	100 mg/kg	5 mL of 20% solution	Seizures, CNS and respiratory depression
Chloroquine	30 mg/kg	1 tab	Seizures, arrhythmia, hypokalemia
Codeine	20 mg/kg	3 tabs	CNS and respiratory depression, bradycardia
Clonidine		1 tab or 1 patch	CNS and respiratory depression, bradycardia
Diphenoxylate (Lomotil)	1.2 mg/kg	2 tabs	CNS and respiratory depression
Hydrocarbons (aspiration)	One swallow		Pneumonitis, CNS depression
Lindane	6 mg/kg	2 tsp of 1% lotion	Seizures, CNS depression
Methyl salicylate (oil of wintergreen)	200 mg/kg	½ tsp	CNS depression, seizures, hypotension
Phenothiazines (chlorpromazine)	20 mg/kg	1 tab	CNS depression, seizures, arrhythmias
Quinidine	50 mg/kg	2 tabs	CNS depression, seizures, arrhythmias
Selenious acid (gun bluing agent)	20 mL	one swallow	CNS depression, arrhythmias, seizures
Sulfonylureas (Glyburide)	1 mg/kg	2 tabs	Hypoglycemia
Theophylline	50 mg/kg	1 tab	Seizures, arrhythmias
Tricyclic antidepressants (Imipramine)	15 mg/kg	1 tab	Seizures, arrhythmias, hypotension

Table 15-3   Delayed Toxicity*

DRUG	ONSET	TOXICITY
Acetaminophen	24–72 h	Hepatic necrosis
Acetonitrile (Acrylic nail remover)	12–24 h	Cyanide toxicity
Aspirin (enteric-coated)	Up to 8–12 h	Seizures, hyperthermia, acidosis, hypotension
Astemizole	Up to 24 h	Ventricular arrhythmias
Calcium channel blockers (sustained-release)	6–12 h	Cardiovascular collapse, brady-caria, hypotension
Diphenoxylate/atropine (Lomotil)	Up to 12–24 h	Respiratory depression
Lithium	6–14 h	Seizures, bradycardia, asystole
MAO Inhibitors	Up to 12 h	Cardiovascular collapse
Methanol	12–24 h	Acidosis, blindness
Mushrooms		
Amanita, Glaerina	6–24 h	Hepatic necrosis
Lepiota	6–24 h	Hepatic necrosis
Gyromitra	6–12 h	Seizures, hepatic necrosis
Cortinarius	2–17 days	Renal failure
Organophoshates (sulfur-containing)	days†	Cholinergic toxidrome, seizures, cardiac arrest
Sulfonylureas		
Chlorpropamide	Up to 48 h	Hypoglycemia
Glipizide/glyburide	Up to 24 h	Hypoglycemia
Thyroid hormone	6 h–11 days	Adrenergic symptoms
Tricyclic antidepressants	Up to 6–24 h‡	Seizures, arrhythmias, cardio-vascular collapse

*In addition, delayed symptoms may occur when medications:

- Form concretions (e.g., theophylline, aspirin, iron, meprobramate, bromides)
- Are packaged in sustained-release formulations (calcium channel blockers, theo-phylline, acetaminophen, lithium)
- Are ingested with medications that slow gastrointestinal motility (anticholiner-gics, opiates).

†Delayed toxicity with sulfur-containing organophosphates (e.g., parathion, chlor-pyriphos) occurs because the compound is stored in adipose tissue and slowly released. Most patients with delayed toxicity have at least mild symptoms within the first 6 h after ingestion.

‡Severe arrhythmias and cardiovascular collapse may occur several days after ingestion if the patient becomes symptomatic. An asymptomatic patient with a normal heart rate at 6 h is unlikely to develop toxicity.

In the critically ill child, symptomatic care must be initiated immediately and the history obtained at the same time. The first priority in the critically ill child is the ABCs (airway, breathing, and circulation), followed by oxygen, IV access, and cardiac monitoring. Empiric therapy of common disorders, such as glucose for hypoglycemia and naloxone for opioid toxicity, can then be considered. After assessment of vital signs and initiation of therapy, the specific toxin may be discerned by physical findings and/or laboratory data and specific care may be rendered.

The Unconscious Patient

1. Assess the patient's respirations. If they are not adequate, perform a jaw lift, insert an oral airway (if tolerated), and suction any secretions. If necessary, intubate the patient, preferably with a cuffed endotracheal tube.
2. Secure a large-bore IV line.
3. Measure the blood pressure and pulse. If the patient has clinical signs of hypoperfusion (poor capillary refill, pallor, cool extremities), give a rapid bolus (20 mL/kg) of normal saline and raise the foot of the bed.
4. Obtain an electrocardiogram (ECG) and attach a cardiac monitor and pulse oximeter.
5. Although it may be clear that the patient is the victim of an overdose or ingestion, assess the pupillary responses, EOMs, GCS, and reflexes and examine the head and neck carefully for evidence of injury while maintaining the cervical spine in a neutral position.
6. Remove the patient's clothing to facilitate the examination, look for signs of trauma, and search for pill containers.
7. Measure the temperature and, if possible, weigh the patient. A soft rectal thermometer probe measures extremes of temperature beyond the ranges of glass or digital thermometers.
8. Obtain an arterial blood gas to assess the adequacy of ventilation and the acid-base status.
9. Obtain blood specimens for a complete blood count, liver function tests, type and hold, pH, electrolytes and glucose, carboxyhemoglobin (if CO poisoning cannot be ruled out by history), an extra red-top tube for other tests that might be needed later, and a finger-stick glucose determination.
10. Give 0.5 g/kg of glucose to any unresponsive patient either empirically or in response to a low bedside-measured glucose.
11. Give naloxone 0.1 mg/kg, up to 2.0 mg (preferably IV, but can be given IM, SC, or ET) either empirically or to correct the miosis and respiratory depression secondary to opioid toxicity. If there is no response within 3 to 5 min, give a second dose. A positive response may last only 30 min, so repeated doses or a continuous IV transfusion may be indicated.
12. Obtain urine by catheter for dipstick examination, urine toxicology, and, in adolescent females, a pregnancy test.
13. If less than 4 h have elapsed since the ingestion, administer a slurry of activated charcoal in water by nasogastric tube (1 g/kg). Add sorbitol only to the first dose of charcoal; additional doses are dangerous in infants and toddlers because the osmotic diarrhea can cause large and rapid fluid shifts that compromise intravascular volume.

The Conscious Patient

1. Measure the vital signs, including temperature and weight.
2. If the patient is alert and stable, try to determine the substance(s) and amounts ingested as well as the time since the ingestion.
3. See no. 13 above.

Once the patient is stable, attempt to ascertain the specific toxicologic diagnosis. If the ingestion was witnessed, determine the specific substance, amount, and time of the ingestion. In addition to the typical historical questions, assess the following:

1. Where was the patient found?
2. Has the patient visited someone recently?
3. Is the patient or anyone else in the house on medication (acutely, chronically, or intermittently)?
4. Is anyone in the house taking any herbal products or home remedies?
5. Is anyone in the house ill now, or has anyone recently had headaches, seizures, or fever?
6. Were there any visitors in the house recently?
7. Were there any pills, pill bottles, or other open containers in the house (including the garbage), or were any unusual odors noticed?
8. Does anyone in the house have a hobby or use unusual chemicals?
9. Was the substance in the original container, or was it transferred into another one?
10. Was there more than one substance in the container?
11. Was the patient given syrup of ipecac, and did the patient vomit?

Perform a complete physical examination (Table 15-4), including assessment of the pupils, mucosal membranes, heart, lungs, abdomen, skin, and a thorough neurologic examination (level of consciousness, pupils, motor reflexes, and gag reflex). Certain poisons manifest consistent and unique sets of vital signs and physical examination findings, grouped into "toxidromes" (Table 15-5). Distinctive odors may help make the diagnosis (Table 15-6).

A comatose patient with symmetric EOMs, pupillary reflexes, and motor responses probably has a toxic-metabolic basis for the coma, although *hypoglycemia* and *toxic alcohols* can cause focal motor deficits.

Table 15-4   Physical Examination Findings

FINDING	DRUGS/TOXIN
Vital Signs	
Increased temperature	Salicylates, amphetamines, anticholinergics, cocaine, theophylline, phencyclidine, tricyclics
Decreased temperature	Barbiturates, phenothiazines, opiates, ethanol, hypotension from any cause
Increased pulse rate	Amphetamines, cocaine, caffeine, anticholinergics, theophylline, hypotension from any cause, hypoglycemia, iron, phenothiazines
Decreased pulse rate	Opiates, barbiturates, digitalis, clonidine, beta blockers, hypothermia, hypoglycemia, increased intracranial pressure, calcium channel blockers
Increased respiratory rate	Salicylates, theophylline, metabolic acidosis, Reye's syndrome
Decreased respiratory rate	CNS depressants, clonidine (early), botulism

Table 15-4 **Physical Examination Findings** *(continued)*

FINDING	DRUGS/TOXIN
Skin	
Cyanosis	Methemoglobinemia, hypoxia
Flushing	Anticholinergics, amphetamines
Diaphoresis	Amphetamines, cocaine, anticholinesterase pesticides, salicylates
Hot, dry skin	Anticholinergics
Piloerection	Opiate withdrawal
Bullae	Carbon monoxide, barbiturates, ethchlorvynol
Pruritis	Vitamin A
Tracks, abscesses, lymphedema, acrocyanosis	Parenteral drug abuse
Eyes	
Miosis	Opiates, cholinesterase-inhibitor pesticides, clonidine
Mydriasis	Amphetamines, cocaine, atropinics, antihistamines, phenylephrine
Conjunctival injection	Direct irritants, cannabis
Nystagmus	Phenytoin, phencyclidine, carbamazepine
Visual disturbances	Botulism, parathion, methanol, digitalis, vitamin A
Neck	
Rigidity	Dystonia from phenothiazines and haloperidol, phencyclidine, strychnine, meningitis
Breath Sounds	
Rhonchi, wheezes	Petroleum distillate aspiration, toxic inhalants, cholinesterase-inhibitor pesticides
Abdomen	
Distention, decreased bowel sounds	CNS depressants (many), anticholinergics, tricyclic antidepressants
Increased bowel sounds	Amphetamines, cocaine, cholinesterase-inhibitor pesticides, drug withdrawal, food poisoning
Tenderness	Alcoholic gastritis, corrosives, salicylates, acetaminophen
Distended bladder	Anticholinergics, tricyclic antidepressants
Neurologic	
Ataxia	Phenytoin, benzodiazepines, sedative hypnotics, solvents, alcohol
Focal signs	Must rule out increased intracranial pressure due to a mass lesion, hypoglycemia
Tremor	Carbon monoxide, parathion, phenothiazines, mercury, ethanol, lithium, arsenic, solvents

Assume that pupillary inequality signifies a *structural intracranial process*. Miosis, on the other hand, strongly suggests an opioid or organophosphate toxicity. Mydriasis with reactive pupils is seen with sympathomimetic toxidromes such as cocaine or amphetamines. Mydriasis with poorly reactive pupils is seen in anticholinergic poisoning.

It is especially important to recognize three toxicologic syndromes, because institution of specific drug therapy may be lifesaving. These are

Table 15-5   Toxidromes

Sympathomimetic

    Findings: Hyperthermia, tachycardia, hypertension, mydriasis, warm/moist skin, agitated delirium

    Causes: Amphetamines, cocaine, phencyclidine, theophylline, opiate withdrawal

Cholinergic

    Findings: SLUDGE (*S*alivation, *L*acrimation, *U*rinary incontinence, *D*iarrhea/*D*iaphoreses, *GI* upset/hyperactive bowel sounds, *E*mesis), miosis, bradycardia, bronchial secretions, seizures, altered mental status, paralysis

    Causes: Betel nut, carbamates, chemical warfare agents (VX, Soman, Sarin), organophosphates, pilocarpine eye drops

Anticholinergic

    Findings: Hyperthermia, tachycardia, hypertension, hot/red/dry skin, mydriasis, unreactive pupils, urinary retention, absent bowel sounds, confusion/hallucinations

    Causes: Antihistamines, atropine, phenothiazines, scopolamine, tricyclic antidepressants

Opioid (narcotic)

    Findings: Miosis, respiratory depression, depressed mental status

    Causes: Codeine, dextromethorphan, fentanyl, heroin, morphine

Table 15-6   Odors

ODOR	TOXIN
Acetone	Aspirin, chloroform, isopropanol, ketoacidosis, methanol
Ammoniacal	Ammonia, uremia
Bitter almonds	Cyanide (silver polish)
Carrots	Cicutoxin
Coal gas	Carbon monoxide
Disinfectants	Creosote, phenol
Eggs (rotten)	Disulfiram, hydrogen sulfide, mercaptans
Fish or raw liver (musty)	Hepatic failure, zinc phosphide
Fruitlike	Amyl nitrite, ethanol, isopropanol
Garlic	Arsenic, dimethyl sulfoxide (DMSO), organophosphates, phosphorus, selenium, thallium
Mothballs	Camphor
Peanuts	*N*-Pyridylmethylurea (Vacor), other rodenticides
Pearlike (acrid)	Chloral hydrate, paraldehyde
Petroleum	Petroleum distillates
Pungent aromatic (vinyl)	Ethchlorvynol (Placidyl)
Shoe polish	Chlorinated hydrocarbons, nitrobenzene
Violets (urine)	Turpentine
Wintergreen	Methylsalicylate

poisonings due to opiates, cholinesterase-inhibiting insecticides, and tricyclic antidepressants (Table 15-5).

Finally, consider a nontoxicologic differential diagnosis (*head trauma, meningitis, cerebrovascular accident, postictal state, posthypoxia, behavioral* or *psychological disorders*), and ask if the patient has been ill or injured or has had headaches, seizures, or fever.

General laboratory testing is rarely helpful in the poisoned patient. Specific levels are available for several medications and are helpful in making treatment decisions (Table 15-7). Always obtain an acetaminophen level after an oral ingestion or if the patient is comatose, since this can be asymptomatic ingestion with significant delayed toxicity. General toxicology screens from the urine and blood are helpful in specific circumstances, but are not routinely indicated.

Acid-base status can be determined from ABG and chemistry panels. The mnemonic "MUDPILES CAT" represents the list of toxins that produce an elevated anion gap with a metabolic acidosis (Table 15-8). The anion gap is calculated by

$$[Na^+] - [(HCO3^-) + (Cl^-)]$$

Table 15-7   Important Drug Levels

DRUG	LEVEL	INTERVENTION
Acetaminophen	Nomogram	N-acetylcysteine
Carbamazepine	60 mg/L	Hemoperfusion
Carboxyhemoglobin	25% (any if pregnant)	Hyperbaric oxygen
Digoxin	15 ng/mL*	Digoxin-specific Fab fragments
Ethanol	Low level	Necessitates search for other toxins
Ethylene glycol	20 mg/dL	Ethanol or fomepizole
	40 mg/dL	Hemodialysis
Iron	500 µg/dL	Deferoxamine
Lithium	4 mEq/L† (acute)	Hemodialysis
Methanol	20 mg/dL	Ethanol or fomepizole
	40 mg/dL	Hemodialysis
Methemoglobin	20%	Methylene blue
Phenobarbital	100 µg/mL	Hemoperfusion
Salicylate	100 mg/dL (acute)	Bicarbonate, hemodialysis
	60 mg/dL (chronic)	Bicarbonate, hemodialysis
Theophylline	80 mg/L	Hemoperfusion or hemodialysis
Valproic acid	1000 mg/L	Hemodialysis

*Treatment with Digoxin-specific Fab fragments is based on symptoms and an elevated potassium (>5.0 mEq/L). However, if the Digoxin level is >2 ng/mL in an overdose, give Fab fragments, regardless of symptoms.

†Treatment with hemodialysis is based on symptoms (severely altered mental status, seizures, arrhythmias). However, a lithium level >4 mEq/L is indicative of severe toxicity and hemodialysis is indicated.

Table 15-8   **Causes of Increased Anion Gap Metabolic Acidosis (Mudpiles CAT)**

Methanol or Metformin	Cyanide
Uremia	Alcohol or Acids (valproic)
Diabetic Ketoacidosis	Toluene or Theophylline
Paraldehyde or Phenformin	
Iron, Isoniazid, or Ibuprofen	
Lactic acidosis	
Ethylene glycol	
Salicylates	

The normal anion gap is typically <12, but use the upper limit of normal set by each laboratory, since this reflects differences in the methods used to calculate the electrolytes.

Order a serum osmolality in cases of suspected poisoning due to ethylene glycol, methanol, or isopropanol. The osmolar gap can be used to approximate serum levels and to determine therapy, such as dialysis. The osmolar gap can be calculated by subtracting the calculated osmolality from the measured osmolality:

$$\text{Osmolar gap} = \text{measured osmolality} - \text{calculated osmolality}$$

$$= \text{measured osmolality} - [(2 \times \text{Na}^+) + (\text{BUN}/2.8) + (\text{glucose}/18) + (\text{ethanol}/4.6)]$$

Including ethanol in the calculated gap increases the likelihood of correctly identifying gaps attributable to methanol, ethylene glycol, or isopropanol.

A normal osmolar gap is +/− 10, while an elevated osmolar gap is consistent with the presence of a toxic alcohol ingestion. However, a normal osmolar gap cannot be used to exclude the diagnosis of a toxic alcohol ingestion.

Radiographic evaluation of the poisoned patient is generally unnecessary; however, the mnemonic CHIPES refers to the tablets that may be seen on abdominal x-ray: chloral hydrate, heavy metals (lead, iron, arsenic), iodides, phenothiazines, enteric-coated medications, and sodium and other elements (calcium, potassium, bismuth). In practice, only the heavy metals are readily visible on abdominal x-rays. "Body packers," who are intentionally transporting illicit drugs wrapped in packages in their intestines, will often have visible oblong densities on x-ray.

Decontamination

If the patient has been exposed to the toxin on the skin, remove all of the patient's clothing, using gloves, and put it in bags. Thoroughly cleanse the skin with copious amounts of water while wearing protection over the mouth, face, and entire skin surface until the chemical is identified.

In the case of ocular exposure to chemicals, thoroughly irrigate the eyes with a minimum of 1 L of saline using a Morgan lens. Most ocular exposures cause an irritant conjunctivitis, but acid, alkali, or hydrofluoric acid can cause chemical ocular burns and abrasions and call for specific therapy. Check the pH of the corneal surface with pH paper prior to and after irrigation and continue irrigation until the pH is approximately 7.0.

There are several safe methods for gastrointestinal (GI) decontamination. Syrup of ipecac has been abandoned because it may cause protracted vomiting and delay charcoal administration.

Gastric lavage involves aspiration of pill fragments from the stomach using a large-bore orogastric tube. In general, gastric lavage may be helpful in adolescents who have ingested a large quantity of lethal toxin less than 1 h prior to arrival. Adolescents can tolerate the larger tubes that are required to evacuate pills and tablets.

Activated charcoal acts as an adsorbent to bind toxins and prevent their absorption into the systemic circulation. It binds to most substances (but not lithium, iron, or caustics). The dose is 1 g/kg. Children tolerate charcoal best if it is mixed with a flavored beverage and served in a covered container with a straw. Do not place a nasogastric tube solely for charcoal instillation unless the ingestion has the potential for severe toxicity.

Multiple doses of charcoal, q 2–4 h, may be necessary for toxins that are ingested in large amounts (i.e., acetaminophen, salicylates, theophylline) in order to supply sufficient charcoal for a 10-to-1 charcoal-to-drug ratio. Thus, a 5 g ingestion of theophylline would require 50 g of charcoal. In addition, multiple doses of activated charcoal may be administered in cases of salicylate, carbamazepine, and phenobarbital poisoning, because the charcoal interrupts enterohepatic and enteroenteric circulation. Use sorbitol only with the first dose of charcoal.

Whole-bowel irrigation may be useful in an ingestion of a sustained-release product or a toxin that is not bound by charcoal. This technique involves instillation of large volumes of polyethylene glycol, a substance that is not absorbed in the GI tract, in order to flush intact pills through and avoid absorption. Instill small quantities at first (adolescent: 250 mL; toddler: 50 mL) and increase the rate to 1 to 2 L/h in an adolescent and 0.5 to 1 L/h in a child via nasogastric tube. Continue until the patient's effluent is clear. It is important to monitor continued peristalsis by periodically auscultating active bowel sounds. Contraindications to WBI include an unprotected airway in a comatose patient, ileus, or GI obstruction, perforation, or significant hemorrhage.

BIBLIOGRAPHY

Anderson IB. Nontoxic or minimally toxic household products, in Olson KR, Anderson IB, Benowitz NL, et al (eds): *Poisoning and Drug Overdose*, 3rd ed. Stamford, CT: Appleton & Lange, 1999, p 240.

Bosse GM, Matyunas NJ: Delayed toxidromes. *J Emerg Med* 1999;17:679–690.

Cisneros L: Lethal single dose ingestions in Pediatrics: a selected review. *Emerg Office Pediatr* 1000;12:172–175.

Emery D, Singer JI: Highly toxic ingestions for toddlers: when a pill can kill. *Pediatr Emerg Med Rep* 1998;3:111–120.

Goldfrank LR, Flomenbaum NE, Lewin NA, et al (eds): *Goldfrank's Toxicologic Emergencies*, (6th ed). Stamford, CT: Appleton & Lange, 1998.

Hoffman RS, Goldfrank LR: The poisoned patient with altered consciousness: controversies in the use of a "coma cocktail". *JAMA* 1995;274:562–569.

Koren G: Medications which can kill a toddler with a tablet or a teaspoon. *Clin Toxicol* 1993;31:407–413.

Krenzelok EP, McGuigan M, Lheur P: Position statement: ipecac syrup. American Academy of Clinical Toxicology; European Association of Poisons Centers and Clinical Toxicologists. *J Toxicol Clin Toxicol* 1997;37:699–709.

Olson KR: Comprehensive evaluation and treatment, in Olson KR, Anderson IB, Benowitz NL, et al (eds): *Poisoning and Drug Overdose,* 3rd ed. Stamford, CT: Appleton & Lange, 1999, pp 1–61.

Pond SM, Lewis-Driver DJ, Williams GM, et al: Gastric emptying in acute overdose: a prospective randomized controlled trial. *Med J Aust* 1995;163:345–349.

Shih RD, Goldfrank LR: Plants, in Goldrank LR, Flomenbaum NE, Lewin NA, et al (eds): *Goldfrank's Toxicologic Emergencies,* 6th ed. Stamford, CT; Appleton and & Lange, 1998, pp 1243–1259.

Sugarman JM, Rodgers GC, Paul RI: Utility of toxicology screen in a pediatric emergency department. *Pediatr Emerg Care* 1997;13:194–198.

Vale JA: Position statement: gastric lavage. American Academy of Clinical Toxicology; European Association of Poisons Centers and Clinical. *J Toxicol Clin Toxicol* 1997;35:711–719.

Weisman RS. Identifying the nontoxic exposure, in Goldfrank LR, Flomenbaum NE, Lewin NA, et al (eds): *Goldfrank's Toxicologic Emergencies,* 6th ed. Stamford, CT: Appleton & Lange, 1998, p 132.

ACETAMINOPHEN

Acetaminophen is a ubiquitous product that, in overdose, can lead to hepatic damage and failure. It is the most common oral ingestant in the United States, a common coingestant, and often found in over-the-counter preparations, particularly cold medicines. It remains a leading cause of poisoning deaths.

Acetaminophen is normally metabolized in the liver by sulfation and glucuronidation. In the overdose setting, these metabolic pathways are saturated and the excess acetaminophen is metabolized by the P450 enzymes to a toxic metabolite called NAPQI (*N*-acetyl-*p*-benzoquinoneimine), which causes centrilobular hepatic necrosis. Rapid diagnosis is necessary, as an antidote N-acetylcysteine (NAC; Mucomyst) effectively prevents toxicity.

Clinical Presentation

In the first hours after an ingestion of acetaminophen, symptoms include nausea, vomiting, and anorexia. This is followed by an asymptomatic latent phase. Between 24 and 48 h after ingestion, subclinical hepatotoxicity occurs, evidenced by elevation of transaminases, bilirubin, and prothrombin time, mild right-upper-quadrant pain, nausea, and vomiting. Over several days, fulminant hepatic failure may develop, with jaundice, renal failure, cerebral edema, and hypotension.

Diagnosis

The potential of an ingestion to cause hepatotoxicity may be predicted by obtaining a serum level 4 h or more after the ingestion. Plot the serum level on the acetaminophen nomogram (Fig. 15-1). If the level appears

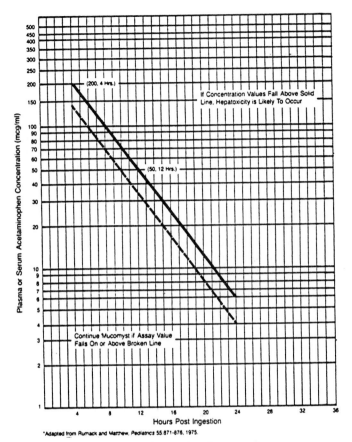

Figure 15-1   Acetaminophen nomogram.

above the "possible hepatotoxicity" line, then immediate therapy with NAC is necessary. NAC is 100% effective in preventing hepatotoxicity if given within 8 h of ingestion.

Toxicity may be predicted less reliably by calculating whether the ingested dose is >150 mg/kg. Toxicity is rare in toddlers because they generally ingest small quantities. However, one 120-mL bottle of children's acetaminophen (160 mg/5 mL) is potentially toxic to a child who weighs <26 kg (approximately 4–6 years old). Toxicity is more common in older children and in intentional overdoses.

ED Management

Immediately administer 1 g/kg of activated charcoal if the ingestion occurred less than 4 h prior to arrival. Although charcoal does adsorb some acetaminophen, it is not the treatment of choice, so do not force the patient to accept a nasogastric tube simply to instill charcoal in an iso-lated acetaminophen ingestion.

NAC is indicated if the serum level is on or above the "possibly hepa-totoxic" line on the nomogram. The oral loading dose is 140 mg/kg, fol-lowed by 70 mg/kg q 4 h for 17 more doses. Oral NAC is foul-smelling and often causes emesis. Dilute it 1:4 in juice or instill it via a nasogastric tube to decrease GI upset. In addition, give an IV antiemetic (metoclo-pramide 0.1 mg/kg, titrating up to 0.5 mg/kg). Intravenous NAC is avail-able in most countries but has not yet been approved for use in the United States. The oral form of NAC can be prepared for intravenous administra-tion, but only in consultation with a toxicologist or Poison Control Center.

If the acetaminophen level will not be available until more than 8 h after ingestion, give a single oral loading dose of NAC while waiting for the level. Patients who arrive 36 h after ingestion require therapy if the acetaminophen level is >10 μg/dL or the aspartate transaminase (AST) is elevated. Treat a patient arriving between 24 and 36 h after ingestion if the acetaminophen level is >10 μg/mL or the AST is elevated at 36 h.

If the time of the ingestion is not known, obtain a serum aceta-minophen level and AST on admission to the ED. If the AST is elevated, admit the patient for a full course of NAC. Alternatively, if the AST is normal but rises over several hours, treat with NAC for a full course. If the AST remains normal, treat with NAC for 24 h and reassess the level after 24 h. If the serum acetaminophen level is <10 μg/mL and the AST is normal, stop the NAC.

Obtain a CBC, electrolytes, liver function tests, prothrombin time, and partial thromboplastin time if the patient has a toxic level or arrives more than 24 h after the ingestion.

Indications for Admission

- Possible acetaminophen toxicity, based on amount ingested (>150 mg/kg) or serum levels
- Suicide attempt or gesture without psychiatric clearance and appro-priate follow-up arranged

BIBLIOGRAPHY

Perry HE, Shannon MW: Efficacy of oral versus intravenous N-acetylcysteine in acetaminophen overdose: results of an open label, clinical trial. *J Pediatr* 1998; 132:149–152.

Pershad J, Nichols M, King W: "The silent killer": chronic acetaminophen toxicity in a toddler. *Pediatr Emerg Care* 1999;15:43–46.

Schiodt FV, Rochling FA, Casey DL, et al: Acetaminophen toxicity in an urban county hospital. *N Engl J Med* 1997;337:1112–1117.

MEDICATIONS FOR THE TREATMENT OF ATTENTION DEFICIT HYPERACTIVITY DISORDER (ADHD)

A variety of medications are used to treat ADHD, including amphetra-mines [methylphenidate (Ritalin), dextroamphetamine (Dexedrine), pemoline (Cylert) and amphetamine (Adderall)], central adrenergic inhibitors (such as guanabenz, clonidine, and guanfacine), and antidepressants (including bupropion).

Clinical Presentation

Amphetamine toxicity consists of a typical sympathomimetic toxidrome (hyperthermia, tachycardia, hypertension, dilated but reactive pupils, and diaphoresis).

The centrally acting andrenergic inhibitors are selective alpha$_2$ agonists, leading to a generalized sympathetic depression including miosis, sedation, coma, hypothermia, hypotension, and bradycardia. Paradoxical hypertension may develop because, early in an overdose, these medications have a preponderance of peripheral alpha stimulation, prior to entry of the drug into the central nervous system (CNS). This paradoxical hypertension is then followed by hypotension.

Bupropion is an antidepressant that blocks reuptake of CNS dopamine and norepinephrine. Toxicity involves a hyperadrenergic state with agitation and seizures, although seizures can also occur with normal therapeutic doses.

Diagnosis

Diagnosis is generally made by history as well as by identifying the signs and symptoms consistent with the appropriate toxidrome.

ED Management

First assess the ABCs. Administer activated charcoal (1 g/kg PO) to a patient who arrives in the ED within 4 h of ingestion. Agitation may lead to acidosis, hyperthermia, and rhabdomyolysis; treat it quickly with midazolam 0.1–0.3 mg/kg IV, 0.2–0.4 mg/kg IM (maximum dose 6–10 mg), or 0.4–0.9 mg/kg PO (maximum dose 20 mg). Aggressively treat severe hyperthermia (>40°C, 104°F) by covering the patient with a wet sheet and applying ice packs to the groin and axillae. The cardiovascular manifestations generally respond to benzodiazepines. However, treat sustained tachycardia and hypertension, despite adequate sedation, with phentolamine (0.02–0.1 mg/kg IV q 10 min) or labetalol (0.25 mg/kg IV q 10 min), and repeat the dose as needed.

The presentation of clonidine, guanabenz, or guanfacine overdose may mimic opioid toxicity, with miosis, sedation, and respiratory depression. Naloxone (0.4–2.0 mg IV) is variably effective because the opioid receptor and the central alpha receptor share a potassium channel in the locus ceruleus. Give up to 10 mg before considering the intervention ineffective.

Indications for Admission

- Abnormal vital signs or mental status
- Suicide attempt or gesture without psychiatric clearance and appropriate follow-up arranged

BIBLIOGRAPHY

Broderick-Cantwell JJ: Case study: accidental clonidine patch overdose in attention-deficit/hyperactivity disorder patients. *J Am Acad Child Adolesc Psychiatry* 1999;38:95–98.

White SR, Yadao CM: Characterization of methylphenidate exposures reported to a regional poison control center. *Arch Pediatr Adolesc Med* 2000;154:1199–1203.

ANTICHOLINERGICS

Anticholinergic poisoning in children may be caused by ingestion of antihistamines, atropine, scopolamine, phenothiazines, antiparkinsonian drugs, mydriatics, jimson weed (*Datura stramonium*), and tricyclic anti-depressants. Antihistamines are commonly found in cold preparations.

Clinical Presentation

The anticholinergic toxidrome must be diagnosed clinically, since laboratory tests are typically not helpful. Symptoms result from peripheral blockade of acetylcholine at the muscarinic receptors and include dry mouth, flushed dry skin, mydriatic and unreactive pupils, blurred vision, constipation, urinary retention, and tachycardia. Central muscarinic blockade causes confusion, disorientation, hallucinations, seizures, and coma.

Symptoms have been described by the mnemonic "Dry as a bone, Mad as a hatter, Red as a beet, Hot as Hades and Blind as a bat."

Diagnosis

Suspect an anticholinergic ingestion in any patient with a change in mental status, hallucinations, coma, arrhythmia, or seizures. On examination, the pupils are usually dilated and unreactive. The presence of confusion, hallucinations, tachycardia, dry mucous membranes, and dry flushed skin also suggests the diagnosis. Obtain blood for a CBC, electrolytes, glucose, and Dextrostix determination and order an ECG.

It is important to differentiate the anticholinergic toxidrome from the *sympathomimetic toxidrome*, as therapy is quite different. Both the anticholinergics and sympathomimetics can cause confusion, agitation, mydriasis, and tachycardia. The pupillary, skin, and abdominal examinations findings may differentiate these toxidromes. Anticholinergics cause large and nonreactive pupils, absent bowel sounds, and red, dry, warm skin. Conversely, sympathomimetics cause large and reactive pupils, with normal or increased bowel sounds and cool, diaphoretic skin.

ED Management

Initiate supportive care and cardiac monitoring, administer activated charcoal if the ingestion is likely to have been within the previous 4 h, and obtain a bedside glucose level. The treatment of coma is supportive. Treat seizures with lorazepam (0.05–0.1 mg/kg slow IV) or diazepam (0.1–0.3 mg/kg slow IV); then if seizures recur, give a loading dose of fosphenytoin (20 mg/kg phenytoin equivalents no faster than 1 mg/min). Wide complex tachycardias may respond to sodium bicarbonate (1 mEq/kg IV).

Physostigmine can be used in pure anticholinergic poisonings such as atropine, scopolamine, diphenhydramine, and jimson weed. Continued seizures, hemodynamic compromise, or severe agitation or hallucinations are indications for its use. Do not use physostigmine merely to arouse a comatose patient. Give a dose of 0.5 mg *slowly* over 5 min. This can be repeated every 15 min until a satisfactory endpoint is achieved. Rapid administration may cause seizures or bradycardia, and an overdose can precipitate a cholinergic crisis (salivation, lacrimation, bradycardia, hypotension, or asystole). Always be prepared to give atropine (one-half the physostigmine dose) to a patient mistakenly treated with physostigmine.

Agitation may be reversed entirely with small doses of physostigmine. Although the potential side effects of physostigmine have made its use less common, it usually causes complete reversal of anticholinergic agitation. This reversal allows confirmation of the diagnosis and also eliminates the need for further invasive diagnostic studies (CT and lumbar puncture). Sedation with benzodiazepines may be effective, although large doses are often necessary.

Indications for Admission

- Lethargy or signs of toxicity (tachycardia, confusion, sedation)
- Coma, arrhythmia, or seizures
- Suicide attempt or gesture without psychiatric clearance and appropriate follow-up arranged

BIBLIOGRAPHY

Chan TY: Anticholinergic poisoning due to Chinese herbal medicines. *Vet Hum Toxicol* 1995;37:156–157.

Myers JH, Moro-Sutherland D, Shook JE: Anticholinergic poisoning in colicky infants treated with hyoscyamine sulfate. *Am J Emerg Med* 1997;15:532–535.

Tiongson J, Salen P: Mass ingestion of jimson weed by eleven teenagers. *Del Med J* 1998;70:471–476.

ANTIDEPRESSANTS

Antidepressants include the tricyclic antidepressants, monoamine oxidase (MAO) inhibitors, selective serotonin reuptake inhibitors (SSRIs), and the atypical antidepressants. Tricyclic antidepressants have a unique toxicity and are discussed on pp 439–440.

MAO inhibitors include tranylcypromine (Parnate), phenelzine (Nardil), isocarboxazid (Marplan) and selegeline (Deprenyl). The enzyme MAO degrades catecholamines in the CNS, liver, and intestine; it also degrades tyramine. Toxicity is related to enhanced catecholamine release.

SSRIs include fluoxetine (Prozac), sertraline (Zoloft), and paroxetine (Paxil). Receptor binding is relatively specific for the serotonin reuptake mechanism; therefore they have less toxicity than their predecessors.

Atypical antidepressants include bupropion (Wellbutrin, Zyban), trazadone, and nefazadone, and they have varied binding to alpha, norepinephrine, and dopamine receptors.

Clinical Presentation

Acute overdose of MAO inhibitors leads to anxiety, flushing, tremor, hyperreflexia, diaphoresis, tachycardia, tachypnea, hyperthermia, agitated delirium, and hypertension. Hypertension may be severe and may lead to intracranial hemorrhage. In severe overdoses, this initial hyperadrenergic crisis may be followed by cardiovascular collapse and multisystem failure. These toxic effects may be delayed for several hours after ingestion, so an asymptomatic patient is still at risk.

MAO inhibitors may lead to a hypertensive reaction when tyramine-rich foods are ingested, since MAO normally degrades tyramine in the intestine. If tyramine-rich foods are ingested while the patient is taking an MAO inhibitor, tyramine may build up and cause release of presynaptic norepinephrine, leading to severe hypertension and adrenergic crisis. Tyramine-rich foods include aged cheese, smoked or pickled meat, and red wine.

Serotonin syndrome may develop in patients who ingest MAO inhibitors with other medications that increase serotonin in the synapse (e.g., SSRIs, meperidine, dextromethorphan). Serotonin syndrome consists of hyperthermia, rigidity, myoclonus, autonomic instability, and mental status changes.

Acute overdose of SSRIs may cause sedation, ataxia, and nystagmus. Serotonin syndrome is possible but quite rare.

The newer, atypical antidepressants also cause sedation and ataxia. Bupropion may cause seizures, even at therapeutic doses. Trazodone may cause priapism as well as hypotension secondary to alpha blockade.

Diagnosis

Suspect an antidepressant overdose in a patient with hypertension, hyperthermia, and mental status changes. Obtain a thorough history from paramedics, and contact family members and friends.

ED Management

Assessment of the adequacy of the ABCs and vital signs is the first priority. Treat severe hypertension secondary to MAO inhibitor toxicity with phentolamine (0.02–0.1 mg/kg IV bolus, repeat q 10 min) and a beta blocker (labetalol 0.25 mg/kg IV over 2 min, repeat q 10 min). Treat hypotension from antidepressants with two fluid boluses (20 mL/kg each), followed by a norepinephrine infusion. Begin with 0.1 μg/kg/min and increase every 5 min (add a 4 mg ampule to 1 L of D_5W to make a solution of 4 μg/mL). Give activated charcoal (1 g/kg PO) to a patient who arrives within 4 h of ingestion. Admit any patient with significant MAO inhibitor ingestion to a monitored setting, because toxicity may occur up to 24 h after ingestion.

Indications for Admission

- Signs of severe toxicity (seizures, vital sign abnormalities)
- All ingestions of MAO inhibitors
- Serotonin syndrome

- Suicide attempt or gesture without psychiatric clearance and appropriate follow-up arranged

BIBLIOGRAPHY

Gill M, Lo Vecchio F, Selden B: Serotonin syndrome in a child after a single dose of fluvoxamine. *Ann Emerg Med* 1999;33:457–459.

Goeringer KE, Raymon L, Christian GD, et al: SSRI safety in overdose. *J Clin Psychiatry* 1998;59(suppl 15): 42–48.

Goeringer KE, Raymon L, Christian GD, et al: Postmortem forensic toxicology of selective serotonin reuptake inhibitors: a review of pharmacology and report of 168 cases. *J Forens Sci* 2000;45:633–648.

ANTIPSYCHOTICS

Antipsychotic medications include the phenothiazines, thiothixines, butyrophenones, and dibenzodiazepines. Drugs of these classes are widely used for the treatment of psychosis as well as emesis. The phenothiazines and butyrophenones include the older antipsychotics such as chlorpromazine (Thorazine), thioridazine (Mellaril), prochlorperazine (Compazine), and haloperidol (Haldol). Although overdose may be common with the antipsychotics, severe toxicity is rare.

Clinical Presentation and Diagnosis

The most common toxicity is a dystonic reaction, with torticollis, opisthotonos, difficulty speaking, facial grimacing, and oculogyric crisis. Onset can be delayed up to days after ingestion and spasm may wax and wane. Ingestions of phenothiazines may produce postural hypotension, sedation, seizures, and an anticholinergic picture (dry mouth, urinary retention, constipation, blurred vision, tachycardia). Massive ingestions of the atypical antipsychotics may produce sedation, myoclonus and tachycardia.

ED Management

Provide supportive care as indicated and administer activated charcoal (1 g/kg) if the ingestion has occurred within 4 h. Diphenhydramine (2 mg/kg IM or IV, 50 mg maximum) and IV or IM benztropine mesylate (toddler: 0.5–1.0 mg; child or adolescent: 1.0–2.0 mg) are both diagnostic and therapeutic for the extrapyramidal symptoms. Prescribe a 2-day course of diphenhydramine (5 mg/kg/day divided qid, 300 mg/day maximum) or benztropine mesylate (toddler: 0.5 mg bid for toddlers; child or adolescent: 1.0 mg bid) to prevent a recurrence of the symptoms.

Treat seizures with lorazepam (0.05–0.1 mg/kg slow IV) or diazepam (0.1–0.3 mg/kg slow IV). Treat orthostatic hypotension with 20 mL/kg of isotonic IV fluid. The management of an anticholinergic syndrome is detailed on pp 406–407.

Follow-up

- Dystonic reaction: next day

Indications for Admission

- Decreased level of consciousness
- Seizures or persistent hypotension
- Suicide attempt or gesture without psychiatric clearance and appropriate follow-up arranged

BIBLIOGRAPHY

Burns MJ: The pharmacology and toxicology of atypical antipsychotic agents. *Clin Toxicol* 2001;39:1–14.

Knight ME, Roberts RJ: Phenothiazine and butyrophenone intoxication in children. *Pediatr Clin North Am* 1986;33:299–309.

Stille CJ: Dystonic reaction to metoclopramide. *Pediatr Rev* 1997;18:63, 64.

BETA AGONISTS

Overdose of beta agonist drugs rarely causes significant toxicity.

Clinical Presentation

Most patients are asymptomatic. Sinus tachycardia, tremor, agitation, and hypokalemia may occur.

Diagnosis

The diagnosis is suggested by the history. There are no specific laboratory tests.

ED Management

Typically, no treatment other than reassurance is required.

Indication for Admission

- Suicide attempt or gesture without psychiatric clearance and appropriate follow-up arranged

BIBLIOGRAPHY

Lewis LD, Essex E, Volans GN, et al: A study of self-poisoning with oral salbutamol-laboratory and clinical features. *Hum Exp Toxicol* 1993;12:397–401.

Rakhmanina NY, Kearns GL, Farrar HC III: Hypokalemia in an asthmatic child from abuse of albuterol metered dose inhaler. *Pediatr Emerg Care* 1998;14:145–147.

BETA BLOCKERS

Beta adrenergic blocking drugs are widely used for the treatment of hypertension, angina, arrhythmias, migraine headaches, and various other conditions. Members of this group include propranolol, atenolol, metoprolol, nadolol, stalol, timolol, pindolol, and acebutolol. Their effect is relaxation of vascular smooth muscle and blockade of the sinus and atrioventricular cardiac nodes.

Clinical Presentation

Symptoms and signs occur within 6 h of overdose unless a delayed-release preparation has been ingested. The most common finding is a decreased heart rate, which may cause sinus, atrioventricular nodal, or ventricular bradycardia. Abnormalities on ECG may include a widened QRS interval, increased PR interval, bundle branch block, and sinus bradycardia. Possible ventricular arrhythmias include various escape rhythms, ventricular tachycardia, and torsades de pointes.

Hypotension and cardiogenic shock can occur. Patients with propranolol overdose are at particular risk for CNS manifestations, including depressed level of consciousness, delirium, coma, and seizures. Other findings are bronchospasm (particularly in patients with asthma), hyperkalemia, and hypoglycemia.

Diagnosis

Consider beta-blocker poisoning in a patient presenting with bradycardia and hypotension. Other cardiotoxic medications, such as *calcium channel blockers* and *digitalis glycosides*, may also cause bradycardia and hypotension. It is rarely necessary to determine serum levels.

ED Management

Initiate supportive care and administer a dose of activated charcoal if less than 4 h have elapsed since the ingestion. Continuously monitor the ECG and blood pressure. Obtain blood for electrolytes and glucose and treat hypotension with a 20 mL/kg bolus of an isotonic fluid (NS or Ringer's lactate). If there is no response, consult a toxicologist and pediatric cardiologist, arrange admission to a pediatric intensive care unit, and begin an isoproterenol infusion (start with 0.1 μg/kg/min and increase every 5–10 min). If isoproterenol fails, use a glucagon infusion (50–150 μg/kg over 1 min, followed by an infusion of 1–5 mg/h). Treat refractory clinically significant bradyarrhythmias with pacing. Hypoglycemia is a particular risk in children; give supplemental glucose (1–2 mL/kg of $D_{50}W$ or 2–4 mL/kg of $D_{25}W$). Correct significant hyperkalemia (>7.0: 0.1 μ/kg regular insulin plus 0.5 g/kg glucose over 30 min). Treat seizures with a lorazepam (0.05–0.1 mg/kg slow IV) or diazepam (0.1–0.3 mg/kg slow IV).

Indications for Admission

- History of beta-blocker overdose unless patient remains asymptomatic for 6 hours after ingestion and the product is not delayed-release
- Suicide attempt or gesture without psychiatric clearance and appropriate follow-up arranged

BIBLIOGRAPHY

Lifshitz M, Zucker N, Zalzstein E: Acute dilated cardiomyopathy and central nervous system toxicity following propranolol intoxication. *Pediatr Emerg Care* 1999;15:262–263.

Reith DM, Dawson AH, Epid D, et al: Relative toxicity of beta blockers in overdose. *J Toxicol Clin Toxicol* 1996; 34:273–278.

Taboulet P, Carious A, Berdeaux A, et al: Pathophysiology and management of self-poisoning with beta-blockers. *J Toxicol Clin Toxicol* 1993; 31: 531–551.

CALCIUM CHANNEL BLOCKERS

Calcium channel–blocking drugs are widely used for the treatment of angina and hypertension. Common agents include verapamil, diltiazem, and nifedipine. Life-threatening poisoning can occur, especially with verapamil. In addition, several calcium channel blockers are now available in sustained-release formulations (Calan SR, Covera HS, Cardizem CD, Carizem SR, Cartia XT, Adalat CC, and Procardia XL).

Clinical Presentation

Toxicity reflects the distribution of calcium channels in the cardiovascular system, including the sinus and atrioventricular nodes, vascular smooth muscle, and cardiac muscle. Overdose causes sinus bradycardia, atrioventricular block, and hypotension. Variable degrees of CNS depression, ranging from drowsiness to coma, may occur. Metabolic effects include hyperglycemia and lactic acidosis. Adynamic ileus can manifest as hypoactive bowel sounds. Of note, serious symptoms have occurred 12 to 18 h after ingestion of a sustained-release preparation.

Diagnosis

Consider a calcium channel blocker overdose in a patient presenting with hypotension and bradycardia. Other cardiotoxic medications, such as *beta blockers* and *digitalis glycosides*, can also cause bradycardia and hypotension.

ED Management

Initiate supportive care and administer a dose of activated charcoal if less than 4 h have elapsed since the ingestion. Continuously monitor the ECG and blood pressure and obtain blood for electrolytes, glucose, CBC, and ABG. If the patient has bradycardia or hypotension, initiate treatment immediately, because these symptoms are often refractory to therapy and are an ominous sign. Consult with a toxicologist and pediatric cardiologist and arrange pediatric ICU admission. Obtain large-bore IV access and give calcium chloride (0.2–0.25 mL/kg IV). Treat hypotension with a 20 mL/kg bolus of isotonic fluid; if there is no response, start a dopamine infusion at 2 to 10 μg/kg/min, increasing to a maximum of 50 μg/kg/min. If that fails, use a glucagon infusion (start with a 50–150-μg/kg bolus over 1 min, followed by an infusion of 1–5 mg/h). Clinically significant bradyarrhythmias that do not respond to the preceding management require pacing.

Since calcium channel blocker toxicity can be so severe, it is important to perform GI decontamination before an ileus or cardiotoxicity can develop. Initiate whole bowel irrigation (WBI) with polyethylene glycol electrolyte lavage solution (COLYTE, GoLYTELY) via a nasogastric tube. For a child less than 6 years old, the dose is 500 mL/h; for an adolescent, 1.5 to 2.0 L/h. Instill small quantities at first (adolescent: 250 mL; toddler: 50 mL), then increase the rate (adolescent 1–2 L/h; child: 0.5–1 L/h). Monitor the patient by periodically auscultating for active bowel sounds. The endpoint of WBI is a clear rectal effluent, which may take several hours to achieve. Gastric lavage and syrup of ipecac are not reliable, the latter may prevent successful WBI.

In view of the potential for a delayed onset of symptoms, admit a patient who has ingested a sustained-release calcium-channel blocker.

Indications for Admission
- History of calcium channel blocker overdose, unless the patient remains asymptomatic for 6 h after the ingestion
- History of sustained-release calcium channel blocker overdose
- Suicide attempt or gesture without psychiatric clearance and appropriate follow-up arranged

BIBLIOGRAPHY

Gleyzer A, Traub S, Hoffman RS: Acute dilated cardiomyopathy and central nervous system toxicity following propranolol intoxication. *Pediatr Emerg Care* 1999;15:262–263.
Proana L, Chiang WK, Wang RY: Calcium channel blocker overdose. *Am J Emerg Med* 1995;13:444–450.

CARBON MONOXIDE

Carbon monoxide (CO) is found in exhaust from combustion engines (automobiles, space heaters, portable gas stoves), cigarette smoke, and in smoke from fires. Carbon monoxide binds to hemoglobin 250 times more avidly than oxygen, which impairs delivery of oxygen to peripheral tissues. In addition, CO binds to myoglobin and mitochondrial cytochrome oxidase, shifts the oxygen hemoglobin dissociation curve to the left, and causes glutamate release and lipid peroxidation in the CNS.

Clinical Presentation

Symptoms of CO intoxication are nonspecific and often misdiagnosed. At low levels, headache, nausea, vomiting, and weakness occur. At higher CO levels, patients develop tachycardia, tachypnea, lethargy, coma, and seizures.

Diagnosis

Obtain a serum carboxyhemoglobin (COHb) level from a venous blood gas (arterial puncture is not necessary). Serum levels correlate poorly with symptoms but may indicate a significant exposure and therefore guide therapy. Ascertain the interval between the end of the exposure and when the level is obtained. If the interval is long or the patient was treated with oxygen before arrival in the ED, he or she may be more severely affected than the COHb level indicates.

ED Management

While waiting for the COHb level, institute treatment with 100% oxygen with a tight-fitting nonrebreathing mask. Hyperbaric oxygen therapy (HBOT) (pp 189–192) is recommended for a patient with a history of unconsciousness after exposure to CO regardless of COHb level, a history of or continued mental status change or other neurologic deficit, cardiac dysfunction or ischemia, a COHb level >25% regardless of symptoms, or for any pregnant woman with a history of CO exposure (regardless of COHb level). The only absolute contraindication to HBOT is an untreated pneumothorax. Cigarette smokers will have an elevated COHb (as high as 10%); pregnant women will have endogenous CO production from hemolysis (less than 10%); and the fetal Hb of neonates will often give false-positive COHb levels (less than 10%).

Follow-up

- Patient treated for CO poisoning: next day

Indications for Admission

- Initial COHb >25%
- Any patient requiring treatment for CO poisoning who has not returned to baseline mental status

BIBLIOGRAPHY

Knobeloch L, Jackson R: Recognition of chronic carbon monoxide poisoning. *WMJ* 1999;98:26–29.
Liebelt EL: Hyperbaric oxygen therapy in childhood carbon monoxide poisoning. *Curr Opin Pediatr* 1999;11:259–264.
Mori T, Nagai K: Carbon-monoxide poisoning presenting as an afebrile seizure. *Pediatr Neurol* 2000;22:330–331.

CAUSTICS

Alkalis frequently cause oropharyngeal injury and serious esophageal ulcerations, while acids typically burn the stomach. Consequences include esophageal perforation with mediastinitis, GI bleeding, gastric ulceration, and stricture. Acids cause coagulation necrosis, which limits penetration of the acid, while alkalis lead to liquefaction necrosis, which can spread. Liquid caustics are more likely than powdered caustics to cause esophageal and stomach burns, with minimal oral burns.

Most caustic ingestions involve alkalis, such as lye, ammonia, oven or drain cleaners, Clinitest tablets, and dishwasher detergents. Household bleach (5% sodium hypochlorite) is not a strong caustic and does not cause significant injury. Acid burns are caused by toilet bowl and drain cleaners, battery fluid, metal cleaners, and industrial acids.

Button batteries are used to power many small consumer products such as watches, pocket calculators, and hearing aids. Ingestion has the potential to cause tissue injury because of leakage of alkali and generation of an external current. For injury to occur, the battery must lodge somewhere within the GI tract. This is extremely uncommon, and most button battery ingestions are inconsequential.

Clinical Presentation

Oropharyngeal pain and drooling are common, and vomiting occasionally occurs. Findings may also include perioral burns, stridor and dyspnea, retrosternal burning, or abdominal pain.

Most patients who ingest button batteries are asymptomatic, but vomiting, abdominal pain, cramps, and bloody stools can occur at any time while the battery remains in the GI tract. Esophageal lodgment is rare because large coin-size batteries are uncommon.

Diagnosis

The presence of oropharyngeal burns does not correlate with esophageal injury, but a serious esophageal injury (second- or third-degree burn) after an alkali ingestion is unlikely in the absence of stridor, vomiting, drooling, or other serious signs. Esophageal injury occurs in approximately 10% of cases of acid ingestion, usually in association with serious gastric damage.

ED Management

A patient with vomiting, drooling, or stridor is at risk of serious esophageal injury. Obtain a CBC, type and cross-match, and a chest x-ray (mediastinal widening indicates mediastinitis). Make the patient NPO, and begin maintenance IV hydration. Do not insert a nasogastric tube or try to neutralize the caustic. Consult with an endoscopist, and arrange endoscopy within 12 to 24 h. Steroid therapy is not recommended.

A patient with a history of possible *alkali* ingestion, with or without oropharyngeal burns but without vomiting, drooling, or stridor, is at low risk of serious esophageal injury. If the chest x-ray is normal and the patient is comfortable and can drink readily, he or she can be sent home if telephone contact is possible. Arrange for immediate endoscopy if a patient who has ingested an *acid* is symptomatic or has oropharyngeal burns.

Chest and abdominal x-rays can locate an ingested button battery. Immediately refer a patient with a battery in the esophagus for endoscopic removal. If the battery is found beyond the esophagus and the patient is asymptomatic, discharge him or her with instructions to return for follow-up in 2 to 3 days.

Follow-up

- Button battery beyond the esophagus: immediately if symptoms develop; otherwise in 2 to 3 days for repeat x-ray.

Indications for Admission

- History of alkali ingestion and vomiting, drooling, or stridor
- History of acid ingestion with oropharyngeal burns, abdominal pain, or other symptoms

- Button battery ingestion with signs of perforation or symptoms of intestinal injury
- Battery lodged in the esophagus
- Battery lodged beyond the esophagus for more than 7 days
- Symptoms of intestinal injury
- Suicide attempt or gesture without psychiatric clearance and appropriate follow-up arranged

BIBLIOGRAPHY

Karjoo M: Caustic ingestion and foreign bodies in the gastrointestinal system. *Curr Opin Pediatr* 1998;10:516–522.

Lamireau T, Rebouissoux L, Denis D, et al: Accidental caustic ingestion in children: is endoscopy always mandatory? *J Pediatr Gastroenterol Nutr* 2001;33: 81–84.

Litovitz T, Schmitz BF: Ingestion of cylindrical and button batteries: an analysis of 2382 cases. *Pediatrics* 1992;89:747–757.

CHOLINERGIC INSECTICIDES

The organophosphate (malathion, parathion) and carbamate (aldicarb, propoxur) insecticides block acetylcholinesterase. The subsequent elevation of acetylcholine in the CNS and peripheral nervous system is responsible for the signs and symptoms of toxicity. Toxicity is usually associated with products formulated for use outdoors or in industrial settings; household "bug bombs" rarely cause significant toxicity, since they contain permethrins, which do not affect cholinesterase. However, cholinergic poisoning can be serious, and specific lifesaving antidotal therapy is available.

Clinical Presentation

Carbamates and organophosphates produce a clinical state of cholinergic excess. Findings include the muscarinic symptoms of salivation, lacrimation, bronchorrhea, bronchospasm, diaphoresis, diarrhea, and miosis; the typical pesticide odor may be apparent. Heart rate may be increased, decreased, or normal. Nicotinic signs and symptoms such as muscle fasciculations, weakness, and paralysis are present, as are CNS effects such as confusion, seizures, and coma. Death is usually due to respiratory failure because of respiratory muscle paralysis, increased pulmonary secretions, and bronchoconstriction. Occasionally the patient may develop hydrocarbon pneumonitis, as these pesticides are commonly formulated in hydrocarbon solutions.

ED Management

Provide supportive care and secure a stable airway. Start an IV, administer activated charcoal if the ingestion is within 4 h of presentation to the ED, and attach an ECG and pulse oximeter. Meticulous respiratory support is critical, and intubation and ventilation are often required.

Atropine therapy is antidotal. The dose is titrated against the patient's response and varies with the specific pesticide ingested. The endpoint is satisfactory gas exchange documented by pulse oximetry and ABGs. Start with 0.01 mg/kg (initial dose is 0.5 mg IV for a toddler; 1.0 mg IV for an adolescent), but be prepared to increase both size and frequency of the doses. Severe cases may require a constant atropine infusion in an ICU.

Pralidoxime is an adjunctive antidote for organophosphate and carbamate poisonings and is indicated when more than 2.0 mg of atropine is required or for nicotinic symptoms, especially muscle weakness. Never use pralidoxime alone, especially for certain carbamates. The dose, given as a bolus, is 25 to 50 mg/kg IV for a child and 1.0 to 2.0 g for an adolescent.

For cutaneous exposure, thoroughly wash the patient with soap and water. The ED staff must take care to protect themselves from exposure by wearing impervious gloves and aprons made with butyl rubber, as most hospital gloves do not prevent the penetration of hydrocarbons.

Indications for Admission

- Presence of any cholinergic clinical findings
- Suicide attempt or gesture without psychiatric clearance and appropriate follow-up arranged

BIBLIOGRAPHY

Lifshitz M, Shahak E, Sofer S: Carbamate and organophosphate poisoning in young children. *Pediatr Emerg Care* 1999;15:102–103.

Rolfsjord LB, Fjaerli HO, Meidel N, et al: Severe organophosphate poisoning in a two-year old child. *Vet Hum Toxicol* 1998; 40:222–224.

Sungur M, Guven M: Intensive care management of organophosphate insecticide poisoning. *Crit Care* 2001;5:211–215.

CLONIDINE

Small children are extremely sensitive to clonidine; toxicity has been reported after ingestion of a single tablet. Clonidine is also available as transdermal patches, which present a unique danger for toddlers; a used patch can contain the equivalent of more than 50 tablets.

Clinical Presentation and Diagnosis

Clonidine is both a peripheral and a central alpha agonist, resulting in peripheral vasoconstriction and central inhibition of sympathetic output. The latter effect usually predominates. A patient may present with the classic opiate triad of *coma, respiratory depression,* and *miosis.* Onset of symptoms can occur very soon after ingestion. Occasionally, a young child is asymptomatic at presentation and suddenly develops apnea. Hypotension is usual, but transient hypertension is occasionally seen early in the course. Hypothermia and bradycardia also occur frequently. There are no specific diagnostic findings or rapidly available tests.

ED Management

Institute supportive care and administer activated charcoal within 4 h of ingestion. Support respirations as indicated. Treat clinically significant bradycardia with atropine (0.01 mg/kg/dose, miminum dose 0.1 mg). Hypertension is usually transient and followed by hypotension, so avoid antihypertensive therapy. Treat hypotension with a fluid challenge of 20 mL/kg of isotonic crystalloid; if this fails, administer a vasopressor such as dopamine, at a rate of 2 to 5 µg/kg/min and titrate against the patient's response. IV naloxone (0.1 mg/kg/dose in children <20 kg; 2 mg/dose in children >20 kg) is variably effective; use a maximum dose of 10 mg before considering it ineffective for reversing mental status depression. However, give naloxone (0.1 mg/kg) to a patient with severe respiratory depression in an attempt to prevent tracheal intubation. Discharge the patient only if asymptomatic for at least 4 h after ingestion.

Indications for Admission

- Coma, respiratory depression, or altered vital signs
- Suicide attempt or gesture without psychiatric clearance and appropriate follow-up arranged

BIBLIOGRAPHY

Broderick-Cantwell JJ: Case study: accidental clonidine patch overdose in attention-deficit/hyperactivity disorder patients. *J Am Acad Child Adolesc Psychiatry* 1999;38:95–98.

Killian CA, Roberge RJ, Krenzelok EP, et al: "Cloniderm" toxicity: another manifestation of clonidine overdose. *Pediatr Emerg Care* 1997;13:340–341.

Nichols MH, King WD, James LP: Clonidine poisoning in Jefferson County. *Ann Emerg Med* 1997;29:511–517.

COLD MEDICINES

Ingestion of cold preparations is common among children because the products are in most households and are available in flavored elixirs. Cold medicines may include any combination of the following: antihistamines, sympathomimetics, acetaminophen, aspirin, dextromethorphan, and guaifenesin. Adolescents seeking the euphoric effects of dextromethorphan and anticholinergics may ingest cold preparations intentionally.

Clinical Presentation

Symptoms depend on the specific contents of the ingested product. Antihistamines such as diphenhydramine, chlorpheniramine, brompheniramine, and triprolidine produce sedation and anticholinergic effects. Newer "nonsedating" antihistamines such as loratadine, fexofenadine, and cetirizine have few sedative or anticholinergic effects and cause almost no toxicity. Anticholinergic symptoms include tachycardia; dilated unreactive pupils; warm, dry, and red skin; decreased bowel sounds; and urinary retention (see Table 15-5).

Sympathomimetics include phenylpropanolamine, pseudoephedrine, ephedrine, and phenylephrine. Phenylpropanolamine (no longer marketed in the United States) and phenylephrine are selective alpha agonists and may cause severe hypertension, leading to intracranial hemorrhage, reflex bradycardia, and AV block. Pseudoephedrine and ephedrine are both alpha and beta agonists and cause a sympathomimetic toxidrome with tachycardia, hypertension, dilated but reactive pupils, and diaphoresis (see Table 15-5).

Dextromethorphan is a codeine analogue that can produce ataxia, nystagmus, and hallucinations. In severe overdose, agitation, dissociation, coma, and respiratory depression may develop. Dextromethorphan can cause a false positive urine immunoassay for phencyclidine (PCP).

Diagnosis

Diagnosis is made by history. Suspect dextromethorphan ingestion in a patient with mild mental status changes and hallucinations.

ED Management

Rarely, toxicity can be severe. Tachycardia may be due to anticholinergic or sympathomimetic mechanisms, but generally no therapy is needed. Treat severe hypertension associated with phenylpropanolamine with phentolamine (0.02–0.1 mg/kg IV; repeat q 10 min as needed). Treat the reflex bradycardia secondary to phenylpropanolamine-induced hypertension by lowering the blood pressure if indicated. Do not use atropine.

See pp 406–407 for the use of physostigmine to reverse anticholinergic symptoms. Always consider occult acetaminophen poisoning, as many preparations contain this drug as an analgesic; evidence of toxicity can be confirmed only by obtaining a drug level.

Administer activated charcoal (1 g/kg PO) to a patient arriving within 4 h of ingestion.

Indications for Admission

- Severe symptoms (hypotension, seizure, sedation)
- Suicide attempt or gesture without psychiatric clearance and appropriate follow-up arranged

BIBLIOGRAPHY

Cetaruk EW, Aaron CK: Hazards of nonprescription medications. *Emerg Med Clin North Am* 1994;12:483–510.

Gunn VL, Taha SH, Liebelt EL, et al: Toxicity of over-the-counter cough and cold medications. *Pediatrics* 2001;108:e52.

Roberge RJ, Hirani KH, Rowland PL III, et al: Dextromethorphan- and pseudoephedrine-induced agitated psychosis and ataxia: case report. *J Emerg Med* 1999;17:285–288.

DIABETIC AGENTS

Diabetic agents include the sulfonylureas [acetohexamide, chlorpropamide (Diabinase), glipizide (Glucotrol), glyburide (Diabeta, Micronase, Glynase), tolazamide (Tolinase), and tolbutamide (Orinase)] and newer agents including the biguanides (metformin and phenformin), and the glitazones (rosiglitazone and pioglitazone).

The sulfonylureas cause hypoglycemia by stimulating pancreatic insulin release as well as enhancing peripheral insulin receptor sensitivity and inhibiting gluconeogenesis. Ingestion of a single pill may cause hypoglycemia in a small child.

Biguanides are unlikely to cause hypoglycemia but have been implicated in lactic acidosis. Metformin has a better safety profile than phenformin, which has been removed from the market.

The glitazones (troglitazone and pioglitazone) are also unlikely to produce hypoglycemia because they do not increase insulin release.

Clinical Presentation

Signs and symptoms of hypoglycemia include pallor, diaphoresis, tachycardia, depressed level of consciousness, and coma.

Diagnosis

Consider oral hypoglycemic ingestion in any patient with hypoglycemia. The differential diagnosis of hypoglycemia is discussed on pp 166–167.

ED Management

Immediately obtain a blood sugar (bedside and venipuncture) if there is a history of possible oral hypoglycemic ingestion. Administer activated charcoal (1g/kg), and start on IV if the patient is symptomatic. Treat hypoglycemia with 1 mL/kg of D_{50}, repeat the blood sugar determination, and give another bolus of D_{50} if hypoglycemia persists. Once the patient is awake, start PO feeds, since 1 mL of D_{50} contains only 4 Kcal, while a candy bar contains as much as 250 Kcal.

If this is unsuccessful, give octreotide to inhibit insulin secretion (25–50 μg SC). The response is usually rapid, but a repeat dose may be required in 12 to 24 h because the half-life of oral hypoglycemics is longer than that of octreotide. Glucagon has a limited effect in children because glycogen stores are minimal in this situation. Urine alkalinization to a pH of 7.0 to 8.0 with sodium bicarbonate (bolus of 1–2 mEq/kg followed by 0.5 mEq/kg/h) is effective only in chlorpropamide ingestions.

Admit normoglycemic patients with a history of significant oral sulfonylurea overdose, because delayed hypoglycemia occasionally occurs. However, do not give prophylactic IV glucose because it complicates discharge decisions; the patient must be euglycemic without sugar supplementation.

It is appropriate to discharge normoglycemic patients with a history of ingestion of a biguanide or glitazone after 4 h of observation.

Indications for Admission

- Hypoglycemia
- History of ingestion of an oral sulfonylurea agent
- Suicide attempt or gesture without psychiatric clearance and appropriate follow-up arranged

BIBLIOGRAPHY

Spiller HA: Management of sulfonylurea ingestions. *Pediatr Emerg Care* 1999; 15:227–230.

Spiller HA, Villalobos D, Krenzelok EP, et al: Prospective multicenter study of sulfonylurea ingestion in children. *J Pediatr* 1997;131:141–146.

DIGOXIN AND CARDIAC GLYCOSIDES

Ingestion of digoxin in children is uncommon and generally occurs when a child has access to an adult relative's medications. Digoxin inhibits the function of the sodium potassium–ATPase pump, leading to bradycardia, hyperkalemia, and ventricular dysrhythmias. The minimum toxic dose is about 0.1 mg/kg. Children are more resistant to the effects of digoxin than adults, so the lethal dose may be up to 20 to 50 times the daily maintenance dose. Cardiac glycosides, or digoxin-like substances, are also found in several plants (rhododendron, foxglove, oleander, lily of the valley, and red squill), but ingestion of these is very rare.

Clinical Presentation

Acute ingestion almost always results in nausea and vomiting. Headache, weakness, confusion and blurry vision may occur. Abnormalities in color vision may be reported. Seizures are rare. Severe ingestions may lead to hyperkalemia, bradycardia, hypotension, and ventricular dysrhythmias. Digoxin causes an increase in automaticity and vagal tone, which leads to bradycardia, high-degree AV block, and ventricular tachycardia and fibrillation. Cardiac toxicity may be more severe in the setting of hypokalemia, hypercalcemia, hypomagnesemia, or with concomitant quinidine use.

Diagnosis

Suspect digoxin overdose when either a previously well patient who lives with someone taking digitalis presents with an arrhythmia or a patient already taking digitalis presents with a new arrhythmia, hyperkalemia, hypotension, CNS depression, or visual disturbance.

ED Management

Give activated charcoal; obtain blood for electrolytes, calcium, and magnesium; and obtain a digoxin level at 4 h post-ingestion to avoid overtreating a predistribution level, which may be high but nontoxic. Examine an ECG for arrhythmias and a prolonged PR interval, and attach a cardiac monitor to follow changes in the rhythm. The classic digoxin-induced dysrhythmias are paroxysmal atrial tachycardia with block or bidirectional ventricular tachycardia. Other common digoxin dysrhythmias are ventricular ectopy, AV blocks, and sinus bradycardia.

Treat clinically significant bradycardia with AV or sinoatrial (SA) block with atropine, 0.01 mg/kg IV (minimum dose 0.1 mg, maximum 0.5 mg). If possible, avoid pacemaker placement, because of an increased risk of ventricular arrhythmias. For ventricular arrhythmias, give phenytoin (2 mg/kg IV slowly over 15 min), which decreases ventricular automaticity without slowing AV conduction. Lidocaine is also effective for ventricular arrhythmias (1 mg/kg IV bolus, then 20–50 μg/kg/min continuous infusion). A life-threatening arrhythmia is an indication for Fab antibody fragments (Digibind). Avoid use of the class Ia (disopyramide, quinidine, procainamide), Ic (propafenone, flecainide, encainide), II (beta blockers such as propranolol and sotalol), and IV (calcium channel blockers such as verapamil, diltiazem, nifedipine) antiarrhythmics as they decrease AV node conduction and may worsen bradycardia.

Treat hyperkalemia aggressively (>5 mEq/L) with the Fab antibody fragments as well as with conventional therapy including $D_5\frac{1}{3}$ NS with 15 mEq/L of sodium bicarbonate. Treat moderate hyperkalemia (6–8 mEq/L) with insulin (0.1 U/kg IV), 200 to 400 mg/kg of glucose IV (4–8 mL/kg of $D_5\frac{1}{2}$ NS), and Kayexalate enemas (1 g/kg); repeat every 4 h. Avoid calcium products in treating hyperkalemia because of concern for a theoretical increase in cardiotoxicity.

Fab antibody fragments specific for digoxin (Digibind) are indicated for ventricular dysrhythmias, refractory bradycardia, potassium >5.0 mEq/L, hypotension, second- or third-degree heart block, and ingestion of ≥10 mg of digoxin by an adolescent or 4 mg by a child. Be cautious in treating a patient who uses digoxin therapeutically, as eliminating the therapeutic effect of the drug by treating only mild elevations of the digoxin level may not be warranted. The dose of Fab antibody fragments is:

$$\text{Number of vials of Fab} = \text{mg ingested} \times 0.8$$

If the serum level is known, the dose is:

$$\text{Number of vials of Fab} = (\text{digoxin level in ng/mL} \times \text{weight in kg}) / 100$$

If neither the dose nor the level is known, give 10 vials empirically. If both are known, treat the level.

Indications for Admission

- Ingestion of >0.1 mg/kg
- New arrhythmia, visual disturbance, headache, CNS depression, hypotension
- Suicide attempt or gesture without psychiatric clearance and appropriate follow-up arranged

BIBLIOGRAPHY

Abad-Santos F, Carcas AJ, Ibanez C, et al: Digoxin level and clinical manifestations as determinants in the diagnosis of digoxin toxicity. *Ther Drug Monit* 2000;22:163–168.

Gittekman MA, Stephan M, Perry H: Acute pediatric digoxin ingestion. *Pediatr Emerg Care* 1999;15:359–362.

Tuncok Y, Hazan E, Oto O, et al: Relationship between high serum digoxin levels and toxicity. *Int J Clin Pharmacol Ther* 1997;35:366–368.

DRUGS OF ABUSE

Adolescents frequently overdose on drugs of abuse such as cocaine, marijuana, and heroin. In addition, teenagers use a unique group of drugs that are quite rare in other age groups, such as MDMA ("Ecstasy"), diphenhydramine, gamma-hydroxy-butyrate (GHB), ketamine, and cold medicines.

Many adolescents who are seen in the ED have taken multiple medications or attempted to commit suicide. Appropriate counseling and psychiatric evaluation are necessary.

Clinical Presentation

Sedative/Hypnotics Sedatives include the benzodiazepines, barbiturates, chloral hydrate, and GHB. These agents cause CNS depression, nystagmus, ataxia and possible respiratory depression. Pupils are generally normal or small and vital signs often remain normal.

Cannabis Cannabis, or marijuana, is the most commonly abused illicit drug in the United States. Most commonly smoked in "joints," or cigarettes, marijuana causes euphoria, conjunctival injection, orthostatic hypotension, and tachycardia. Uncommonly, patients may experience palpitations, anxiety, paranoia, and hallucinations.

Opioids Opioids include heroin, morphine, codeine, meperidine, hydromorphone, fentanyl, oxycodone, hydrocodone, dextromethorphan, and methadone. In recent years, abuse of oxycodone (generally ground up and insufflated) and dextromethorphan (in cold medications) have become popular as drugs of abuse among teenagers. Opioids bind to specific opiate receptors in the CNS and cause euphoria, CNS depression, miosis, and bradycardia. Severe intoxication may lead to coma, respiratory depression, pulmonary edema, and aspiration.

Hallucinogens Hallucinogens include lysergic acid diethylamide (LSD), phencyclidine (PCP), 3,4-methylenedioxymethamphetamine ("Ecstasy"), and mescaline (peyote) and psilocybin (hallucinogenic mushrooms or "'shrooms"). Several other methamphetamine derivatives exist and are commonly abused by teenagers such as "Eve," MDA, and PMA. These products bind to central serotonin and dopamine receptors and produce hallucinations, visual illusions, and sympathomimetic effects. Medical care is sought when a user exhibits unusual behavior or experiences a "bad trip." Rarely, severe sympathomimetic reactions, including fatal hyperthermia, can occur. PCP may cause aggressive behavior as well as seizures. MDMA causes destruction of serotoninergic neurons and may cause severe depression and memory loss for weeks or permanently.

CNS Stimulants Stimulants include cocaine and crack cocaine, amphetamines, phenylpropanolamine (no longer marketed in the United States), pseudoephedrine, phenylephrine, and ephedrine. Pseudoephedrine is commonly found in cold preparations. Phenylephrine and ephedrine are commonly found in over-the-counter weight-loss medications. Ephedra alkaloids are found in the herbal product ma huang and "natural" diet agents. These produce tachycardia, hypertension, dilated but reactive pupils, diaphoresis, hyperthermia, and agitated delirium (agitation, confusion, and paranoia). With severe intoxication, seizures, coma, arrhythmias, and myocardial infarction may become evident. Intracranial hemorrhage has been reported, particularly with phenylpropanolamine.

Diagnosis

The diagnosis is often made through information obtained from friends, family members, and the patient. If this is not possible or helpful, ask the paramedics if drug paraphernalia was found at the scene (patients from a "rave" party or club are more likely to ingest MDMA, GHB, ketamine, or cold preparations).

A thorough physical examination will provide enough information to direct therapy and disposition (Table 15-5). The patient must be fully undressed and the clothes checked for drugs or paraphernalia. Note the presence of "track marks," or fresh needle-sticks. Lethargy implies a CNS depressant or an opioid, whereas agitation suggests a CNS stimulant. Large, reactive pupils and diaphoresis imply sympathomimetic drugs. Small pupils may be seen with the sedative/hypnotics, opioids, and PCP. Paranoia and tachycardia may occur with the hallucinogens.

ED Management

The priorities in the treatment of severe intoxications are the ABCs, followed by treatment of grossly abnormal vital signs. Treat severe hyperthermia ($>40°C$, 104°F) with aggressive cooling measures (p 188) until the temperature is below 38°C (100.4°F). Drug-related hyperthermia, in contrast to environmental hyperthermia, can continue in the hospital and must be treated immediately. Hyperthermia may lead to rhabdomyolysis, myoglobinuria, renal failure, and death. If the patient has respiratory depression or is in a coma, obtain a bedside glucose evaluation and give a trial of naloxone (0.4–2.0 mg IV). If a second dose of naloxone is necessary, start a naloxone drip (two-thirds of the bolus dose per hour). Doses up to 2 mg are generally effective, but up to 10 mg may be necessary for some opioids, particularly propoxyphene. Naloxone may precipitate acute withdrawal, but this is not life-threatening and occurs only in chronic abusers. Be prepared for a potentially combative patient; do not treat withdrawal with opioids, as the withdrawal symptoms will resolve over 30 min to 1 h.

Although flumazenil is a benzodiazepine antagonist, it is not recommended in the overdose setting because it may induce seizures in patients who coingest epileptogenic medications or are chronic benzodiazepine abusers. Safer therapy is careful observation and endotracheal intubation if necessary. Infants and children are less likely to be habituated to benzodiazepines, and flumazenil may be used more safely in the setting of an established benzodiazepine overdose in this population.

Treat seizures with lorazepam (0.05–0.1 mg/kg slow IV) or diazepam (0.1–0.3 mg/kg slow IV). If necessary, sedate the patient with benzodiazepines (diazepam or lorazepam, p 474). In PCP ingestions, haloperidol (5 mg IM) is a useful adjunct.

Gastric decontamination with orogastric lavage and activated charcoal may be useful in certain situations. Multiple doses of charcoal (1 g/kg PO q 3 h for four doses) may help decrease the serum level of phenobarbital by adsorbing drug from the enterohepatic and enteroenteric circulation. Urinary alkalinization (p 437) will increase renal excretion of phenobarbital after overdose.

Indications for Admission

- CNS or respiratory depression
- Ventricular arrhythmia
- Opiate overdose requiring naloxone treatment
- Suspected opiate or CNS depressant withdrawal
- Suicide attempt or gesture without psychiatric clearance and appropriate follow-up arranged

BIBLIOGRAPHY

Schwartz RH, Miller NS: MDMA (Ecstasy) and the rave: a review. *Pediatrics* 1997;100:705–708.

Shannon M, Albers G, Burkhart K, et al: Safety and efficacy of flumazenil in the reversal of benzodiazepine-induced conscious sedation. The Flumazenil Pediatric Study. *J Pediatr* 1997;131:582–586.

Suner S, Szlatenyi CS, Wang RY: Pediatric gamma hydroxybutyrate intoxication. *Acad Emerg Med* 1997;4:1041–1045.

ETHANOL

Ethanol is a commonly abused drug and is the most common coingestant in suicidal ingestions. Ethanol is found in alcoholic beverages as well as colognes, after-shaves, food flavorings (vanilla extract), mouthwash, and some medicinal preparations.

Clinical Presentation

Mild intoxication causes euphoria, ataxia, nystagmus, nausea, and aggressive behavior. Moderately intoxicated patients may have aggressive behavior, vomiting, and slurred speech. With severe intoxication, patients may develop respiratory depression, aspiration, miosis, hypothermia, coma, seizures, and rhabdomyolysis. Young children are at high risk of hypoglycemia.

Diagnosis

The diagnosis is usually made by history. The smell of alcohol may be present on the patient's clothing and breath. Consider ethanol intoxication in any patient with nystagmus, ataxia, confusion, or sedation. However, sedation may be from other sedative/hypnotic medications like *benzodiazepines* or *barbiturates*, and these drugs are often coingestants.

Obtain an ethanol level if alcohol toxicity is suspected. Ethanol levels correlate loosely with intoxication. However, experienced drinkers can tolerate higher levels of ethanol without symptoms.

ED Management

Management of the intoxicated patient depends on the severity of intoxication. If there is CNS depression, give naloxone (0.1 mg/kg, up to 2.0 mg) and obtain a bedside glucose elevation. Protect the airway (if necessary), secure IV access, obtain serum electrolytes, CBC, and a serum ethanol level, and give a dextrose-containing fluid. Gastric decontamination is generally ineffective and therefore not indicated.

A patient who is mildly intoxicated requires an ethanol level for confirmation, a careful physical examination to rule out organic causes of confusion (such as head injury), and observation, with frequent reassessments, until the mental status has returned to baseline. The mental status of an intoxicated patient gradually and consistently improves. However, obtain a CT scan of the head if the mental status does not improve, the ethanol level is inconsistent with the mental status, or there are signs of head trauma. An intoxicated patient is at higher risk for falls; therefore the mental status changes attributed to alcohol may represent intracranial pathology.

The observation may be performed at home if the parents are reliable and the patient is alert.

Indications for Admission

- Intoxicated preadolescent with an unstable home environment
- Alcohol level >250 mg/dL
- Focal neurologic findings
- Suicide attempt or gesture without psychiatric clearance and appropriate follow-up arranged

BIBLIOGRAPHY

Lamminpaa A: Alcohol intoxication in childhood and adolescence. *Alcohol* 1995; 30:5–12.

Lamminpaa A, Vilska J, Korri UM, et al: Alcohol intoxication in hospitalized young teenagers. *Acta Paediatr* 1999;82:783–788.

Tovey C, Rana PS, Anderson DJ: Alcohol intoxication in a toddler. *J Accid Emerg Med* 1998;15:69–70.

TOXIC ALCOHOLS (ETHYLENE GLYCOL, METHANOL, AND ISOPROPANOL)

The toxic alcohols include ethylene glycol, methanol, and isopropanol, as well as benzyl alcohol and propylene glycol. Ethylene glycol can be found in antifreeze (up to 95%) and is generally ingested unintentionally by children because of its sweet taste. Methanol is found in solvents, windshield-wiper fluid, and duplicating fluids. Isopropanol is the main ingredient in rubbing alcohol (70%) and is also found in solvents and disinfectants.

These alcohols may be ingested unintentionally by children or as an alcohol substitute by adolescents. All three cause intoxication similar to that from ethanol, as well as gastritis. Isopropanol is metabolized to acetone, a CNS depressant, and produces toxicity similar to that due to ethanol in children. Methanol is metabolized to formic acid and ethylene glycol is metabolized to glycolic, glyoxylic, and oxalic acids. These "toxic metabolites" may produce an anion-gap metabolic acidosis, which can lead to renal failure and death.

Clinical Presentation and Diagnosis

Ethylene glycol toxicity occurs in two distinct stages. Within the first 3 to 4 h, there is inebriation, with ataxia, nystagmus, nausea, and euphoria. At this stage, the ethylene glycol level is high and the osmolar gap is elevated, but there is no acidosis. As the ethylene glycol is metabolized into toxic metabolites, the patient develops an anion-gap metabolic acidosis leading to tachypnea, tachycardia, hypotension, renal failure, cerebral and pulmonary edema, and seizures. In this acidemic stage, the ethylene glycol levels and the osmolar gap may be lower, but acidosis is present.

Methanol produces a similar two-stage toxicity. The initial intoxication is not as pronounced as with ethylene glycol or ethanol. As the methanol is metabolized, an anion-gap metabolic acidosis develops, with tachypnea, tachycardia, visual changes, blindness, seizures, and death.

Isopropyl alcohol produces a more pronounced inebriation than that due to ethanol. In the first few hours, euphoria, nausea, and vomiting predominate. Laboratory studies reveal an elevated osmolar gap without metabolic acidosis. Metabolism of isopropanol to acetone leads to CNS depression and a distinctive ketone odor.

ED Management

Lethal oral doses of ethylene glycol and methanol-containing compounds are very small, approximately 1.5 mL/kg. For any potential ingestion, obtain a CBC, electrolytes, ethanol, measured osmolality, and, if possible, a specific alcohol level. Calculate the osmolality and subtract it from the measured osmolality to determine the osmolar gap (p 400). Elevation of the osmolar gap may be indicative of a toxic alcohol ingestion, but it can also be secondary to ethanol, IV contrast (osmotic contrast), mannitol, acetone, ketoacidosis, or chronic (not acute) renal failure. If the laboratory is unable to perform levels of the specific toxic alcohols, approximate them by multiplying the osmolar gap by the following conversion factors: ethanol, 4.6; ethylene glycol, 6.2; isopropyl alcohol, 6.0; and methanol, 3.2. For example, if the osmolar gap is 20, the estimated ethylene glycol level is 124 mg/dL.

Treatment of methanol and ethylene glycol toxicity involves blocking the production and enhancing the clearance of toxic metabolites. Hemodialysis is the mainstay of therapy, allowing clearance of both the alcohol and the acidosis. Gastric decontamination is generally not beneficial, because alcohols are rapidly absorbed. Sodium bicarbonate may be used to treat the metabolic acidosis if the pH is <7.2.

Inhibiting the enzyme alcohol dehydrogenase with either ethanol or fomepizole blocks production of the toxic metabolites. Indications for ethanol or fomepizole are suspicion of methanol or ethylene glycol ingestion with one of the following: methanol or ethylene glycol >20 mg/dL, an osmolar gap >10 mosm/L, and a metabolic acidosis. Indications for hemodialysis are methanol or ethylene glycol >40 mg/dL, an osmolar gap >20 mosm/L, renal failure, or metabolic acidosis.

To treat with ethanol, use a 10% solution and give an IV loading dose of 10 mL/kg, followed by 1 to 2 mL/kg/h. An ethanol level of 100 mg/dL is sufficient to block most of the metabolite production. Serum ethanol levels and bedside glucose checks must be performed frequently. Ethanol may also be given via nasogastric tube, but this can cause a severe gastritis.

Fomepizole also blocks alcohol dehydrogenase and is approved by the FDA for the treatment of both methanol and ethylene glycol ingestions in adults. Its advantages are that there are no levels to monitor, and it does not cause gastritis or hypoglycemia. The loading dose is 15 mg/kg IV over 30 min, followed by 10 mg/kg q 12 h for four doses. The dosing must be adjusted during hemodialysis to allow for clearance of fomepizole.

Indications for Admission

- Toxic levels of ethylene glycol, methanol, or isopropanol
- CNS depression, nausea, hypoglycemia, tachycardia, or other serious symptoms of alcohol ingestion
- Suicide attempt or gesture without psychiatric clearance and appropriate follow-up arranged

BIBLIOGRAPHY

Barceloux DG, Krenzelek EP, Olson K, et al: American Academy of Clinical Toxicology Practice Guidelines on the Treatment of Ethylene Glycol Poisoning. Ad hoc Committee. *J Toxicol Clin Toxicol* 1999;37:537–560.

Brent J, McMartin K, Phillips S, et al: Fomepizole for the treatment of ethylene glycol poisoning. Methylpyrazole for toxic alcohols study group. *N Engl J Med* 1999;340:832–838.

Shannon M: Toxicology reviews: fomepizole—a new antidote. *Pediatr Emerg Care* 1998;14:170–172.

HYDROCARBONS

Hydrocarbons are organic compounds such as camphor, motor oil, gasoline, kerosene, mineral seal oil, pine oil, phenol, carbon tetrachloride, and naphtha. The main toxicity of hydrocarbons is aspiration pneumonitis, which can occur with all products except those with very high viscosity (motor oil and petroleum jelly). The halogenated and aromatic hydrocarbons can cause systemic toxicity including coma, seizures, and arrhythmias. Pine oil may produce severe CNS depression and carbon tetrachloride may cause hepatotoxicity.

Clinical Presentation

Most patients who ingest hydrocarbons are asymptomatic. CNS depression may occur within the first few hours. Pulmonary symptoms consistent with chemical pneumonitis (cough, tachypnea, hypoxia, and dyspnea) may be delayed up to 4 to 6 h. Hepatotoxicity from carbon tetrachloride develops over several days.

Diagnosis

Determine the type of hydrocarbon ingested. Have a family member return home and bring the container to the ED. If the chemical is unfamiliar, call the Poison Control Center or the manufacturer for assistance.

ED Management

Once the specific hydrocarbon has been identified, a decision must be made whether to perform gastric decontamination. In general, gastric lavage or activated charcoal is rarely necessary for pediatric hydrocarbon ingestions. Gastric lavage is indicated for ingestions of more than 1 mL/kg of a hydrocarbon that has significant systemic toxicity. A mnemonic to identify when gastric decontamination is recommended is CHAMP: *C*amphor, *H*alogenated hydrocarbons (carbon tetrachloride), *A*romatic (benzene, phenol), *M*etals (lead, selenium, cadmium, iron), and *P*esticides. Do not induce emesis or perform gastric lavage if the hydrocarbon does not have significant systemic toxicity because of the high risk of aspiration chemical pneumonitis.

The type of hydrocarbon ingested is a useful determinant in predicting toxicity. Wood-derived hydrocarbons such as pine oil can cause pulmonary edema and pneumonitis without aspiration because they are absorbed in the GI tract. Petroleum-derived hydrocarbons such as gasoline do not have this property. Therefore it is usually safer to leave them undisturbed in the GI tract, as discussed above.

Observe the patient for CNS depression, seizures, and respiratory complaints for 4 to 6 h. If symptoms occur, admit the patient. Obtain a chest radiograph only if the patient develops respiratory symptoms; a baseline chest radiograph is not necessary for an asymptomatic patient.

Inhalation or ingestion of hydrocarbons with systemic toxicity may lead to a sensitization of myocardial cells to catecholamines. Therefore continuously monitor the ECG and avoid catecholamines, such as epinephrine, if possible.

Indications for Admission

- Ingestion of hydrocarbons with significant systemic toxicity, such as heavy metals, insecticides, aniline dyes, pine oil, and camphor
- Pulmonary signs or symptoms
- Suicide attempt or gesture without psychiatric clearance and appropriate follow-up arranged

BIBLIOGRAPHY

Flanagan RJ, Ruprah M, Meredith TJ, et al: An introduction to the clinical toxicology of volatile substances. *Drug Saf* 1990;5:359–383.

Mekinda Z, Azad M, Alard S, et al: Acute hydrocarbon pneumonia. *JBR-BTR* 2000;83:18.

Vale JA: Position statement: gastric lavage. American Academy of Clinical Toxicology; European Association of Poisons Centers and Clinical Toxicologists. *J Toxicol Clin Toxicol* 1997;35:711–719.

INHALANTS

Inhalation of solvents has become popular among adolescents because these substances are ubiquitous and inexpensive. Examples of volatile inhalants include toluene (found in model glue and spray paints), trichloroethane (found in typewriter correction fluid and spot removers), and nitrates (found in incense and used as aphrodisiacs).

Clinical Presentation

Inhalation produces rapid euphoria and light-headedness and may cause CNS depression or hallucinations. Hydrocarbon inhalation can lead to sensitization of the myocardium to catecholamines, leading to arrhythmias and "sudden sniffing death." However, the myocardium is sensitized to catecholamines for approximately 5 to 15 min after inhalation, so this is generally not a concern in the ED.

Diagnosis

An inhalant abuser rarely arrives in the ED with complaints involving the inhalation. Occasionally a novice user will complain of transient light-headedness or a patient will show evidence of abuse, such as spray paint on the skin around the nose. Consider inhalant abuse in an adolescent with ventricular arrhythmias or sudden cardiac arrest.

ED Management

Supportive care and education is all that is necessary.

Indications for Admission

- Ventricular arrhythmias
- Suicide attempt or gesture without psychiatric clearance and appropriate follow-up arranged

BIBLIOGRAPHY

Committee on Substance Abuse and Committee on Native American Child Health: inhalant abuse. *Pediatrics* 1996;97:420–422.

McGarvey EL, Clavet GJ, Mason W, et al: Adolescent inhalant abuse: environments of use. *Am J Drug Alcohol Abuse* 1999;25:731–741.

Young SJ, Lengstaff S, Tenenbein M: Inhalant abuse and the abuse of other drugs. *Am J Drug Alcohol Abuse* 1999;25:371–375.

IRON

Iron is the leading cause of fatal poisoning in children. It is readily available for the treatment of anemia and in prenatal and multivitamins. Most adult iron formulations contain 60 to 90 mg of elemental iron per pill, and children's formulations generally contain 12 to 18 mg per pill. Ferrous gluconate is 12% elemental iron (32 mg Fe per 325 mg tablet), ferrous fumarate is 33% (100 mg Fe per 325 mg tablet), and ferrous sulfate is 20% (65 mg Fe per 325 mg tablet). Most pediatric multivitamins have 4 to 15 mg of elemental iron per tablet.

Clinical Presentation

Iron toxicity results from both direct GI injury and diffuse cellular toxicity; it presents in five stages. In the initial phase (first 6 h), GI symptoms predominate, with vomiting, hematemesis, abdominal pain, diarrhea, and hematochezia. During the next few hours, there may be a period in which the symptoms abate (stage II). During the third stage, at 6 to 24 h after ingestion, systemic toxicity occurs, sometimes followed by severe hepatotoxicity (stage IV). Signs and symptoms include hypotension, hepatic failure, shock, seizures, metabolic acidosis, coagulopathy, and hyperglycemia. Stage V is gastric outlet or intestinal stricture, which may occur 4 to 6 weeks after the ingestion.

Diagnosis

The diagnosis of iron overdose is easily overlooked if the history does not suggest the possibility of ingestion. *Gastroenteritis*, especially from *Salmonella* and *Shigella*, and *acute hepatitis* are common misdiagnoses.

Clinically significant iron toxicity is possible if the history suggests that more than 20 mg/kg of elemental iron was ingested or the patient is symptomatic (abdominal pain, vomiting, or diarrhea). Obtain a serum iron concentration at the expected peak, 2 to 6 h after ingestion. The peak iron level predicts toxicity, but the total iron-binding capacity is not a reliable marker.

Elevation of the white blood cell count >15,000/mm^3 and glucose >150 mg/dL often occur in patients who are iron-toxic but cannot be used to rule out toxicity. Abdominal radiographs may help to identify pills that are radiopaque; however, x-rays are normal in a patient who has ingested liquid or children's formulations.

ED Management

When it is absolutely certain that an asymptomatic patient has ingested <20 mg/kg, he or she may be discharged to reliable parents. For all other patients, obtain an abdominal radiograph and serum iron level.

If a significant number of tablets are seen on the radiograph, decontaminate the gut by whole-bowel irrigation (WBI) with polyethylene glycol electrolyte lavage solution (COLYTE, GoLYTELY), using a nasogastric tube. See pp 401–402 for the procedure for using WBI. Contraindications to WBI include an unprotected airway in a comatose patient, ileus, or GI obstruction, perforation, or significant hemorrhage. Gastric lavage and syrup of ipecac are not reliable, and the latter may prevent successful WBI. Activated charcoal does not adsorb iron significantly and is not recommended unless there is a coingestant. Oral deferoxamine, sodium bicarbonate, and phosphate lavage are unsafe.

Provide supportive care as indicated. Start an IV, and pay special attention to perfusion and acid-base status. Large amounts of IV fluid and bicarbonate are frequently required.

Obtain a serum iron level 2 to 6 h after ingestion; if it is >500 μg/dL, initiate deferoxamine therapy (15 mg/kg/h IV, 6.0 g/day maximum). Other indications for deferoxamine therapy include shock, intractable vomiting, or severe acidosis. Correct intravascular volume deficits before instituting chelation therapy, because deferoxamine in the presence of decreased renal blood flow can lead to acute renal failure. Obtain blood for a CBC, electrolytes, coagulation profile, BUN, creatinine, liver function tests, and type and hold before instituting chelation therapy.

Indications for Admission

- Serum iron >500 μg/dL
- Signs or symptoms of iron toxicity
- Suicide attempt or gesture without psychiatric clearance and appropriate follow-up arranged

BIBLIOGRAPHY

Fine JS: Iron poisoning. *Curr Probl Pediatr* 2000;30:71–90.
McGuigan MA: Acute iron poisoning. *Pediatr Ann* 1996;25:33–38.
Moris CC: Pediatric iron poisonings in the United States. *South Med J* 2000;93: 352–358.

MOTHBALLS

Mothballs can be composed of two different chemicals, *para*-dichlorobenzene, which is relatively nontoxic, and naphthalene, which can cause sedation and seizures as well as severe hemolysis in G-6-PD–deficient patients.

Clinical Presentation

In most cases the patient is asymptomatic. However, a patient who ingests naphthalene may develop lethargy, sedation, and seizures within hours of ingestion. The onset of hemolysis in a G-6-PD–deficient patient may be delayed for up to 24 to 48 h. Weakness, pallor or jaundice, dark urine, and oliguria may occur.

Diagnosis

When the chemical nature of the mothball is unknown, try dissolving a sliver in absolute ethanol: para-dichlorobenzene (nontoxic) dissolves, while naphthalene does not. In addition, an x-ray of the mothball can differentiate the two, as para-dichlorobenzene is radiopaque whereas naphthalene is not. Another method for identifying the type of mothball is to get a large amount of salt and make a concentrated salt solution. Naphthalene mothballs float in this solution, but para-dichlorobenzene does not.

Hemolysis can be documented with serial hematocrit determinations (decreasing), the peripheral smear (fragmented red cells), and a urinalysis (dipstick positive for blood and bilirubin but no RBCs seen). If the patient is symptomatic, a low level on a G-6-PD quantitative assay (not a qualitative screen) confirms that the child is at risk. In the presence of hemolysis, young RBCs, which do contain G-6-PD enzyme, predominate, so a qualitative screen may be falsely reassuring.

ED Management

Give activated charcoal and determine the patient's G-6-PD status if the mothball contains naphthalene or if the ingredients are unknown. If the mothball is known to be para-dichlorobenzene, then charcoal and gastric decontamination are not necessary. For asymptomatic patients, no further workup is needed. Instruct the family to return at once if pallor, jaundice, lethargy, or dark urine is noticed. If sedation or seizures develop, admit the patient to a monitored setting for supportive care and close observation.

If the patient is symptomatic, obtain a CBC, type and cross-match, urinalysis, electrolytes, BUN, and creatinine. If hemoglobinuria is present, institute alkaline diuresis with $D_5\frac{1}{2}$ NS and sodium bicarbonate (1 mEq/kg q 4 h, infused over 30 min) to maintain a urine output of 3 to 6 mL/kg/h, using furosemide (1 mg/kg IV) if necessary. Give small transfusions (5 mL/kg) of packed red cells to maintain the hematocrit at about 80% of normal.

Indications for Admission

- Suspected naphthalene ingestion in a patient known to be G-6-PD–deficient
- Sedation
- Seizures
- Evidence of intravascular hemolysis
- Suicide attempt or gesture without psychiatric clearance and appropriate follow-up arranged

BIBLIOGRAPHY

Santucci K, Shah B: Association of naphthalene with acute hemolytic anemia. *Acad Emerg Med* 2000;7:42–47.

Weintraub E, Gandhi D, Robinson C: Medical complications due to mothball abuse. *South Med J* 2000;93:427–429.

NONSTEROIDAL (NONSALICYLATE) ANTI-INFLAMMATORY DRUGS

Nonsteroidal anti-inflammatory drugs (NSAIDs) are widely used for the treatment of pain, arthritis, and dysmenorrhea. Among the many agents in this category, ibuprofen and naproxen are nonprescription, and ibuprofen is readily available as a pleasant-tasting liquid.

NSAIDs inhibit cyclooxygenase, thereby decreasing prostaglandin synthesis and thus inflammation. However, inhibition of prostaglandin synthesis and elevation of leukotriene synthesis may also disrupt the gastric mucosa and decrease renal blood flow, leading to toxicity. Nonetheless, overdoses of NSAIDs rarely produce serious consequences.

Clinical Presentation

Mild symptoms such as epigastric pain, nausea, and vomiting are the rule, although lethargy and drowsiness sometimes occur. Very large overdoses of ibuprofen can result in metabolic acidosis. Mefenamic acid, oxyphenbutazone, phenylbutazone, and piroxicam overdose can cause seizures and metabolic acidosis.

Diagnosis

The history suggests the diagnosis. Elevation of liver transaminases, metabolic acidosis, and hypoprothrombinemia may occur with massive overdoses of ibuprofen, mefenamic acid, and the enolic acids (oxyphenbutazone, phenylbutazone, and piroxicam).

ED Management

Typically, no interventions are required unless very large amounts (>400 mg/kg for ibuprofen) have been ingested. In such a case, administer activated charcoal, monitor the level of consciousness, and obtain an ABG. Treat seizures secondary to mefenamic acid and the enolic acids with lorazepam (0.05–0.10 mg/kg slow IV) or diazepam (0.1–0.3 mg/kg slow IV).

Indications for Admission

- Decreased level of consciousness, metabolic acidosis, or seizures
- Suicide attempt or gesture without psychiatric clearance and appropriate follow-up arranged

BIBLIOGRAPHY

Kim J, Gazarian M, Verjee Z, et al: Acute renal insufficiency in ibuprofen overdose. *Pediatr Emerg Care* 1995;11:107–108.
Wolfe TR: Ibuprofen overdose. *Am J Emerg Med* 1995;13:375.
Zecca TC: Management of ibuprofen overdose. *Pediatr Rev* 1997;18:107.

RAT POISON

The vast majority of commercial rat poisons are long-acting warfarin-like (superwarfarin) products such as brodifacoum, although, historically, rat poisons have been made of arsenic, thallium, strychnine, red squill and other compounds. Newer poisons that are still in use include bromethaline and zinc phosphide in industrial settings. In view of the varied toxicity of this eclectic group of compounds, it is crucial to identify the rat poison ingested when one is evaluating a poisoned patient.

The long-acting warfarin products inhibit hepatic synthesis of the vitamin K–dependent coagulation factors (II, VII, IX, and X). Anticoagulation occurs approximately 2 to 3 days after ingestion, as new synthesis is impared but existing functional factors remain. As the existing factors are consumed, elevation of the prothrombin time and International Normalized Ratio (INR) occurs.

Clinical Presentations

Most patients who ingest one of the superwarfarin products are asymptomatic on presentation and remain asymptomatic. However, significant toxicity is more common in a small child, who may be able to ingest enough poison to produce anticoagulation.

If ingestion was days prior to presentation, there may be bleeding problems, such as ecchymosis, bleeding gums, melena, hematemesis, or hematuria.

Overdose experience with bromethaline is extremely limited, but it has caused cardiovascular collapse in laboratory animals.

Diagnosis

The diagnosis is generally made by history. Send a family member to retrieve the product, as identification of the product is absolutely necessary.

ED Management

If the product is confirmed as a superwarfarin product and the ingestion was recent (<4 h), give activated charcoal (1 g/kg PO). There is no need to obtain blood tests. Discharge the patient and arrange for follow-up in 48 h for a coagulation profile. Instruct the family to return earlier for any bleeding problems.

If the patient develops a coagulopathy, give vitamin K_1, 10 mg/day divided q 6 to 8 h. Increase the dose as needed, up to 125 mg/day, to maintain a normalized INR. The vitamin K_1 may be needed for more than 1 month. If the INR >9.0 or there is evidence of severe bleeding, give fresh frozen plasma (FFP).

Follow-up

- 48 h after a significant ingestion, for coagulation studies

Indications for Admission

- Coagulopathy
- Suicide attempt or gesture without psychiatric clearance and appropriate follow-up arranged

BIBLIOGRAPHY

Chia JD, Friedenberg WR: Superwarfarin poisoning. *Arch Intern Med* 1998;28: 158:1929–1932.

Mullins ME, Brands CL, Daya MR: Unintentional pediatric superwarfarin exposures: do we really need a prothrombin time? *Pediatrics* 2000;105:402–404.

Travis SF, Warfield W, Greenbaum BH, et al: Spontaneous hemorrhage associated with accidental brodifacoum poisoning in a child. *J Pediatr* 1993;122:982–984.

SALICYLATES

Aspirin (acetylsalicylic acid) is in many nonprescription analgesics and cold preparations. In addition, the active ingredient in the skin liniment, oil of wintergreen, is methylsalicylate (7.0 g/5 mL). The acute toxic dose is 150 mg/kg, or about two baby aspirin tablets per kilogram. A large number of salicylate tablets can form a concretion in the GI tract, resulting in prolonged absorption and toxicity. Chronic overmedication and sustained-release preparations can cause more serious toxicity at a lower serum level.

Clinical Presentation

Mild poisoning causes tinnitus, abdominal pain, vomiting, and hyperpnea (respiratory alkalosis). With larger doses, marked hyperpnea, fever, lethargy, dehydration, metabolic acidosis, and hypo- or hyperglycemia occur. Severe poisoning leads to coma, seizures, severe metabolic acidosis, oliguria, pulmonary edema, and death. An unusual presentation is acute behavior change, including confusion, agitation, hallucinations, or psychosis.

Diagnosis

In the past, the Done nomogram was used to predict toxicity in an acute ingestion, but it is now considered unreliable. The minimum toxic level at 6 h is 45 mg/dL; 65 mg/dL causes a moderate poisoning, 90 mg/dL is serious, and 120 mg/dL is often lethal. However, toxicity is unlikely at any level in the absence of signs of metabolic acidosis, especially hyperpnea.

An ABG and serum electrolytes will demonstrate a respiratory alkalosis early after overdose. In toddlers, an increased anion-gap acidosis may develop at the same time or slightly later, and hypo- or hyperglycemia may occur. Adolescents usually present with signs of metabolic acidosis.

Salicylate poisoning can be confused clinically with *diabetic ketoacidosis* (glucose usually >300 mg/dL, polyuria), *influenza* (myalgias, symptoms of upper respiratory infection), *pneumonia* (rales, infiltrate on chest x-ray), *gastroenteritis* (diarrhea more common), *ketotic hypoglycemia* (starvation, no acid-base disturbance unless postictal), *Reye's syndrome* (elevated serum ammonia), or a *primary neuropsychiatric disturbance*. Other causes of an increased anion gap are (the mnemonic MUDPILES) *methanol poisoning, uremia, DKA, paraldehyde, phenformin, iron, isoniazid, ethanol* and *ethylene glycol poisoning*, and *lactic acidosis* (shock, idiopathic).

ED Management

Provide supportive care as needed, administer activated charcoal (<4 h of ingestion, or anytime if there are symptoms of delayed gastric emptying of the salicylate), secure an IV, and obtain blood for ABG, electrolytes, glucose, a salicylate level, PT, and CBC. Also obtain a salicylate level at 6 h postingestion. Consider the possibility of coingestion of acetaminophen, and obtain a level at 4 h postingestion or with the 6-h salicylate level (see Acetaminophen, pp 402–404).

If the patient has an altered mental status, give 0.5 g/kg of dextrose IV and maintain the serum glucose level at approximately 150 mg/dL. If the patient is dehydrated or in shock, give a bolus of 20 mL/kg of isotonic crystalloid (NS or Ringer's lactate). If adequate urine output (1 mL/kg/h) is not established, give a second bolus. Once there is satisfactory urine output, infuse D_5W with 132 mEq/L bicarbonate and 20 to 40 mEq/L of potassium chloride (add three 50-mL ampules of sodium bicarbonate solution to 1 L of D_5W) at twice the maintenance rate. The goal is a urine output of 3 mL/kg/h with a pH ≥ 7.5. Salicylate reabsorption in the kidney tubules is inhibited at an alkaline urine pH, so the ionic form of salicylate is "trapped" in the urine. Begin treatment before the 6-h salicylate level is obtained.

Carefully monitor the serum potassium, since it is lowered by both sodium bicarbonate administration and hyperventilation. A serum potassium in the high normal range is necessary for achieving an alkaline diuresis, otherwise hydrogen ions will acidify the urine in exchange for retaining potassium.

Hemodialysis is indicated for an acute salicylate level >100 mg/dL, severe acidosis, oliguria or anuria, pulmonary edema, intractable seizures, or progressive deterioration despite appropriate therapy regardless of the salicylate level. Hemodialysis may be indicated for chronic toxicity with a serum level >60 mg/dL in association with lethargy, mental status changes, or acidosis. Multiple doses of activated charcoal (1 g/kg q 3 h × 4) may decrease serum half-life but is not as effective as hemodialysis. If hemodialysis is not available, exchange transfusion is an alternative.

Avoid mechanical ventilation if possible. A salicylate-toxic patient compensates for metabolic acidosis with significant tachypnea. Decreasing the respiratory rate to "normal" with mechanical ventilation may lead to severe acute acidosis, seizures, arrest, and death. If intubation is necessary, pretreat with boluses of bicarbonate and set the ventilator to a high respiratory rate.

Indications for Admission

- Salicylate level >45 mg/dL 6 h after an acute ingestion
- Signs and symptoms of salicylism in a patient taking salicylates chronically
- Suicide attempt or gesture without psychiatric clearance and appropriate follow-up arranged

BIBLIOGRAPHY

Candy JM, Morrison C, Paton RD, et al: Salicylate toxicity masquerading as malignant hyperthermia. *Paediatr Anaesth* 1998;8:421–423.

Chan TY: The risk of severe salicylate poisoning following the ingestion of topical medicaments or aspirin. *Postgrad Med J* 1996;72:109–112.

Ishihara K, Szerlip HM: Anion gap acidosis. *Semin Nephrol* 1998;18:83–97.

THEOPHYLLINE

Theophylline is a methylxanthine used in the treatment of asthma, neonatal apnea, and congestive heart failure. It enhances catecholamine release and inhibits phosphodiesterase. There are numerous, usually sustained-release preparations that contain theophylline (Theo-dur, Slo-bid, Theo-bid).

While the therapeutic range is 10 to 20 mg/L, there is little risk of life-threatening toxicity after acute overdose until a serum level of 80 mg/L is reached. The minimum toxic dose of theophylline is about 20 mg/kg.

Clinical Presentation

Vomiting, agitation, tremors, and tachycardia are possible with a therapeutic serum level. Large doses can cause SVT, PVCs, ventricular tachycardia, hypertension, seizures, and coma. The more serious clinical findings rarely occur without any preceding minor symptoms; the seizures may be particularly difficult to treat and can develop into status epilepticus.

Diagnosis

If a theophylline overdose is suspected, obtain a serum level. In general, the peak level occurs within 3 to 4 h after ingestion. However, if a sustained-release preparation is ingested, the serum level may continue to rise for up to 12 to 16 h or more. Obtain serial levels every 2 h until it is clear that the level is decreasing.

ED Management

Provide supportive care as needed, secure an IV, obtain blood for a theophylline level, and continuously monitor the heart rate and rhythm. If there are active bowel sounds, give activated charcoal (1 g/kg PO q 3 h) to decrease the serum theophylline level. Add sorbitol to the first dose of charcoal, and treat vomiting with an antiemetic (metoclopramide s0.1 mg/kg IV).

Charcoal hemoperfusion, performed in an ICU, is the treatment of choice for a patient with a severely elevated level, coma, seizures, or a severe arrhythmia (ventricular tachycardia). The level at which charcoal hemoperfusion is recommended depends on the patient's age and history of chronic theophylline therapy. In children without a history of theophylline use, a level of 80 mg/L is an indication. If hemoperfusion is unavailable, give multiple-dose activated charcoal and schedule hemodialysis.

Indications for Admission

- Coma, seizures, ventricular tachycardia
- Initial theophylline level >30 mg/L
- Suicide attempt or gesture without psychiatric clearance and appropriate follow-up arranged

Bibliography

Cantrell FL: Treatment of theophylline overdose. *Am J Emerg Med* 1997;15:547.

Shannon MW: Comparative efficacy of hemodialysis and hemoperfusion in severe theophylline intoxication. *Acad Emerg Med* 1997;4:674–678.

Shannon M: Life-threatening events after theophylline overdose: a 10-year prospective analysis. *Arch Intern Med* 1999;159:989–994.

TRICYCLIC ANTIDEPRESSANTS

Common tricyclic antidepressants include imipramine (Tofranil), amitriptyline (Elavil), and doxepin (Sinequan). The pathophysiology of tricyclic toxicity includes direct myocardial (quinidine-like) depression, inhibition of norepinephrine uptake, and anticholinergic activity. Toxic doses vary with specific drugs.

Clinical Presentation

Clinical toxicity from tricyclic antidepressants includes anticholinergic effects (tachycardia, confusion), peripheral alpha blockade (hypotension), sodium channel blockade (widened QRS), GABA inhibition (seizures), and acidosis. Mental status changes can range from combativeness, delirium, and hallucinations to lethargy and coma. The patient is typically tachycardic and transient hypertension may occur early, but hypotension is more frequent. Tachyarrhythmias are common; ventricular arrhythmias are the primary cause of death. Changes in pupillary size are inconsistent, and hyperpyrexia can also occur.

Diagnosis

Suspect a tricyclic overdose in a patient presenting with an acute change of mental status, seizures, abnormal vital signs, or an arrhythmia. Attach a cardiac monitor, and if the QRS is widened (>100 ms), it is likely that a tricyclic has been ingested. Toxicity can also be predicted by a rightward axis in the terminal 40 ms of the QRS complex. This manifests as QRS widening with an R wave in aVR that generally exceeds 3 mm in amplitude.

ED Management

Initiate supportive care, administer activated charcoal if ingestion was within 4 h of presentation (do not give repeated doses), and continuously monitor the ECG. If the QRS interval is greater than 100 ms, give 1 to 2 mEq/kg of sodium bicarbonate IV over 2 min and repeat every 5 min until the QRS narrows to <10 ms. Start a bicarbonate drip and titrate the serum pH to 7.45 to 7.55.

Do not treat hypertension, which is usually transient, since hypotension frequently follows. Treat hypotension with a 20 mL/kg bolus of an isotonic crystalloid NS, Ringer's lactate). If that is unsuccessful, give norepinephrine (0.1–0.2 μg/kg/min IV) and titrate the dose against the patient's response. Treat seizures with lorazepam (0.05–0.1 mg/kg IV) or diazepam (0.1–0.3 mg/kg slow IV). If seizures recur, give a loading dose of fosphenytoin, 20 mg/kg phenytoin equivalents by slow IV push over 10 to 15 min (see Seizures, pp 470–476).

It is not necessary to treat supraventricular arrhythmias, but treat life-threatening ventricular arrhythmias with lidocaine (p 40) or phenytoin. Electrical pacing may be needed. Do not use physostigmine, as asystole has been reported.

Consult a toxicologist and cardiologist, and admit a symptomatic patient to an ICU, where continuous cardiac monitoring and close nursing supervision can be provided, until the patient is symptom-free for 12 h.

Indications for Admission

- Any signs or symptoms of tricyclic overdose
- History of possible tricyclic overdose unless 6 h have elapsed and the patient has remained asymptomatic with normal vital signs, a normal mental status, and no changes on ECG monitoring
- Suicide attempt or gesture without psychiatric clearance and appropriate follow-up arranged

BIBLIOGRAPHY

Harrigan RA, Brady WJ, ECG abnormalities in tricyclic antidepressant ingestion. *Am J Emerg Med* 1999;17:387–393.

James LP, Kearns GL: Cyclic antidepressant toxicity in children and adolescents. *J Clin Pharmacol* 1995;35:343–350.

McFee RB, Caraccio TR, Mofenson HC: Selected tricyclic antidepressant ingestions involving children 6 years old or less. *Acad Emerg Med* 2001;8:139–144.

CHAPTER 16

Neurologic Emergencies

Bonnie Bunch

ACUTE ATAXIA

Ataxia is caused by disorders affecting the cerebellum, vestibular apparatus, bilateral frontal lobes, or posterior column sensory input into the cerebellum. Ataxia manifests as an unsteady, reeling, wide-based gait or truncal instability (titubation). Dysmetria, tremor, slow, dysrhythmic "scanning" speech, and nystagmus may also be present. Although intoxications (alcohol, benzodiazepines, anticonvulsant medications) and viral infections are the most likely causes (Table 16-1), always consider trans-

Table 16-1   Etiologies of Acute Ataxia

Parainfectious acute cerebellar *ataxia*	*Transverse myelitis*
Mumps	Tumors
Measles	Posterior fossa
Varicella	Brainstem
Cytomegalovirus	Spinal cord
Enteroviruses	
Epstein-Barr virus	*Weakness*
	Guillain-Barré syndrome
	Myasthenic syndromes
Toxic-metabolic disturbances	
Drug toxicity/poisons	*Ischemic or vascular events*
Ethanol	Cerebellar infarct
Anticonvulsants	Arteriovenous malformation
Benzodiazepines	Sickle cell anemia
Antihistamines	Vasculitis
Inborn errors of metabolism	
Hypoglycemia	*Trauma*
	Posterior fossa hematoma
Infection	Intraaxial (cerebellar)
Meningitis	Extraaxial (subdural or epidural)
Encephalitis	

verse myelitis, meningitis, hydrocephalus, or a mass lesion (posterior fossa, brainstem, or spinal cord).

Clinical Presentation

Parainfectious Acute Cerebellar Ataxia   Acute cerebellar ataxia most often occurs days to weeks after a viral infection such as varicella. Typically, a 1- to 3-year-old presents with a short history (hours to days) of incoordination, unsteady gait, or tremor. The mental status and the rest of the examination are normal. The well appearance of the child helps distinguish this syndrome from encephalitis and meningitis. The ataxia may precede or follow the appearance of an exanthem. The cerebrospinal fluid (CSF) may be normal, or there may be a mild pleocytosis or elevation of the protein. The prognosis is good; recovery is rapid (often within days, usually within 4–6 weeks), but as many as 10–20% of patients have sequelae of variable severity.

Meningitis   Ataxia, with or without fever, may be the first sign of bacterial or viral meningitis (pp 366–369). Other meningeal signs (nuchal rigidity, Kernig's and Brudzinski's signs) may be present.

Encephalitis   A viral infection affecting the brainstem can present with ataxia and cranial nerve abnormalities. There is minimal effect on the level of consciousness unless higher cortical structures are also involved. Common agents are echovirus, adenovirus, and coxsackievirus. CSF findings are consistent with viral meningitis (pleocytosis without significant protein elevation or hypoglycorrhachia).

Posterior Fossa Tumor   A posterior fossa tumor can present with the insidious onset of headaches, vomiting, and ataxia.

Transverse Myelitis   Transverse myelitis is a presumed parainfectious inflammation at a specific level of the spinal cord. It may present initially with ataxia, back or neck pain, and paresthesias, followed by the rapid development of weakness at and below the level of the lesion.

Ingestion   Poisoning is a common cause of ataxia in toddlers. The most common agents are anticonvulsants, benzodiazepines, tricyclic antidepressants, phenothiazines, and alcohol. In addition, there may have been an unintentional overdose of medications, such as dilantin, carbamazepine, phenytoin, or antihistamines, including topical diphenhydramine.

Guillain-Barré Syndrome   In the Miller-Fisher variant of Guillain-Barré syndrome, ataxia is accompanied by ophthalmoplegia (usually diplopia). This may be followed by areflexia, an ascending weakness, and autonomic symptoms (flushing, pulse and blood pressure changes, gastrointestinal symptoms). Classically, the CSF demonstrates cytoalbuminogenic dissociation (elevated protein without pleocytosis).

Diagnosis

Attempt to ascertain the time of onset of the symptoms (chronic ataxia usually results from *tumors, metabolic disorders,* or *hereditary ataxias*) and whether there was any antecedent trauma, viral illness, rash, or toxin exposure. Inquire about the possibility of *recreational drug use, ingestion,* or *overuse of prescription and nonprescription medications* (anticonvulsants, sedatives, tranquilizers, or antihistamine preparations). Specifically inquire about over-the-counter medications, including topical diphenhydramine, which may cause intoxication if applied to a large surface area.

Pertinent physical examination findings include a typical exanthem (*varicella, measles*), the odor of alcohol on the breath (*intoxication*), or fever and meningeal signs (*meningitis*).

A careful neurologic exam is necessary to confirm the presence of ataxia, search for associated findings, and rule out a *posterior fossa mass lesion*. Note the head circumference, and carefully examine the fundi (disk margins, presence of spontaneous venous pulsations) for evidence of intracranial hypertension. However, in toddlers the sutures may split before eyeground changes appear. Other evidence of a posterior fossa tumor may include neck stiffness, head tilt, cranial nerve palsies (facial weakness, ophthalmoplegia), or long-tract findings (hemiparesis, spasticity, extensor plantar responses). Tone and reflexes may be diminished in the ataxic patient, but consider *Guillain-Barré syndrome* if the patient is areflexic. Check for a sensory level, suggestive of a spinal cord lesion (*transverse myelitis, tumor*).

Acute Cerebellar Ataxia   In acute cerebellar ataxia, there are no meningeal signs, the sensory examination is normal, and although tone may be somewhat diminished, there is no focal weakness. In most of the disorders listed in Table 16-1, the lethargy associated with the ataxia helps to distinguish these entities from acute cerebellar ataxia.

Vertigo   It can be difficult to distinguish an unsteady gait or stance secondary to the loss of balance associated with vertigo from ataxia. This is particularly true in children who may be unable to articulate a sense of motion or spinning. Nausea, vomiting, and nystagmus usually accompany vertigo, which can be provoked or worsened by changes in head position.

ED Management

If the child is lethargic, immediately assess the airway, breathing, and cardiovascular functions, give oxygen, and obtain intravascular access. If there is papilledema, focal neurologic findings, or bradycardia, hypertension, and hyperpnea (Cushing's triad), begin treatment for increased intracranial pressure (pp 468–470) and arrange for an emergency noncontrast CT scan to rule out an expanding posterior fossa lesion. If you suspect meningitis, obtain a blood culture and give meningitic doses of IV antibiotics (p 368) before obtaining the CT scan.

After the CT scan has documented no evidence of increased intracranial pressure or mass effect, perform a lumbar puncture, including a measurement of the opening pressure. Obtain serum electrolytes for comparison of the glucose with the CSF glucose and, if intoxication is suspected, a serum osmolality (increased with ethanol). In cases of suspected ingestion or drug overdose, obtain a blood level of the drug (e.g., alcohol, phenytoin, phenobarbital, carbamazepine).

Indication for Admission

- Acute ataxia until the cause has been established and the course stabilized

BIBLIOGRAPHY

Fenichel GM: *Clinical Pediatric Neurology,* 3rd ed. Philadelphia: Saunders, 1997, pp 230–252.
Maggi G, Varone A, Aliberti F: Acute cerebellar ataxia in children. *Childs Nerv Syst* 1997;13:542–545.
Nussinovotch M, Soen G, Volovitz B, et al: Acute cerebellar ataxia associated with varicella. *J Fam Pract* 1995;40:494–496.

ACUTE HEMIPARESIS AND STROKE

Acute hemiparesis is a rare event during childhood. The numerous causes can be grouped into a few etiologic categories, including thrombotic and embolic events, hemorrhage, trauma, mass lesions, and the idiopathic syndrome of acute infantile hemiplegia (Table 16-2).

Clinical Presentation

In the mildest form, acute hemiparesis presents as a tendency for the patient to adopt the decorticate posture. This entails shoulder adduction; flexion of the elbow, wrist, and fingers; pronation of the hand; extension of the knee; and eversion and plantarflexion of the foot. In young infants, mild hemiparesis may be manifest by an asymmetric startle response or absent grasp reflex on the affected side. Older infants and toddlers may demonstrate a hand preference (not normally established before 2½–3 years of age). More severe lesions can cause hemiplegia. While acute lesions may cause flaccidity, long-standing hemiparesis is usually accompanied by hyperreflexia, spasticity, and extensor plantar reflexes (corticospinal tract signs).

Intracranial Hemorrhage   An intracranial hemorrhage typically has a sudden onset and rapid evolution. Headache, vomiting, and obtundation are common, and there may be other signs of increased intracranial pressure, such as hypertension, bradycardia, hyperpnea, and papilledema. Seizures may also occur early in the course.

Acute Infantile Hemiplegia   Acute infantile hemiplegia presents with sudden weakness and altered mental status. The motor deficit persists for minutes to days and is often followed by seizures and slowed mentation. The typical patient is under 3 years of age and was previously well.

Table 16-2 Etiologies of Acute Hemiparesis in Childhood

Thrombotic events	*Head trauma*
Posttrauma/inflammation arterial occlusion	
Penetrating oral trauma	*Embolic events*
Tonsillectomy	Subacute bacterial endocarditis
Posttraumatic dissection	Prosthetic valves
Carotid artery	Atrial myxoma
Posterior circulation	Posttraumatic (fat or air embolus)
Vertebral artery	
Venous thrombosis	*Intracranial hemorrhage*
Dehydration	Arteriovenous malformation rupture
Cyanotic heart disease with polycythemia	Aneurysm (rare in prepubertal children)
Infections	Venous angioma
Meningitis	
Mastoiditis	*Blood dyscrasia*
Encephalitis	Hemorrhage into a tumor
Sinusitis	
Sickle cell anemia	*Mass Lesion*
Collagen vascular disease	Abscess
Systemic lupus erythematosus	Trauma
Polyarteritis nodosa	Cyanotic heart disease
Pregnancy or puerperium	Neurofibroma
Idiopathic occlusion intracranial carotid	Neoplasm
	*Hemiplegic migraine**
	*Acute infantile hemiplegia**

*Diagnosis of exclusion

Diagnosis

In general, determining the cause of the hemiparesis can be deferred to the inpatient setting. However, inquire about the rate of onset of the weakness and the occurrence of seizures, fever, *intraoral* or *head trauma,* infections (*upper respiratory, sinusitis, mastoiditis*), or change in mental status. Ask about past or associated medical conditions (*sickle cell disease, cardiac malformations, lupus, coagulopathies, neurofibromatosis, seizure disorder*). Consider the possibility of *nonaccidental trauma,* particularly in an infant or toddler.

On physical examination, check for nuchal rigidity; if it is present, suspect an infectious process (*meningitis, encephalitis*) or a *subarachnoid hemorrhage.* Examine the skin for *neurofibromas* and café-au-lait spots, check for cyanosis, and look for signs of head or neck trauma. Auscultate the head and neck for a bruit and the chest for a cardiac murmur.

Perform a thorough neurologic examination. Assess the mental status. A limited unilateral, nonexpanding, structural hemispheric lesion does not in itself cause a change in mental status. If the patient is lethargic, consider *hemorrhage, stroke, bilateral disease, metabolic defect, infectious disease,* or *postictal state.*

ED Management

Management takes priority over etiologic diagnosis. Perform a quick survey to assess the adequacy of the airway, breathing, and cardiovascular function, and obtain a complete set of vital signs. Check the extraocular movements, the pupils for equality of size and reactivity, and the fundi for papilledema, and assess the level of consciousness. See pp 468–470 for the management of patients with evidence of increased intracranial pressure. Secure an IV with normal saline and obtain blood for a complete blood count, platelet count, prothrombin time and partial thromboplastin time, sickle prep (if patient's status is unknown), erythrocyte sedimentation rate, Dextrostix, liver function tests, electrolytes, arterial blood gas, Lyme titer, and culture (if the patient is febrile).

Immediately consult a pediatric neurologist or neurosurgeon, and arrange for a noncontrast CT scan of the head. If there is no evidence of a structural lesion (tumor, acute infarct, hematoma) or increased intracranial pressure on the scan, perform a lumbar puncture (including opening pressure) and obtain specimens for cell count, protein and glucose, culture, and Gram's stain.

The management of sickle cell disease (pp 319–323), encephalitis (pp 332–335), meningitis (pp 366–369), and headache (pp 456–461) is discussed elsewhere.

Indication for Admission

• Acute hemiparesis or hemiplegia.

BIBLIOGRAPHY

deVeber G, Roach ES, Riela A, et al: Stroke in children: recognition, treatment, and future directions. *Semin Pediatr Neurol* 2000;7:309–317.

Fenichel GM: *Clinical Pediatric Neurology,* 3rd ed. Philadelphia: Saunders, 1997, pp 253–266.

Roach ES: Etiology of stroke in children. *Semin Pediatr Neurol* 2000;7:244–260

ACUTE WEAKNESS

Although acute weakness is uncommon in childhood, it usually heralds a significant neurologic disorder. The possibility of rapid progression to respiratory collapse makes the onset of acute weakness a true neurologic emergency until the cause and course have been established.

Clinical Presentation and Diagnosis

The history is vital to defining the underlying process. Determine the time of onset, progression, pattern of weakness (unilateral; bilateral; hemi-, di-, para-, or quadriparetic; flaccid versus spastic) and associated systemic features. A history of fever or a viral prodrome suggests an infectious or parainfectious origin.

Guillain-Barré Syndrome   Guillain-Barré syndrome, or acute demyelinating polyneuropathy, is usually a postinfectious or postinfluenza vaccination phenomenon. It is characterized by premonitory vague sensory symptoms or pain, ascending motor weakness, depressed or absent deep tendon reflexes, and sparing of bowel and bladder sphincters. The weakness is often asymmetric at onset but becomes symmetric as the disease progresses. Examination of the CSF early in the course may show a mild pleocytosis, but later the classic finding is cytoalbuminogenic dissociation: striking elevation of the protein without pleocytosis. About 10% of patients have significant respiratory, cardiac, and/or autonomic dysfunction, which may be sudden in onset and unrelated to the degree of motor weakness.

Myasthenia Gravis Myasthenia gravis is an autoimmune disorder that causes weakness by blocking the acetylcholine receptor at the neuromuscular junction. The most common initial presentation is ptosis and diplopia or blurry vision due to extraocular muscle weakness. There may also be generalized muscle weakness, which may be rapidly progressive and lead to respiratory compromise, necessitating intubation. Deep tendon reflexes are usually preserved.

Tick Paralysis A toxin released by dog and wood ticks prevents the release of acetylcholine at nerve endings, causing a rapidly progressive (12–48 h) generalized paralysis. The deep tendon reflexes are depressed or absent. There is no sensory loss, but dysesthesias may be present. In contrast to Guillain-Barré syndrome, there is no elevation of the CSF protein. The symptoms resolve quickly once the tick is removed.

Botulism Botulism-induced weakness (pp 329–330), resulting from release of exotoxin, is characterized by a fairly rapid progression of cranial nerve dysfunction (diplopia, ptosis, pupillary dilatation, dysarthria, dysphagia) and weakness.

Polio Poliomyelitis presents with asymmetric paralysis, signs of meningeal irritation, and a normal sensory examination. Typically, there is a history of a brief febrile illness, followed by a few days of recovery. The patient then has recurrent fever accompanied by weakness, lethargy, and irritability. Pain in the affected limbs is a prominent feature. The CSF shows a pleocytosis with protein elevation. The paralytic syndrome may also be caused by other enteroviruses (echovirus, coxsackievirus). There may be a history of incomplete or inadequate immunization.

Diphtheria The neurologic manifestations of diphtheria may begin during the acute illness, but most often they occur several weeks to months after the onset of the acute membranous pharyngitis. Diphtheria produces a flaccid limb paralysis, which may be accompanied by muscle tenderness and may be preceded by extraocular muscle weakness, ptosis, dysphagia, and a stocking-glove sensory loss. The CSF may show an elevated protein without pleocytosis. As with polio, there may be a history of incomplete or inadequate immunization.

Spinal Cord Pathology Spinal cord pathology can produce acute weakness with either paraplegia or quadriplegia. *Trauma* is the most likely cause. Patients with *Down's syndrome* or *rheumatoid arthritis* are particularly susceptible to C1 to C2 subluxation, which can result in quadriparesis. The presence of fever and vertebral tenderness strongly suggests a *spinal epidural abscess*, which is a neurosurgical emergency. *Myelitis*, an inflammatory process of the spinal cord, may result in para- or quadriparesis and loss of pain and temperature sensation below the site of inflammation. Weakness can also be caused by demyelinating lesions, such as those associated with *multiple sclerosis, spinal cord infarction* (most common in the thoracic levels), or hemorrhage secondary to *arteriovenous malformation.*

Metabolic Causes   Metabolic causes (*hypokalemia, hypo-* and *hypercalcemia, hypo-* and *hyperthyroidism*) are rare in childhood and usually have associated systemic manifestations. Episodic paralysis, particularly during rest after exercise, suggests *periodic paralysis*, especially if there is a positive family history.

Other Causes   Acute or subacute weakness with a rash, fever, and myalgias suggests an inflammatory process such as *dermatomyositis, polymyositis*, or *systemic lupus erythematosus*. Certain toxins, especially the anticholinesterase-inhibiting insecticides (*organophosphates, carbamates*), cause acute weakness.

Psychogenic Causes   Consider psychogenic causes when the history and physical examination fail to suggest an organic origin and the neurologic examination shows neurophysiologic inconsistencies. There may be a history of a stressful precipitating event or situation.

ED Management

Perform a careful neurologic examination to define the extent and pattern of weakness and any associated sensory findings (particularly a sensory level). Ask about dysphagia, bladder fullness, constipation, or incontinence of urine or stool. Percuss the lower abdomen for a distended bladder, and check the rectal tone. Examine the skin for a rash or a tick (often found hidden in hairy areas). Observe the patient's respiratory efforts, and document the adequacy of ventilation with an ABG or pulse oximetry.

Obtain a urinalysis, CBC, electrolytes, and glucose and, if the patient is febrile, a blood culture and ESR. A lumbar puncture is indicated, particularly if *Guillain-Barré* syndrome is suspected, but it can be delayed until after consultation with a pediatric neurologist.

The management of the *trauma* victim is detailed on pp 649–658. If there is any history of trauma, the patient with weakness must be maintained in neutral position. Obtain the appropriate spine films (cervical, areas of tenderness), and consult with a neurosurgeon and a pediatric neurologist.

If *myasthenia* is suspected, perform a Tensilon (edrophonium chloride) test under the direction of a pediatric neurologist. Edrophonium is a rapid-acting cholinergic drug. Perform the test with the child on a cardiorespiratory monitor in a setting where personnel and equipment for resuscitation are readily available. Have a syringe with atropine (1 mg) available as hypersensitive subjects can develop severe cholinergic reactions. The dose of edrophonium chloride is 0.04 mg/kg (maximum 1 mg <34 kg; 2 mg ≥ 34 kg). Give one-tenth of the total dose IV, and flush the line with NS. The patient may experience a feeling of warmth or a stinging sensation near the IV site, but if there are no serious autonomic effects, give the rest of the dose and assess the effect over the next 5 to 10 min. Assess the improvement of ptosis and extraocular muscle weakness, not generalized weakness, to evaluate the effectiveness of the drug. The effects of edrophonium dissipate within 10 to 15 min. Alternatively, test patients with ptosis by applying a cold pack to the lids; it will lessen the ptosis of myasthenia.

Arrange for psychological counseling if the weakness is determined to be *psychogenic*.

Indication for Admission

- Acute weakness of any origin except psychogenic

BIBLIOGRAPHY

Anlar B: Juvenile myasthenia: diagnosis and treatment. *Paediatr Drugs* 2000; 2:161–169.

Evans OB, Vedanarayanan V: Guillain-Barré syndrome. *Pediatr Rev* 1997;18: 10–16.

Fenichel GM: *Clinical Pediatric Neurology,* 3rd ed. Philadelphia: Saunders, 1997, pp 176–204.

BREATHHOLDING

Breathholding spells typically begin between 6 and 18 months of age and in 90% of cases disappear by 6 years. Most patients have no more than one attack per month, although 10% of affected children will have two or more per day. In 25% of cases, there is a positive family history of breathholding. Although the physiologic basis of breathholding is unclear, the episodes are not associated with an increased risk of epilepsy.

Clinical Presentation

Breathholding spells are brief, lasting about 30 s. The episodes are preceded by crying, which may be due to anger, frustration, fear, or pain. The child cries briefly, then stops breathing and loses consciousness. There may be a brief postictal period of confusion.

Breathholding spells are divided into two types, pallid and cyanotic, depending on the patient's color change. An individual child generally has only one type of spell. A *cyanotic* spell follows a frustrating event in which the child cries briefly, then develops apnea, cyanosis, and loss of consciousness. Rigid limbs and opisthotonos may be seen.

A *pallid* spell has a rapid onset after a frightening event or occipital trauma. The child starts crying, stops breathing, loses consciousness, and becomes pale and limp. Clonic jerks may be noted at the end of the episode.

Diagnosis

The diagnosis is made from the history, as the patient usually appears well and back to baseline by arrival in the ED. Breathholding spells are most often confused with *seizures.* Before a convulsion, there is sometimes an external precipitating factor, sustained crying, or cyanosis. Occasionally, spells may be confused with *syncopal episodes.* Fainting is very unusual in young children, however, and is not usually associated with rigidity or opisthotonos.

ED Management

If the history of the event is typical and a thorough neurologic exam yields normal results, reassure the family about the benign nature of the episode (no risk of epilepsy). Instruct the parents to be consistent in disciplining the child and not to allow him or her to derive secondary gain from the episodes (try not to pick up the child).

If the history is unusual or unclear, obtain a CBC, Dextrostix, electrolytes, glucose, and calcium, and perform an electrocardiogram (ECG) and rhythm strip (see Syncope, pp 59–62, and Cyanosis, pp 50–52). If a seizure cannot be ruled out from the history, ask about a family history of epilepsy, examine the skin for café-au-lait or ash-leaf spots, and schedule an electroencephalogram (EEG).

Follow-up

- Frequent (≥ 1/day) breathholding spells: pediatric neurology follow-up in 2 to 4 weeks

Indication for Admission

- Cyanotic episode that cannot be confidently diagnosed as a breath-holding spell

BIBLIOGRAPHY

Breningstall GM: Breath-holding spells. *Pediatr Neurol* 1996;14:91–97.
DiMario FJ Jr: Prospective study of children with cyanotic and pallid breath-holding spells. *Pediatrics* 2001;107:265–269.
Evans OB: Breath-holding spells. *Pediatr Ann* 1997;26:410–414.

COMA

While there is no universally standard terminology to describe the states of arousal between normal mental status and coma, one helpful scheme uses the following definitions, in order of decreasing level of arousal:

Lethargy
Lethargy implies difficulty in maintaining the aroused state. Although the patient is able to respond appropriately when addressed, without continual stimulation he or she lapses back into a somnolent state.

Obtundation
The obtunded patient responds to verbal or tactile stimuli with cerebral alerting but does not make fully appropriate responses.

Stupor
The stuporous patient responds with cerebral alerting only to painful stimuli.

Coma
Coma is a state of supreme unresponsiveness in which the patient appears as if asleep, yet does not respond to external or internal stimuli. Coma may result from medical (toxic-metabolic) causes or structural lesions. Distinguishing between metabolic causes and mass lesions is critical, as structural causes of coma may require emergency neurosurgical intervention, while metabolic coma can usually be managed medically.

Toxic-Metabolic   These derangements depress the cerebral hemispheres and often brainstem structures as well. They may be due to endogenous toxins (uremia, liver failure, respiratory failure, DKA) or exogenous toxins (salicylates, tricyclics, sedatives, carbon monoxide, narcotics, anticonvulsants), cerebral hypoxia or hypoperfusion, or hypoglycemia. Also, subclinical seizure activity (nonconvulsive status) may resemble coma.

Structural   Structural causes may be divided into supratentorial and sub- or infratentorial lesions.

Supratentorial mass lesions   These exert compressive forces on the cerebral hemispheres as well as brainstem structures. Large lesions of the dominant hemisphere alone can induce coma. In children, the most common mass lesion leading to coma is intracranial bleeding and swelling due to head trauma. Tumors, spontaneous hemorrhages, and ischemic strokes are rare.

Subtentorial mass lesions.   These destroy or compress core brainstem structures, such as the ascending reticular activating system, and may produce hydrocephalus and increased intracranial pressure.

Clinical Presentation and Diagnosis
Several elements of the physical examination help to distinguish structural from metabolic causes of coma. These include the pupillary responses, the extraocular movements (EOMs), and the motor response to pain. Changes in the respiratory pattern may also help localize the level of the lesion, but they are more difficult to interpret.

Asymmetry of pupillary response, EOMs, or the motor response to pain suggest a structural lesion. Fixed pupils are also more likely with a structural lesion. However, the earliest stage of central herniation can produce small, sluggish pupils indistinguishable from those seen in many metabolically induced coma states. Therefore, evidence of a structural origin (history or signs of trauma), other focal deficits with symmetric pupils, or signs of progressive deterioration cannot be ignored. The few medical states that can produce fixed pupils (Table 16-3) must always be considered when the pupils are nonreactive. In addition, focal neurologic findings may be seen in any metabolic encephalopathy (uremia, hypercalcemia, hepatic encephalopathy, and especially hypoglycemia), as these metabolic derangements may provoke signs and symptoms of previously subclinical lesions.

Absent EOMs or motor responses or symmetric posturing may be due either to structural lesions or to profound metabolic coma. Progression from purposeful motor responses to posturing and then to flaccidity suggests a structural lesion.

The EOMs can be tested with the doll's-eyes maneuver or, when head or neck injury is suspected, with cold-water vestibular stimulation with the head in the midline position. Intact doll's eyes are manifest by transient conjugate deviation away from the direction of rapid head rotation. Intact cold caloric responses are manifest by conjugate deviation of the eyes toward the stimulated ear. Absent EOMs on testing with the doll's-eyes maneuver may also indicate an awake patient. Never perform cold caloric stimulation on a patient who is awake, as it causes severe vertigo, nausea, and vomiting.

The *presence* of asymmetric (lateralizing) findings on examination helps to make the diagnosis of a structural lesion, but the *absence* of asymmetry does not rule out a structural lesion, particularly in the case of midline lesions.

Table 16-3   Toxic-Metabolic Causes of Fixed Pupils

Cause	*Pupils*	*Diagnosis/Characteristics*
Anoxia	Fixed, dilated	Antecedent history of shock, cardiac or respiratory arrest, etc.
Anticholinergics (tricyclics, atropine)	Fixed, dilated	Tachycardia, QRS>0.12 s Warm, dry skin
Cholinergics (organophosphates)	May be small with barely perceptible reflex	Diaphoresis, vomiting, incontinence
Opiates (heroin)	Very small with barely perceptible reflex	Needle marks History of overdose
Hypothermia	May be fixed	History of exposure
Barbiturates Glutethimide	May be midsized or dilated and fixed	History of overdose

Nonconvulsive status is suggested by subtle findings such as eye deviation, nystagmus, or changes in tone.

ED Management

If there is a history or suspicion of head trauma, assume that there has been cervical spinal trauma. Immobilize the neck and treat appropriately until cervical trauma has been definitively ruled out (pp 641–644).

The priority is stabilization of the vital signs. Initial blood tests include a CBC, electrolytes, blood urea nitrogen (BUN), Dextrostix and glucose, and an ABG. If the cause is unknown, a serum osmolality, PT, PTT, LFTs, and various toxicologic levels (barbiturates, alcohol, aspirin) may be useful. Save an additional red-top tube for future analysis. Give 100% oxygen and establish IV access. Give all patients naloxone (0.1 mg/kg), and if the Dextrostix is <80 mg/dL or if it was not obtained, give IV glucose (2 mL/kg of D_{25}) for diagnostic and therapeutic purposes.

See pp 461–467 for the management of *head trauma*.

When the cause of the coma is unknown and the vital signs are stable, treatment can be directed by the results of the coma examination as outlined above. If structural coma is suspected, management is as described for head trauma, including an emergency CT scan to identify the lesion. If metabolic coma is suspected, the situation is generally less urgent. A key exception is the patient with suspected *meningitis* (pp 366–369), who requires a lumbar puncture and appropriate antibiotics immediately following the CT. If the CT is delayed, give the antibiotics prior to obtaining CSF. The general approach to medical coma requires supporting the vital signs and correcting abnormalities in acid-base and electrolyte status. A *toxic ingestion* may require GI decontamination and supportive therapy (pp 401–402).

Indication for Admission

- Coma

BIBLIOGRAPHY

Fenichel GM: *Clinical Pediatric Neurology,* 3rd ed. Philadelphia: Saunders, 1993, pp 47–76.
Gemke RJ, Tasker RC: Clinical assessment of acute coma in children. *Lancet* 1998;351:926–927.
Kirkham FJ: Non-traumatic coma in children. *Arch Dis Child* 2001;85:303–312.

FACIAL WEAKNESS

The most common presentation of seventh cranial nerve dysfunction in children is a peripheral facial palsy. The lesion is in the facial nerve nucleus or the peripheral nerve distal to the nucleus, so both the upper and lower halves of the face are affected (including the frontalis muscle). Causes of a peripheral seventh nerve palsy include trauma, infections (Lyme disease, varicella, otitis, mastoiditis, parotitis, infectious mononucleosis), parainfectious phenomena (associated with Guillain-Barré syndrome), and neoplasms (neurofibromatosis, cerebellopontine angle tumors). A peripheral facial palsy of unknown origin is termed a Bell's palsy.

A central facial palsy affects only the lower half of the face, sparing the frontalis muscle. It is secondary to a lesion in the contralateral cerebral hemisphere, most commonly caused by stroke, demyelinating disease, or tumor.

Clinical Presentation

With the exception of acute trauma, most peripheral facial palsies evolve over 24 to 48 h, and they may be preceded or accompanied by pain around or behind the ear. The pain can be quite severe and may be the presenting complaint. The patient may complain of asymmetry of the face, weakness of the facial muscles, hyperacusis, excessive tearing of the ipsilateral eye, alteration of taste, or difficulty eating or drinking. Often there may also be a complaint of a feeling numbness or tingling over the affected side of the face.

A central facial palsy is not accompanied by hyperacusis or alteration of taste. In contrast to a peripheral seventh nerve palsy, wrinkling of the forehead and elevation of the eyebrow are unaffected. With a vascular origin, the onset may be acute.

Diagnosis

To determine if the weakness is peripheral or central, note whether the patient can wrinkle the forehead. Acute trauma and congenital causes of facial weakness can almost always be ruled out from the history and by inspection.

Perform a careful neurologic exam to rule out other neurologic origins (*Guillain-Barré syndrome*). Test the cranial nerves, motor strength, and deep tendon reflexes. Check for an accompanying hemiparesis, particularly in an infant or nonambulatory child. If there is a central facial palsy, examine for aphasia, which can be manifest by mutism. This may be difficult to determine in a shy or uncooperative child.

Examine the external auditory canals and tympanic membranes for signs of infection (*otitis, mastoiditis*, or vesicular lesions associated with *herpes simplex*).

On physical examination, look for a rash (Lyme disease, *varicella*, herpes), café-au-lait spots (*neurofibromatosis*), and generalized adenopathy and splenomegaly (*infectious mononucleosis*).

If the patient has a history of a recent tick bite or lives in an area where *Lyme disease* (pp 362–366) is endemic, perform a lumbar puncture if there is a history of headache or if other cranial nerve deficits are noted. The lumbar puncture may be deferred in the absence of headache, stiff neck, and neurologic deficits other than the facial palsy.

Bell's palsy is a diagnosis of exclusion if no other cause of a peripheral seventh nerve palsy is evident.

ED Management

If the patient has eye pain or discomfort, perform a fluorescein test (pp 489–495) to rule out a corneal abrasion. For the affected eye, give artificial tears (one to two drops qid), Lacri-lube at bedtime, and an eye patch to be worn at night to prevent drying of the cornea. If the patient cannot cover the entire cornea with a blink, patch the eye and refer him or her to an ophthalmologist. Do not permit the patient to wear contact lenses. Advise the patient to report any ocular discomfort immediately (possible corneal abrasion).

If *Lyme disease* is suspected, obtain blood for a Lyme titer and treat for 3 weeks with either amoxicillin (<8 years old: 40 mg/kg/day divided tid) or doxycycline (≥8 years old: 100 mg bid). CSF pleocytosis in *Lyme disease* is an indication for IV antibiotics (ceftriaxone 100 mg/kg/24 h divided q 12 h [maximum 4 g in 24 h]). The management of *otitis media* (pp 121–126), *mastoiditis* (pp 126–127), *Guillain-Barré syndrome* (pp 446–449), *infectious mononucleosis* (pp 352–354), *head trauma* (pp 461–467), and *increased intracranial pressure* (pp 468–470) is discussed elsewhere. The presence of facial nerve weakness does not usually alter the treatment of the problem. If otitis media associated with a facial nerve palsy does not improve after 2 days of oral antibiotics, arrange for tympanocentesis, culture the middle-ear fluid, and admit the patient for IV antibiotics (cefuroxime, 100 mg/kg/day divided q 8 h).

If the patient is seen within 48 h of the onset of a peripheral facial weakness and the most likely diagnosis is idiopathic *Bell's palsy*, give a 5- to 7-day course of prednisone (2 mg/kg/day, maximum 60 mg). Steroids have not been shown to affect the long-term prognosis for resolution of the palsy, but they may relieve associated pain. If there is no improvement noted within 3 weeks, refer the patient to a neurologist for electromyography.

If the weakness is central and is clearly of new onset, consult a pediatric neurologist and obtain a CT scan of the head.

The prognosis varies with the severity of the initial palsy; approximately 80% of patients recover completely, generally within 2 months, and improvement usually begins within 1 to 2 weeks of diagnosis.

Follow-up

• Peripheral weakness, including Lyme disease: 2–3 days, to check the affected eye and the laboratory tests

Indication for Admission

• Acute facial nerve palsy associated with progressive weakness, evidence of a mass lesion, CNS infection, intracranial hypertension, acute trauma, or other neurologic signs

BIBLIOGRAPHY

Guerrissi JO: Facial nerve paralysis after intratemporal and extratemporal blunt trauma. *J Craniofac Surg* 1997;8:431–437.

Riordan M: Investigation and treatment of facial paralysis. *Arch Dis Child* 2001; 84:286–288.

HEADACHE

There are many causes of headache in childhood (Table 16-4); fortunately, most are benign, such as migraine and tension-type or chronic daily headache. However, a number of life-threatening illnesses that may present with headache must be eliminated from consideration before the patient is discharged from the ED.

Clinical Presentation

Although the following clinical entities are discussed individually, bear in mind that many patients have headaches that do not easily fit into one particular category. Also, a child may have two or more types of headache, such as chronic tension-type headaches in a patient who also has migraines.

Common Benign Causes of Headache
Migraine   Migraine is the most common type of headache in children of any age. Among prepubertal children, the incidence of migraine is equal in boys and girls, while among adolescents and adults, more females are affected. In 70 to 90% of cases, there is a family history of migraine in a first-degree relative. Migraine attacks may be triggered by stress, exercise, head trauma (which may be so insignificant that it is forgotten), skipping meals, particular foods, drugs, strong sunlight or odors, hormonal changes associated with the menstrual cycle and pregnancy, and possibly by allergies. The frequency varies from once a year to several times a week. The duration of migraine headache is at least 2 to 3 h in older adolescents but may be as short as 30 min in young children. Patients with migraine are frequently treated with antibiotics for "sinus headache" before the diagnosis of migraine is finally considered.

Table 16-4   Etiologies of Headache

Common benign causes of headache	Infection-related causes of headache
Migraine	Sinusitis
Migraine without aura (common)	Dental infection
Migraine with aura (classic)	Systemic infection
Less common migraine syndromes	Group A *streptococcus*
Hemiplegic migraine	*Mycoplasma pneumoniae*
Ophthalmoplegic migraine	Influenza
Basilar artery migraine	Viral ("aseptic") meningitis
Cyclic vomiting	Lyme disease
Acute confusional migraine	Meningitis
Chronic tension-type headache	
Stress-related	*Headache due to increased ICP*
Visual abnormalities*	Brain abscess
Exo-/esophoria causing	Brain tumor
convergence difficulty	Head trauma
Posttraumatic headache	Pseudotumor cerebri
	Carbon monoxide poisoning

*Not caused by uncorrected refractive errors

Migraine without aura Migraine without aura (previously called *common migraine*) is not preceded by any visual, olfactory, or somato-sensory aura and is usually bilateral. The headache is described as pulsating or throbbing, may be paroxysmal in onset or arise in the setting of a preexisting tension-type headache, and may be accompanied by photophobia, phonophobia, nausea, vomiting, and a desire to sleep or rest in a quiet, dark room.

Migraine with aura Migraine with aura, or classic migraine, is preceded by an aura (most commonly a visual aura of scintillating lights, scotomata, blurry vision, visual hallucinations, or, rarely, an alteration of perception of time and body image known as the "Alice-in-Wonderland" syndrome). The headache is usually unilateral, although it may alternate sides. If the headache is always on the same side, there is more concern about the possible presence of an underlying structural lesion.

Migraine variants Migraine variants may present with hemiplegia, ophthalmoplegia, ptosis, an acute confusional state, or episodes of vomiting. These manifestations may or may not be accompanied by headache and are diagnoses of exclusion. The neurologic deficits are transient in most cases, but there have been reports of patients who eventually have strokes in the vascular distribution suggested by the deficit.

Chronic Tension-Type Headache This category of headache includes the headaches formerly known as "muscle contraction headache," "tension headache," and "psychogenic headache." The headaches are generally prolonged, may be waxing and waning in intensity, and are not preceded by an aura or accompanied by any neurologic deficits. The pain is described as dull, achy, or tight and usually begins in the occipital region; however, it may move anteriorly to the vertex or the frontal region. The headaches typically occur in the late afternoon or evening and are relieved by mild analgesics such as acetaminophen. Unlike migraines, these headaches rarely interrupt normal activities. They may be triggered by a recent emotional or traumatic event and may be associated with personality changes, as evidenced by poor school performance, sleep disturbances, aggression, lack of energy, and self-deprecatory behavior.

Heterophorias An exo- or esophoria that forces the patient to continually exert effort to converge the eyes may cause headache. Typically, the onset is in the afternoon or evening after concentrated visual activity. Unlike heterotropia (constant misalignment of the eyes), heterophorias may be difficult to appreciate on physical examination without specific testing. Pure refractive errors such as myopia are usually not associated with headache.

Temporomandibular Joint Dysfunction (TMJD) Disorders of temporomandibular joint function may present with headache. Patients with bruxism and habitual gum chewers are at increased risk. The headache of

TMJD may be associated with jaw or ear pain and locking of the jaw or inability to open the mouth.

Posttraumatic Headache   Early-onset posttraumatic headache is common after minor head trauma. The headache may initially be isolated to the area of impact but often becomes generalized and may be associated with vomiting and/or somnolence. There are no focal neurologic deficits or signs of increased intracranial pressure (ICP), but the patient may have amnesia for the events surrounding the trauma. Headache with onset minutes to days after significant head trauma may be due to an epidural or subdural hematoma. Worrisome signs are a decreasing level of consciousness, projectile vomiting, and symptoms of increased ICP (bulging fontanelle, split sutures, unequal pupils, sixth nerve palsy, hypertension with bradycardia and changes in respiratory pattern). Head trauma (pp 461–467) and increased ICP (pp 468–470) are discussed elsewhere.

Occasionally, posttraumatic headache may continue for prolonged periods (weeks to years). The headache may be a migraine, triggered by head trauma in a susceptible person. Psychogenic factors or the possibility of secondary gain may be involved.

CO poisoning   (pp 189–192) is infrequent, although it commonly causes headache, as well as fatigue and irritability, and may affect several family or group members simultaneously.

Infection-Related Causes of Headache
Sinusitis   The headache of sinusitis (pp 139–140) may be referred to the upper teeth, the cheek, or the frontal or retroorbital area. There may be cough, mucopurulent nasal discharge, fever, and facial pain and tenderness. Often the pain occurs in the early morning and is accentuated by leaning forward.

Dental Infection   A dental infection (pp 65–67) causes pain in the cheek or mandibular area as well as producing temporal headaches. The infected tooth or gum may be sensitive upon percussion or manipulation.

Systemic Infection   Systemic infections, such as group A streptococcal infection, influenza, EBV and mycoplasmal pneumonia, can cause a headache in addition to other symptoms (fever, sore throat, cough, coryza, conjunctivitis, or myalgias). Early Lyme disease (pp 362–366) may present with headache in addition to arthralgias, lethargy, and behavioral changes.

Meningitis   The headache of bacterial meningitis is generalized, constant, often described as "throbbing all over," and associated with fever, toxicity, nuchal rigidity (in older children), and other meningeal signs. Viral meningitis causes a similar presentation, usually during summertime epidemics. At any age, the absence of nuchal rigidity does not rule out meningitis, particularly early in the course of infection.

Headache Caused by Increased Intracranial Pressure
Brain Abscess   A child with a brain abscess may present with a nonspecific headache, usually accompanied by fever. Vomiting, diplopia, seizures (focal, partial complex, or generalized convulsions), and altered mental status may be present. Predisposing factors are congenital heart disease with right-to-left shunting and ethmoid or frontal sinusitis that has been unresponsive to therapy.

Brain Tumor   The headache of a brain tumor is intermittent initially but very quickly increases in frequency and severity. It is often present in the very early morning hours and may awaken the child from sleep (lying supine slows the drainage of CSF increasing intracranial pressure). There may be associated projectile vomiting in the absence of abdominal pain or ataxia. Localization may be difficult, especially in the case of midline lesions. Occipital headache may indicate a posterior fossa lesion, although the pain is frequently referred to a frontotemporal location. Thus, frontal headache may accompany either a supratentorial or a posterior fossa tumor.

Pseudotumor Cerebri   Patients with pseudotumor cerebri can present with intermittent headaches, vomiting, blurred vision, papilledema, and occasionally diplopia. However, there is no alteration in the level of consciousness or intellectual functioning.

Ventriculoperitoneal (VP) Shunt Obstruction   See pp 478–479.

Diagnosis

Despite the wide spectrum of causes, most childhood headaches are due to one of the common benign causes listed in Table 16-4. With the exception of children whose headaches are accompanied by severe nausea and vomiting, these patients are afebrile; appear awake, alert, and nontoxic; and have normal physical and neurologic examinations. Although only a small minority of headaches in children are secondary to some serious intracranial process, these conditions must always be considered.

Obtain a complete description of the headaches, including onset, triggering factors, duration, location, quality, usual time of day they occur, what (if anything) makes the pain better or worse, and whether the severity and frequency are increasing. This information may be difficult to elicit, especially if the child is less than 8 to 10 years old. Avoid suggesting possible descriptive terms to the preschool child, who may agree that all apply, even if they are mutually exclusive. Ask about recent emotional stress, personality changes, head trauma, changes is speech or gait, warning signs (aura), family history of migraines, medications, and associated symptoms, including fever, nausea or vomiting, photophobia or visual disturbances, rash, nasal discharge or cough, and possible tick or carbon monoxide (CO) exposure.

Measure the blood pressure and perform a complete physical examination, looking for fever, split sutures, bulging fontanelle, facial tenderness, gingival swelling, dental caries and tooth percussion sensitivity, otitis media, nuchal rigidity and meningeal signs, and signs of a systemic infection. A thorough neurologic exam is necessary, including ophthalmoscopy. Asymmetry of the pupils, EOMs, or motor response suggests a structural abnormality such as a *brain tumor* or *abscess* or a *subdural* or *epidural hematoma* (see Coma, pp 450–453). Finally, check the visual acuity and visual fields.

ED Management

The priority is expeditious diagnosis and treatment of a CSF infection or increased ICP. The management of a suspected mass lesion, meningitis, head trauma, pseudotumor cerebri, sinusitis, systemic infection, and dental infection is discussed elsewhere in the appropriate sections.

Indications for CT of the head are listed in Table 16-5. A urinalysis, CBC, blood glucose, or carboxyhemoglobin level may be indicated, based on the clinical presentation. Obtain a shunt series, CT scan, and neurosurgical consultation for a child with a VP shunt and severe headache.

The ED treatment of chronic tension-type headaches is limited to oral analgesics (acetaminophen 15 mg/kg q 4 h, ibuprofen 10 mg/kg q 6 h) and reassurance that a serious disease process is not present. Refer the patient to a primary care setting, where the stresses contributing to the headaches can be addressed.

Migraines

Migraines can be chronic and debilitating. For that reason, avoid treating with narcotics and other habit-forming drugs and give only mild analgesics (as above). Brief (10- to 15-min) exposure to 100% oxygen may be helpful if the headache is incapacitating. In addition, give an IV or PR dose of metoclopramide (0.1 mg/kg by slow IV push, maximum 10 mg), which will relieve the headache and associated vomiting. A dystonic reaction or akathesia, although rare, is possible even at minimal doses. Consult a neurologist if the headache does not respond to these measures.

The newer injectable drugs for acute migraine (dihydroergotamine, sumatriptan and related "triptan" agents) are not approved for use in children, although they may benefit adolescents older than 18 years of age. Refer a child with frequent or intractable migraine to a primary care setting or a pediatric neurologist. The ED is not an appropriate site for instituting therapy with ergotamines or prophylactic agents such as propranolol, verapamil, or amitriptyline.

Table 16-5   Indications for Computed Tomography in Patients with Headache

Focal neurologic abnormality
Papilledema
Recurrent morning headache
Persistent vomiting
Paroxysmal onset of excruciating headache
Head trauma with focal neurologic signs or lethargy

Ask the family or patient to keep a headache diary. For each headache, record the time of onset, duration, location, quality, exacerbating and remitting factors, and note any other associations that may help to identify the type of headache, its temporal pattern, and triggers. Have the parents of young children record any spontaneous complaints of headache, but advise them to avoid eliciting spurious complaints by asking the child if he or she has a headache. Have the patient or family take the diary to the follow-up appointment.

Follow-up
- Migraine requiring ED treatment (other than acetaminophen or ibuprofen): 2 to 3 days. Otherwise, primary care follow-up in 1 to 2 weeks

Indications for Admission
- Focal neurologic findings
- Intracranial hypertension
- Meningitis
- Acute confusional state
- Headache associated with frontal sinusitis with air-fluid level
- Severe headache after head trauma
- Newly diagnosed mass lesion

BIBLIOGRAPHY

Linder SL, Winner P: Pediatric headache. *Med Clin North Am* 2001;85:1037–1053.
Molofsky WJ: Headaches in children. *Pediatr Ann* 1998;27:614–621.
Singh BV, Roach ES: Diagnosis and management of headaches in children. *Pediatr Rev* 1998;19:132–136.

HEAD TRAUMA

Head trauma is a very common injury in childhood, accounting for 76% of trauma admissions and 70% of trauma deaths. Head trauma can result from a fall from a window or a bicycle or motorcycle and from automobile accidents. Consider child abuse (shaking, whiplash injuries) in infants and young children. Always consider the possibility of associated cervical spine injury (pp 641–644) in a patient with head trauma.

Clinical Presentation

Most pediatric head trauma victims do not suffer serious injury, although soft tissue swelling or laceration is common. The most common scenario is a toddler who runs into an object or falls from his or her own height. Occasionally the patient is sleepy but fully arousable; however, the neurologic examination is otherwise normal.

A less obvious presentation is the young afebrile infant with a full fontanelle who is lethargic or vomiting. The baby may be a "shaken infant," with or without other physical evidence of abuse (pp 543–547).

Serious signs and symptoms include persistent headache, repeated episodes of vomiting, ataxia, blurred vision, altered level of consciousness, focal neurologic signs, seizures, a compound skull fracture, or evidence of increased intracranial pressure.

Contact seizures occur at the moment or within seconds of the head trauma. Although frightening to observers, contact seizures are of no clinical significance. In contrast, early posttraumatic seizures occur 1 min to 1 week after the head trauma, whereas late posttraumatic seizures occur 1 week or more after the injury. About 25% of children with early posttraumatic seizures develop late seizures, and nearly 75% of children with late posttraumatic seizures develop epilepsy. Almost 100% of patients with penetrating head trauma eventually have epilepsy. Specific brain injuries include the following:

Concussion   This is a brain injury that is not demonstrable by radiographic studies but may be associated with transient confusion or loss of consciousness.

Contusion   A cerebral contusion is an area of focal edema, with or without hemorrhage, that can be seen on CT scan. There is usually loss of consciousness, and there may be focal deficits.

Epidural Hematoma   An epidural hematoma results from a tear in one of the meningeal arteries (middle meningeal is the most common site) or meningeal or diploic veins. A temporoparietal skull fracture is present in up to 75% of children with epidural hematomas. The classic presentation is a concussion followed by a lucid interval and then loss of consciousness associated with signs of increased ICP. However, this classic presentation occurs only about one-third of the time; many cases will have no history of loss of consciousness or a lucid interval. With a large epidural hematoma, there may be ipsilateral pupillary dilatation and, less commonly, contralateral decerebrate posturing.

Subdural Hematoma   With a subdural hematoma, there is tearing of the bridging veins between the cerebral cortex and the dura, with compression of the underlying brain. These lesions are often associated with more widespread shear injury to the brain and have high morbidity and mortality rates. A subdural hematoma can present with coma or seizures, or it may develop more slowly and be associated with nonspecific signs and symptoms of increased ICP. It is most common in infancy and in young children. The presence of a subdural hematoma suggests child abuse.

Diffuse Axonal Injury   This serious injury is produced when shearing forces generated by rapid acceleration-deceleration cause disruption of myelin and tearing of long axonal fibers. Very young children can also exhibit visible tears in the white matter. A CT scan reveals diffuse brain swelling, which develops over 24 to 48 h, but no mass lesions.

Basilar Skull Fracture   Common fractures of the base of the skull include longitudinal or transverse fractures of the petrous portion of the temporal bone and fractures of the cribriform plate. Suspect petrous fractures when there is hemotympanum, Battle's sign, CSF otorrhea or rhinorrhea, facial palsy, or hearing loss. Hemorrhage in the nose or naso-pharynx, CSF rhinorrhea, or anosmia suggest fracture through the cribriform plate. Basilar skull fractures are rarely seen on plain film; if they are suspected, noncontrast CT with thin cuts through the area of interest are necessary.

Diagnosis

The treatment of a serious head injury takes priority over obtaining the history and performing a complete physical examination. Determine the nature of the trauma, including whether the patient lost consciousness or cried immediately. Ask about vomiting, seizures, recollection of the event, activities both before and after the injury, and past medical problems (seizure disorder, neurologic handicap). Once the patient is medically stabilized, obtain a developmental history. Many victims of severe head trauma have a history of behavioral or developmental problems.

Perform a complete physical examination, including vital signs. Look for scalp lacerations and hematomas, a depressed skull fracture, and evidence of a basilar skull fracture (retroauricular or periorbital ecchymoses, hemotympanum, serous or serosanguineous rhinorrhea or otorrhea). Consider the possibility of cervical spine injury in every case (pp 641–644), and check for sources of bleeding and other major injuries (see Multiple Trauma, pp 649–658).

Head trauma per se does not cause hypotension except in very young infants or patients with serious scalp lacerations. Hypotension demands an immediate, thorough evaluation of the rest of the body (particularly the chest, abdomen, pelvis, and thighs) for sources of blood loss. Tachycardia, particularly in association with a narrowed pulse pressure, suggests impending shock (pp 18–22).

Hypertension and bradycardia associated with slow or irregular respirations (Cushing's triad) indicate increased intracranial pressure. Treatment must be instituted at once (see pp 468–470). Very young children may not exhibit the full Cushing's triad. Hypertension may not develop or may be a late finding shortly before herniation.

Perform a careful neurologic examination, paying careful attention to the signs of structural coma (pp 451–453): asymmetry of pupillary responses, EOMs, or motor response. Examine the cranial nerves, perform ophthalmoscopy (for papilledema, loss of spontaneous venous pulsations, or retinal hemorrhage), and test the reflexes, strength, sensation, and coordination, comparing one side with the other.

Test fluid draining from the ear or nose for glucose. CSF has glucose in it; mucus does not. If the fluid is bloody, touch it with a piece of filter paper. Formation of two concentric rings suggests that CSF is mixed with the blood.

The Glasgow Coma Scale (GCS) indicates the initial severity of the head injury and facilitates monitoring of changes in the patient's status (Table 16-6). A modified GCS has been developed for preverbal children (Table 16-7).

Table 16-6   Glasgow Coma Scale*

	Score
Eyes open	
Spontaneously	4
To speech	3
To pain	2
None	1
Best verbal response	
Oriented	5
Confused	4
Inappropriate words	3
Incomprehensible sound	2
None	1
Best motor response	
Obeys	6
Localizes	5
Withdraws	4
Abnormal flexion	3
Abnormal extension	2
None	1

*Total GCS is the sum of the scores of the three parts.

Table 16-7   Modified Glasgow Coma Scale*

	Score
Eyes open	
Spontaneously	4
To speech	3
To pain	2
None	1
Best verbal response	
Coos and babbles	5
Irritable cries	4
Cries to pain	3
Moans to pain	2
None	1
Best motor response	
Normal spontaneous movements	6
Withdraws to touch	5
Withdraws to pain	4
Abnormal flexion	3
Abnormal extension	2
None	1

*Total GCS is the sum of the scores of the three parts.

The neurologic exam, the nature of the injury, and the age of the patient determine the need for skull x-rays. Since CT scans provide information about the skull and, more important, the underlying brain, skull radiographs are rarely needed. If a depressed skull fracture is suspected (trauma caused by a sharp, high-velocity object; large scalp hematoma preventing palpation of the skull below), obtain an x-ray tangential to the area in question. Skull x-rays may not be needed to rule out a linear compound fracture in a patient with a scalp laceration, since these wounds are explored under local anesthesia.

Risk assignment based on GCS monitoring and clinical exam may help guide further management (Table 16-8).

ED Management

The priorities are securing the airway, maintaining vital signs, stabilizing the cervical spine, and treating increased ICP. Serial examination of the patient, preferably by the same health care provider, is essential to the early detection of evolving injuries.

First, assess the airway and adequacy of ventilation and stabilize the cervical spine (if that was not done in the field) with a rigid neck collar. Since a patient with a depressed level of consciousness may have inadequate ventilation despite respiratory movements, obtain an ABG, monitor oxygen saturation, and give 100% oxygen if the patient is not fully awake and alert. Intubate any patient with a GCS ≤8, using in-line stabilization of the cervical spine, the jaw thrust/chin lift maneuver and rapid sequence intubation (see pp. 6–8). Examine the chest for the presence of bilateral breath sounds and signs of respiratory distress.

Table 16-8   Risk Assignment Based on GCS and Clinical Exam

Low-risk injuries (GCS = 15)

   Asymptomatic
   Mild headache
   Dizziness
   Short-term vomiting (duration <4 h)
   Normal neurologic examination

Moderate-risk injuries (GCS = 9–14)

   History of loss of consciousness
   Progressive headache
   Persistent vomiting (duration ≥4 h)
   Early posttraumatic seizure
   Associated injuries (long bone fracture, contusion of internal organs)
   Altered mental status (including drug or alcohol intoxication)
   Suspected child abuse
   Basilar skull fracture

High-risk injuries (GCS <9)

   Depressed level of consciousness
   Penetrating injury to brain
   Focal neurologic examination

Next, measure the vital signs at least every 15 min, more frequently in patients with severe head trauma or an abnormal pulse or blood pressure. Secure a large-bore IV in any patient with hypotension or a GCS <15. The treatment of hypotension with 20-mL/kg boluses of isotonic crystalloid and packed red cell transfusions takes precedence over concerns about increased intracranial pressure. Once a normal BP is maintained, infuse $D_5\frac{1}{2}NS$ at a KVO (keep vein open) rate.

A patient with a depressed skull fracture, penetrating head trauma, focal neurologic findings, or an early posttraumatic seizure is at risk for the development of seizures. Give a loading dose of IV fosphenytoin (20 mg phenytoin equivalent) slowly over 30 min. Give nafcillin (150 mg/kg/day divided q 6 h) to a patient with a compound skull fracture before debridement, but do not give antibiotics routinely to a patient with a basilar skull fracture.

GCS <8 or GCS ≥8 but Worsening   Immediately intubate the patient and call for neurologic and neurosurgical consultations. Hyperventilate the patient to a PCO_2 of 30 to 35 mmHg, keep the head in the midline and the bed elevated to 30 degrees, and restrict fluids to NS at a KVO rate. If there is pupillary asymmetry or decorticate posturing, give mannitol (0.5–1 g/kg) as an IV push. Arrange for an immediate CT scan (see Increased Intracranial Pressure, pp 468–470).

GCS 9–14   Insert a large-bore IV for access and repeat the GCS every 15 min. Arrange for an urgent CT. Admit the patient for close observation if the GCS remains less than 15 during the first hour in the ED.

GCS = 15   If the child has not vomited and has a normal examination, he or she may be sent home if the parents can follow instructions and, if necessary, return immediately. Loss of consciousness in the absence of other neurologic signs or symptoms is not an indication for a CT scan. If there is persistent vomiting or dizziness, arrange for a CT scan or admit the patient for observation and serial neurologic examinations. Regardless of whether the CT scan is normal, if the parents are anxious, do not discharge a patient until he or she has returned to baseline status.

Admit a patient with a basilar skull fracture if a CSF leak is suspected, there are associated neurologic findings, or the parents are anxious. If there is associated CSF leakage, elevate the head of the bed to 30 degrees and consult with neurosurgery. A patient with CSF otorrhea or rhinorrhea is at risk for bacterial meningitis (10%), but prophylactic antibiotics are not indicated. Most CSF leaks resolve spontaneously within 7 to 10 days.

Follow-up

- GCS = 15: Next day. Instruct the parents to return immediately if the patient cannot be aroused or has diplopia, unsteady gait, several episodes of vomiting, or a headache unresponsive to ibuprofen or acetaminophen.

Indications for Admission

- GCS <15
- Early posttraumatic seizure (not a contact seizure)
- Compound or depressed skull fracture
- Persistent vomiting, dizziness, or abnormal neurologic findings in the ED
- Basilar skull fracture

BIBLIOGRAPHY

Committee on Quality Improvement, American Academy of Pediatrics, Commission on Clinical Policies and Research, American Academy of Family Physicians: The management of minor closed head injury in children. *Pediatrics* 1999;104:1407–1415.

Quayle KS: Minor head injury in the pediatric patient. *Pediatr Clin North Am* 1999;46:1189–1199.

Schutzman SA, Barnes P, Duhamie AC, et al: Evaluation and management of children younger than two years old with apparently minor head trauma: proposed guidelines. *Pediatrics* 2001;107:983–993.

IMPLANTABLE DEVICES

A number of implantable devices for treatment of chronic neurologic disorders are coming into use in children and may be encountered during pediatric ED visits. These include vagus nerve stimulators (VNS) for the treatment of intractable seizures and intrathecal baclofen pumps (IBP) for spasticity. When a patient with one of these devices presents to the ED, consult a physician experienced in the use of the device.

Vagus Nerve Stimulator   The VNS consists of a small pulse generator implanted under the skin, usually on the left side in the infraclavicular region. Electrodes are wrapped around the left vagus nerve, and pulses are transmitted in a retrograde fashion to the brain. The generator is programmed to emit pulses at specific intervals, with characteristics defined by the physician. A magnet, provided to the patient, can be moved once across the pulse generator to produce an extra pulse in the event of a seizure. The pulse generator can be stopped from firing by taping the magnet on top of the pulse generator and leaving it there.

A patient with the VNS may not have an MRI with a body coil, although MRI of the head using a transmit-and-receive head coil may be performed. Reprogram the current amplitude to 0 mA before the MRI, and reset after the procedure. Also, do not bring the patient's magnet into the MRI suite. Diathermy is also absolutely contraindicated, although diagnostic ultrasound can be performed.

Problems associated with the VNS include hoarseness; cough; pain in the throat, neck, or GI tract; vomiting; and, rarely, cardiac arrhythmias or asystole. The device may also become infected, especially within the 3 months following implantation.

Intrathecal Baclofen Pump (IBP)   The IBP consists of a medication pump and reservoir medication implanted under the skin, usually in the flank, with a small catheter threaded into the intrathecal space. Although the manufacturer warns that the U.S. Food and Drug Administration has not approved performance of MRI on patients with the pump, MRIs have been performed successfully under the supervision of an experienced physician. Turn the pump off before the procedure (and restart afterwards).

Problems with the IBP include decreased delivery of baclofen, with severe spasticity (due to empty reservoir, kinking or migration of the catheter); occasional overdose of baclofen, characterized by hypotonia, lethargy, and depressed respiratory drive; or infection of the pump. If the pump is empty, use oral baclofen or a benzodiazepine, although neither is as effective.

BIBLIOGRAPHY

Armstrong RW, Steinbok P, Cochrane DD, et al: Intrathecally administered baclofen for treatment of children with spasticity of cerebral origin. *J Neurosurg* 1997; 87:409–414.
Binnie CD: Vagus nerve stimulation for epilepsy: a review. *Seizure* 2000;9:161–169.
Kita M, Goodkin DE: Drugs used to treat spasticity. *Drugs* 2000;59:487–495.

INCREASED INTRACRANIAL PRESSURE

An increase in the volume of any intracranial compartment (blood, CSF, or parenchyma) can cause an elevation in intracranial pressure (ICP), a true neurosurgical emergency. Head trauma is the most common cause of increased ICP in children. Although the onset of increased ICP is usually acute, onset may be delayed in patients with subdural or epidural hematomas. Other causes are brain tumor, meningitis (see pp 366–369), hemorrhage from a vascular malformation, intracerebral abscess, pseudotumor cerebri, and shunt obstruction (see pp 478–479) in a patient with hydrocephalus. Intracranial hypertension is also the major life-threatening complication of Reye's syndrome.

Clinical Presentation

Lethargy is an important finding in a patient with increased ICP. A patient with a GCS less than 9 or a falling GCS after head trauma requires an immediate evaluation for intracranial hypertension.

A patient with increased ICP may complain of early-morning headache and vomiting or headaches of recent onset that have become more frequent and severe. A verbal child may complain of blurry vision, frank diplopia, or intermittent loss of vision. Altered mental status, a change in personality (constant crying or irritability in an infant), neck pain, and a head tilt are also suggestive of increased ICP. Papilledema is a highly specific but insensitive finding in the first 24 h of acutely increased ICP.

In an infant, increased ICP causes irritability, vomiting, widening of the sutures, an increasing head circumference, a full or bulging fontanelle, and possibly "sunsetting" of the eyes.

Clinical signs of imminent cerebral herniation include a deteriorating level of consciousness, unequal pupils (the dilated pupil is usually on the same side as the herniation), asymmetric EOMs, and decorticate (flexor-early) or decerebrate (extensor-late) posturing. Abnormal respirations, bradycardia, and hypertension (Cushing's triad) occur with severely increased ICP.

Diagnosis

Any patient who has suffered significant head trauma is at risk for increased ICP. Always ask about persistent vomiting or visual or behavioral changes. Check the pupillary responses, EOMs, and level of consciousness. Perform a careful ophthalmoscopic examination and a sensory and motor examination, comparing one side of the body with the other. Coma can be due to *metabolic causes* (see pp 451–453), but typically the pupils are equal and reactive and there are no focal findings.

Congenital anisocoria, the use of *mydriatic drops*, or *traumatic mydriasis* or *iritis* can cause pupillary inequality. These are always diagnoses of exclusion in a patient with lethargy or any other signs suggesting increased ICP.

The evaluation of headaches is discussed on pp 456–461. Morning headaches or headaches that are increasing in frequency and intensity are worrisome. However, headaches in an alert patient with no other abnormal neurologic findings are most likely to be *psychogenic, tension*, or *migraine headaches*.

ED Management

If increased ICP is suspected, immediately arrange for a CT scan and notify a neurosurgeon and a neurologist to assist in further management. See pp 465–466 for the treatment of head trauma.

If the patient has an altered level of consciousness but does not have unequal pupils, bradycardia, hypertension, or decorticate or decerebrate posturing, continuously monitor the heart rate and blood pressure and assess the adequacy of ventilation with an ABG. Secure an IV and give NS at a KVO rate. However, if the patient is hypotensive, restoration of a normal BP takes priority over treatment of the increased ICP and is required in order to maintain adequate cerebral perfusion pressure. Always keep the patient's head in the midline and, unless he or she is in shock or has a cervical spinal injury, elevate the head of the bed 30 degrees. Provide 100% oxygen, and intubate any patient who is hypoxic, hypercarbic (Pco_2 >40 mmHg), stuporous, comatose, or is leaving the ED for diagnostic procedures (so that monitoring will be difficult).

If the patient has signs of markedly increased ICP (unequal pupils, bradycardia and hypertension, abnormal posturing), employ all available modalities to lower the ICP while a neurologist and neurosurgeon are summoned. These include immediate intubation and hyperventilation to a Pco_2 of 30 to 35 mmHg (if the patient is intubated, increase the rate of ventilation) and, if a mass lesion is suspected, the administration of IV mannitol (0.5–1 g/kg) and dexamethasone (0.2 mg/kg up to 16 mg). When giving mannitol, insert a urinary bladder catheter. Limit the IV fluid rate to KVO unless the patient is in shock.

To avoid further increasing the ICP, it is preferable to perform intubation under controlled circumstances (see Rapid Sequence Intubation, pp 7–8). As soon as intubation has been accomplished, insert a nasogastric tube (orogastric tube if the patient has sustained head trauma), aspirate the stomach contents, and connect the tube to suction.

Order a shunt survey if there is a suspected shunt obstruction. If a shunt infection is suspected, arrange for a neurosurgeon to tap the reservoir to obtain CSF for culture, cell count, and chemistries.

Indication for Admission

- Intracranial hypertension

BIBLIOGRAPHY

Friedman DI: Pseudotumor cerebri. *Neurosurg Clin North Am* 1999;10:609–621.
Larson GY, Goldstein B: Consultation with the specialist: increased intracranial pressure. *Pediatr Rev* 1999;20:234–239.
Stocchetti N, Rosszi S, Buzzi F, et al: Intracranial hypertension in head injury: management and results. *Intensive Care Med* 1999;25:371–376.

SEIZURES

Although more than 5% of children will have at least one seizure, most seizures are either benign febrile convulsions or breakthrough seizures in a patient known to have epilepsy. The priorities are to identify and treat status epilepticus appropriately and to rule out life-threatening causes such as meningitis, severe head trauma, intracranial bleeding, the long-QTc syndrome (LQTS), or a metabolic derangement.

Clinical Presentation and Diagnosis

Some types of seizures, such as generalized convulsions, are easily recognized, while other types are less familiar and subtler in appearance. Common features of seizures include rhythmic jerking movements of the head or limbs, changes in tone, fixed staring with or without deviation of the eyes, myoclonic jerks, nystagmus, and unresponsiveness.

Infants, and neonates in particular, tend to have multifocal clonic seizures or more subtle types of seizure activity, including tongue thrusting and lip smacking. In infants, posturing and "funny" movements that are not accompanied by either eye deviation or alteration in vital signs are usually not seizures.

Other nonepileptic paroxysmal events—such as syncope, migraine, movement disorder, and "pseudoseizures"—may be mistaken for seizures. These can usually be differentiated with a careful history. *Syncope* (pp 59–62) is rare in very young children and is often preceded by a stressful event, giving rise to a vasovagal reaction. Syncope may be preceded by light-headedness or nausea. Also, a syncopal episode secondary to LQTS may present as a first afebrile seizure.

Confusion or a decreased level of consciousness may accompany *migraine*, but headache is usually the most striking feature. *Movement disorders* disappear in sleep and are not associated with a decreased level of consciousness. In contrast, seizure activity frequently arises during sleep or shortly after awakening and often causes a change in level of alertness.

Pseudoseizures are also known as nonepileptic or hysterical seizures. The diagnosis may be not be clear unless the patient is known to have had previous attacks, as many patients also have true seizures. Suspect pseudoseizures in an unresponsive patient by holding the patient's hand above his or her face and allowing it to fall. A patient with pseudoseizures (in a pseudo postictal state) will never hit his or her face with the falling hand; in a truly postictal patient the hand will fall onto the face. Occasionally, the differentiation of pseudoseizures from true epileptic seizure cannot be made in the ED, and extended monitoring with continuous EEG and closed-circuit television may be necessary.

For the purposes of evaluation and management in the ED, seizures are divided into status epilepticus, febrile seizures, first unprovoked seizure, and breakthrough seizures without regard to the actual appearance of the seizure or its formal classification.

Status Epilepticus

Status epilepticus is defined as either a single seizure lasting longer than 15 min or a series of seizures without a return to baseline mental status between each episode. If the seizure started at home and has not stopped before arrival in the ED, the patient is most likely in status. The term *status epilepticus* refers only to the duration of the seizure and does not imply anything about the cause, prognosis, or type of seizure activity. Generalized tonic-clonic status, partial complex status, and febrile status are the most frequent types of status.

The most common cause of status is low antiepileptic drug levels in a child with documented epilepsy. Other predisposing factors in patients known to have epilepsy are fever, vomiting, and intercurrent infections. Less commonly, status is symptomatic of an acute encephalopathic process such as CNS infection (meningitis, encephalitis), metabolic disturbance (hypoxia, hypoglycemia, hyponatremia, hypocalcemia), intoxication or poisoning (cocaine, theophylline, tricyclic antidepressants, amphetamines, camphor), mass lesion, or head trauma.

Children generally tolerate status epilepticus well, although there may be hypoxia and hypercarbia with metabolic and respiratory acidosis significant enough to require intubation and mechanical ventilation. Increased cerebral oxygen consumption and cerebral blood flow occur and may cause intracranial hypertension, leading to exacerbation of brain damage if the seizure is due to trauma or spontaneous intracranial hemorrhage. Physical injury and vomiting with aspiration are additional hazards. Therefore, treat status epilepticus as quickly as possible, but avoid the overuse of sedating antiepileptic drugs, which may exacerbate respiratory depression or alteration of mental status.

Febrile Seizure

A febrile seizure occurs in 2 to 5% of otherwise normal children between 6 months and 6 years of age. The seizure occurs during the course of a febrile illness that does not involve the CNS. The characteristics of febrile seizures are noted in Table 16-9.

Meningitis must be ruled out. This is often possible during the history and physical examination of older children. However, young children can

Table 16-9   Characteristics of Febrile Seizures (Age 6 Months to 6 Years)

	Family history in 10%
	No CNS involvement

Simple	*Complex*
Brief (<15 min)	Prolonged duration
Generalized	Focal (before, during, after)
Single event	Multiple occurrences within 24 h
	Febrile status epilepticus
	Patient with prior CNS dysfunction
	Patient with prior developmental delay

have meningitis without the typical signs (stiff neck, headache, Kernig's and Brudzinski's signs). Therefore a lumbar puncture is indicated for any febrile patient less than 12 months of age unless he or she has an identified source of fever, appears well, and is functioning in a normal baseline fashion. Be particularly cautious with infants who are too young to sit, as clinical assessment may be difficult.

About two-thirds of patients have only one febrile seizure episode. Of patients who have a second episode, about one-half to two-thirds will have three or more febrile seizures. Recurrences are more likely in children less than 18 months of age at the time of the first seizure and those who have febrile seizures with temperatures less than 40°C (104°F). Simple febrile seizures and febrile status epilepticus do not indicate an increased risk of epilepsy. However, some children who are eventually diagnosed with epilepsy do present initially with seizures in the setting of a febrile illness.

First Unprovoked Seizure
An unprovoked seizure is one that is not associated with fever, infection, trauma, ingestion, metabolic abnormality, or any other identifiable cause. The first such episode can sometimes be the initial presentation of epilepsy.

Breakthrough Seizure
A breakthrough seizure occurs in a patient taking chronic antiepileptic drugs. The most common cause is low antiepileptic drug level secondary to noncompliance (particularly common in teenagers), inability to obtain the needed medication(s), having outgrown the drug dose(s), or a change in the patient's metabolism of the drug(s). Antibiotics, birth control pills, and other drugs metabolized through the hepatic P450 system may reduce antiepileptic drug levels. In contrast, erythromycin may lead to an increased level of carbamazepine (Tegretol), and any new medication that is protein-bound may displace phenytoin (Dilantin) from protein-binding sites and lead to transient toxicity. Adding a second antiepileptic agent can also change other drug levels. Finally, a febrile illness or any other type of stress can lower the child's seizure threshold.

ED Management

The priorities are evaluation and stabilization of the patient's airway and vital signs, termination of ongoing seizure activity, prevention of recurrent seizures, diagnosis of CNS infection, and determination of the cause of the seizure. If the patient has seizure activity in the ED, document the features of the seizure, including any focal movements, gaze deviation, presence and direction of nystagmus, and alteration in autonomic function.

Obtain a complete history, including an accurate description of the seizure and how and where it started. Ask about any "aura" at the onset of the seizure, the time of day, and the patient's activity at the time of the seizure (particularly whether the seizure had its onset in sleep or early morning), the duration of the seizure, and the postictal state. Inquire about medications taken, family history of epilepsy or other neurologic or neurocutaneous disorders, developmental history, and past medical history. On physical examination, check the skin for neurocutaneous stigmata, perform a thorough general and neurologic examination, including a complete mental status examination appropriate to the patient's age, and assess the patient's developmental status.

Once it is clear that the patient did have a seizure and is not in status epilepticus, the ED workup and management are directed by the answers to the following questions:

1. Is this a first seizure, or is there a history of seizures? If there have been previous seizures, is this seizure similar with regard to type of activity, duration, and frequency?
2. Is the patient taking antiepileptic drugs? Has the child "outgrown" the dose, or has there been a problem with adherence to the drug regimen?
3. Is the patient febrile? Is this a febrile seizure in an otherwise normal child with a fever and an infection that does not involve the CNS? Is this a child with an underlying neurologic disorder who has seizures when febrile?
4. Is there evidence of meningitis?
5. Could the seizure have been provoked by something other than fever, such as hypoxia, hypoglycemia, ingestion of cocaine or another drug, electrolyte abnormality, or head trauma? Has the patient had previous syncopal episodes, raising the possibility of LQTS?

Status Epilepticus

Assess the airway, breathing, and circulation before proceeding with treatment. Suction the oral cavity, apply a face mask with 100% oxygen over the nose and mouth, and monitor the vital signs and oxygen saturation. Secure an IV with D$_5$NS (at KVO if the vital signs are stable), and obtain blood for laboratory tests as indicated by the history. These may include blood for antiepileptic drug levels, serum toxicology screen, CBC, electrolytes, glucose, calcium, and magnesium. If acute exposure to lead is a possibility, also obtain a lead level. Always obtain a rapid Dextrostix estimate of the serum glucose and an extra red-top tube. If the child is febrile and appears toxic, obtain a blood culture. If the cause of the seizure is not clear, obtain a urine drug screen which includes cocaine metabolites.

Protocol for Treatment of Status Epilepticus
While monitoring the blood pressure, ECG, and respiratory status, give

1. Lorazepam, 0.05 to 0.1 mg/kg, maximum 1 to 2 mg, slow IV over 2 min (preferred), IO, PR, or intrabuccally. Alternatives include diazepam 0.1 to 0.3 mg/kg given slow IV over 2 min (maximum 5–10 mg) IO or PR and midazolam 0.05 to 0.2 mg/kg slow IV over 2 min IO or IM (maximum dose 5 mg). Respiratory depression and hypotension may occur. Do not give lorazepam or diazepam IM because of erratic absorption. Repeat the dose if the seizure does not stop within 5 min.
2. Fosphenytoin, 20 mg/kg phenytoin equivalents IV (preferred) or IO given by slow push over 10 to 15 min. Alternatively, give phenytoin, 20 mg/kg IV by slow push over 20 to 30 min. If the seizure does not stop within 5 min after the dose is complete, proceed to step 3 and contact a pediatric neurologist. Fosphenytoin has significant advantages over phenytoin. It can be given quickly with much less risk of cardiac arrhythmia or asystole. As the pH is ~8 (as opposed to ~13 for phenytoin), it is much less likely to cause extensive tissue necrosis in case of extravasation. Fosphenytoin can be diluted in NS or dextrose-containing fluids to concentrations from 1:2 to 1:25 as convenient, while phenytoin is compatible only with NS. However, do not give fosphenytoin IM for status epilepticus because of slow absorption.
3. Phenobarbital, 20 mg/kg IV. Phenobarbital can cause respiratory depression and hypotension, especially if given in combination with benzodiazepines. If there is any sign of respiratory depression or if the patient does not have good airway protection reflexes (gag and cough), prophylactic intubation prior to administration of phenobarbital is recommended. If the seizure does not stop, consider steps 4 and 5 and contact a pediatric intensivist or anesthesiologist.
4. Pentobarbital coma, in intensive care unit.
5. General anesthesia, in intensive care unit.

If the seizure activity is stopped by lorazepam, the patient usually needs no further antiepileptic medication. This includes a patient with febrile status or breakthrough seizures due to low antiepileptic drug levels that can be adjusted once the patient returns to baseline.

For the rare patient who does not have a history of epilepsy and does not respond to lorazepam or diazepam, check the electrolytes and obtain an ABG. A patient with a metabolic or hypoxic basis for the status needs correction of the underlying problem and usually does not require treatment with anticonvulsants. Treat hyponatremic seizures with water restriction and NS (see Hyponatremia, pp 168–170). If needed, give hypertonic (3%) saline (2–4 mL/kg IV push). Correction of the sodium to 125 mEq/L is generally sufficient to stop seizures. Avoid a rapid correction to a "normal" sodium. Treat hypertensive seizures with IV labetalol (0.25 mg/kg over 10 min). (see Hypertension, pp 609–611).

Fever with irritability or lethargy is an indication for a blood culture and a lumbar puncture once the seizure has been terminated. It is essential that the child's respiratory status be stable before a lumbar puncture is attempted. If there is apnea or hypoventilation or there are signs of increased ICP such as papilledema or posturing, give antibiotics and delay the procedure. If the Dextrostix reading is low (<80 mg/dL), give an IV push of 0.5 g/kg glucose (2 mL/kg of D_{25}) after obtaining blood for glucose and insulin levels. Obtain urine to check for ketones if the patient was hypoglycemic.

A patient with evidence of focality (except for known stable neurologic deficits without new findings) or increased ICP on neurologic exam must undergo immediate CT scanning (see Increased Intracranial Pressure, pp 468–470). However, a patient with generalized seizures with no residual defects does not require radiographic imaging in the ED. An EEG is indicated for a patient with new-onset status epilepticus with focal features or focal neurologic deficits or if the onset of seizure activity was unwitnessed, but it is more useful if deferred until after the immediate postictal period. An EEG is indicated in the ED when there is reason to suspect subclinical status epilepticus (subtle seizure activity that continues after convulsive status epilepticus has been treated).

Febrile Seizures

A patient with a febrile seizure lasting more than 15 min has status epilepticus; treat as described above. For most children with febrile seizures, vigorous antipyresis with acetaminophen (15 mg/kg q 4 h) and/or ibuprofen (10 mg/kg q 6 h) is usually sufficient to prevent recurrences. Consult a neurologist to consider treatment with antiepileptic drugs for a patient whose seizures are unusually severe, frequent, or accompanied by aspiration or a need for intubation.

A patient with a febrile seizure without focality may be discharged from the ED when all infectious disease issues have been resolved, his or her condition has returned to baseline status, and the family has an adequate supply of antipyretics, with instructions for their use.

First Unprovoked Seizure

Long-term antiepileptic drug treatment for a first-time unprovoked seizure in an otherwise normal child may be postponed until the child has a second or third seizure. Defer these decisions to the primary medical provider or pediatric neurologist. Metabolic derangements are rare, although the likelihood increases in younger children and infants. For an older child who appears well and has returned to a normal neurologic baseline following a seizure, routine electrolyte, calcium, and magnesium determinations are seldom helpful. However, if the patient has a history of syncopal episodes or a family history of arrhythmia, syncope, sudden death, or deafness, obtain an ECG and rhythm strip to rule out LQTS (see Syncope, pp 59–62).

A patient with a new-onset unprovoked seizure without focality may be discharged from the ED when his or her condition has returned to baseline status, arrangements for appropriate follow-up have been made, and the immediate concerns of the child and family have been addressed.

Breakthrough Seizure

If the patient is known to have had a recent therapeutic anticonvulsant level, give an extra dose of that medication rather than a full loading dose. For example, give 5 mg/kg of either fosphenytoin, phenytoin, or phenobarbital IV over 15 to 20 min. Do not give either drug IM. If there are subsequent seizures, treat as for status epilepticus, as described above. Valproic acid, but not carbamazepine, is now available in IV form. Use the same dose as for oral administration, over 1 h. Valproic acid syrup can also be given PR as a retention enema, using the oral dose.

A patient with a history of epilepsy and breakthrough seizures may be discharged from the ED when his or her condition has returned to baseline status, there is a therapeutic antiepileptic drug level, and the patient has an adequate supply of all necessary anticonvulsant medications.

Follow-up
- Febrile or first unprovoked seizure: next day
- Breakthrough seizure: 2 to 3 days to recheck anticonvulsant levels

Indications for Admission
- Status epilepticus
- Increasing number of breakthrough seizures or new types of seizures in a known epileptic
- Focality or evidence of increased intracranial pressure
- CNS infection
- Structural lesion (trauma, tumor, hemorrhage)
- Patient does not return to baseline mental status within 1 to 2 h of the seizure

BIBLIOGRAPHY

American Academy of Pediatrics. Provisional Committee on Quality Improvement, Subcommittee on Febrile Seizures: Practice parameter: long-term treatment of the child with simple febrile seizures. *Pediatrics* 1999;103:1307–1310.
Bebin M: The acute management of seizures. *Pediatr Ann* 1999;28:225–229.
Hanhan UA, Fiallos MR, Orlowski JP: Status epilepticus. *Pediatr Clin North Am* 2001;48:683–694.
Sabo-Graham T, Seay SR: Management of status epilepticus in children. *Pediatr Rev* 1998;19:3069.

SLEEP DISORDERS

Clinical Presentation and Diagnosis

Nightmares, night terrors, and sleepwalking can occur with enough frequency to bring a patient to the ED.

Nightmares Nightmares are frightening dreams that occur during rapid-eye-movement (REM) sleep. The child is easily arousable or awakens spontaneously and typically has a good recall of the dream. Nightmares are fairly common in children beginning at about age 3, but it is important to obtain a careful medication history, since withdrawal from minor tranquilizers, anticonvulsants, and sedative-hypnotics can be associated with nightmares.

Night Terrors   Night terrors occur within 2 h of falling asleep, most often in children 3 to 8 years old. The child will be frightened and crying inconsolably. In contrast to a nightmare, it is very difficult to arouse the patient. Signs of autonomic arousal are common, including increased heart rate, pupillary dilatation, sweating, and combativeness. After a few minutes, the child will return to sleep and will have little if any recall of the episode. A patient with night terrors frequently also has somnambulism (see below). Night terrors are easy to confuse with nightmares or *nocturnal seizures*. A thorough history is of primary importance in making the diagnosis.

Somnambulism   Somnambulism, or sleepwalking, occurs in 1 to 6% of the population (particularly boys), and there is often a positive family history. The child will be out of bed, often performing some sort of purposeful behavior, and may even respond somewhat to verbal commands, although there is usually no recall of the event when the patient is fully awake. Somnambulism can be confused with *psychomotor seizures*, which do not occur exclusively at night.

Take a careful history of the event, and review the patient's general health status and medication history. Ask about recent stresses in the child's life.

ED Management

Nightmares   Occasional nightmares are of little concern. Recurrent episodes, especially if a particular dream occurs frequently, may be indicative of stress or emotional upset that requires further attention.

Night Terrors   Generally, a patient "outgrows" night terrors, so that reassurance is all that is needed. However, frequent recurrences suggest underlying stress. If nocturnal seizures cannot be ruled out (episodes also occur during the day or more than 2 to 3 h after falling asleep), order a sleep-deprived EEG.

Somnambulism   Sleepwalking is difficult to prevent and, once it begins, may continue into adulthood. Advise the parents to secure the child's area to prevent injury during sleepwalking (protect stairways, doors, windows).

Follow-up

- Primary care follow-up in 2 to 4 weeks

BIBLIOGRAPHY

Laberge L, Tremblay RE, Vitaro F: Development of parasomnias from childhood to early adolescence. *Pediatrics* 2000;106:67–74.

Ohayon MM, Guilleminault C, Priest RG: Night terrors, sleepwalking, and confusional arousals in the general population: their frequency and relationship to other sleep and mental disorders. *J Clin Psychiatry* 1999;60:268–276.

Vgontzas AM, Kales A: Sleep and its disorders. *Annu Rev Med* 1999;50:387–400.

VENTRICULOPERITONEAL SHUNTS

The survival of premature infants has led to a significant increase in the number of patients with ventriculoperitoneal (VP) shunts. A VP shunt places a patient at risk for malfunction, leading to increased ICP, infection, and in some cases low-pressure headache due to overdraining of the CSF.

Clinical Presentation

While the presentation may be dramatic, with signs of increased ICP or CNS infection, the parent may note only that the child "looked just like this the last time he or she had a shunt problem." Although most parents will mention that the patient has a shunt, occasionally this part of the patient's history may be forgotten, particularly if the shunt has been functioning well for a long time or if the presenting complaints are primarily referable to the abdomen.

Shunt Malfunction   Proximal (intracranial) obstruction can be caused by CSF protein, choroid plexus, or embedding of the tube in the brain parenchyma. Distal obstruction to CSF flow may result from the formation of an abdominal pseudocyst around the end of the shunt. Malfunction may also result from disconnection or kinking of elements of the shunt, leading to symptoms of shunt obstruction. Proximal obstruction causes headache, vomiting, neck pain, lethargy, sixth nerve palsy, persistent downward gaze ("sunsetting" eyes), and feeding intolerance (see Increased Intracranial Pressure, pp 468–470). If the obstruction is distal, the patient may also have nausea, abdominal pain, and a distended abdomen.

Shunt Infection   Meningitis and ventriculitis present with fever, irritability or lethargy, meningismus, and signs of increased ICP. Infection is most likely to occur in the first 3 months after placement of the shunt, secondary to contamination at the time of the procedure. A late infection is due to hematogenous spread. Occasionally, a patient may develop peritonitis, followed by an ascending infection of the shunt.

Low-Pressure Headache   While newer shunts have antisiphoning devices and may have programmable valves to allow for adjustment of the opening pressure of the valve, an older patient may have a shunt without these devices. The shunt may intermittently overdrain, with subsequent tension on the dura and other pain-sensitive structures, causing nausea and severe headache. On CT scan, the ventricles appear slit-like. This syndrome is annoying but not life-threatening; consult with the neurosurgeon.

Diagnosis

Perform a thorough evaluation for shunt problems if a patient with a VP shunt has headache, lethargy, vomiting, or abdominal pain. Inspect the overlying skin along the entire course of the shunt for erythema, erosions, or induration, which may suggest a source of infection. Evaluate for possible obstruction by depressing the subcutaneous reservoir. Inability to depress the reservoir suggests distal obstruction, while if the reservoir is depressible but does not refill within 10 s, there may be obstruction proximal to or within the one-way valve at the cranial end of the reservoir. If an obstruction is suspected, obtain a noncontrast CT of the brain and compare it with previous studies to determine whether there has been an increase in the size of the ventricular system. However, an unchanged CT does not rule out obstruction, particularly in cases where the patient has been shunted for a long time and the ventricles are no longer compliant. Also obtain a shunt series (a series of plain films that show the full extent of the shunt) to rule out malfunction due to disconnection or kinking of the elements of the shunt.

If a distal obstruction is suspected, obtain an abdominal ultrasound to look for a pseudocyst or fluid collection.

If infection is suspected, consult a neurosurgeon to obtain a specimen of CSF for cell count and culture. Although a lumbar puncture can be attempted in any patient except those with meningomyelocele (in which case the location of spinal cord elements is unclear), the procedure is often unsuccessful because of alterations in CSF flow due to the presence of the shunt. Most shunts can be tapped directly by inserting a butterfly needle through the skin into the reservoir under sterile conditions.

ED Management

Assess the airway, breathing, and cardiovascular functions, and, if necessary, give oxygen and obtain IV access. Consult a neurosurgeon to assess shunt function and, if necessary, tap or externalize the shunt. In the event of papilledema, focal neurologic findings, bradycardia, or hypertension, begin treatment for increased ICP (pp 468–470) while arranging for radiologic assessment of the shunt.

If the patient has Cushing's triad or asymmetry of the pupils, suggesting that herniation is imminent, summon a neurosurgeon to insert a spinal needle through the bony defect along the track of the intracranial portion of the shunt catheter into the ventricle and allow CSF to drain out. Follow the neurologic examination carefully before and during this procedure. If a shunt infection is suspected, obtain appropriate blood and urine cultures and begin antibiotic treatment (vancomycin 60 mg/kg/day divided q 6 h) *only* if the patient is unstable or the shunt cannot be tapped within a reasonable amount of time. *Staphylococcus epidermidis* and *S. aureus* are the most common organisms.

Indication for Admission

- All patients in whom there is evidence or strong clinical suspicion of shunt infection or malfunction

BIBLIOGRAPHY

Dias MS, Li V: Pediatric neurosurgical disease. *Pediatr Clin North Am* 1998; 45:1539–1578.

Goeser CD, McLeary MS, Young LW: Diagnostic imaging of ventriculoperitoneal shunt malfunctions and complications. *Radiographics* 1998;18:635–651.

Madikians A, Conway E Jr: Ventriculoperitoneal shunt problems in pediatric patients. *Pediatr Ann* 1997;26:613–620.

CHAPTER 17

Ophthalmologic Emergencies

Caroline Lederman and Martin Lederman

ANATOMY

A thorough knowledge of anatomy is required in order to adequately evaluate the eye and related structures (Fig. 17-1).

The eye is protected by the lids and surrounding orbital bones. The most anterior part of the eye is the tear film layer covering the cornea (clear front portion of the eye). The corneal margin, where the cornea meets the sclera, is referred to as the limbus. The conjunctiva is a thin membrane covering both the white sclera (where it is called the bulbar conjunctiva), and the inside of the lids (where it is referred to as the palpebral conjunctiva). Because the bulbar and palpebral conjunctivae join in the superior and inferior fornix (the area where they join is known also as a cul-de-sac), objects such as foreign bodies and contact lenses cannot slip behind the eye and be lost.

Behind the cornea is the anterior chamber, which is approximately 1 to 2 mm in depth and is filled with clear aqueous. The aqueous circulation begins in the ciliary body, located behind the iris, and flows through the pupil and out through the trabecular meshwork, located in the angle between the iris and the peripheral cornea.

The iris contains a circular constrictor muscle and radial dilator muscles, each controlling the circular pupil.

Behind the iris plane lies the crystalline lens, which functions as the focusing mechanism of the eye. It is kept in place and controlled by fine suspensory ligaments (zonules), which form an attachment from the lens to the ciliary body.

The inner volume of the eye is filled with a clear gel, the vitreous body. Lining the inner sclera is the retina, a fine network of nerves and blood vessels, which are the first receptors of the visual pathway.

The bony orbit surrounds, supports, and protects the globe. The orbit is filled with connective tissue, blood vessels, fat, and the six extraocular muscles that control eye movement.

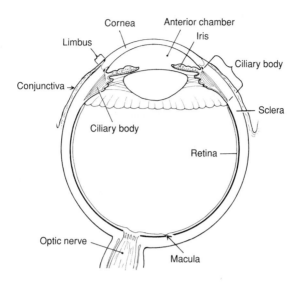

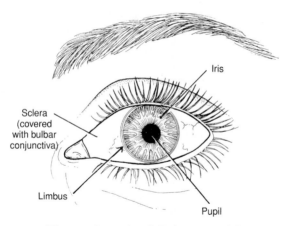

Figure 17-1   *A* and *B.* Anatomy of the eye.

EVALUATION

Visual Acuity   Except for chemical injury, when immediate flushing is indicated, the adequate examination of the eye begins with an evaluation and recording of its sensory function, i.e., visual acuity. While parts of the following eye examination can be omitted when appropriate, an assessment of visual acuity should always be done.

The standard Snellen chart at 20 ft is best, but other distances may be used as long as that distance is noted. The numerator of the Snellen fraction denotes the distance from the chart and the denominator is an arbitrary number given to each line. A smaller denominator refers to a smaller letter (optotype), i.e., a letter on the "20" line is half the size of a letter on the "40" line and 10 times smaller than a letter on the "200" line. Thus, 20/200 means that a letter on the "200" line was correctly identified at 20 ft and 4/40 (its equivalent) means that the "40" line letter (five times smaller) was correctly identified at 4 ft (five times closer).

Charts using other symbols have been constructed for preliterate children. Other methods can be used if a chart is not available, such as counting fingers at a specified distance, hand motions at a specified distance, observed eye closure when a light is directed in the eye (light rejection), or reading a newspaper headline at some distance. It is important to check each eye separately using a sterile gauze pad to occlude the non-tested eye and then to check both eyes together, with and without glasses. Test the "good" eye first in order to reduce anxiety.

Assuming that there are no other life- or organ-threatening injuries, evaluate the eyes in a systematic manner, starting from the most anterior aspect of the eye to the most posterior. Look first at the lids and surrounding structures, palpate the bony orbital rim, assess the tears, look at the anterior aspect of the eye (including the conjunctiva, cornea, and sclera), and assess ocular mobility with a finger (not a bright light) moving in all positions of gaze (up, down, left, right, and oblique). Note the depth and clarity of the anterior chamber, and observe pupillary motility and quality. In a semidarkened room at a distance of 1 to 2 ft, use the ophthalmoscope with the lens set to sharply define iris markings (usually black or plus 1 or 2) and assess the clarity and symmetric color of the pupils. Use the ophthalmoscope to evaluate the retina, noting the sharpness and color of the optic nerve, vascular pattern, foveal reflex, and retinal contour. Finally, palpate the globes if a penetrating injury is not suspected.

DECREASED VISION

Decreased vision can be caused by life-threatening intraocular or intracranial tumors, eye-threatening diseases (trauma, iridocyclitis, pseudotumor cerebri, glaucoma, retinal detachment), or minor conditions (corneal foreign body, conjunctivitis, tearing). In addition, decreased vision may be a functional complaint.

Clinical Presentation

The most common cause of an acute decrease in vision is ocular trauma, particularly a corneal abrasion. The priority is to rule out a life-threatening or eye-threatening condition.

Diagnosis

Unless there is an obvious ruptured globe or chemical injury, the evaluation of the eyes starts with a determination and description of visual acuity, preferably as a numeric function.

For infants and preverbal children, describe the vision in both eyes first, then in each eye separately. The sleeping infant reacts to bright light directed into each eye with further eyelid closure ("light rejection") if the eye and vision sense are intact. Absence of light rejection or asymmetric light rejection suggests vision loss in one or both eyes. The preverbal child follows objects of interest, such as toys (avoid shining a bright light in the awake child's eyes), by fixing centrally on the object and following it. Test each eye separately, using the examiner's or parent's thumb as an occluder. For an older child, a Snellen chart that has been calibrated at 20 ft is most accurate, especially if the light is constant and reproducible and the examining area is quiet. Testing can be done at a distance of 5 to 10 ft, although using shorter testing distances may miss subtle differences between the eyes. In the absence of a Snellen chart, ask the patient to count fingers held a few feet away or check the patient's ability to read a newspaper headline at a set distance. The testing distance must be noted.

ED Management

Treat the chief complaint or primary illness. Indications for immediate ophthalmologic evaluation include suspicion of an eye-threatening disease or tumor, a sleeping infant who does not reject light, an awake infant who does not follow with either or both eyes, and asymmetry in the vision testing results, particularly if there has been ocular trauma.

Indications for Admission

- Eye-threatening disease
- Intraocular or intracranial tumor

BIBLIOGRAPHY

Calhoun JH: Eye examinations in infants and children. *Pediatr Rev* 1997;18:28–31.
Day S: History, examination and further investigation, in Taylor D (ed): *Pediatric Ophthalmology,* 2nd ed. Malden, MA: Blackwell Science, 1997, pp 77–92.
Repka MX: Refraction in infants and children, in Nelson LB, Harley RD (eds): *Harley's Pediatric Ophthalmology,* 4th ed. Philadelphia: Saunders, 1998, pp 112–114.

EXCESSIVE TEARING

Tears are produced immediately after birth, but the volume increases after the sixth week. Excess tearing is very common and is secondary to either excess production or insufficient drainage. Excess production is usually due to irritation, infection, foreign body, trauma, iritis, or glaucoma. Insufficient drainage is caused by a stenotic or blocked lacrimal system, usually at the level of the nasolacrimal duct, which conducts tears from the lacrimal sac into the nose.

Clinical Presentation

Excess Production
Tearing due to excess production is often accompanied by conjunctival injection in older children, but redness is usually absent in the newborn. Lid swelling and nasal discharge are common.

Congenital Glaucoma (Elevated Intraocular Pressure)   Congenital glaucoma is accompanied by excess growth of the eye (buphthalmos), photophobia, loss of vision, and tearing, with discharge at the nares. The clarity of the cornea may be reduced, with obscuration of the iris markings. Glaucoma may be unilateral or bilateral, and there may be a positive family history.

Iritis   Iritis is accompanied by photophobia, ciliary flush, a small pupil with diminished response, and decreased visual acuity. It is uncommon in infancy, except after eye trauma.

Insufficient Drainage

Dacryostenosis (Nasolacrimal Duct Obstruction)   Dacryostenosis is the most common ophthalmologic cause of excess tearing in infancy, usually presenting in the first 3 months of life. A persistent mucoid or mucopurulent discharge is usually present, in addition to recurrent conjunctivitis. Nasolacrimal duct obstruction may be accompanied by dermatitis of the lids due to the chronic infection, but there is no nasal discharge or photophobia (distinguishing dacryostenosis from congenital glaucoma). Digital pressure on the distended lacrimal sac at the side of the nose causes reflux of mucoid or mucopurulent material into the palpebral fissure.

Dacryocystitis   Acute dacryocystitis is a suppurative infection of the lacrimal sac. It presents with tenderness and swelling of the lacrimal sac as well as erythema and swelling of the overlying skin. There is usually a history of nasolacrimal duct obstruction.

Diagnosis

The priority is to rule out *excessive tear production* as the cause before diagnosing nasolacrimal duct obstruction. Photophobia, eyelid closure (blepharospasm), ciliary flush, and nasal discharge suggest excessive production.

Consider a *foreign body* if the tearing started suddenly, especially if it is accompanied by pain and blepharospasm. The diagnosis of *glaucoma* is confirmed by evaluation of the intraocular pressure. Consider *iritis* after trauma.

The diagnosis of *nasolacrimal duct obstruction* is suggested by constant tearing beginning in the second or third month of life, associated with concurrent eye discharge and conjunctivitis. There may be swelling of the lacrimal sac with reflux of material from the punctum when pressure is applied. *Dacryocystitis* is likely if there is erythematous swelling of the lacrimal sac. Discharge from the punctum is rarely present.

ED Management

The management of excessive tearing secondary to a foreign body (pp 491–494) or conjunctivitis (pp 495–499) is detailed elsewhere. Glaucoma and iritis require immediate ophthalmologic consultation.

Dacryostenosis   In most cases, dacryostenosis clears spontaneously by 6 to 12 months of age. Treatment consists of massage of the lacrimal sac three times a day to express the contents. Using the pad of a clean finger, direct the massage from the area of the medial canthal ligament down the side of the nose to the level of the nostril. Refer the patient to an ophthalmologist for evaluation if the condition does not clear by the sixth month, especially if there have been frequent infections.

Dacryocystitis   After obtaining a culture of any material in the palpebral fissure, treat acute dacryocystitis with oral antibiotics. Use 30 mg/kg/day of cefadroxil (divided bid) or 50 mg/kg/day of cephalexin (divided qid or tid). Topical ophthalmic antibiotics (bacitracin, erythromycin, sulfacetamide, or polymyxin-trimethoprim) four times a day, along with warm compresses, are useful as adjunctive therapy. Probing of the nasolacrimal duct may eventually be necessary in order to avoid recurrence.

Follow-up

- Dacryocystitis: in 2 to 3 days if there is no improvement

Indications for Admission

- Congenital glaucoma
- Dacryocystitis unresponsive to outpatient management

BIBLIOGRAPHY

Ballard EA: Excessive tearing in infancy and early childhood. The role and treatment of congenital nasolacrimal duct obstruction. *Postgrad Med* 2000;107: 149–154.

Campolattaro BN, Lueder GT, Tychsen L: Spectrum of pediatric dacryocystitis: medical and surgical management of 54 cases. *J Pediatr Ophthalmol Strabismus* 1997;34:143–153.

Robb RM: Tearing abnormalities, in Isenberg SJ (ed): *The Eye in Infancy,* 2nd ed. St. Louis: Mosby-Year Book, 1994, pp. 248–253.

EYELID INFLAMMATION

The eyelids can be affected by dermatologic conditions that also involve the skin elsewhere. However, the eyelids may appear inflamed because of more serious infections such as preseptal and orbital cellulitis.

Clinical Presentation and Diagnosis

Preseptal and Orbital Cellulitis   The orbital septum connects to both the periosteum of the orbital bones and the tarsal plates of the lid and separates the lid structures from the orbital contents. Infections can spread from contiguous structures or be blood-borne from distant sites. The organisms most frequently implicated are *S. aureus, S. pyogenes,* and *S. pneumoniae. H. influenzae* type B is no longer a common pathogen.

Both preseptal (or periorbital) cellulitis and orbital cellulitis present with lid swelling, erythema, and pain. Preseptal cellulitis can arise from a break in the skin (insect bite, laceration), trauma, dacryocystitis, chalazion, stye, or sinusitis. The vision is usually normal.

Orbital cellulitis is characterized by the diagnostic triad of proptosis, limitation of motion, and pain on motion. Vision may be decreased and, in severe cases, there may be an afferent pupillary defect (APD). (To assess for APD, shine a bright light on each pupil for a few seconds, alternating back and forth. Normally there is a consensual response, with both pupils constricting when one eye is illuminated. With APD however, both pupils gradually dilate, rather than constrict, when the affected eye is illuminated.) The patient appears toxic, with fever and lethargy. Most often, the sinuses are involved and there is a history of a recent upper respiratory infection. CT scan is indicated if the differentiation between preseptal and orbital cellulitis is in doubt.

Hordeolum   A hordeolum, or stye, is an infection of a sebaceous gland of the lid (gland of Zeis). It usually presents as a localized erythematous swelling of the lid margin, although the entire lid may be affected. The area is tender, and the abscess may point at the base of a lash. Several styes may be present simultaneously.

Chalazion   A chalazion is a granulomatous swelling of the other sebaceous gland of the lid (meibomian gland). It begins as a firm, painless, ovoid swelling within the lid itself. There may be multiple chalazia. Secondary infection leads to increased swelling and pain, with the abscess pointing onto either the skin surface or the conjunctival side of the lid.

Blepharitis   Blepharitis is inflammation of the margin of the lid, usually secondary to *Staphylococcus aureus* infection. Blepharitis is often chronic and may lead to the development of styes and chalazia. Typically, the lid margins are erythematous, crusted, and swollen, and there may be an associated conjunctivitis. Pruritus, burning, tearing, blurry vision, and loss of lashes are common complaints.

Seborrheic Dermatitis   Seborrheic dermatitis is an erythematous or crusting eruption with overlying yellowish greasy scale. Affected areas can include the eyelids and eyelashes in addition to the scalp, postauricular areas, ears, and neck. Conjunctivitis is uncommon in the absence of blepharitis.

Herpes Simplex   Herpes simplex is a viral infection that can affect the eyelids as primary or secondary disease. It presents with grouped vesicles on an erythematous base. The surrounding skin and lips may also be affected, and there may be associated conjunctivitis, keratitis, and preauricular lymphadenopathy. Recurrences are common.

Varicella   The characteristic papular, vesicular, and crusting rash of varicella may affect the eyelids and surrounding skin. Conjunctivitis can be present, particularly if the lid margin is affected. Photophobia, iritis, pupillary abnormalities (irregular or sluggishly reacting), and loss of vision are worrisome but rare findings. Zoster causes pain in the affected area, followed by swelling of the eyelids. Several days later, the characteristic vesicles develop.

Molluscum Contagiosum   Molluscum appear as 1 to 5 mm flesh-colored umbilicated papules, usually associated with similar lesions on the periorbital skin. Patients are usually asymptomatic, although involvement of the lid margins can produce a concomitant conjunctivitis.

Parasitic Infestation   The crab louse (*Phthirus pubis*) can infest the eyelids. The infestation is pruritic, and lice and ova, or "nits" (tiny white dots), can be seen attached to the lashes and eyebrows. Severe conjunctivitis can result.

ED Management

Preseptal and Orbital Cellulitis   Mild preseptal cellulitis can be treated on an outpatient basis with oral amoxicillin-clavulanate [45 mg/kg/day of amoxicillin (200/28.5, 400/57) divided bid]. However, if orbital cellulitis cannot be ruled out, obtain a CT scan of the orbits. If orbital involvement is confirmed, admit the patient and treat with IV antibiotics (nafcillin 150 mg/kg/day divided q 6 h *and* cefotaxime 100 mg/kg/day divided q 8 h), and consult with an ophthalmologist. Obtain blood cultures prior to giving IV antibiotics, and perform a lumbar puncture if meningeal or cerebral signs are present. Consult an otolaryngologist if there is sinus involvement.

Hordeolum and Chalazion   Treat hordeola and infected chalazia with warm (not hot) compresses for 3 to 5 min three times a day. Apply about ½ cm of an ophthalmic antibiotic ointment (e.g., erythromycin, bacitracin) three times daily after the compress. Treat an associated blepharitis (see below) to prevent recurrence. Usually a hordeolum disappears within a week. Refer the patient to an ophthalmologist if improvement does not occur within 2 or 3 days. A chronic chalazion may remain for weeks to months and does not require excision as long as the patient's vision is unaffected.

Blepharitis   Blepharitis is a chronic disorder, and treatment is directed toward keeping the disease under control. Use warm-water compresses to loosen the scales at the base of the lashes. The scales can then be removed with an applicator stick moistened with diluted baby shampoo. Apply erythromycin or bacitracin ophthalmic ointment three times daily to reduce bacterial overgrowth.

Seborrhea   Treat seborrhea with gentle cleansing with diluted baby shampoo to remove the crusts. Shampoo the scalp every other day with a keratolytic shampoo (Sebulex, Zetar, Head and Shoulders). Ophthalmologic referral is needed before treatment with topical corticosteroids.

Herpes Simplex   If conjunctivitis is present or keratitis is suspected, refer the patient immediately to an ophthalmologist for topical antiviral therapy.

Consider oral antiviral therapy (acyclovir 80 mg/kg/day divided qid, maximum 800 mg qid) for frequent recurrences.

Varicella and Zoster   Varicella and zoster eyelid infections do not require treatment unless intraocular or corneal involvement is suspected. If the patient demonstrates ciliary flush, photophobia, pupillary abnormalities, or visual loss, refer to an ophthalmologist immediately.

Molluscum Contagiosum   Molluscum is usually a self-limited disease, so no treatment is necessary unless the lesions are cosmetically unacceptable, increase in number, or occur at the lid margin and are associated with conjunctivitis. Refer to an ophthalmologist for incision and curettage.

Lice   Treat pediculosis with applications of a bland ophthalmic ointment (Lacri-Lube) to the base and length of the lashes three times daily. Repeat at weekly intervals to kill the emerging lice. Defer forceps removal of lice and nits to an ophthalmologist. Check for and treat pubic lice, and thoroughly wash clothing and bedding. Sexual abuse must be considered.

Follow-up

- Chalazion, blepharitis, seborrhea, and lice: primary care follow-up in 1 to 2 weeks.
- Preseptal cellulitis: 24 hours

Indications for Admission

- Orbital cellulitis
- Preseptal cellulitis if no improvement on oral antibiotics

BIBLIOGRAPHY

Donahue SP and Schwartz G: Preseptal and orbital cellulitis in childhood. A changing microbiologic spectrum. *Ophthalmology* 1998;105:1902–1905.

Herpetic Eye Disease Study Group: Oral acyclovir for herpes simplex virus eye disease: effect on prevention of epithelial keratitis and stromal keratitis. *Arch Ophthalmol* 2000;118:1030–1036.

Lederman C, Miller M: Hordeola and chalazia. *Pediatr Rev* 1999;20:283–284.

Ostler HB, Ostler MW: *Diseases of the External Eye and Adnexa: A Text and Atlas.* Baltimore, Williams & Wilkins, 1993, pp 11–66.

Uzcategui N, Warman R, Smith A, Howard CW. Clinical practice guidelines for the management of orbital cellulitis. *J Pediatr Ophthalmol Strabismus* 1998; 35:73–79.

OCULAR TRAUMA

Consider ocular trauma in cases of sudden reduction of vision, blepharospasm (uncontrollable closure of one or both eyes), facial trauma, and high-velocity projectile injury. In the setting of multiple trauma, delay the search for and treatment of ocular injuries only until more serious priorities have been addressed. If trauma to the eye is suspected, however, apply a protective shield until it can be adequately evaluated. Eye trauma may also be the presentation of child abuse.

Clinical Presentation

Lid Lacerations   Lid lacerations, particularly if vertical, are easily seen. However, a search for lid lacerations is required in all cases of facial trauma. There may also be an associated injury to the underlying globe. Vertical lacerations through the lid margin result in wide gaping of the wound because of the circular nature of the orbicularis oculi muscle. Lacerations through the medial one-sixth of the lower lid margin may be associated with a severed canaliculus.

Ruptured Globe   Always suspect a ruptured or lacerated globe in cases of blunt facial trauma or when there is an eyelid laceration. The findings may be subtle and can include reduction of vision, subconjunctival hemorrhage, swelling of the conjunctiva, deformity or obvious laceration of the cornea or sclera, shallowing or absence of the anterior chamber, deformity of the iris, cataract, softness of the globe, and extrusion of intraorbital contents. Iris tissue may plug the perforation, so the only finding may be a distorted pupil (peaked, pointed, pulled to one side, or flattened on one side). Staining the tears with fluorescein can help diagnose a subtle perforation of the cornea because the clear aqueous stream leaking from the perforation will be more obvious in the fluorescein (Seidel test). Do not use an open solution of fluorescein because of possible bacterial contamination, particulary with *Pseudomonas aeruginosa*.

Hyphema   Blunt or penetrating trauma can cause a hyphema (an anterior-chamber intraocular hemorrhage). The findings can be subtle, particularly in the supine patient, if small amounts of blood are mixed with the aqueous humor. Look for obscuration of the iris markings. Larger quantities of blood are more obvious and cast a reddish glow on the iris. In the upright patient, the blood settles because of gravity, and a blood-aqueous level can be seen. The vision is reduced, the conjunctiva hyperemic, and the pupil often irregular and pointed. Pain is almost always present.

A dangerous rise in intraocular pressure may result, especially in patients with sickle cell disease or trait. Rebleeding can occur, usually within the first 5 days after the injury. It is associated with the sudden onset of pain, increased intraocular pressure, and eventual opacification of the cornea.

Corneal and Conjunctival Abrasions   Superficial abrasions of the conjunctiva and cornea present with pain that can be severe, photophobia, conjunctival hyperemia, and tearing. The vision is variably affected. An abrasion can often be seen as an irregularity of the normally smooth surface of the globe or as a shadow cast on the iris when a light is directed into the eye.

Fluorescein dye instilled into the cul-de-sac will stain areas of epithelial cell loss and glow bright yellow-green under a cobalt blue or Wood's lamp. A subtle perforation of the cornea can be diagnosed when fluorescein staining reveals clear aqueous leaking from the perforation site (Seidel test). Do not use an open solution of fluorescein because of possible bacterial contamination, particulary with *P. aeruginosa.*

Foreign Bodies   Superficial foreign bodies present with poorly localized discomfort. Vision is variably affected, but tearing, photophobia, and blepharospasm are common. Lid eversion may be required for the object to be seen, and magnification may be needed if the object is transparent. A foreign body can adhere to the conjunctiva of the upper lid at the edge of the tarsal ridge and cause a vertical linear abrasion of the superior cornea. There may be one or more foreign bodies.

Intraocular foreign bodies may present with variable signs of ocular irritation. The expected findings of decreased visual acuity, irritation, pain, and signs of penetration may be absent, so a high index of suspicion is required. The history is very important in establishing the diagnosis.

Orbital Fracture   Fracture of the floor or walls of the orbit can injure the extraocular muscles or surrounding tissues and result in limitation of ocular motion and diplopia. Enophthalmos or, rarely, proptosis can result. Fracture of the floor of the orbit can result in injury to the infraorbital nerve, with resultant hypesthesia in the lower lid and cheek. Air may be introduced subcutaneously from the affected sinus, causing crepitus. Injury to the ciliary ganglion causes dilation of the pupil and loss of accommodation (ability to focus), so that near vision is more affected than distance vision.

Burns   Thermal and chemical burns can cause both immediate and delayed damage. Burns due to acids coagulate and denature surface proteins but generally do not penetrate the eye, whereas alkali burns penetrate and damage internal ocular structures. In addition to the globe, the skin of the face and lids may be affected. Presentation depends on the extent of the injury but may include blepharospasm, tearing, photophobia, decreased visual acuity, conjunctival swelling, hyperemia or ischemia, loss of corneal clarity, and variable pain.

Iris Tears   Tears of the iris occur after blunt or penetrating injuries to the eye. The muscles of the iris are circular and radial, so a tear in the iris can cause deformity in its size, shape, and motility. Despite the highly vascular content of the iris, hyphema after an iris tear may not occur.

Retrobulbar Hemorrhage   A retrobulbar hemorrhage causes acute proptosis, chemosis, variable subconjunctival hemorrhage, decreased vision, pain, reduced corneal clarity, glaucoma, and limitation of ocular motion. It can occur after blunt or penetrating injury and may lead to loss of vision because of central retinal vessel occlusion.

Traumatic Iritis   Traumatic iritis is due to exudation of protein and inflammatory cells into the aqueous humor and can occur after any injury to the eye. It is characterized by decreased vision, photophobia, conjunctival hyperemia [particularly in a halo fashion around the corneal limbus (ciliary flush)], and miosis with pupillary inequality (the affected pupil smaller).

Child Abuse   Child abuse victims may present with injury to the face and eyelids, subconjunctival hemorrhage, hyphema, pupillary abnormalities, eye movement abnormalities, papilledema, and retinal hemorrhages.

Diagnosis

A thorough history and determination of visual acuity in each eye with and without glasses are the first steps in the evaluation of all cases of possible ocular injury *with the exception of chemical (especially alkali) burns to the eye, which require immediate lavage.* Ascertain the precipitating event, the nature of the implicated vehicle or substance, the time of the injury, any visual loss or disturbance in either eye, onset of pain and injection, presence of light intolerance, and any previous trauma or other ocular difficulty.

Check vision with a standard Snellen chart (see pp 482–483). Test the uninjured eye first in order to reduce anxiety. Unless there is a suspected ruptured globe, place one drop of an anesthetic in the eye (e.g., proparacaine 0.5%) to reduce the pain and aid in the evaluation. Make a note about the eye tested (it is customary to test the right eye first), the vision test used, the distance from the object of regard to the examined eye, and the result.

Examine the face, lids, lashes, and brows. Look for ptosis and deformity of the lid and surrounding orbit. Observe the extraocular movements, look for strabismus, and note any complaint of diplopia, limitation of movement, or pain caused by movement. Examine the palpebral and bulbar conjunctiva, and look for evidence of laceration, localized injection, or foreign body.

To evert the upper lid, hold an applicator stick horizontally at the midportion of the lid. Grasp the lid lashes with the thumb and forefinger of the other hand and evert, using the applicator stick to help form a hinge. Look for foreign bodies at the ridge formed by the top of the tarsal plate or lodged deep in the upper or lower fornix (junction of bulbar and palpebral conjunctivae).

Check the clarity of the cornea, and look for laceration, particularly at the corneoscleral junction. Suspect a ruptured globe if the anterior chamber is shallower or deeper than that of the other eye or if the pupil is distorted.

A hyphema can be as obvious as a definite aqueous-blood level in the anterior chamber or as subtle as a faint red tinge to the iris. It may be visible only on magnification with a biomicroscope (slit lamp). Pupillary distortion and pain often accompany a hyphema.

An abrasion can be delineated with fluorescein dye. Instill the fluorescein into the cul-de-sac. The dye will adhere to areas of epithelial cell loss and fluoresce bright yellow-green under a cobalt blue or Wood's lamp.

Use the red reflex of light from the direct ophthalmoscope illuminating the pupil to estimate and compare the clarity of the ocular media. In a darkened room, set the dial of the ophthalmoscope to zero, stand 12 to

18 inches away from the patient's eyes, and direct the light beam so that the two pupils are equally illuminated and can be viewed through the aperture of the instrument (you may have to change the dial setting of the ophthalmoscope to focus on the iris). A shadow of a corneal abrasion or cataract may be illuminated in the red pupillary reflex, and there can be a difference in the color and brightness of the reflex. Use the ophthalmoscope to examine the optic nerve head for papilledema and the retina for hemorrhage, tears, or detachment.

The diagnosis of a foreign body may require ultrasound or x-ray, but avoid magnetic resonance imaging (MRI) if a magnetic foreign body is suspected.

To evaluate a possible orbital fracture and compare the position of the eyes, stand above and behind the patient and sight down the forehead. With the patient's eyes open, compare the position of the most forward point of each cornea. With the patient's eyes closed, compare the most anterior point of the upper lid. Palpate the orbital rim for any irregularity.

ED Management

For eye injuries in which the integrity of the eye is not assured, avoid increasing intraocular pressure, and do not manipulate the eyes. Have the patient rest supine and avoid excessive movement. Tape a protective shield from forehead to cheekbone over the injured eye until a definitive diagnosis can be made. Avoid a bulky pad under the shield to prevent pressure on the globe. Topical cycloplegics are not necessary in the initial evaluation of the patient, but topical anesthesia can be very helpful with chemical burns and foreign bodies.

Lid Lacerations   Refer the patient to an ophthalmologist if there is a vertical laceration through the lid margin or the laceration affects the nasal one-sixth of the lower lid and may therefore damage the tear excretory apparatus. Always check for injuries to the underlying globe.

Ruptured Globe   Immediately refer the patient to an ophthalmologist. Delay radiographs to search for foreign bodies until after the evaluation. Do not remove pigmented material from the surface of the globe, as it may represent intraocular contents. Use a protective shield without a pad, and place the patient supine, with the head of the bed elevated 30 degrees.

Hyphema   Refer immediately to an ophthalmologist. Put the patient at rest in a quiet area, use a protective shield, and avoid excessive manipulation. Do not give aspirin or ibuprofen, which may prolong the bleeding time, and test for sickle cell disease when appropriate.

Corneal Abrasion   Treat with a topical ophthalmic antibiotic (e.g., sulfacetamide, polysporin-trimethoprim, erythromycin) three times daily for 1 to 2 days. Occlusive dressings are often removed by young children and are optional in small superficial abrasions. If an occlusive dressing is used, instill two drops of a topical anesthetic, followed by a topical antibiotic. Avoid repeated instillation of topical anesthetics because they interfere with healing and can cause keratitis. Refer the patient to an ophthalmologist the next day if the abrasion is large, pain or photophobia is still present, vision is affected, or the eye remains red. Small corneal abrasions often heal within a day. If the pain seems out of proportion to the size of the abrasion or if there is corneal haze around the abrasion, consider corneal ulcer and refer immediately to an ophthalmologist.

Foreign Bodies   Superficial corneal and conjunctival foreign bodies may be irrigated off the anesthetized eye with a forceful stream of sterile saline or other ocular irrigating solution (Dacriose). A swab can be used to remove or loosen a foreign body and the remainder irrigated off the eye. Check for multiple foreign bodies. Treat any remaining corneal or conjunctival abrasion as above. Refer the patient immediately if the foreign body cannot easily be removed or there is a retained rust deposit.

Intraocular and intraorbital foreign bodies require an immediate ophthalmologic consultation. Apply a protective shield.

Orbital Fracture   Refer any patient with an orbital (blowout) fracture to an ophthalmologist, particularly if there is enophthalmos, limitation of motion, diplopia, pupillary inequality, or hypesthesia in the area of the infraorbital nerve. Obtain Waters' and Caldwell views, and look for an air-fluid level in the maxillary antrum and for orbital emphysema. A computed tomography (CT) scan is not routinely indicated unless limitation of motion is noted. Antibiotics are not necessary, but advise the patient to avoid blowing the nose until the follow-up visit. The ophthalmologist must evaluate the patient within 5 days and arrange surgical repair within 7 to 14 days after the injury.

Burns   Chemical burns require immediate lavage with 1 to 2 L of sterile saline, although tapwater is preferable to any delay. Use a topical anesthetic and lid retractors. A Morgan lens (a clear plastic scleral shell with cannula attached) will deliver irrigation to the eye more thoroughly. Sweep the fornices with applicator sticks to remove foreign bodies, and check the pH of the tears with litmus paper 30 min after irrigation is complete to be sure that neutralization has occurred. Normally tears are approximately neutral (pH 7). Do not use an irrigant of opposite pH to the caustic chemical, as more damage will occur. Consult an ophthalmologist immediately.

Thermal burns are rarely isolated to the lids or globe except in cases of cigarette burns, which are treated as simple abrasions with antibiotic ointment. More extensive burns of the face also require an ophthalmologic evaluation of the eye and lid function.

Traumatic Iritis   Refer immediately to an ophthalmologist for evaluation of the globe and treatment with topical cycloplegics.

Retrobulbar Hemorrhage   Immediate ophthalmologic evaluation is necessary for treatment with pressure-lowering drugs (intravenous mannitol), surgery (lateral canthotomy), and intravenous steroids.

Follow-up

- Corneal abrasion: opthalmology the next day
- Hyphema: ophthalmology the next day if adherence assured
- Orbital fracture: within 5 days with ophthalmology

Indications for Admission

- Ruptured globe
- Hyphema if adherence with follow-up visits and bed rest cannot be assured
- Lid laceration requiring surgical repair in operating room
- Intraocular foreign body
- Orbital fracture if compliance with follow-up care cannot be assured
- Retrobulbar hemorrhage

BIBLIOGRAPHY

Coody D, Banks JM, Yetman RJ, et al: Eye trauma in children: epidemiology, management, and prevention. *J Pediatr Health Care* 1997;11:182–188.

Grant WM, Schuman JS: *Toxicology of the Eye*, 4th ed. Springfield, IL: Charles C Thomas, 1993.

Kivlin JD, Simons KB, Lazoritz S, Ruttum MS: Shaken baby syndrome. *Ophthalmology* 2000;107:1246–1254.

Kuhn F, Morris R, Witherspoon CD, et al: Standardized classification of ocular trauma. *Ophthalmology* 1996;103:240–243.

THE RED EYE

The conjunctiva is normally transparent. When it is inflamed, the numerous fine blood vessels become engorged; hence the term pink eye. Inflammation is most often secondary to infection. Organisms include bacteria (*Staphylococcus aureus, Streptococcus viridans, S. pneumoniae, Haemophilus influenzae,* enterococci, *Neisseria gonorrhoeae, Chlamydia trachomatis*) and viruses (herpes simplex, adenovirus, enterovirus).

Conjunctival hyperemia can be secondary to keratitis (superficial corneal inflammation) or uveitis (inflammation of the iris and ciliary body). Keratitis is most often caused by ocular trauma or infection (adenovirus, herpes, *Chlamydia*). The anterior uvea can be inflamed by trauma, infection (Lyme disease, tuberculosis, varicella), a corneal foreign body, or JRA.

Other causes of a red eye are allergy and reaction to dust, smoke, foreign bodies, chemicals, and other irritants. Conjunctival hyperemia can also accompany serious acute conditions such as orbital cellulitis, erythema multiforme, and Kawasaki disease.

Clinical Presentation and Diagnosis

Conjunctivitis   Inflammation of the bulbar and palpebral conjunctival mucous membranes produces vascular engorgement, appearing as diffusely distributed, discrete red vessels. Although itching or a "sandy" sensation is frequently noted, there is no ocular pain, and photophobia, if present, is mild. Visual acuity is normal. On examination, a discharge ranging from mucous and crusting to frank pus may be present, along with lid edema and erythema. The perilimbal area (immediately adjacent to the outer edge of the cornea) is spared.

A *viral* etiology is suggested by a watery or mucoid discharge during a URI, especially if there is preauricular adenopathy or an associated pharyngitis (adenovirus pharyngoconjunctival fever). *Herpes simplex* can be diagnosed from viral culture or with immunofluorescence.

A *bacterial* cause is more likely if there is a purulent eye discharge with or without otitis media.

Allergy is suggested by a seasonal (spring or autumn) watery or mucoid discharge, edema, pruritus, multiple creases on the lower lid, and cobble-stoning of the palpebral conjunctiva. However, there is wide overlap in the clinical picture among the causes.

Neonatal conjunctivitis was more frequent when silver nitrate prophylaxis was used. A purulent discharge in the first week of life suggests gonococcal or chlamydial infection, but a definite diagnosis cannot be made without confirmatory tests. Gram-negative intracellular diplococci and polymorphonuclear neutrophil leukocytes (PMNs) are found on Gram-stained smears of eye discharge caused by *N. gonorrhoeae;* the organism can be grown on nonselective chocolate agar with incubation in 5 to 10% carbon dioxide or on specialized culture media. Moisten the swab with saline before the culture is done.

Chlamydia trachomatis is diagnosed with cell culture of conjunctival scrapings, immunoglobin antibody titers, monoclonal antibody antigen tests on conjunctival smears, or enzyme-linked immunosorbent assay (ELISA). Obtain the specimen from the lower palpebral conjunctiva by scraping with a sterile spatula.

Do not use a topical anesthetic in obtaining a scraping or a sample of the discharge for culture, as the preservatives in the anesthetic can interfere with growth.

Corneal Disease (Keratitis)   Corneal involvement is generally accompanied by conjunctival hyperemia which extends to the edge of the cornea. Pain, photophobia, and decreased vision are common. Diagnose a disruption of the corneal epithelium by fluorescein staining of the cornea, followed by illumination with a cobalt blue or Wood's light. Areas of epithelial disturbance or loss will fluoresce a bright yellow-green in the middle of the yellow fluorescein. Do not use an open solution of fluorescein because of the frequency of bacterial contamination, particularly with *P. aeruginosa.*

Uveitis   Inflammation of the interior pigmented vascular structures of the eye can be associated with conjunctival hyperemia. The presentation is variable and may include photophobia, reduced vision, pain on reading, conjunctival hyperemia, ciliary flush (a pink halo of dilated episcleral vessels that surround the cornea), and pupillary miosis.

Erythema Multiforme   Erythema multiforme major (pp 95–97) is characterized by skin and mucous membrane involvement (Stevens-Johnson syndrome). There may be a purulent conjunctival discharge or membrane formation with adhesions between the bulbar and palpebral conjunctiva.

Kawasaki Disease   Consider Kawasaki disease (pp 360–362) in a patient with some combination of fever, cervical lymphadenopathy, stomatitis, rash, and edema of the peripheral extremities; transient conjunctivitis without discharge accompanies the fever.

ED Management

The determination of visual acuity is of paramount importance; any acute reduction is an indication for immediate ophthalmologic referral. Evidence of intraocular involvement includes severe photophobia or ocular pain, vascular engorgement at the limbus (corneoscleral junction), and pupillary abnormalities. Always inquire about a history of ocular trauma.

Conjunctivitis   In general, bacterial cultures are not needed. Treat with a topical ophthalmic antibiotic, either one drop three times daily of a solution (ciprofloxacin, ofloxacin, polymyxin B/trimethoprim, 10% sulfacetamide, tobramycin) or three times daily application of an ointment (bacitracin, erythromycin, gentamicin, polymixin B/bacitracin, 10% sulfacetamide, tobramycin). The antibiotics will rapidly treat most uncomplicated bacterial cases and prevent secondary bacterial infection if the etiology is viral. *Do not prescribe steroid preparations without ophthalmologic consultation.* Continue treatment for 5 days or for 2 days after clinical resolution. Instruct the parent to gently wipe away any crust with a warm, damp gauze pad or cotton ball before instilling the antibiotic. Meticulous hygiene (no shared towels or washcloths) and frequent handwashing are also necessary, and advise the patient to discard any eye makeup. Refer the patient to an ophthalmologist if there is persistent infection, severe photophobia or pain, or visual complaints.

With *neonatal conjunctivitis*, consider the presence of gram-negative diplococci in PMNs to be diagnostic of *gonococcal conjunctivitis* until cultures are available. Admit the infant and treat with one dose of ceftriaxone (25 to 50 mg/kg, maximum 125 mg) IM or IV; a single dose of cefotaxime (100 mg/kg IV or IM) is an acceptable alternative. Isolate the infant for 24 h, and remove any discharge with frequent sterile saline irrigations, taking care to avoid splashing the pus into the caregiver's eyes. Test the infant for concomitant infection with *Chlamydia*, *Treponema pallidum*, and HIV.

If the Gram's stain in an infant 1 to 12 weeks of age with a purulent discharge reveals PMNs but few organisms and antigen detection, culture, and serologic testing for *Chlamydia* are not available, treat for presumed chlamydial conjunctivitis with oral erythromycin (50 mg/kg/day divided q 6 h) for 2 weeks to avoid systemic complications such as pneumonitis. Topical ophthalmic antibiotics are optional; use erythromycin ointment four times daily for 3 days.

If testing for *Chlamydia* is available, treat with erythromycin ointment pending test results. Oral, but not topical, erythromycin is associated with pyloric stenosis in infants less than 3 months of age. Reserve the oral antibiotic for confirmed cases of *Chlamydia* conjunctivitis.

Treat *allergic conjunctivitis* with one drop four times daily of an antihistamine (levocabastine, naphazoline/antazoline, naphazoline/pheniramine) and a mast cell stabilizer (lodoxamide). Alternatively, use a nonsteroidal anti-inflammatory drug (NSAID), such as ketorolac, alone. Combination drugs (mast cell stabilizer plus H_1 antagonist plus NSAID) have recently been introduced (see Table 17-1). Do not give topical steroids. If there is no improvement in 7 days or the symptoms worsen, refer the patient to an ophthalmologist.

Refer all cases of *keratitis* and *uveitis* to an ophthalmologist immediately. The treatment of *erythema multiforme* (pp 95–97) and *Kawasaki disease* (pp 360–362) is detailed elsewhere.

Follow-up

- Conjunctivitis: 4 days if no improvement

Indications for Admission

- Stevens-Johnson syndrome
- Gonococcal conjunctivitis

Table 17-1   Topical Ophthalmic Antiallergics

ANTIALLERGICS	MECHANISM OF ACTION	DOSING
Ketorolac (Acular)	Nonsteroidal anti-inflammatory drug (NSAID)	1gtt qid
Levocabastine (Livostin)	H_1 antagonist	1 gtt qid (shake well)
Lodoxamide (Alomide)	Mast cell stabilizer	1–2 gtts up to qid for up to 3 mos
Cromolyn (Crolom)	Mast cell stabilizer	1–2 gtts regularly q 4–6 h
Naphazoline/ Pheniramine (Naphcon-A)	Antihistamine/ vasoconstrictor	1–2 gtts up to qid
Naphazoline/ Antazoline (Vasocon-A)	Antihistamine/ vasoconstrictor	1–2 gtts up to qid
Ketotifen (Zaditor)	Mast cell stabilizer/ H_1 antagonist/	1 gtt q 8–12 h
Nedocromil (Alocril)	Mast cell stabilizer	1–2 gtts bid
Olopatadine (Patanol)	Mast cell stabilizer/ H_1 antagonist	1 gtt bid

BIBLIOGRAPHY

Nakanisji AK, Soltau JB: Common viral infections of the eye. *Pediatr Ann* 1996; 25:5452–5454.

Tabbara KF, Hyndiuk RA (eds): *Infections of the Eye.* 2nd ed. Boston, Little, Brown, 1996.

THE WHITE PUPIL (LEUKOCORIA)

Light entering the eye is absorbed by the pigmented interior and does not leave in sufficient quantity to illuminate the pupil. If an opacity exists in the normally clear optical media, light will reflect off the opacity and be seen in the pupil as a white reflection (leukocoria).

The most common causes of leukocoria are cataracts, infections (syphilis, toxocariasis, toxoplasmosis, tuberculosis), intraocular hemorrhage, retinopathy of prematurity, detached retina, retinoblastoma, coloboma, and persistent hyperplastic primary vitreous. Therefore opacities can represent static conditions that interfere with vision (cataracts), active diseases that can lead to visual difficulties (early retinal detachment), or life-threatening illnesses (retinoblastoma).

Clinical Presentation and Diagnosis

Examine both pupils, using a direct ophthalmoscope set at zero at a distance of 12 to 18 in. from the eye. Normally, the red reflex is symmetric and the pupil size equal. If there is an opacity in the media, all or part of the pupil will appear dark or off-white instead of red. Depending on the extent of the abnormality, the eyes and/or pupils may be asymmetric in size. There may be no pupillary light response, or it may be slower than in the opposite eye.

Leukocoria can be unilateral or bilateral. If unilateral disease is suspected, covering the "good" eye will upset a small child, while covering the affected eye will not change the child's behavior.

ED Management

Consult an ophthalmologist immediately whenever leukocoria is suspected.

Indication for Admission

- Any case of leukocoria if prompt outpatient evaluation and follow-up cannot be assured

BIBLIOGRAPHY

Abramson DH, Frank CM, Susman M, et al: Presenting signs of retinoblastoma. *J Pediatr* 1998;132:505–508.

Canzano JC, Handa JT: Utility of pupillary dilation for detecting leukocoria in patients with retinoblastoma. *Pediatrics* 1999;104:e44.

Lee YC, Kim HS: Clinical symptoms and visual outcome in patients with presumed congenital cataract. *J Pediatr Ophthalmol Strabismus* 2000;37:219–224.

CHAPTER 18

Orthopedic Emergencies

Ronald L. Mann
- Eric Small (contributor—Back Pain; Rehabilitation of Sports Injuries)
- Katherine J. Chou (contributor—Splinting)

ARTHRITIS

Arthritis results from synovial inflammation due to infectious and non-infectious causes (Table 18-1). The hallmarks of arthritis are joint swelling, pain, and limitation of motion. In contrast, arthralgia is pain or tenderness *without swelling.*

Acute bacterial arthritis or septic arthritis is a true orthopedic emergency that requires prompt diagnosis and treatment. Pyarthrosis can be devastating because of the risk of necrosis and subsequent growth arrest.

Acute rheumatic fever, juvenile rheumatoid arthritis, systemic lupus erythematosus, Henoch-Schönlein purpura, and Crohn's disease are the most common noninfectious causes of arthritis.

Clinical Presentation

By definition, an arthritic joint presents with a combination of swelling, erythema, increased warmth, pain, and decreased range of motion. The

Table 18-1   Etiologies of Arthritis

Infectious	*Rheumatic diseases*
Infants: group B *Streptococcus*	Acute rheumatic fever
Toddlers, young children:	Juvenile rheumatoid arthritis
Staphylococcus	Systemic lupus erythematosus
H. influenzae type B	Inflammatory bowel disease
Pneumococcus	
Lyme disease	*Vasculitis*
Viruses (rubella, hepatitis B,	Henoch-Schönlein purpura
Epstein-Barr virus)	Serum sickness
Mycoplasma pneumoniae	
Tuberculosis	*Malignancies*
Kawasaki disease	Leukemia
	Neuroblastoma
Trauma	

patient may limp or refuse to use the affected extremity. The affected joint has a decreased range of motion as the patient holds it in the position that maximizes the joint's volume. The hip is flexed, abducted, and slightly externally rotated; the knee and elbow are flexed; and the ankle is held in plantarflexion.

Septic Arthritis   Septic arthritis (pp 529–531) is most common in children 1 to 3 years of age. It is almost always monoarticular; the knee (41%) and the hip (23%) are the joints most frequently infected. The onset is usually abrupt, with fever of 38 to 40°C (100.4 to 104°F) and systemic toxicity. However, young infants may appear well and be afebrile, despite not moving the affected extremity. Typically the joint is erythematous, swollen, and painful, and the patient resists any passive movement of the affected joint. Gonococcal arthritis can be migratory and monoarticular or pauciarticular. Adolescents with gonococcal infection may have tenosynovitis and rash (erythematous, hemorrhagic, papular, or vesiculopustular) rather than a vaginal discharge or urethritis.

Lyme Disease   Ninety percent of Lyme disease occurs in the Northeast, northern Midwest, and Northwest, most commonly in the summer and early fall. Monoarticular Lyme arthritis occurs in the early disseminated stage of the illness, several weeks to months after the tick bite or the appearance of the distinctive eruption (erythema migrans), if it occurs. The typical "Lyme knee" is swollen and tender, but warmth and erythema are notably absent. Migratory arthritis may also occur, but polyarthritis is uncommon. The arthritis can last weeks to months and can be recurrent.

Acute Rheumatic Fever (ARF)   ARF typically presents with a migratory polyarthritis and fever. Pain is subacute and insidious. Other clinical findings may include rash (erythema marginatum), subcutaneous nodules, murmur, fever, tachycardia out of proportion to the fever, chorea, and a prolonged PR interval on the ECG.

Systemic Lupus Erythematosus (SLE)   SLE may present with symmetric arthritis of both large and small joints. Symptoms are generally insidious and recurrent, and the pain is usually more severe than the clinical findings. Other associated findings may be a butterfly rash, alopecia, polyserositis, fever, and nephritis (microscopic hematuria and proteinuria).

Inflammatory Bowel Disease   Associated findings may include weight loss, failure to thrive, bloody diarrhea, and erythema nodosum.

Juvenile Rheumatoid Arthritis (JRA)   There are three major types of JRA: pauciarticular (four or fewer large asymmetric joints, uveitis); polyarticular (five or more small or large symmetric joints); and systemic (arthritis similar to polyarticular type, spiking fevers, evanescent salmon-pink macular rash, uveitis, lymphadenopathy, hepatosplenomegaly). Persistence of the arthritis (>6 weeks) and its nonmigratory nature distinguish JRA from ARF.

Henoch-Schönlein Purpura (HSP)   HSP presents with some combination of arthritis, purpuric rash of the buttocks and lower extremities, abdominal pain, hematuria, and hematochezia. The rash is essential for making the diagnosis.

Serum Sickness   Serum sickness causes arthritis, fever, urticaria, and lymphadenopathy 1 to 3 weeks after exposure to foreign proteins, including drugs (sulfonamides, penicillin, phenytoin) and infectious agents (hepatitis B virus, Epstein-Barr virus).

Malignancies   Malignancies cause arthritis either by cellular infiltration of the synovium or by causing a sympathetic effusion. Weakness, weight loss, bleeding, fever, and pallor may also be present.

Hemophilia   Hemarthrosis presents as monoarticular swelling, pain, and decreased range of motion in the absence of erythema or fever. The typical history of trauma may not always be elicited.

Diagnosis

Inquire about a history of fever, rash, upper respiratory infection (URI), time of onset of the symptoms, antecedent trauma, tick bites, and similar previous episodes. On examination, document that arthritis is present, and not merely *arthralgias, myalgias, sprains*, or *bruises*. With arthritis, the joint is erythematous, warm, swollen, and tender, with a decreased range of motion. Compare the affected joint with the contralateral side to confirm the presence of joint fluid.

Monoarticular Arthritis   Consider monoarticular arthritis to be infectious. Obtain a CBC with differential, ESR, blood culture, and two additional red-top tubes in the event that septic arthritis is ruled-out. Obtain an x-ray of the affected joint, and arrange for immediate arthrocentesis if a joint effusion is documented. The only exceptions to performing arthrocentesis are a *traumatic effusion* (unless indicated for pain relief), *Lyme disease* (joint not erythematous), *HSP*, and a known *autoimmune disorder*. Culture of the joint fluid is critical; inoculate the specimen into a blood culture bottle. A Gram's stain and cell count on the joint fluid are also necessary. Send the remainder of the fluid for complement levels if septic arthritis seems unlikely. Interpretation of the results of joint fluid analysis is summarized in Table 14-1.

A swollen, tender, nonerythematous knee is highly suggestive of *Lyme disease*. In addition to the tests outlined above, obtain a Lyme titer. Arthrocentesis is not necessary if septic arthritis can be confidently ruled out on clinical grounds or erythema migrans was diagnosed in the recent past.

Polyarticular Arthritis   Inquire about hepatitis exposure, weight loss, aspirin and drug use, change in bowel habits, and vaginal or urethral discharge. Perform a compete physical examination, looking for petechiae, rash, pharyngitis, lymphadenopathy, hepatosplenomegaly, and, in an adolescent, vaginal or urethral discharge (if the history is positive). A history of migratory arthritis suggests *ARF* or, in adolescents, *gonococcal arthritis.* Consider *Lyme arthritis* if the patient is from an endemic area and there is a history of a tick bite or a rash consistent with erythema migrans.

Obtain a complete blood count (CBC) with differential, ESR, ASLO, FANA, complement (C3, C4, CH50), rheumatoid factor, and urinalysis. Hematuria occurs in *HSP, serum sickness,* and *SLE,* and hematochezia is seen in *inflammatory bowel disease* and *HSP.*

Suspect that an adolescent with mono- or pauciarticular arthritis associated with tenosynovitis, pustules, or necrotic lesions has *gonococcal arthritis.* Obtain genital, rectal, and pharyngeal cultures for gonorrhea in addition to cultures of the joint fluid and blood.

Migratory Polyarthritis   True migratory polyarthritis (especially of the knees, ankles, elbows, and wrists) is highly suspicious for *ARF.* Tachycardia may be out of proportion to the fever. Obtain a chest x-ray to look for cardiomegaly and an ECG to identify a prolonged PR interval.

ED Management

Septic arthritis is an emergency, since significant joint destruction may occur in a short time. Unless septic arthritis can be reliably ruled out, joint drainage is necessary to remove the organism's debris and enzymes, which can destroy articular cartilage. As soon as joint fluid and blood cultures have been obtained, secure an IV and admit the patient for IV antibiotics and surgical drainage. While staphylococci continue to be the most common organism, use the synovial fluid Gram's stain and the patient's age to guide the choice of antibiotic (p 531).

After the appropriate blood tests have been obtained, afebrile, well-appearing patients with multiple (but not migratory) joint involvement may be evaluated as outpatients, if the parents are reliable.

See pp 362–366 for the treatment of Lyme arthritis. Reevaluate the patient in 72 h.

Follow-up

- Afebrile patient with nonmigratory polyarthritis: Primary care follow-up within 1 week
- Lyme arthritis: 2 to 3 days. Change to IV ceftriaxone if there is no improvement

Indications for Admission

- Suspected septic arthritis, rheumatic fever, malignancy
- Arthritis associated with weight loss, systematic toxicity, or severe pain
- Migratory polyarthritis
- Follow-up not certain

BIBLIOGRAPHY

Adebajo AO: Rheumatic manifestations of infectious diseases in children. *Curr Opin Rheumatol* 1998;10:79–85.

Ansell BM: Rheumatic disease mimics in childhood. *Curr Opin Rheumatol* 2000; 12:445–447.

Schaller JG: Diagnosis and management of rheumatic diseases in adolescence. *Adolesc Med* 1998;9:1–10.

BACK PAIN

In contrast to adults, low back pain is a relatively uncommon complaint in children. However, back pain in a prepubertal child is particularly concerning and may indicate significant underlying pathology.

Etiologies of pediatric back pain can be classified as mechanical (musculoskeletal/orthopedic), medical (infection, masses, systemic disease), and miscellaneous (reflex sympathetic dystrophy, fibromyalgia). Of note, idiopathic scoliosis is not a cause of pediatric low back pain.

Clinical Presentation

Mechanical Conditions
Spondylolysis and Spondylolisthesis   Spondylolysis and spondylolisthesis are the most common causes of back pain in children over 10 years of age. *Spondylolysis* is a defect in the pars interarticularis, a bony process on the posterior spine, possibly secondary to repetitive stress. This defect may take the form of a fracture, stress fracture, or sclerotic change and is most common at L5. A symptomatic pars defect is more likely to occur with activities that involve lumbar hyperextension, such as dance, figure skating, football, tennis, and weight training.

A patient with spondylolysis generally complains of low back pain worsened by activity, often associated with tight hamstrings and buttock pain. Spondylolysis may become complicated by *spondylolisthesis*, which is a forward slippage of one vertebra upon another (usually L5 on S1). The physical examination may be normal, although there may be a palpable step-off in the lower lumbar region and tight hamstrings with limited forward flexion.

Disk Injury   The intervertebral disk is a gelatinous substance that provides shock absorption to the spine and allows for a smooth range of motion. A disk may be injured (bulging) or herniated; the most common sites are L4-L5 and L5-S1. Affected patients are usually older than 10 years of age and complain of back pain with or without sciatica (pain down the back of the thigh). Physical examination findings include decreased lumbar lordosis, limited forward flexion, paraspinal muscle spasm, and a positive straight leg–raising test (p 508).

Lumbar Sacral Sprain   This is an injury or tearing of the ligaments and/or muscle fibers (interspinous or paraspinal) that connect one vertebra to another or support a vertebra. A common mechanism of injury is a sudden twisting motion; a patient who is inflexible and overweight is more likely to suffer from this type of injury. This variety of injury can occur in children who carry heavy backpacks.

Scheuermann's Kyphosis   Excessive kyphosis in either the thoracic or lumbar regions is a frequent cause of back pain in adolescents. The patient has poor posture and complains of dull pain over the deformity, which is worsened by activity. On examination, the kyphosis is obvious, accentuated by bending forward, and persists despite the patient's conscious efforts to stand erect.

Medical Etiologies

Infection   Orthopedic infections, including diskitis and osteomyelitis (pp 527–529), can cause back pain. *Diskitis* usually occurs in children younger than 10 years of age and may present with fever, malaise, low back pain, difficulty walking, and associated hip or abdominal pain. On physical examination, there may be tenderness over the involved disk, decreased range of motion, and pain with hip flexion. While the erythrocyte sedimentation rate (ESR) is usually elevated, the white blood cell count (WBC) is generally normal. The blood culture is sometimes positive, most often for *Staphylococcus aureus*.

Vertebral osteomyelitis presents similarly to diskitis but is more common in the older child. Typically, both the WBC and ESR are elevated and the blood culture is positive in about 50% of cases (usually *S. aureus*).

In addition, various nonorthopedic infections, such as *pyelonephritis* and *pancreatitis*, can also present with low back pain.

Rheumatologic Diseases   *Ankylosing spondylitis* is a spondyloarthropathy involving the sacroiliac joints and lumbar spine. It is most common in boys under 8 years of age, and the majority of affected patients are HLA B27 positive. The patient may experience transient arthritis of large joints, followed by back involvement later in the disease course. Pain in the lower back, hips, and thighs is associated with morning stiffness that is relieved by movement. There may also be an acute iridocyclitis and/or aortitis. The spinal involvement begins in the sacroiliac joints and ascends progressively to involve the rest of the spine, including the cervical vertebrae. In contrast, *JRA* affects the cervical spine, but spares the lumbar spine.

A patient with irritable bowel disease: (*Crohn's disease* or *ulcerative colitis*) may have associated spondylitis similar to ankylosing spondylitis. The patient may present with low back pain prior to the onset of gastrointestinal symptoms.

Tumor   A tumor is a particular concern in children under 4 years of age with back pain. The majority of cases are benign, including osteoid osteomas, eosinophilic granulomas, and unicameral bone cysts. However, possible malignancies include Ewing's sarcoma, neuroblastoma, and metastatic lesions. A history of nighttime pain, pain not associated with activity, or a painful scoliosis raises the concern of a tumor.

Miscellaneous Conditions

Reflex Sympathetic Dystrophy (RSD)   The hallmark of this syndrome is severe pain associated with autonomic dysfunction (swelling, edema, skin color changes, mottling). RSD may occur in the back after a trauma, fall, or collision. The initial injury may be a sprain or disk injury, with ongoing pain out of proportion to what is expected for the original injury (allodynia, dysesthesias).

Fibromyalgia   This condition is defined as chronic musculoskeletal pain (>6 months duration) associated with trigger points and nonspecific symptoms (sleep disturbance, headache, irritable bowel, weakness, swelling or stiffness in the morning). A child may present with severe lower and upper back pain.

Diagnosis

History   A thorough history is essential in determining whether the patient's back pain requires urgent or immediate intervention. Ascertain the onset of the pain, its timing, severity, and radiation, as well as factors that alleviate or trigger it. Inquire about sports participation, including the intensity of the involvement and the initiation of any new sports, and ask specifically about trauma. Ask about the child's activity level since the onset of symptoms; back pain that forces the child to refrain from usual activities requires a thorough evaluation.

Determine whether the pain is related to sleep or resting in bed. Specific difficulty in moving from side to side in bed may suggest a *disk problem* or *lumbar sprain*. Importantly, any patient awakened and kept awake by back pain must be thoroughly evaluated for a *tumor, infection,* or *inflammatory condition*. In contrast, back pain from *overuse syndromes, muscle pain, Scheuermann's disease,* or *spondylolysis* (with or without spondylolisthesis) usually improves with rest.

In addition, always check for the presence of systemic symptoms, such as fever, malaise, or irritability. A positive history for ankle or foot weakness, changes in bowel or bladder function, and/or an altered gait is suggestive of *neurologic impairment*. Ask about medications or therapies already tried, including chiropractic manipulation and acupuncture.

Physical Examination   Have the patient undress down to his or her underwear and observe the gait and posture. Note any muscle asymmetry and signs of splinting; assess the back for a midline defect or lesion such as a tuft of hair or hemangioma. Check carefully for tenderness by palpating over the vertebrae, spinous processes, vertebral spaces, and interspinal ligaments as well as the shoulders and paraspinal muscles.

For the lumbar spine, check forward flexion, lateral rotation, lateral bending, and extension. The forward bend test helps reveal any deformities of the spine; low back pain increased by hyperextension suggests *spondylolysis* and *spondylolisthesis*.

Look for quadriceps and hamstring asymmetry, which can result from a low back problem. Check the strength of hip flexion, extension, abduction, and adduction as well as flexion of the quadriceps (knee flexion), hamstrings (knee extension), and feet and ankles (plantarflexion/dorsiflexion, inversion, eversion).

A *straight leg–raising test* will frequently be positive in patients with *disk herniation.* For the straight leg–raising test, have the patient lie supine, grasp the ankle, and, with the knee held in extension, bring the leg upward to assess range of flexion of the hip joint. Note the angle and location of any elicited pain. Then repeat the maneuver and dorsiflex the foot as the painful angle is neared; this should aggravate the pain. Radiating pain in the back indicates sciatic nerve irritation and a herniated disk.

Perform a complete neurologic examination, paying particular attention to symmetry, muscle strength, and deep tendon reflexes (knee jerk, ankle jerk). Also check for signs of meningeal irritation (Kernig's and Brudzinski's signs).

Radiologic Studies   Unless it is clear that *minor trauma* is the cause of the back pain, obtain anteroposterior and lateral radiographs of the spine; oblique lumbar spine views are also needed if *spondylolysis* is suspected. Obtain a technetium-99m (^{99m}Tc) bone scan if a febrile patient has an examination that is consistent with *diskitis* or *osteomyelitis* but the plain films are normal. A CT scan can further define spinal pathology located by bone scan and a fine-cut CT scan (1- to 3-mm cuts) is useful in diagnosing and evaluating spondylolysis. Obtain an MRI for any abnormal neurologic findings. The MRI is a valuable tool in evaluating *spinal cord tumors, tethered cord, disk herniation, diskitis,* and other spinal pathology, but clinically insignificant disk herniation or degenerative disk disease may be overread.

Laboratory Studies   If a medical cause is suspected, order a CBC, serum electrolytes, ESR, and a blood culture. If a rheumatologic cause is suspected, further laboratory evaluation may include antinuclear antibodies (ANA), rheumatoid factor, and HLA B27 screening.

ED Management

The priority is to identify conditions requiring immediate treatment, including mass lesions, diskitis, or osteomyelitis. If the patient has any of the clinical features outlined in Table 18-2, arrange for immediate radiologic evaluation (see above) and consultation with a neurologist and/or orthopedist.

Table 18-2   Clinical Features of Back Pain Requiring Immediate Evaluation

Age < 4 years
Pain for >1 month
Systemic symptoms: fever, lethargy, irritability
Point tenderness over spine or intervertebral space
Pain triggered by usual activities
Pain awakens patient from sleep
Neurologic abnormalities: foot or ankle weakness, changes in bowel or
    bladder function, altered gait, abnormal deep tendon reflexes or Babinski
    reflex, asymmetric strength, meningeal signs

If an older child with back pain for less than 1 month appears well, has a normal neurologic examination, and does not have point tenderness, nighttime pain, or restriction of daily activities, refer him or her to a primary care provider, orthopedist, or sports medicine specialist for follow-up within 1 week. In general, appropriate management for these patients includes referral to a physical therapist, avoidance of the offending activity (usually hyperextension), and, occasionally, a back brace. Bed rest has virtually no role in the management of back pain. Encourage the patient to walk and go to school as soon as possible. Reserve ibuprofen (10 mg/kg q 6 h) for acute pain (sprains, fractures, disk injuries).

Follow-up

- Within 1 week; patient to return immediately for worsening pain, especially at night, neurologic symptoms, or systemic symptoms

Indications for Admission

- Osteomyelitis or diskitis
- Suspected tumor

BIBLIOGRAPHY

King HA: Back pain in children. *Orthop Clin North Am* 1999;30:467–474.
Mason DE: Back pain in children. *Pediatr Ann* 1999;28:129–138.
Micheli LJ, Wood R: Back pain. *Arch Pediatr Adolesc Med* 1995;149:15–18.

FRACTURES, DISLOCATIONS, AND SPRAINS

Skeletal injuries account for 10 to 15% of all injuries in children; 15% of these affect the physis, or growth plate. Always consider the possibility of child abuse in young children presenting with skeletal injuries.

Clinical Presentation and Diagnosis

Obtain a complete history, including the mechanism of the injury, location of maximal pain, previous orthopedic or rheumatologic problems (fractures, dislocations, joint pain or swelling), chronic medical problems (rickets, renal failure, liver disease, malignancy), and drug use (phenytoin can produce a rickets-like picture). For open fractures, ascertain the patient's tetanus status and whether the trauma occurred in a dirty environment (farm and field injuries pose a risk of clostridial infections).

On physical examination, focus on the area(s) of pain and tenderness as well as the joints above and below the suspected injury. However, perform a complete examination, looking for associated and/or additional traumatic injuries.

Begin the examination by assessing the neurovascular status of the affected extremity. Palpate the pulses; check the warmth, capillary filling, and active motion of the fingers or toes; and evaluate sensation, using the uninjured limb for comparison. The presence of any of the "six P's" (pain, pulselessness, pallor, paralysis, paresthesias, and painful passive motion) distal to the fracture site suggests neurovascular compromise. The presence of a pulse does not assure adequate circulation; however, assume that absence of a pulse means compromise.

Inspect the extremity and compare it with the uninjured side, looking for asymmetry, swelling, abrasions, ecchymoses, and deformity. Significantly displaced fractures and dislocations may cause an obvious deformity. Swelling and ecchymosis may be present or may develop over several hours. Check for point tenderness, which is often, but not always, associated with a fracture. In some cases, the pain may not be well localized, but it usually is present in the affected bone.

Next, evaluate the joints. Have the patient attempt an active range of motion of the injured joint, using the other side for comparison. If the child is unable to complete a full range of motion, gently perform a passive examination of joint mobility.

Suspect an orthopedic injury if there is a history of significant trauma (fall from height, motor vehicle accident, etc.) or if the patient complains of pain after an injury. However, the cause may have been unwitnessed or not noticed, so that an injury is not suspected until significant swelling becomes apparent. Toddlers and young children may present with crying after an unwitnessed fall. In addition, children can self-splint injuries, particularly buckle fractures of the distal forearm, so that the discomfort may appear minimal.

Fracture
A fracture is a break in the continuity or architecture of a bone. Describe a fracture by the skin integrity (open or closed) overlying the site of the injury; the name of the bone; the location within the bone (intraarticular, distal, proximal, or midshaft); the character of the fracture (comminuted, spiral, greenstick, transverse, oblique); and the direction of displacement (nondisplaced, displaced 10 degrees, dorsally angulated, etc.). The clavicle, radius, and ulna are the most frequently fractured bones in children.

A fracture usually presents with point tenderness, ecchymosis, and swelling after an episode of trauma. An infant or toddler, however, may merely refuse to use the affected limb, which is neither swollen nor markedly tender, or the patient may suddenly refuse to walk. Significant blood loss, leading to shock, can occur with a fracture of the femur or pelvis.

Open Fracture   An open or compound fracture communicates with the outside environment by means of a puncture or laceration through the skin.

Pathologic Fracture   A pathologic fracture can occur in areas of bone weakness. Causes include rickets, bone cysts, osteogenesis imperfecta, and malignancies.

Buckle Fracture   A buckle or torus fracture is caused by compression of the metaphysis in a young child's bone. There is disruption of at least one side of the cortex but no visible fracture line.

Greenstick Fracture   A greenstick fracture, which usually involves the diaphysis, occurs when an angulated force breaks one but not both sides of the cortex.

Complete Fracture   A complete fracture is a through and through (displaced or nondisplaced) break of the cortex.

Epiphyseal Injury   Determining whether a growth plate is injured is critical. Although many growth plate injuries do not result in growth arrest, serious deformity and disability can result from such injuries, despite optimal medical care. The Salter-Harris classification scheme of epiphyseal injury (Fig. 18-1) is useful for describing the fracture. This system correlates well with the degree of injury and is useful in treatment and prognosis.

Dislocation

A dislocation is a complete disruption of the normal articular relationships of a joint. A dislocated joint appears deformed, with a limited, painful range of motion. The most common sites are the shoulder (anterior), metacarpophalangeal (MCP) joints, interphalangeal (IP) finger joints (p 517), and patella. Posterior elbow and knee dislocations are rare, but they are significant because of the risk of vascular compromise.

Subluxation

A subluxation is an incomplete dislocation. A subluxed joint may appear normal but will have a limited, painful range of motion as with a dislocated joint. The most common bone subluxed is the radial head of a toddler ("nursemaid's elbow").

Sprain

A sprain is a disruption of a ligament. Young children are more likely to have physeal fractures than sprains because of the relative weakness of the physis compared with the surrounding ligaments. Joint injuries, dislocations, and ligamentous injuries are therefore less common in the young child. Sprains occur more frequently in the adolescent with closed or closing growth plates. Sprains of the knees and ankles are the most common sports-related injuries.

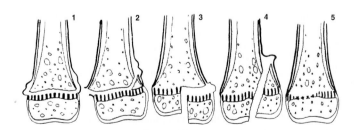

Figure 18-1   The Salter-Harris classification of growth plate
fractures. (Adapted with permission from Salter RB,
Harris WR: Injuries involving the epiphyseal plate.
J Bone Joint Surg 1963;45A:587.)

Sprains present as joint swelling, with ecchymosis and tenderness over the affected ligament. Usually there is a clear history of trauma. There may be pain on palpation over the ligament without any instability (grade I), increased joint laxity upon stress (grade II), or total joint instability (grade III).

Strain
In contrast to a sprain, a strain is an injury to the musculotendinous unit.

Radiographs

Confirm a fracture or dislocation with radiographs, including standard anteroposterior and lateral views to assess the presence and nature of a fracture. Although CT, MRI, and bone scans are helpful in making a detailed assessment of a fracture or dislocation, these are not the primary means of making the diagnosis.

AP and lateral x-rays are indicated if there is an obvious deformity, point tenderness, or marked swelling or ecchymosis. Splint the extremity first, and obtain views that include the joints above and below the site of injury. If the radiologist or orthopedist is experienced in interpreting pediatric films, comparison views of the uninjured extremity are not routinely indicated (with the exception of the elbow). Obtain oblique views if a "toddler's fracture" is suspected.

When viewing the radiographs, carefully follow the cortex, looking for any discontinuity, which is diagnostic of a fracture. Evaluate the growth plates and joints for displacement, disruption, or widening.

The differentiation between sprains and Salter I epiphyseal injuries can be difficult, as both can present with minimal swelling over the growth plate and normal radiographs. However, growth plate injuries are more common in young children, while sprains are more likely in adolescents. With a sprain, the ligament is tender and the joint may be lax, while Salter I injuries cause tenderness over the growth plate. Do not stress the ankle when there is tenderness over the lateral malleolus, because a nondisplaced Salter I fracture may deteriorate into a more serious injury.

A number of fractures are suspicious for child abuse: metaphyseal (bucket-handle), rib (especially posterior), scapular, spinous process, and sternal fractures. Other injuries that are associated with inflicted trauma include epiphyseal separations, vertebral body fractures and subluxations, digital fractures, complex skull fractures, and multiple fractures, especially if bilateral or in various stages of healing. Common lesions that have a low specificity for abuse include subperiosteal new bone formation, clavicular fractures, fractures of long bone shafts, and linear skull fractures.

ED Management

Time is critical with neurovascular compromise, open fractures, and joint sepsis. These orthopedic emergencies demand prompt intervention to avoid complications and possible loss of a limb.

After stabilization of vital signs and assessment of nonorthopedic injuries, the priority is assessment of the neurovascular status of the injured extremity. As discussed above, the presence of any of the "six P's" suggests neurovascular compromise and is an indication for immediate orthopedic consultation. If orthopedic consultation is not immediately available, place the extremity in longitudinal traction and align any gross deformities.

If there is an open fracture, priorities before obtaining radiographs are as follows: obtain a culture of any exposed bone or soft tissues; cover the wound with sterile dressings; start an IV; give the first dose of an antibiotic (nafcillin 40 mg/kg, cephalothin 25 mg/kg, or clindamycin 10 mg/kg if the patient is penicillin-allergic); and give tetanus toxoid unless there is documentation of adequate immunization.

Pain relief is the next priority. Splint the extremity in a physiologic position, elevate it, and apply ice to minimize swelling. Splints can be made from any firm material and tape. Give acetaminophen (15 mg/kg PO), ibuprofen (10 mg/kg PO), or codeine (0.5 mg/kg PO [maximum 60 mg]). For a patient with severe pain, give morphine, 0.1 mg/kg IV or IM.

Obtain radiographs after the initial assessment is conducted.

Fractures   Definitive treatment ranges from a simple sling to complex surgical reconstruction. In general, most nondisplaced extremity fractures can be treated with in situ immobilization with a cast or splint. Immediately refer all displaced fractures and growth plate fractures to an orthopedist. These usually require reduction to an anatomic position, followed by immobilization. If the patient must travel to see an orthopedist, splint the extremity in a physiologic position to avoid further displacement of the fracture.

Dislocations   Reduce a finger dislocation promptly, with axial traction, after finger-block anesthesia. See below for the reduction of a glenohumeral dislocation. Elbow, hip, and knee dislocations are at risk of neurovascular compromise and therefore require orthopedic consultation.

Contusions and First-Degree Sprains   Treat with RICE therapy: *rest, ice* (for 24–48 h), *compression* (with an elastic bandage), and *elevation* (to reduce swelling). Advise that activities can be resumed as tolerated. Most minor injuries will resolve over 5 to 7 days. Instruct the patient to follow up if there is no improvement.

Severe Sprains   A second- or third-degree sprain requires splinting for several weeks. In the ED, apply any of the commercially available splints or a Jones dressing (alternating layers of Webril and ace bandages). Give crutches if the patient has a severe sprain of a lower extremity.

Cast Care   After casting, arrange for orthopedic follow-up. Instruct the patient to keep the extremity elevated, move the fingers or toes, keep the cast dry, and avoid putting any objects into the cast. Advise the family to check for pain out of proportion to the injury, color change of the distal extremity, and numbness or tingling. These signs suggest excessive cast tightness or neurovascular compromise and require an immediate return to the ED.

THE MOST COMMON OR SIGNIFICANT
ORTHOPEDIC INJURIES

Upper Extremity

Clavicle

Clavicular fractures are particularly common in newborns (5 per 1000 births). They are associated with a breech or difficult delivery but may not be noticed until about 1 week of age, when a grossly obvious callus (swelling) is found in the area of the fracture. In older children, they are caused by a fall on an outstretched hand or by a direct blow and present with crepitus, swelling, and tenderness. In some cases, a tender or nontender swelling is noted 7 to 10 days after an injury. Most clavicular fractures heal with minimal supportive treatment. Either immobilize the arm with a sling or apply a figure-of-eight clavicular splint. A full return of function requires 3 to 4 weeks.

Following blunt trauma, a patient with a posterior dislocation of the clavicle may present with isolated clavicular or diffuse shoulder pain. Dysphonia, dyspnea or difficulty swallowing may also be present if the distal fragment is displaced posteriorly, pressing on the trachea or esophagus. Plain radiographs are not useful, but a CT scan is diagnostic. If the injury is on the left side, a CT with contrast is necessary to rule out an injury to the arch of the aorta. Insert an IV with $D_5\frac{1}{2}NS$ at a maintenance rate and obtain preoperative blood tests (CBC, type and crossmatch). Admit the patient to a PICU for close monitoring and arrange for reduction in the operating room with a cardiothoracic team on standby.

Acromioclavicular Joint

The acromioclavicular joint, at the lateral end of the clavicle, can be injured by a direct blow or a fall onto the joint. Most injuries are simple sprains, although in some cases the clavicle may be displaced superiorly and require reduction. Otherwise, treat with a sling.

Shoulder

Shoulder dislocations are rare in childhood, as the proximal humeral epiphysis is weaker than the shoulder joint capsule. As the growth plate closes, shoulder dislocations can occur with a fall on an outstretched hand, forced abduction of an externally rotated arm, or a posterior blow to an elevated, abducted arm. Anterior dislocation is the most common, presenting with the arm held slightly abducted and in external rotation, with a squared-off appearance to the shoulder. There may be numbness and tingling of the arm. The recurrence rate approaches 90% after an initial dislocation in a teenager.

Reduce an anterior shoulder dislocation with the Stimpson method. After providing adequate sedation and muscle relaxation (diazepam 0.2 mg/kg/dose IM or IV to 10 mg) (p 621), have the patient lie prone on a stretcher, with the affected arm hanging down. Application of a 5 to 10 lb weight to the arm will cause gradual reduction over 15–30 min.

Proximal Humerus

Injuries to the proximal humerus usually involve the growth plate, occurring during a fall onto an outstretched arm. Neurovascular compromise is rare. This area has tremendous remodeling potential, so growth disturbances are uncommon. Angulations up to 30 degrees and displacement of up to 50% may not require reduction. Treat with a sling and immobilization. More significantly displaced fractures require reduction.

Humeral Shaft   These fractures are less common than proximal and distal humeral fractures. They can be associated with a unicameral bone cyst of the humerus. Carefully assess the radial nerve (wrist dorsiflexion), which may be injured as it passes close to the bone in the distal half of the shaft. Treat with closed reduction and neurovascular checks before and after reduction.

Elbow Injuries
Fractures about the elbow are the second most common type in children. If there is an obvious deformity, do not test passive range of motion because of the risk of displacing the fracture. Splint the extremity and obtain radiographs, including comparison views. Otherwise, check flexion, extension, supination, and pronation. To test for ligamentous stability of the medial and lateral collateral ligaments, cup the elbow in one hand and hold the wrist in the other, ask the patient to flex the elbow a few degrees, and then apply varus and valgus stress, looking for opening of the sides of the joint. Compare both elbows. Have the patient extend the elbow and make a fist.

Since a child's elbow is a maze of growth centers, comparison views of the uninjured elbow are mandatory. If a fracture is suspected, obtain true AP and lateral x-rays, looking for the "fat-pad sign" indicative of intra-articular effusion. The posterior fat pad lies deep in the olecranon fossa and is not normally visible when the elbow is flexed. When the joint capsule is distended by blood or an effusion, however, the posterior fat pad is pushed out and seen as a triangular lucency posterior to the elbow. The anterior fat pad may be seen in the normal elbow, but consider it abnormal when it protrudes (sail sign).

The collateral circulation about the elbow is usually sufficient to maintain circulation even if the brachial artery is disrupted. However, do not overflex the elbow to the point of diminished circulation. Minimize swelling with a splint and ice packs.

Supracondylar Fractures   Fractures of the distal end of the humerus pose a high risk of neurovascular compromise. There is a 1% chance of vascular insult, and 7 to 10% of displaced supracondylar fractures result in radial or median nerve injuries. These injuries occur in the distal humerus, above the elbow joint, so there is no growth plate injury. They account for about two-thirds of elbow fractures and typically occur in children under 10 years of age who fall on an outstretched arm with either a hyperextended elbow or a dorsiflexed hand and a flexed elbow. Supracondylar fractures may present with ischemic pain in the forearm from injury to the brachial artery. An attempt to extend the fingers may cause considerable pain. This is a more reliable sign of ischemia than the presence or absence of the radial pulse. Prompt orthopedic intervention is required to prevent a Volkmann's contracture.

Treat nondisplaced fractures with in situ immobilization; these heal well. Displaced fractures require accurate anatomic reduction and immobilization, often necessitating pin fixation by an orthopedist. Treat significant swelling with overhead traction and careful neurovascular assessment.

Fractures of the Lateral and Medial Condyles and Epicondyles   These represent Salter IV fractures involving both the growth plate and the elbow joint. The lateral epicondylar fracture is one of the few types of pediatric fractures that may proceed to nonunion. Radiographs may not reveal the true extent of the displacement; an arthrogram may be required. Suspect a fracture if there is instability on valgus and varus stress. Treat nondisplaced fractures with immobilization, but displaced fractures require surgery for precise anatomic reduction.

Fractures of the Proximal Radius   These can also occur from a fall onto an outstretched arm. Characteristic findings are pain over the radial head and decreased forearm pronation and supination. On examination, decreased forearm rotation is the most common finding. Neurovascular compromise is unusual. However, obtain radiographs of the ipsilateral elbow, as a second fracture or dislocation may be missed if only the deformed area is x-rayed. In the absence of excessive displacement, treat symptomatically with either a sling or a splint.

Nursemaid's Elbow (Radial Head Subluxation)   This is a common problem that may be recurrent, but it can be managed without radiographs or orthopedic consultation. It occurs when a young child's (1–3 years of age) arm is suddenly pulled while the elbow is extended and the arm pronated. The arm may be tugged as the child steps off a curb, or the child may be swung by the forearm. The toddler with a nursemaid's elbow is comfortable but refuses to actively flex the elbow, preferring an extended, internally rotated position. There is no swelling and minimal tenderness around the elbow or wrist unless passive flexion of the elbow is attempted.

To reduce a nursemaid's elbow, cup the elbow in one hand and the wrist in the other. Rapidly flex the elbow while simultaneously supinating the forearm. Usually a click is felt, and, within 10 to 15 min (sometimes longer) the child actively flexes the elbow.

Forearm and Wrist Fractures
These are the most common fractures of childhood (45% of the total) and are usually caused by falls. About 75% occur in the distal third of the forearm and most others in the middle third. Over one-half are greenstick fractures presenting with pain and swelling without significant deformity.

Treat a nondisplaced fracture with splinting or casting. A displaced fracture requires closed reduction and casting under sedation. Use a long arm cast for a midshaft fracture, but a short arm cast will suffice for a distal fracture. In patients under 10 years of age, the forearm and wrist will remodel with no lasting deformity if proper reduction is achieved.

Hand Fractures

Carpal fractures are unusual in children; the scaphoid (navicular) is the most commonly fractured carpal bone. They are caused by a fall on an outstretched hand. Carpal fractures present with pain in the wrist but little deformity or swelling. These fractures may occur without definite radiologic abnormalities. Point tenderness at the bottom of the anatomic snuff box suggests a fracture of the navicular, as does pain in the snuffbox with axial loading of the thumb, regardless of the radiographic findings.

The lunate is the most frequently dislocated as well as the second most frequently fractured carpal bone. With the wrist flexed, palpate the base of the third metacarpal, then proceed proximally. Pain suggests fracture of the lunate or capitate. Confirmation of a dislocation of the carpal bones (usually a lunate or perilunate dislocation) requires careful examination of a true lateral radiograph of the wrist and carpus.

Metacarpal fractures are usually the result of fighting. The neck of the fifth metacarpal is most often affected (boxer's fracture). The patient may present 1 to 2 days after the injury with swelling of the dorsum of the hand and decreased range of motion. In the absence of significant displacement, treat with a hand-and-wrist splint.

Finger Fractures and Injuries

Most finger fractures are simple injuries of the distal phalangeal shaft. They are commonly seen in toddlers who get a finger caught in a door. A subungual hematoma is often associated with the fracture. Splint the fractured digit in a functional position [45 degree metacarpal (MP) flexion, with 20 degree flexion at the proximal interphalangeal (PIP) and distal interphalangeal (DIP) joints] and buddy-tape to the adjacent digit for added stability. If there is a displaced phalangeal fracture with more than 20 degrees of volar angulation, reduction is indicated. Use a dorsal splint to immobilize a fractured digit, maintaining the hand joints at 45 degrees of flexion and ensuring that the rotational alignment of the digits is preserved. Injuries to the base of the thumb may require a thumb spica cast, and significantly unstable fractures may require pin fixation.

Finger dislocations are easily recognized from the deformity of the digit. The most frequently dislocated MCP joint is the second. The patient presents with the finger slightly supinated and shortened, overlapping the adjacent finger. Distal IP dislocations are secondary to hyperextension. Proximal IP dislocations are commonly called "jammed fingers." Patients present with a painful swollen finger. Reduce finger dislocations with simple traction; finger-block anesthesia may be required. Afterward, splint for 7 to 10 days.

Lower Extremity

Pelvic Fractures

Fractures of the pelvis are rarely isolated, occurring most often in a multiple trauma victim who has pain with movement or palpation of the pelvis. There may be associated injuries to the viscera and bladder or a vaginal or rectal laceration. There may be a large hematoma superficially beneath the inguinal ligament or in the scrotum (Destot's sign), a bony promi-nence or a large hematoma as well as tenderness on rectal examination (Earle's sign), or a decreased distance from the greater trochanter to the pubic spine on the affected side with a lateral compression fracture (Roux's sign). If there is any suspicion of a pelvic injury, obtain pelvic x-rays as part of a multiple trauma workup. Most pelvic fractures are stable, so treatment is directed toward fluid resuscitation and hemody-namic stabilization.

Hip Fractures

Hip fractures are rare, occurring with significant high-energy trauma. In 30% of cases, there are associated injuries. Observe how the patient holds the leg while lying supine. The affected leg is shortened and externally rotated, while the hip may be flexed. Compare the skinfolds of young patients; asymmetry can occur with dislocation or fracture. Obtain AP and lateral radiographs. Prompt surgical reduction is required to prevent avas-cular necrosis, especially with fractures of the femoral neck and hip dislo-cation. A delay in treatment can cause permanent deformity.

Fractures of the Femoral Shaft

Femoral fractures are easily identified, presenting with swelling, defor-mity, and tenderness in the thigh. Look for other injuries, such as ipsilat-eral hip dislocation, femoral neck fracture, epiphyseal injury, tibial fracture, and fracture of the contralateral femur. While a fracture of the femoral shaft can occur with falls and play, suspect child abuse in a patient under 2 years of age.

Treatment varies with the patient's age. In general, children under 6 years of age require a spica cast. Older children and adolescents are treated with either internal fixation, or delayed casting after traction. If there are no concerns about abuse, a young child in a spica cast can be discharged with outpatient follow-up.

Knee Injuries

The knee is a common site of sports injuries, especially in football players and skiers. The history of the mechanism of injury, including the position of the knee and foot at the time and whether there was any contact, helps suggest the most likely diagnosis. The patient may complain of pain or swelling or may be limping or unable to bear weight. A sensation of "tightness" behind the knee suggests a small effusion.

It is quite common for an acutely injured knee to be so swollen and painful that an examination is impossible. In this situation, obtain radio-graphs to rule out a fracture and aspirate the joint to relieve some of the pain. Utilize the RICE protocol with a knee immobilizer, and refer the patient to an orthopedist for definitive diagnosis and treatment.

Knee Sprains   Knee sprains are rare in young children; they occur more frequently in adolescents with closed or closing growth plates. The medial collateral ligament (MCL) is the most common site of sprain, caused by a lateral blow to the knee in football players and skiers. Injuries of the ante-rior cruciate ligament (ACL) can occur without contact by abrupt deceleration maneuvers, jumping, missed landing, or "cutting" maneuvers such as those seen in basketball, football, or tennis. Injuries to the lateral collateral ligament (LCL) and posterior cruciate ligament (PCL) are much less common.

After the initial evaluation of the injured extremity, check the integrity of the knee ligaments. For each ligament, assess the range of motion and whether there is a definite endpoint, using the other side as a reference. With the patient supine, the hip extended, and the knee at 0 degrees (fully extended), place one hand above the ankle and the other on the lateral aspect of the distal femur. Abduction of the lower leg then causes valgus knee stress, testing the MCL. Place the upper hand on the medial aspect of the distal femur and adduct the lower leg (varus stress, LCL). If there is instability, stop the examination; if the knee is not unstable, repeat the examination at 30 degrees of flexion. MCL sprains cause medial pain; LCL injuries result in pain on the lateral side of the knee.

Next, test the cruciate ligaments by performing Lachman's test. With the knee flexed to 20 degrees, stabilize the femur with one hand and draw the tibia downward with the other. A sharp endpoint indicates integrity of the ACL. Then flex the hip to 45 degrees and the knee to 90 degrees with the foot flat on the table. Sit on the patient's toes, place four fingers of both hands on either side of the patient's calf and your thumbs on the femoral condyles, and pull the tibia forward (anterior draw, ACL), feeling for a definite endpoint. Then push it backward (posterior draw, PCL). With tears of the ACL, the patient or bystanders may report having heard a "pop" or "snap," the patient refuses to bear weight, and swelling begins almost immediately. Treat knee sprains with a knee immobilizer and crutches.

Meniscal Injuries   Meniscal injuries occur on weight bearing with the foot externally rotated, pushing off, often during squatting and twisting (baseball catchers); injuries to the lateral meniscus are uncommon. Meniscal injuries present with painful ambulation and inability to extend the knee fully. To evaluate the menisci, perform McMurray's test. While the knee is hyperflexed, rotate it internally and externally by applying torque at the ankle. Palpate over the medial and lateral joint lines; clicking or grinding reflects a positive test.

Patellar Dislocation   A lateral patellar dislocation is most common in adolescent girls. It can be caused without contact by an acute, strong contraction of the quadriceps muscles or by a direct blow to the knee. A ripping sound is often reported by the patient, and the knee is held semiflexed, appears deformed, and cannot be straightened. Patellar dislocation is obvious when the patella is lateral to the joint and the anterior aspect of the knee appears concave and empty. Since knee extension causes patellar relocation, however, the patient can arrive in the ED complaining of knee pain with no obvious deformity. The patellar apprehension test is useful if relocation has occurred. Slightly flex the knee and prepare to push the patella laterally. The patient will become anxious and stop the procedure. Reduction can usually be achieved by manipulating the patella medially while the knee is extended. Apply a knee immobilizer and give the patient crutches. Consult an orthopedist if reduction is unsuccessful.

Knee Fractures   Intraarticular fractures of the knee are uncommon with sports injuries. However, pain, deformity, decreased range of motion, and fluid in the knee joint suggest the possibility. The distal femoral growth plate (which can be displaced, leading to growth disturbance), tibial tubercle, tibial spine, and proximal tibial metaphysis are the most common areas fractured. Fractures of the patella are uncommon, resulting from a forceful blow directly to the knee.

Perform a careful neurovascular examination to ensure that the popliteal vessels are intact. If there is neurovascular compromise, apply gentle longitudinal traction in line with the extremity. Comparison x-rays are helpful in assessing the degree of displacement of the tibial tubercle and tibial spine. Treatment of tibial fractures usually consists of closed reduction, but fractures of the distal femoral epiphysis usually require surgical reduction and fixation.

Tibial and Fibular Fractures

These are most frequently caused by motor vehicle accidents and falls from height. Many are greenstick-type fractures. Spiral fractures of the tibia, caused by rotational force on a foot that is fixed, are a common sports injury. Pain and swelling occur with nondisplaced tibial fractures but may not be seen in isolated fibular fractures. Treat tibial fractures with long leg casting.

A toddler's fracture is a nondisplaced fracture of the distal diaphysis of the tibia or fibula. It most commonly occurs between 9 months and 3 years of age, sometimes without a history of significant trauma. The child presents with a limp, and the initial radiograph may show a faint line in the tibial shaft. A callus can be seen on repeat films 1 week later. If a toddler's fracture is missed, however, it will heal without sequelae.

Isolated fibular fractures are rare; careful examination and radiographs are necessary to rule out any displacement. An isolated, nondisplaced fibular fracture requires supportive specific therapy only.

Ankle Injuries

Ankle injuries are among the most common in all age groups. Fortunately, most are simple sprains caused by inversion or eversion. They present with a decreased range of motion and local swelling around the malleoli. For a lateral sprain caused by inversion, obtain radiographs to rule out a fracture of the distal fibula and treat with RICE therapy and ankle support for 2 to 3 weeks. Medial ankle injuries can involve the distal tibial growth plate, with a risk of growth arrest. The epiphysis must be reduced, and careful follow-up is necessary. However, growth disturbances are common. Preadolescents with partly closed growth plates can have fractures through the remaining growth plate and into the joint (triplane fracture). Usually, operative reduction is required.

Careful clinical evaluation can identify a patient with an ankle injury who does not require radiographs. A set of adult guidelines, the Ottawa ankle rules, suggest that an ankle fracture is very unlikely if, in the absence of bony tenderness at the posterior edge or tip of the malleolus, the patient can bear weight for at least four steps. However, a Salter I fracture may be missed in a child with open epiphyses.

Evert and invert the foot while palpating the medial and lateral malleoli. Ligamentous tenderness without point tenderness over a malleolus suggests a sprain.

Foot Injuries
Tarsal and Metatarsal Injuries   These most commonly occur secondary to a direct blow to the foot. Ninety percent of foot fractures occur in the metatarsals, presenting with pain and swelling. Treat with a padded support dressing and protected weight bearing with crutches. A common error is mistaking the growth center of the first metatarsal (located proximally) for a fracture; the growth centers of the other metatarsals are located distally. Fractures of the base of the fifth metatarsal are common injuries, but they can be confused with secondary ossification centers. This fracture most commonly occurs with inversion injury and presents with point tenderness and mild swelling.

Metatarsal Stress Fractures   These occur in patients who have recently become physically active, such as adolescents beginning to participate in sports. The usual complaint is pain on weight bearing, with less discomfort at rest. Swelling is minimal, but localized tenderness is marked. Anterior, lateral, and oblique x-rays are normal early, but callus formation can be seen after 2 to 3 weeks. Treat with rest and avoidance of the offending activity.

Tarsometatarsal Dislocation   A dislocation of the tarsometatarsal joint can occur when violent plantarflexion of the forefoot occurs if the foot is in the "tiptoe" position (foot used to brake a fall from a bicycle or motorcycle). These dislocations are generally accompanied by fractures of the metatarsal shaft or neck. The patient presents with swelling of the dorsum of the foot overlying the tarsometatarsal joints, with marked pain and tenderness and inability to bear weight. Often, a deformity is not present because of the high rate of spontaneous reduction. Reduction with immobilization or pinning is required.

Fractures of the Phalanges of the Foot   These are rare in young children but more common in adolescents. They are caused by direct trauma secondary to being hit by a falling object or to kicking a hard object. The patient presents with pain, swelling, and occasionally deformity. Treat with alignment and buddy taping.

Indications for Orthopedic Consultation
- Compound, complete, or pathologic fracture
- Displaced fracture requiring reduction
- Growth plate (Salter) injury
- Grade II or III sprain
- Suspected neurovascular compromise
- Specific fractures: supracondylar, pelvic, hip, femoral
- Specific dislocations: shoulder, patellar, tarsometatarsal

Follow-up

- Fracture treated with casting: immediately for pain out of proportion to the injury, color change of the distal extremity, and numbness or tingling; otherwise as per orthopedist
- Injury treated with sling, splint, or immobilizer: immediately for unremitting pain; otherwise 1 to 2 weeks
- Nursemaid's elbow: 24 h if the child is not moving the arm in a normal fashion
- Hip fracture, in spica cast: orthopedist in 1 week

Indications for Admission

- Posterior clavicular dislocation
- Proximal humerus fracture with >50 degrees of displacement
- Supracondylar fracture
- Displaced fracture of the medial or lateral elbow epicondyle
- Fracture of the femoral neck
- Triplane ankle fracture
- Tarsometatarsal dislocation
- Fracture requiring open reduction
- Displaced fracture requiring external immobilizer
- Compound fracture of a long bone
- Unremitting pain
- Significant blood loss

BIBLIOGRAPHY

Della-Giustina K, Della-Giustina DA: Emergency department evaluation and treatment of pediatric orthopedic injuries. *Emerg Med Clin North Am* 1999;18: 895–922.

England SP, Sundberg S: Management of common pediatric fractures. *Pediatr Clin North Am* 1996;43:991–1012.

Jones K, Weiner DS: The management of forearm fractures in children: a plea for conservatism. *J Pediatr Orthop* 1999;19:811–815.

Kleinman PK: *Diagnostic Imaging of Child Abuse,* 2nd ed. New York: Mosby, 1998.

Lyon RM, Street CC: Pediatric sports injuries: when to refer or x-ray. *Pediatr Clin North Am* 1998;45:221–244.

LIMP

Limp in children is most often secondary to trauma. Other causes are infections, connective tissue disorders, and sickle cell disease (Table 18-3). In addition, if the pain can be localized to either the hip or knee joint, there are specific age-related disorders to consider.

Clinical Presentation

Trauma

The etiology may be a minor trauma, such as a sore from an ill-fitting shoe or a foreign body in the sole of the foot. However, there may be a more serious injury, such as a fracture, sprain, or dislocation with ecchy-

Table 18-3 Etiologies of Limp

Infections	*Trauma*
Osteomyelitis	Soft-tissue injury (bruise)
Septic arthritis	Fracture
Lyme disease	Dislocation
Intervertebral diskitis	Sprain
Viral infections	Foreign body
Hip diseases	*Other causes*
Transient synovitis	Henoch-Schönlein purpura
Legg-Calvé-Perthes disease	Inflammatory bowel disease
Slipped capital femoral epiphysis	Serum sickness
	Acute rheumatic fever
Knee diseases	Systemic lupus erythematosus
Osgood-Schlatter disease	Sickle cell disease
Painful patella syndrome	
Osteochondritis dissecans	

mosis, swelling, localized tenderness, decreased range of motion, ligamentous laxity, or obvious deformity.

Infections

Osteomyelitis   Osteomyelitis (pp 527–529) causes fever and limp or unwillingness to use the extremity. Point tenderness is typical, with or without overlying cellulitis.

Septic Arthritis   Septic arthritis (pp 529–531) presents with the sudden onset of fever and limp or complete unwillingness to move the leg. There is erythema, increased warmth, and tenderness over the affected joint, and the patient resists passive range of movement. The hip is most commonly affected; it is maintained in flexion, external rotation, and abduction.

Lyme Disease   In the first stage (early localized) of Lyme disease (pp 363–364), there may be arthralgias and the patient may favor one extremity over the other. Fever, lethargy, and headache may occur, along with the pathognomonic rash, erythema migrans. Frank arthritis (especially of the knee) is a manifestation of the subsequent early disseminated stage. The joint is swollen and tender but not warm or erythematous.

Intervertebral Diskitis   Intervertebral diskitis is an infectious or inflammatory disease occurring primarily in 2- to 7-year-olds. The patient may present with limp, back pain, refusal to sit or walk, irritability, and low-grade fever. Physical examination findings include localized tenderness directly over the spine, paravertebral muscle spasm, and limited straight-leg raising.

Hip Diseases
With hip diseases, the pain may be in the groin or anterior thigh, or it may be referred to the anteromedial aspect of the knee.

Transient Synovitis   Transient synovitis is a benign, self-limited, inflammatory hip disease that occurs predominantly in 3- to 8-year-olds. There is an acute or gradual onset of limp and either hip or referred knee pain. Fever is variable and the child does not appear toxic, but may have a URI. The hip is held in mild flexion, external rotation, and abduction, but there is no erythema or increased warmth. Abduction and internal rotation are limited by pain at the extremes of motion. Transient synovitis is a diagnosis of exclusion and must be distinguished from an early septic arthritis of the hip.

Legg-Calvé-Perthes Disease   Legg-Calvé-Perthes disease, or osteochondrosis of the femoral head, usually occurs in 4- to 9-year-old boys. There is a gradual onset of limp and pain in the hip, groin, or medial knee. Abduction and internal rotation of the hip are limited. The radiographic findings may be confused with avascular necrosis associated with corticosteroid use, sickle cell disease, or Gaucher's disease.

Slipped Capital Femoral Epiphysis   A slipped capital femoral epiphysis (SCFE) is a displacement of the normal relationship between the femoral head and neck. Ten to 20% of cases are bilateral; some are associated with hypothyroidism. The typical patient is an obese adolescent who presents with a limp and subacute or chronic groin pain, which may be referred to the anterior thigh or knee. The hip is held in flexion and external rotation. Passive hip flexion may accentuate the external rotation deformity, while internal rotation and abduction may be limited.

Knee Diseases
Although there are a number of specific disorders that affect the knee, the course of the obturator nerve can cause hip diseases to present with knee pain. Therefore examine the hips carefully in all patients with knee pain.

Osgood-Schlatter Disease.   Osgood-Schlatter disease, or apophysitis of the tibial tuberosity, is a self-limited disorder that usually occurs in physically active adolescents. The patient presents with a gradual onset of limp, especially after exercise. On examination, there is unilateral or bilateral tenderness and swelling over the tibial tuberosity, but the knee joint is otherwise normal.

Painful Patella Syndrome (Chondromalacia Patella).   Typical findings of painful patella syndrome include patellar pain after activity, episodes of buckling (but not locking), and crepitance and tenderness on palpation of the patellar articular surface.

Osteochondritis Dissecans   With osteochondritis dissecans, an area of bone, usually on the lateral aspect of the medial femoral condyle, develops ischemic necrosis and subsequent fracture. A piece of bone and cartilage may then break loose into the joint. This causes intermittently painful limp after exercise, buckling, locking, and a tender medial femoral condyle. It is most common in adolescent boys.

Other Causes
Arthritis   Arthritis (nonseptic) presents with swelling, erythema, tenderness, decreased range of motion, and increased warmth of single or multiple joints (pp 501–505). Associated findings may include fever, rash, heart murmur, generalized adenopathy, and hepatosplenomegaly.

Sickle Cell Disease   Sickle cell bone infarcts (pp 319–323) can cause diffuse bone pain with tenderness and limp. Associated findings may include fever, jaundice, abdominal pain, and, in younger children, swelling of the dorsum of the hands and feet (dactylitis).

Diagnosis

The priority is the prompt diagnosis of a septic arthritis, osteomyelitis, or SCFE. Inquire about trauma, rate of onset (acute versus chronic), similar previous episodes, medical history, fever, and location and radiation of the pain. Have the child undress from the waist down, then first evaluate the neurovascular status of the extremity. Next, look for erythema, warmth, and tenderness, and put the joint through complete active and passive ranges of motion. Thoroughly examine the hip of any child with a complaint of knee pain. Flex and extend the hip from 0 degrees to maximal flexion. While the hip is flexed, check internal and external rotation. Pain on rotation may be the first sign of hip disorders.

Unless it is clear that the cause of the limp is *minor trauma*, obtain standard AP and lateral x-rays of the suspicious areas. If the limp is associated with decreased hip range of motion, obtain AP pelvic and frog-leg lateral radiographs of both hips. Possible findings include fractures, *SCFE* (on the frog-leg view), joint space widening (*septic arthritis*, *Legg-Calvé-Perthes disease*), increased density of the femoral epiphysis (Legg-Calvé-Perthes disease), or subchondral bone fragmentation (*osteochondritis dissecans*). An MRI is needed to diagnose early Legg-Calvé-Perthes disease. X-rays of the knee are not needed when *Osgood-Schlatter disease* is suspected, and the films are normal in *painful patella syndrome*.

If the limp is associated with back pain, consider *diskitis*, particularly if the patient is febrile. Obtain plain x-rays and arrange for an MRI scan.

Obtain a CBC, ESR, *Lyme* titer (in endemic areas), and a blood culture when fever and/or constitutional symptoms are found and there is no definite history of trauma. Leukocytosis, a shift to the left, and a markedly increased ESR (>60 mm/h) may occur in inflammatory conditions such as septic arthritis, *osteomyelitis*, and diskitis. With *synovitis*, the ESR is elevated, but usually <60 mm/h.

ED Management

It may be impossible to make a specific diagnosis of the cause of a limp. If the fever is not high, the WBC and ESR are normal, and the radiographs are unremarkable, the patient may be discharged with close follow-up. Many such children have a minor injury without fracture or a self-limited synovitis. Give instructions to the parents and/or patient to return at once if there is high fever or an inability to ambulate or bear weight. Aspiration of a joint is indicated if the patient is unable to bear weight and has a fever ($>38.9°C$, $102°F$), elevated ESR (>60 mm/h), and elevated WBC ($>15,000$/mm^3).

Infection

If septic arthritis or osteomyelitis is suspected, refer the patient immediately to an orthopedist for aspiration of joint fluid or subperiosteal pus. Intravenous antibiotics are then indicated. The treatment of septic arthritis (pp 529–531), osteomyelitis (pp 527–529), and Lyme disease (pp 362–366) are detailed elsewhere. Since diskitis is difficult to distinguish from osteomyelitis, admit the patient for bed rest and IV nafcillin (150 mg/kg/day divided q 6 h).

Hip Diseases

Transient Synovitis   Patients who are afebrile, with a normal WBC and an ESR under 60 mm/h, may be treated at home with bed rest and acetaminophen (15 mg/kg q 4 h) or ibuprofen (10 mg/kg q 6 h) until the symptoms have resolved completely (in 3–5 days). For more severe symptoms, consult an orthopedist and admit the patient for bed rest and skin traction until the range of motion is normal.

SCFE   Immediately obtain orthopedic consultation, as minor trauma can cause complete displacement of the femoral epiphysis. Weight bearing must be discontinued and the patient placed at rest. Obtain thyroid function tests in addition to a CBC.

Legg-Calvé-Perthes   Although no emergency treatment is required, refer these patients to an orthopedist so that a comprehensive plan of treatment can be arranged.

Knee Diseases

Osgood-Schlatter Disease   Treat with aspirin or ibuprofen (as above) and limitation of activity until the acute symptoms resolve (in 2 to 6 weeks); then increase the activity level slowly.

Painful Patella Syndrome   The treatment is the same as for Osgood-Schlatter disease. In addition, recommend quadriceps strengthening exercises (straight-leg raising).

Osteochondritis Dissecans   Refer patients with suspected osteochondritis dissecans to an orthopedist, since treatment usually requires immobilization or possibly surgery.

Follow-up

- Transient synovitis: 3 to 5 days if symptoms have not resolved

- Legg-Calvé-Perthes, osteochondritis dissecans: orthopedist in 1 to 2 weeks
- Osgood-Schlatter, painful patella syndrome: primary care follow-up in 2 to 4 weeks

Indications for Admission

- Slipped capital femoral epiphysis
- Possible septic arthritis, osteomyelitis, diskitis
- Transient synovitis with fever, leukocytosis, ESR >60 mm/h, or markedly decreased range of motion

BIBLIOGRAPHY

Adebajo AO: Rheumatic manifestations of infectious diseases in children. *Curr Opin Rheumatol* 1998;10:79–85.

Do TT: Transient synovitis as a cause of painful limps in children. *Curr Opin Pediatr* 2000;12:48–51.

Leet AI, Skaggs DL: Evaluation of the acutely limping child. *Am Fam Physician* 2000;61:1011–1018.

OSTEOMYELITIS

Osteomyelitis is a bacterial bone infection caused by organisms introduced hematogenously or by direct spread from a contiguous local focus. *Staphylococcus aureus* is by far the most common agent. Group B *Streptococcus* and enteric bacteria occur more often in young infants, whereas children with hemoglobinopathies (sickle cell disease) are at risk for *Salmonella* infections. The usual site is the metaphysis, especially of the distal femur and proximal and distal tibia. In the newborn, the proximal humerus is a common location.

Clinical Presentation

The usual presentation in a child or adolescent is pain with point tenderness at a long-bone site and a decreased range of motion in the adjacent joints. Swelling, erythema, and warmth are generally not seen unless the infection has spread to the subcutaneous tissues. The patient may be febrile and often refuses to bear weight on the limb, holding it as motionless as possible. With vertebral osteomyelitis, there is chronic back pain with spasms of the paraspinal muscles.

An infant may occasionally have nonspecific signs, such as fever, irritability, and vomiting, but more often there is swelling and tenderness of the affected area. The infection spreads to contiguous structures in muscles and joints more often than in an older patient because of the relatively thin cortex and loose periosteum. Seventy percent of neonates with osteomyelitis have an associated septic arthritis.

Diagnosis

The diagnosis of osteomyelitis is clinical. The typical combination of fever, point tenderness, and unwillingness to use an extremity is not invariably seen, but when present is highly suggestive of osteomyelitis.

An elevated ESR is the most common abnormal blood test; the WBC may also be elevated. Aspiration of the pus from the bone and positive blood cultures confirm the diagnosis.

Radiographic studies are helpful, as plain films and CT scan may show soft tissue changes and swelling as early as 3 days after onset of symptoms. However, routine x-rays do not show bone changes until 10 to 20 days after the onset of the infection. A ^{99m}Tc phosphate bone scan can detect bone changes earlier than plain films, and prior aspiration of the bone does not affect results. MRI is very sensitive in detecting osteomyelitis after the first 24 to 36 h.

Trauma can cause pain, swelling, and limitation of movement. Usually there is a positive history, the x-rays may be diagnostic (fracture), and the ESR and CBC are normal. *Cellulitis* of a distal extremity can be mistaken for a manifestation of osteomyelitis. However, there is no point tenderness over the bone.

Sickle cell disease (pp 319–323) can cause pain that may be secondary to infection or vasoocclusive crisis. Distinguishing between the two may be difficult, although the pain of a crisis tends to recur in the same sites, can be felt in several locations at once, and often resolves with IV hydration. Pain in a single bone that has not been affected in the past suggests a possible osteomyelitis.

Other considerations include *bone tumor, Caffey's disease* (infantile cortical hyperostosis), and *Langerhans' cell histiocytosis.* All of these can be excluded by x-rays.

ED Management

When osteomyelitis is suspected, obtain a blood culture, CBC, ESR, and x-rays of the extremity. Needle aspiration is essential to drain the pus and provide specimens for culture and Gram's stain. If no pus is obtained, send marrow for culture and Gram's stain. Surgical drainage is often recommended if frank pus is obtained during needle aspiration. It will also exclude a sickle cell vasoocclusive crisis when the clinical picture is unclear. If available, a ^{99m}Tc phosphate bone scan usually confirms the diagnosis (increased uptake at the site), although it may be normal early in the illness.

Admit a patient with osteomyelitis and treat with an IV penicillinase-resistant antistaphylococcal drug (nafcillin, 150 mg/kg/day divided q 6 h). Provide *Salmonella* coverage for a patient with a hemoglobinopathy (sickle cell disease): ceftriaxone 100 mg/kg/day divided q 12 h. Treat a neonate with nafcillin (150 mg/kg/day divided q 6 h) and cefotaxime (150 mg/kg/day divided q 8 h). The doses may need to be adjusted for patients in the first week of life.

Indication for Admission

- Osteomyelitis

BIBLIOGRAPHY

Oudjhane K, Azouz EM: Imaging of osteomyelitis in children. *Radiol Clin North Am* 2001;39:251–266.

Waagner DC: Musculoskeletal infections in adolescents. *Adolesc Med* 2000;11: 375–400.
Wall EJ: Childhood osteomyelitis and septic arthritis. *Curr Opin Pediatr* 1998;10: 73–76.

SEPTIC ARTHRITIS

Septic arthritis is a bacterial infection involving a joint. The bacteria usually enter the joint space by hematogenous spread but can also enter through direct inoculation or direct extension from a contiguous site (osteomyelitis).

Staphylococcus aureus is the most common etiology. The incidence of *H. influenzae* has decreased dramatically secondary to vaccination, but it can still occur in inadequately immunized children under 2 years of age. Children with functional or anatomic asplenia are at particular risk for encapsulated organisms such as *Salmonella* and *Streptococcus pneumoniae. Neisseria gonorrhoeae* can cause septic arthritis in newborns or sexually active adolescents. Less common causes of septic arthritis include *Pseudomonas aeruginosa, Enterobacter, Bacteroides*, and *Campylobacter fetus. Serratia* species and *Corynebacterium pyogenes* can cause septic arthritis in immunocompromised patients with malignancies.

Clinical Presentation

Pain and fever are common presentations in septic arthritis, along with swelling, tenderness, and erythema. However, these findings may be absent, particularly in an infant who may manifest only fever, irritability, and poor feeding. An older child tends to present with limp, joint swelling, and inability to flex or extend a joint.

On examination, the affected joint is swollen, tender, warm, and erythematous. There is limitation of range of motion and pain on movement. The patient usually holds the joint in a position of minimal hydrostatic pressure. For the hip, this is moderate flexion with slight abduction and external rotation. The knee and elbow are held in flexion, the ankle in plantar flexion position, and the shoulder abducted and rotated.

Diagnosis

Rapid diagnosis of septic arthritis is essential, as significant destruction of the joint may occur over a short period of time. Consider a monoarticular arthritis to be septic until proved otherwise.

If there are signs of monoarticular arthritis (erythema, swelling, or decreased range of motion) or polyarticular involvement associated with evidence of gonococcal infection (rash, tenosynovitis), immediately obtain AP and lateral x-rays of the involved joint. For the hip, add a frog-leg view.

Although monoarticular joint involvement may also occur after *trauma*, a history of injury can usually be elicited. Toxic or *transient synovitis* (pp 524–526) causes less severe joint findings on physical examination than septic arthritis, and the x-rays are usually normal. *Acute rheumatic fever* classically causes a migratory polyarthritis with other features of the disease; the response to aspirin is dramatic. *Rheumatoid arthritis* tends to have a more gradual onset, with milder findings, in more than one joint. *Osteomyelitis* (pp 527–528) can cause a sympathetic effusion in the nearest joint. On examination there is point tenderness, usually in the metaphysis, while with septic arthritis maximal pain is elicited in the joint. *Legg-Calvé-Perthes* disease and *slipped capital femoral epiphysis* (pp 524–526) cause limp and decreased range of motion. The patient is afebrile and does not appear toxic. Other diagnoses to consider include *viral arthritis, mycobacterial* and *fungal arthritis, bacterial endocarditis, leukemia, deep cellulitis, serum sickness, ulcerative colitis, granulomatous colitis, Henoch-Schönlein purpura*, and *metabolic diseases* affecting the joints.

ED Management

Immediate arthrocentesis is indicated if septic arthritis is suspected. Because joint fluid may be bacteriostatic, the organism frequently does not grow in culture. Therefore it is imperative that the joint fluid be analyzed by Gram's stain and cell count. Collect the joint fluid in a heparinized syringe to prevent clotting and send the specimen for leukocyte count, glucose, viscosity, and its ability to form a mucin clot. Interpretation of the results is summarized in Table 18-4. In a normal joint, a mucin clot is formed when glacial acid is added to joint fluid immediately after aspiration while the specimen is being stirred with a stirring rod. A "white rope" precipitates around the stirring rod, leaving a clear supernatant. In septic arthritis, glacial acid produces a solution resembling curdled milk.

Obtain a CBC, ESR, glucose, and multiple blood cultures. Typically, the WBC count is elevated ($>$15,000/mm^3) with a shift to the left, and the ESR is increased ($>$30 mm/h). Peripheral blood cultures for the causative organism are positive in 35 to 40% of cases. If gonococcal arthritis is suspected, culture the pharynx, rectum, and cervix or urethra.

After the joint fluid is evaluated, admit the patient for IV antibiotics. Treat patients above 2 years of age with a semisynthetic antistaphylococcal drug (nafcillin 150 mg/kg/day divided q 6 h); if the patient is below age 2, use cefuroxime (100 mg/kg/day divided q 8 h) to cover *H. influenzae*.

If gonococcal infection is likely, use IV or IM ceftriaxone 50 mg/kg/day (1 g/day maximum) once daily or cefotaxime 100 mg/kg/ day IV (1 g/day maximum) divided q 8 h for 7 days with nafcillin (as above) until the diagnosis is confirmed.

Because antibiotics achieve such high concentrations in the joint fluid, direct infusion is not necessary and may be contraindicated with certain antibiotics that are capable of evoking an intense inflammatory reaction. Septic arthritis in the hip of a child is a medical emergency because of the high risk for permanent hip damage, the hip must be surgically drained.

Indication for Admission

- Suspected septic arthritis

BIBLIOGRAPHY

Matan AJ, Smith JT: Pediatric septic arthritis. *Orthopedics* 1997;20:630–635

Shetty AK, Gedalia A: Septic arthritis in children. *Rheum Dis Clin North Am* 1998; 24:287–304.

Wall EJ: Childhood osteomyelitis and septic arthritis. *Curr Opin Pediatr* 1998;10: 73–76.

Table 18-4 Synovial Fluid Findings

DIAGNOSIS	COLOR	CLARITY	VISCOSITY	MUCIN CLOT	WBC/mm³	% PMNs
Normal	Straw	Transparent	High	Good	<200	<25
Traumatic arthritis	Straw to bloody to xanthochromic	Transparent to turbid	High	Good	<2000	<25
					Few to many RBCs	
Rheumatic fever	Yellow	Slightly cloudy	Low	Good	10,000–12,000	50
Rheumatoid arthritis	Yellow to greenish	Cloudy	Low	Poor	15,000–20,000	75
Tuberculosis arthritis	Yellow	Cloudy	Low	Poor	25,000	50–60
Septic arthritis	Grayish or bloody	Turbid or purulent	Low	Poor	80,000–200,000	75

Adapted with permission from Holander JL, McCarthy DI: *Arthritis and Allied Conditions*, 8th ed. Philadelphia: Lea & Febiger, 1972. p. 72.

531

SPLINTING

Many simple, nondisplaced fractures can be managed solely with splinting. Splinting is also useful in the treatment of ligamentous injuries, soft tissue injuries and infections, and joint infections.

General Procedure of Splint Application

Equipment
1. Cotton padding (Webril) between the fingers or toes to prevent maceration and against the skin, to be covered by plaster or fiberglass
2. Plaster of Paris or prefabricated fiberglass rolls
3. Ace bandages

Splint Application
Wrap cotton padding around the affected limb; be sure to separate the fingers or toes. Dip the plaster or fiberglass into a basin of room-temperature water until no bubbles are seen; then roll or "squeegie" the slab until excess water is removed. Smooth the plaster to avoid wrinkles, and apply it to the affected limb in the position desired. Roll a layer of Webril, followed by an Ace bandage, over the splint. Smooth and mold the splint with the palms of both hands, taking care to avoid using fingertips or applying excessive force (Fig. 18-2).

As the splint hardens, heat will be generated and the splint will shrink slightly. After the splint hardens and before the patient is discharged, per-

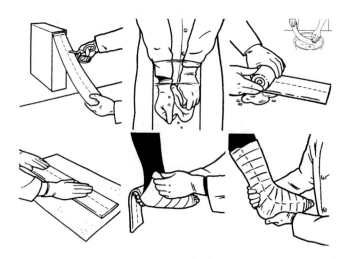

Figure 18-2   Splint application. (From Roberts JR, Hedges JR: *Clinical Procedures in Emergency Medicine*, 3rd ed. Philadelphia: Saunders, 1997, with permission.)

form a careful neurovascular examination of the fingers or toes. Instruct the patient and family about rest, ice, and elevation in the first 24 h, and arrange appropriate follow-up to check the injury and remove the splint at the appropriate time.

Suggested Lengths of Immobilization

Contusion or abrasion	1–3 days
Mild sprain	5–7 days
Soft tissue laceration	5–7 days
Fracture	As per orthopedist
Tendon laceration	As per orthopedist or plastic surgeon

Commonly Used Splints
Volar Splint   Use the volar forearm splint (Fig. 18-3) for a wrist sprain, soft tissue injury, or laceration. The splint extends from the distal aspect of the metacarpals to the proximal aspect of the forearm, leaving the phalanges and elbow free. Apply the splint along the volar surface of the arm with the wrist in a neutral or slightly hyperextended (10 to 20 degree) position.

Gutter Splint   Employ a gutter-type splint (Fig. 18-4) for a metacarpal fracture, such as a fracture of the neck of the fifth metacarpal (boxer's fracture. Use a radial gutter splint to immobilize the second and third fin-

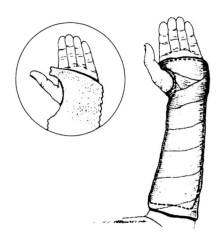

Figure 18-3   Volar forearm splint. (From Roberts JR, Hedges JR: *Clinical Procedures in Emergency Medicine*, 3rd ed. Philadelphia: Saunders, 1997, with permission.)

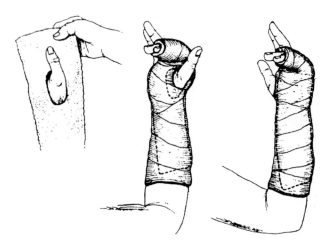

Figure 18-4　Gutter splint. (From Roberts JR, Hedges JR: *Clinical Procedures in Emergency Medicine,* 3rd ed. Philadelphia: Saunders, 1997, with permission.)

gers and an ulnar gutter splint to immobilize the fourth and fifth fingers. Separate the fingers with gauze or Webril, apply the plaster along either the radial or ulnar aspect of the forearm, and wrap it around the two fingers to be immobilized. Flex the MCP joints to 90 degrees and the IP joints to 10 to 20 degrees; place the wrist in the neutral position or hyperextend it slightly (10 to 20 degrees).

Thumb Spica　Apply a thumb spica splint (Fig. 18-5) for a scaphoid fracture, an ulnar collateral ligament injury (gamekeeper's thumb), or a stable fracture of the thumb. Apply the splint along the radial aspect of the forearm and wrap it around the thumb, extending to the thumbnail. Keep the wrist in a neutral or slightly hyperextended position (10 to 20 degrees) and the thumb abducted and slightly flexed (10 to 20 degrees).

Posterior Arm Splint　Use a long posterior arm splint (Fig. 18-6) for a reduced dislocation of the elbow, a nondisplaced radial head or midshaft forearm fracture, a wrist sprain or fracture, or a soft-tissue injury or laceration around the elbow. Apply the plaster to the posterior aspect of the upper arm and forearm, extending to the midpalmar area. Flex the elbow to 90 degrees and place the wrist in a neutral or slightly hyperextended (10 to 20 degree) position. Put the arm in a sling after the splint is applied.

Posterior Leg Splint　Employ a short posterior leg splint (Fig 18-7) for an ankle sprain or a fracture of the foot, ankle, or distal fibula. Apply a short leg splint from the head of the metatarsals to the midcalf, with the

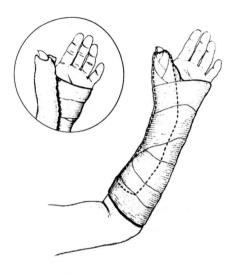

Figure 18-5   Thumb spica splint. (From Roberts JR, Hedges JR: *Clinical Procedures in Emergency Medicine*, 3rd ed. Philadelphia: Saunders, 1997, with permission.)

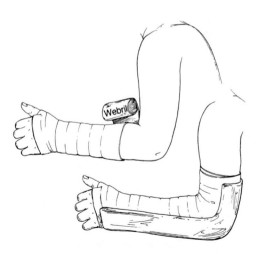

Figure 18-6   Posterior arm splint. (From Roberts JR, Hedges JR: *Clinical Procedures in Emergency Medicine*, 3rd ed. Philadelphia: Saunders, 1997, with permission.)

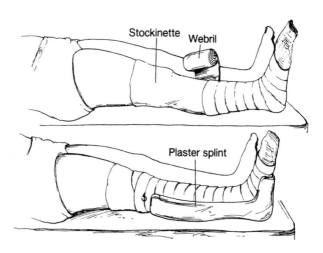

Figure 18-7   Posterior leg splint. (From Roberts JR, Hedges JR: *Clinical Procedures in Emergency Medicine*, 3rd ed. Philadelphia: Saunders, 1997, with permission.)

ankle in as close to a neutral position as possible. Use a long posterior leg splint for knee injuries, with the plaster extended to the midthigh and the knee in extension.

Finger Splint   Perform a careful examination of the injured finger and review the radiographs to determine the presence of a rotational or unacceptably angulated deformity, growth plate injury, or collateral ligament injury, all of which require orthopedic consultation.

A simple phalangeal fracture or a reduced interphalangeal dislocation may be managed with splinting alone. A soft tissue injury or laceration will also benefit from finger splinting. Dynamic splinting, or "buddy taping" (Fig. 18-8), permits movement at the MP joint and slight movement at the IP joints. Splint the injured finger to the adjacent finger, or "buddy," to provide support.

An alternative splint is the foam-backed aluminum splint (Fig. 18-9), which may be cut and bent to fit. It is preferably applied to the dorsal surface of the finger, which preserves dexterity more effectively than splints applied to the volar surface. The splint should immobilize as few joints as possible; measure it to include only one joint above and one joint below the injury. Place the finger in the position of function or slightly flexed (10 to 20 degrees) at the IP joints. Two-finger injuries require specific splinting techniques (see pp 533–534) and not simple buddy taping or dorsal splinting.

Mallet Finger   The mallet finger is caused by a rupture of the extensor tendon at the DIP joint. Splint the finger only over the dorsal aspect of the

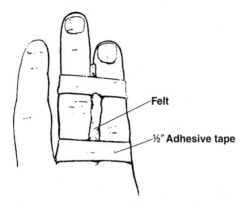

Figure 18-8   Dynamic splinting. (From Roberts JR, Hedges JR: *Clinical Procedures in Emergency Medicine*, 3rd ed. Philadelphia: Saunders, 1997, with permission.)

DIP in full extension or slight hyperextension. The splint must remain for at least 8 weeks, and the finger must not be flexed at any time during that period.

Boutonnière Deformity   The boutonnière deformity is a rupture of the central slip of the extensor digitorum communis tendon, resulting in the PIP "buttonholing" through the torn extensor hood. Splint the finger only over the dorsal aspect of the PIP in full extension or slight hyperextension.

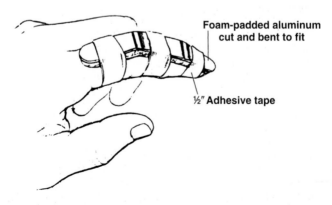

Figure 18-9   Foam-backed aluminum splint. (From Roberts JR, Hedges JR: *Clinical Procedures in Emergency Medicine*, 3rd ed. Philadelphia: Saunders, 1997, with permission.)

Keep the splint in place for at least 4 weeks; the finger must not be flexed during that time.

BIBLIOGRAPHY

Fleisher GR, Ludwig S (eds): *Textbook of Pediatric Emergency Medicine,* 4th ed. Baltimore: Williams & Wilkins, 1997, pp 1886–1891.
Roberts JR, Hedges JR (eds): *Clinical Procedures in Emergency Medicine,* 3rd ed. Philadelphia: Saunders, 1997.

REHABILITATION OF SPORTS INJURIES

As a rule of thumb, the amount of time necessary for proper rehabilitation (Tables 18-5 and 18-6) from an injury is about half the time spent not participating in sports since the injury. For example, if an athlete has refrained from competition and sports for 4 weeks, about 2 weeks of rehabilitation will be needed. Early referral to professional rehabilitation (physical therapist, athletic trainer) will hasten a more complete recovery and facilitate an earlier return to competition. In any case, there are four stages of rehabilitation:

Stage One: Early Mobilization and Restoration of Range of Motion (ROM)
The goals are to decrease pain and inflammation and to begin to reestablish the range of motion. Early mobilization can limit disabling swelling and muscle atrophy and minimize the loss of range of motion in the joint. While a small degree of soreness is generally acceptable, more significant pain is an indication that the patient must reduce his or her level of activity. For moderate to severe injury, give anti-inflammatory medication (ibuprofen 10 mg/kg q 6 h) to control swelling and pain and recommend nonimpact activities such as swimming and biking to keep the muscles moving.

Various therapeutic modalities that may be used during stage one include ultrasound, electronic stimulation, icing, and whirlpool. These stimulate blood flow and repair damaged tissue, which then lessen the pain and swelling.

Stage Two: Strength, Balance, and Flexibility Training
The goals are almost full strength and complete range of motion. In this stage, the athlete begins a progressive resistance program. Exercise frequency is increased to several times a day, and while therapy often focuses on one particular muscle group, it is necessary that the complementary muscles be strengthened as well.

Stage Three: Sport-Specific Training
The goal of stage three is to have the athlete perform sport-specific tasks encompassing strength, balance, and flexibility. Once the patient demonstrates that he or she can perform sport-specific skills, participation in the sport can be resumed, with proper precautions.

Sport-specific skills for a running sport include running, cutting (changing directions at various speeds), and jumping. Examples include the following:

Table 18-5 Rehabilitation of Acute Injuries

	ANKLE SPRAIN	HIP FLEXOR INJURY	SHOULDER DISLOCATION	PATELLAR DISLOCATION
Missed time	2–8 weeks	3–12 weeks	4–12 weeks	4–12 weeks
Stage I	ROM: plantar/dorsiflex eversion/inversion Stationary biking as soon as possible	Gentle stretching and ROM Stationary biking as soon as possible	Light ROM (not above head) Pendulum exercises	Leg lifts and isometric exercises No bending of the knee
Stage II	Biking advancing to treadmill Resistance band exercises Calf stretches One-legged balance and cutting drills	Leg lifts and hurdler's stretch Stationary biking Walking on treadmill	Resistance band exercises Free weights Arm raises	Begin ROM: Straight leg raises with weights Progress as tolerated One-legged balance drills
Stage III	Running on treadmill or padded surface Kicking, jumping	Running on treadmill Running, kicking, and jumping Soccer, basketball, and tennis drills	Throwing balls Tennis serves	Walking/running on treadmill Start jumping and cutting drills Start sport specific skills
Stage IV	Continue resistance band exercises and balance drills	Continue leg lifts Continue stretches tid-qid, before and after sports	Continue resistance band exercises and free weights	Continue leg lifts and wall squats
Equipment/ Bracing*	Crutches for several days Ankle strap/brace	None	Sling for comfort (<7 days)	Knee immobilizer/crutches or 4–6 weeks, then neoprene knee brace with patella cut out

*The equipment is not the treatment but rather an adjunct to the primary treatment, the rehabilitation (therapy).
Adapted from Small, E: *Kids & Sports*. New York. Newmarket Press, 2002.

Table 18-6 Rehabilitation of Chronic (Overuse) Injuries

	SHIN SPLINTS	SHOULDER TENDINITIS	SEVER'S DISEASE	OSGOOD-SCHLATTER DISEASE
Missed time	No running for 2–6 weeks	50% decrease in activities (swimming, tennis serving, baseball pitching)	1–6 weeks	1–6 months
Stage I	Calf stretching, stationary biking, swimming, water running	Upper extremity stretching Internal/external rotation Arm raises After 1–2 weeks: bent over arm raises	Calf stretching qid Toe raises Swimming, biking	Icing over tender bone Biking
Stage II	Resistance bands, toe raises Toe walking/heel walking One-legged balance drills Begin walking on treadmill, progress to speed walking, then running		One-legged balance drills Scrunching towel Walking progressing to running	Leg lifts in three directions
Stage III	Increase resistance bands, toe raises, and stretches Progress to running	Add 10–20% activity per week Continue exercises (internal/ external rotation, bent-arm raises)	Sport-specific skills: cutting, jumping, and kicking	Add 10–20% activity per week
Stage IV	Continue toe raises, calf stretches	Continue at least two of four exercises	Continue calf stretches and resistance band	Continue stretches and leg lifts
Equipment/ Bracing*	Over-the-counter orthotics (custom-made only if no response)	None	Heel cushions, heel lifts or over-the-counter orthotics	Osgood-Schlatter band Neoprene knee brace with patella cut-out

*The equipment is not the treatment but rather an adjunct to the primary treatment, the rehabilitation (therapy).
Adapted from Small, E: *Kids & Sports*, New York, Newmarket Press, 2002.

- Intense running, with muscle endurance being rebuilt using a skiing machine, bike, stair or stepping machine, or treadmill
- Agility drills, such as running figure eights and zigzag patterns
- Balance and strength exercises such as hopping and jumping
- For an upper-body sport activity, light tosses from 3 to 5 ft and one- and two-handed basketball passes

Stage Four: Maintenance
The goal is to improve upon strength and sport-specific skills, so that the injured body part is stronger and more functional than prior to the injury. Stage four is a maintenance program, so no new exercises are given. Instead, the program entails increasing the number of repetitions and weight on the various exercises.

CHAPTER 19

Psychological and Social Emergencies

Stephen Ludwig and Joel Fein
- Olga Jimenez and Madeline Garcia-Bigelow
  (contributors—Chart Documentation in Child Abuse;
  Medical Testimony and Court Preparation)

PHYSICAL ABUSE

Physical abuse is defined as nonaccidental physical injury to a child by acts of commission or omission on the part of the parents or others. There has been an alarming increase in reported cases of child abuse throughout the United States in the past three decades. In all states, health professionals are now legally required to report their suspicions of abuse to their state child protection services (CPS) or police.

Clinical Presentation and Diagnosis

Determination of suspected abuse is based on a compilation from five data sources: (1) history, (2) physical examination, (3) laboratory and radiographic information, (4) observation of parental interaction, and (5) a detailed family social history.

In examining any child with an injury, be suspicious of abuse if the history reveals an unusual delay in seeking medical care, the parents' explanation of the injury is not compatible with the physical findings, the cause of the injury is unknown or "magical," or there is a history of similar episodes. Parents may be reluctant to give information, or their reaction may be inappropriate to the seriousness of the injuries. Other worrisome signs are a lack of primary care (no immunizations, no source of health care), a history of parental mental illness or substance abuse, and high levels of family stress.

While examining the child, maintain a high index of suspicion for abuse or neglect if the child's weight is below the third percentile for age and there is poor personal hygiene, lack of adequate clothing, behavioral disturbance (especially undue compliance with the examiner), or an abnormal interaction between the parent and child (unwarranted roughness or extreme aloofness).

Remove all the child's clothing and examine the skin carefully for contusions, abrasions, burns, and lacerations in various stages of resolution. Any bruise on a child who is not yet cruising is unusual. Certain skin lesions are typical for specific types of abuse, such as circular cigarette burns; human bite marks; J-shaped curvilinear or loop-shaped marks from a wire, cord, or belt; circumferential rope burns; "grid" marks from an electric heater; and symmetric scald burns on the buttocks or extremities. Other dermatologic manifestations are cutaneous signs of malnutrition (decreased subcutaneous fat, increased creases), scalp hematomas, and signs of trauma to the genital area.

Fractures are suggested by the child's refusal to bear weight or move an extremity, gross deformity, or soft tissue swelling and point tenderness over an extremity. However, most metaphyseal chip fractures are not associated with deformity. Neurologic manifestations may include retinal hemorrhages, inexplicable irritability, coma, or convulsions. Finally, an acute abdomen, poisoning, or any traumatic injury that cannot be explained may in fact represent child abuse of some type.

The differential diagnosis of the abused child includes conditions with skeletal involvement: *accidental trauma, osteogenesis imperfecta, Caffey's disease, scurvy, rickets, birth trauma*, and *congenital infection*. Diseases with dermatologic manifestations include bleeding disorders (*idiopathic thrombocytopenic purpura, leukemia, hemophilia, von Willebrand disease), recurrent pyodermas*, and *scalded skin syndrome. Sudden infant death syndrome* and *accidental poisonings* may be mistaken for child abuse. The most common clinical problem is the differentiation between accidental and nonaccidental trauma.

ED Management

If there is any fracture or other suggestion of abuse in a child under 2 years of age, obtain a complete skeletal survey for trauma. For older patients, if the physical examination suggests a fracture, obtain specific x-rays. Order other radiologic studies, such as computed tomography (CT) of the head or magnetic resonance imaging (MRI), as indicated by the nature of the injuries.

If the parents deny any knowledge of the cause of skin bruises, obtain a complete blood count (CBC) with differential, platelet count, prothrombin time (PT), partial thromboplastin time (PTT), and a bleeding time. The differential diagnosis and other possible laboratory studies are shown in Table 19-1.

Physicians and other health care workers are required to report the *suspicion* of abuse. Use the information gathered in the assessment phase to determine the level of concern. Notify the CPS or police by telephone if abuse or neglect is suspected. Generally, the CPS is required to initiate action in all cases reported and may not refuse to accept a referral made in good faith by a competent reporter. Usually, a physician, nurse, or social worker must complete a report within 48 h. However, do not delay reporting if there are other children at home, as up to 20% will also have been abused.

The CPS worker must evaluate the case and decide whether the child can safely return home or must go to a temporary shelter or foster placement. Hospitalize the child if medical care is needed or if that is the only option for providing a safe environment. Arrange appropriate follow-up for patients who do not require hospitalization. Notify the parents about

Table 19-1 Differential Diagnosis and Abnormal Laboratory Studies to Support a Diagnosis

FINDINGS	DIFFERENTIAL DIAGNOSIS	DISTINGUISHING FEATURES AND TESTS
Bruising (extensive or deep)	Trauma ITP Hemophilia Von Willebrand disease Henoch-Schönlein purpura Purpura fulminans Ehlers-Danlos syndrome	Physical examination Decreased platelets Increased PT, PTT Increased bleeding time Rash on lower extremities; rule out sepsis; normal platelet count Clinical appearance (findings of sepsis); decreased platelet count Joint hyperextensibility
Dehydration	Renal or prerenal	Increased BUN, creatinine, urine specific gravity Prerenal: BUN/creatinine >20:1
Failure to thrive	Organic or nonorganic	History, physical examination; abnormal studies based on symptoms
Abdominal pain	Trauma Tumor Infection	Hematuria; increased liver enzymes Increased amylase; abdominal ultrasound; abnormal urinalysis Increased WBC, ESR; abdominal ultrasound
Fractures (multiple or in various stages of healing)	Trauma Osteogenesis imperfecta Rickets Hypophosphatasia Leukemia Previous osteomyelitis or septic arthritis Neurogenic sensory deficit	Blue sclerae; x-ray: decreased bone density Decreased calcium; increased phosphorus, alkaline phosphatase; x-ray: cupping at ends of long bones, widened metaphysis Decreased alkaline phosphatase; x-ray: abnormal bone mineralization Abnormal peripheral smear; bone marrow biopsy Increased WBC, ESR, CRP; positive culture Detailed neurologic examination

Table 19-1 Differential Diagnosis and Abnormal Laboratory Studies to Support a Diagnosis (*Continued*)

FINDINGS	DIFFERENTIAL DIAGNOSIS	DISTINGUISHING FEATURES AND TESTS
Metaphyseal/ epiphyseal lesions	Trauma	X-rays: consistent mechanism of injury
	Scurvy	X-rays: periosteal elevation; nutritional history
	Rickets	(See above)
	Menkes' syndrome	Decreased copper, ceruloplasmin; hair analysis
	Syphilis	Abnormal serology (VDRL)
	Little League elbow	History of use
	Birth trauma	Neonatal history
Subperiosteal ossification	Trauma	X-ray; biopsy
	Osteogenic malignancy	(See above)
	Syphilis	No metaphyseal changes
	Infantile cortical hyperostosis	Dramatic clinical response to aspirin
	Osteoid osteoma	(See above)
	Scurvy	
CNS injury	Trauma	CT and/or MRI scan
	Aneurysm	CT and/or MRI scan
	Tumor	MRI scan

KEY: BUN, blood urea nitrogen; CRP, C-reactive protein; CT, computed tomography; ESR, erythrocyte sedimentation rate; ITP, idiopathic thrombocytopenic purpura; MRI, magnetic resonance imaging; PT, prothrombin time; PTT, partial prothrombin time; WBC, white blood count your intention to report and/or hospitalize the child. If the parents refuse to allow hospitalization, it may be necessary to have law enforcement officials intervene. In most states, hospital personnel may place a child under temporary protective custody without either parental consent or a family court order, although it is the responsibility of the CPS worker to decide whether the child can be placed in the custody of a relative or guardian.

Working with the families of abused children can be a difficult experience. Avoid an accusatory attitude, as most of these parents love their children and deserve a supportive approach. Keep the parents informed and involved, and emphasize that the goal of all concerned is to keep the child safe and, when possible, the family together. Explain the role of the social worker and supportive services, and assure confidentiality. Careful documentation is critical (see pp 550–554); the record will be needed for legal reference.

Follow-up

- Patient discharged home or to a shelter: primary care follow-up in 1 week

Indications for Admission

- Medical care required
- Extent of injury uncertain
- Needed protection unavailable through community resources

BIBLIOGRAPHY

American Academy of Pediatrics Section on Radiology: Diagnostic imaging of child abuse. *Pediatrics* 2000;105:1345–1348.

Ludwig S, Kornberg A: *Child Abuse and Neglect: A Medical Reference,* 2nd ed. New York: Churchill Livingstone, 1991.

Reece RM, Ludwig S: *Child Abuse: Medical Diagnosis and Management.* New York: Lippincott Williams & Wilkins, 2001.

SEXUAL ABUSE

Sexual abuse is the exposure of a child to sexual stimulation inappropriate for his or her age, cognitive development, or position in the relationship. The legal definition is nonconsensual sexual contact. *Incest* is legally defined as marriage or intercourse (oral, anal, genital) with a person known to be related as an ancestor, descendant, brother, sister, uncle, aunt, nephew, or niece. *Rape* is legally defined as nonconsensual sexual intercourse; a person having legitimate access to the child is the typical perpetrator.

Clinical Presentation

A number of signs, symptoms, and behavioral changes may signal the possibility of sexual abuse, including difficulties in school, a sudden change in behavior, fears, unwillingness to go to certain places, enuresis and encopresis, sleep disturbances, running away, and attempted suicide.

Sexual abuse victims may exhibit seductive or regressive behavior. More specific complaints include difficulty walking or sitting and genital trauma, discharge, pain, or itching. A sexually transmitted disease (STD) in a child under the age of 12 is sexual abuse until proven otherwise. Consider sexual abuse in girls who become pregnant.

Diagnosis

Maintain a high index of suspicion in order to identify sexual abuse promptly. Ensure privacy for the patient and whoever accompanies the child, and keep the number of staff members involved to a minimum. Because sexual abuse usually evokes intense feelings, it requires effort to maintain objectivity.

The key to establishing the diagnosis in these cases is careful history taking. Use language that is appropriate for the child's age, and ask specifically about all types of sexual contact. It may be helpful to use anatomically correct dolls or pictures to encourage the child to describe the sexual contact in as much detail as possible. Try to ascertain when the last sexual activity occurred and what the child has done since the assault (changed clothes, bathed, urinated, defecated). Assure the child that he or she was right to reveal information about the sexual abuse.

Consent for physical examination is often an issue. However, consent from the minor (regardless of age) is all that is required, since the examination also serves to rule out STD. Do not force the patient if the examination is refused.

If the abuse has occurred within the preceding 72 h, be aggressive in terms of evidence collection. If the patient has not changed clothes since the sexual activity, have him or her undress on a sheet and save all clothing for legal evidence. If the child has changed clothes but not bathed, collect only the underwear. If the child has pubic hair, comb it onto a paper towel and seal the towel, combings, one plucked pubic hair, and the comb in a labeled envelope. These samples may be used for DNA evidence. Perform a complete and careful physical examination looking for bite marks, scratches, bruises, or other signs of physical injury or illness, and note the child's Tanner stage of pubertal development.

In most cases, the revelation of sexual abuse occurs long after the actual contact. If sexual contact has not occurred within 72 h and there are no physical complaints (e.g., bleeding, discharge), refer the patient to a specialized sexual abuse center.

With prompt revelation, a careful genital examination is necessary. Perform a perineal-genital examination in young children in the frog-leg, supine, or knee-chest prone position. Using a saline-moistened cotton Q-tip, swab any areas of possible seminal fluid deposition and placed it on a labeled slide to air-dry. In girls, spread the labia with two fingers to examine the hymenal ring, the introitus, and the area between the labia majora and minora. If there are no acute signs of pelvic injury in the prepubertal girl, a speculum examination is not necessary. If there are obvious signs of physical injury (bleeding, lacerations), consult with a pediatric gynecologist or surgeon about the need for pelvic examination under anesthesia.

Table 19-2   Possible Laboratory Studies in Sexual Abuse

Neisseria gonorrhoeae cultures: oropharynx, vagina/urethra, rectum
Chlamydia trachomatis cultures: vagina/urethra, rectum
Clothing, hair, fingernail scrapings, and other physical evidence
Serum pregnancy test (if appropriate)
HIV testing (depending on the locale and nature of the abuse)
Stool test for occult blood (in cases of anal penetration)
If contact occurred within 72 h:
    Detection of sperm: obtain specimens from the mouth/vagina/rectum,
       place the swabs in saline, then dry mount on slide
    Determination of blood group: saliva

In boys, examine the penis and scrotum for bruises, swelling, teeth marks, erythema, or other signs of trauma. In both boys and girls, spread the buttocks with both hands to examine the anus and perineal area. If there are obvious signs of physical injury or severe pain, anoscopy or sigmoidoscopy is indicated, under anesthesia if necessary.

Table 19-2 lists the specific laboratory evaluation of a sexually abused child. Obtain cultures for *Neisseria* and *Chlamydia* from the cervix (postmenarchal), vagina (premenarchal), urethra, rectum, and pharynx if the symptoms of an STD are present. Examine vaginal specimens for the presence of *Trichomonas*. Obtain wet preps from all affected areas to look for sperm: mouth, up to 6 h after assault; rectum and vagina, up to 24 h. If a speculum examination is performed, obtain a Pap smear and ask the hospital laboratory to specifically note the presence of sperm. Immotile sperm are present up to 2½ weeks after intercourse. Obtain a pregnancy test for all pubertal females. HIV testing may be indicated (at 1 month, 6 months, and 1 year after contact) in areas of high incidence or if the perpetrator has any risk factors for HIV infection.

ED Management

If the alleged perpetrator is a family member or someone with family-like contact with the child, report the suspected sexual abuse to the CPS. It is not the responsibility of the ED staff to determine whether the abuse actually occurred. In many jurisdictions, child sexual abuse is also reported to the police. Make careful documentation, in writing, of all findings on the physical examination; diagrams and drawings are very useful. Take photographs of any bruises or other evidence of physical injury. Label all specimens taken for evidence, and place them in evidence envelopes to be logged and secured by the security department of the hospital or given directly to the police. Assure that the chain of legal evidence is unbroken.

Give treatment for gonorrhea and chlamydial infections as outlined in Table 11-2 (Sexually Transmitted Diseases, pp 286–293) to all adolescent and prepubertal victims with signs of infection, and arrange for HIV prophylaxis (see pp 347–352).

Offer a postcoital contraceptive to the postmenarchal adolescent girl who is seen within 72 h. Lo-Ovral (0.3 mg norgestrel, 0.03 mg ethinyl estradiol), 4 tablets at once and 4 tablets 12 h later, is an efficacious regimen that has few side effects (nausea and vomiting).

Reassure the child that his or her body is not harmed, that he or she was not responsible for the sexual assault, and that you believe the patient and will do everything to protect him or her from further assault. Some victims and parents may need reassurance that the encounter will not alter the child's sexual preference in the future.

Follow-up

- Within 1 to 2 days, with a skilled psychotherapist or child abuse specialist
- With a physician in 2 weeks (for repeat cultures) and in 6 weeks (to obtain a VDRL)

Indications for Admission

- Sexual abuse that occurred very near the home or when the patient's family is unable to provide the necessary support when alternative placement is not possible
- Active vaginal or rectal bleeding

BIBLIOGRAPHY

American Academy of Pediatrics Committee on Child Abuse and Neglect: Guidelines for the evaluation of sexual abuse of children: subject review. *Pediatrics* 1999;103:186–191.

Atabaki S, Paradise JE: The medical evaluation of the sexually abused child: lessons from a decade of research. *Pediatrics* 1999;104:178–186.

Christian CW, Lavelle JM, DeJong AR, et al: Forensic evidence findings in prepubertal victims of sexual assault. *Pediatrics* 2000;106:100–104.

Swanston HY, Tebbutt JS, O'Toole BI, et al: Sexually abused children 5 years after presentation: a case-control study. *Pediatrics* 1997;100:600–608.

CHART DOCUMENTATION IN CHILD ABUSE

Medical professionals caring for abused children may be subpoenaed to testify in court, where information in the patient's chart is subjected to close scrutiny; meticulous documentation is therefore mandatory. In addition, as court proceedings may not begin for several months to years after the initial evaluation, details entrusted solely to memory may be forgotten. The medical record must be legible and, if possible, typed. In addition, documentation of physical evidence need not be limited to written descriptions and drawings; photographs, videotapes, and computer technology are appropriate means of preserving evidence of physical findings.

Verbal Evidence

The principal diagnostic component of the child abuse assessment lies in the history obtained from the parent, the primary caretaker, or the child suspected of being abused. Interview each parent and the patient separately. Always document the time and place of the interview, who was present, and whether a translator was utilized. If a translator was involved, document his or her name and the language spoken.

In interviewing a child, use appropriate interviewing techniques, including nonleading and nonsuggestive questions and language suitable for the child's age and developmental stage. Basic nonleading questions usually begin with "who," "what," "when," "where" or "why"; these types of questions allow the patient the freedom to describe details of what happened without jeopardizing the integrity of the interview. For example, if the patient discloses that her stepfather touched her inappropriately, a leading follow-up question might be "Did he touch you on your vagina?" In contrast, a nonleading question might be "Where did he touch you?" or "Can you point to where he touched you?" Write the patient's statements down verbatim; do not correct grammatical errors or paraphrase the child's remarks. Use quotations as often as possible. Ask the child the name he or she uses to identify body parts and make a notation (for example, "child identified 'pee pee' as the name she uses for her vagina").

Statements made by a child are often considered "hearsay"—a statement made out of court offered into evidence in order to establish the truth of the matter asserted in the statement. In other words, the child's words are offered in court to prove that what the child said is actually the truth. Generally, hearsay statements are not admissible in court, although there are exceptions to this rule. The two pertinent exceptions to the hearsay rule are the *"excited utterance"* exception and the *"medical diagnosis or treatment"* exception. Documentation of the features that allow a statement to qualify as a hearsay exception increases the chances the child's words will be admissible in court.

The *excited utterance* exception is a hearsay statement that relates to a stressful event. Three requirements are necessary for a statement to fall under this exception: the child must have experienced a stressful event, the child's statement must be associated with the event, and the child must still be experiencing the emotions caused by the event. Document in the chart the type of stressful event; the amount of time that passed between the event and when the child first made the statement; the child's speech, spontaneity, and emotions; what questions led to the disclosure; and what was the first secure opportunity the child had to disclose.

The *medical diagnosis or treatment* exception relates to the belief that people are honest with medical professionals and that the information provided is therefore trustworthy. Under this exception the information obtained in the medical history (including chief complaint, review of systems, past medical history, and the child's description of the cause of injury) are admissible in court. Ensure that the patient understands the importance of providing accurate information and that the purpose of the interview and examination is to provide diagnosis or treatment. In some states this exception also applies to mental health professionals providing treatment services.

It is also important to document the characteristics of the patient's statements that enhance their reliability, including the child's advanced knowledge of anatomy, description of distinctive details of sexual acts (e.g., taste, color, or smell of the ejaculate), and changes in the child's behavior (emotions displayed when the statement was made).

Documentation of the Medical History

Obtain a thorough medical history. Include in the chart any medical condition, surgery, or previous injury that could explain the child's current findings. In evaluating injuries, take into account the patient's developmental stage and document whether the interviewer or another objective observer was able to corroborate the information provided. Note the presence of specific symptoms (e.g., vaginal bleeding, discharge) and nonspecific symptoms (e.g., enuresis, encopresis) related to the abuse. Include in the family history any hereditary condition that could potentially explain the child's injuries (e.g., parent with history of osteogenesis imperfecta). Include any pertinent social information, including who lives in the home with the child and who has been identified as the alleged offender. This information will help to determine whether it is safe for the patient to go home.

Documentation of the Physical Examination

A thorough and complete physical examination is indicated for all children and adolescents suspected of being abused or neglected. Include the following in the medical record:

- Growth parameters. These are especially important in evaluating a child for failure to thrive and possible neglect. Chart current values on a growth curve and compare them with previous measurements.
- Documentation of any marks, bruises, burns, bites, scars, and/or other lesions suggestive for abuse. Describe their pattern, shape, location, size, and color.
- All positive findings and any pertinent negative findings (e.g., no retinal hemorrhages noted in a child with suspected inflicted head trauma).

It is essential to describe genital findings in a precise manner. Refer to guidelines published by the American Professional Society on the Abuse of Children for standardized language to describe normal, variants of normal, and abnormal pediatric genital findings. Use the clock face to describe the location of the injury. The 12 o'clock position is anterior (urethra being 12 o'clock), the 6 o'clock is posterior, following a clockwise rotation. The anal examination can be performed in the lateral decubitus, supine, or knee-chest position.

Document the following about the anogenital examination:

- Position in which the patient was examined (e.g., supine, knee-chest).
- Tanner stage.
- Any use of magnification (colposcope or other magnifying instrument).
- Whether medical findings were photographed or videotaped (see below, under "photographic documentation").
- A description of each anatomic structure (labia, clitoris, vestibule, hymen, fossa navicularis, posterior fourchette, vagina). Mention the presence or absence of lesions, bruises, petechiae, etc. (for ex-

ample, "hymen with a tear at 6 o'clock, the tear extends to the fossa navicularis").

- A description of the shape of the hymen (crescentic, annular, redundant, etc.). Make note of the presence of warts, bruises, tears, petechiae, and/or ecchymoses (e.g., "hymen crescentic in shape with an acute complete transection at 6 o'clock, few petechiae noted at 3 and 5 o'clock"). Avoid terms like *virginal* or *intact*.
- Body or genital diagrams demonstrating the site and type of injury.
- Documentation of any anal tags, fissures, bruises, lacerations, scars, rashes, discharge, bleeding, and/or other lesions. Note the normal variants of the anal examination so that these are not confused with abnormal findings.
- For the male genitalia, a description of the penis and scrotum, noting the presence of circumcision and any hematomas, lacerations, scars, ecchymoses, rashes, discharge, erythema, and/or other lesions.

Photographic Documentation
Documentation of medical findings with photographs is an essential element of the child abuse evaluation. Photographs allow clinicians an opportunity for later review of the medical findings; in some cases additional information, initially overlooked, may be found. If a second opinion is sought, the photos can be reviewed instead of having the child endure repeated examinations. In court, photographs provide a visual impact that may surpass the best-written chart. In addition, photographs can be used to compare examinations over time.

Before taking a picture, explain to the child in simple language what is going to happen, who will see the pictures, and why pictures are being taken. Label the photographs, at minimum, with the patient's medical record number and the date the photograph was taken. Full documentation of the date, patient's name, identification number, date of birth, and the name of the photographer is preferable. Photograph the child's face, and take as many pictures as needed of each injury. Include a measuring device to document the size of the lesion (if not available, place an object with known measurement, such as a penny, next to the part being photographed). A standardized color bar captured in the photo may be useful for color comparison. Nevertheless, photographs do not substitute for body diagrams and a detailed description of the injury. Each institution must have a policy for photographing, storing, releasing, and handling pictures.

Documentation of Laboratory and Radiologic Tests
Document the results of all laboratory tests performed. If cultures for sexually transmitted diseases (STDs) are taken, document the type of culture and the site from which it was obtained (e.g., vagina, rectum). At the present time, cultures are still the gold standard for evaluating STDs in children suspected of being abused. Follow the Centers for Disease Control/American Academy of Pediatrics (CDC /AAP) recommendations for testing children and adolescents in the context of sexual abuse. Also include in the report any radiographic and/or CT scan interpretations. A skeletal survey, looking for previous fractures, is indicated in all cases of suspected physical abuse in children below 2 years of age.

Impression and Plan
For the impression and plan:

- Indicate clearly the disclosure of abuse and findings of the physical examination. Avoid using phrases such as "alleged sexual assault" or "rule out abuse." It is important to note that a normal genital or anal examination does not exclude sexual abuse and that most sexually abused children do not have medical findings.
- List any medications prescribed, including indications, length of treatment, and potential side effects.
- State the names of the child protective worker and detectives or police officers involved, if any.
- In sexual assault cases, note the name and badge number of the police officer who receives the forensic evidence (rape kit). It is of utmost importance to maintain the chain of evidence at all times. In those cases when collected evidence is not immediately handed to police, follow hospital policy for storing the evidence.
- If other providers were consulted, state their recommendations clearly in the chart.
- Arrange an appointment for medical follow-up to discuss results of tests performed in the ED, repeat certain tests, or repeat a physical examination after any injuries are treated. Document if a referral has been made to a specialized program for a sexual or physical abuse evaluation. In most cases of child sexual abuse, a detailed genital examination can be deferred until a later date in a more appropriate setting. Consult the hospital's child protection team.
- Offer a follow-up mental health appointment to all abused children and their families.
- Work together with the child protective and law enforcement agents to establish the safest environment for the child. A representative for child protective services will determine whether the child may stay at home or should be placed in foster care temporarily.

BIBLIOGRAPHY

American Academy of Pediatrics, Committee on Child Abuse and Neglect: Guidelines for the evaluation of sexual abuse in children: subject review. *Pediatrics* 1999;103:186–191.

Limbos MA, Berkowitz CD: Documentation of child physical abuse: how far have we come? *Pediatrics* 1998;102:53–58.

Socolar RR, Champion M, Green C: Physicians' documentation of sexual abuse of children. *Arch Pediatr Adolesc Med* 1996;150:191–196.

MEDICAL TESTIMONY
AND COURT PREPARATION

The testimony of a medical provider can be among the most critical pieces of evidence supplied to the court in cases of child abuse and maltreatment. Attorneys rarely have the luxury of providing the court with eyewitness accounts of the incident in question. Therefore the testimony of the medical provider who cared for the child may prove to be pivotal in the final determination of the matter before the court.

Medical providers are mandated reporters of suspected child abuse and maltreatment. As such, they have both an ethical and legal responsibility to participate in and cooperate with any investigatory and/or court process. Medical providers may be subpoenaed to testify in two distinct venues. One such venue is Family Court (civil case), where the focus will be on determining the safe placement of the child; alternatively, the case may be tried as a criminal matter, in which the court will make a factual determination and decide upon a verdict of guilty or not guilty. In either case, the role of the medical provider remains essentially the same.

Expert Qualification

A medical provider may testify at trial as an expert in the field of child abuse only after being qualified to do so by the court. The expert brings his or her experience and knowledge to the case and as such plays an important role in helping the court reach a proper verdict. In order to qualify a person as an expert, the court must be shown that the individual has knowledge and experience outside the realm of the average layperson. Having been qualified at previous trials does not automatically ensure one's qualification at future court proceedings.

It is essential that the provider prepare in advance to ensure that the qualification process is completed without incident. The provider must make available his or her most current curriculum vitae, which will serve as a vital source of information for both the attorneys and the court. Other aspects of the medical provider's pretrial preparation for qualification include reviewing all questions that he or she will be asked by the subpoenaing attorney, as well as any hypothetical questions that may arise, and reviewing and explaining any technical terminology that may be used in the trial. In addition, the potential expert must be prepared to discuss his or her practical experience in the field and all authored publications, including why and how they differ from other respected publications and treatises.

Proper preparation is also crucial in readying the provider for cross-examination by opposing counsel. At this juncture, cross-examination will be limited to questions about the medical provider's experience and knowledge in the field; the purpose of this cross-examination will be either to prevent the qualification of the provider or to ensure that the witness is, in fact, an expert in the field. At the end of this portion of the proceeding, the court will be asked to deem the provider an expert.

Factual Witness

A second distinct function of medical testimony is to elicit factual evidence, including details of patient interviews and/or medical procedures performed by the provider. Not uncommonly, the only witness to the alleged incident is the victim; in such cases, the medical provider's testimony can substantially influence the outcome of the case. Detailed documentation of the interview with the patient is therefore crucial. The provider must show documentation not only of the patient's exact statements but also of the circumstances surrounding the disclosure. More credibility and weight may be given to the medical provider's testimony if he or she is able to provide extensive details of the interview (see Chart Documentation in Child Abuse, pp 550–554).

Part of any cross-examination will be to discredit the testimony by attempting to show that the patient's statements were, in fact, tainted. The fewer the details documented by the provider, the more likely that opposing counsel will be able to weaken the case by injecting doubt into the minds of the court or jury. Cross-examination is distinctly different in nature from a direct examination, in which a witness is allowed relative freedom to explain any findings and observations. During cross-examination, opposing counsel may attempt to discredit and/or confuse the witness with a barrage of questions. It is within a witness' purview to request that an attorney repeat or rephrase any question that is not understood. The role of the witness is simply to state the facts as they are known, in as clear and direct a manner as possible, while preserving the integrity of the testimony. Despite his or her personal feelings, a witness must remain as unbiased and unprejudiced as possible. It is the role of the attorney, not the witness, to object when there is an evidentiary or legal problem; the judge will then determine whether the objection is sustained or overruled.

Impact of Documentation on Court Proceedings

The notes and observations of a mandated reporter may be called into question during a court proceeding. Therefore it is crucial for medical providers always to document interviews with the patient in a way that preserves details for future possible court testimony. Medical providers must be especially careful in interviewing children, asking only open-ended and nonleading questions (see p 551).

In addition to documenting details of the actual disclosure, medical providers' records must include the circumstances in which the patient first presented to medical care, how, when and where the disclosure was made, who was present at the time of the disclosure, the physical state of the patient (i.e., nervous, calm, shifting in seat, eyes downcast, etc.), and observations of any family members present with the child. Information that may not seem pertinent at the time of the initial interview with the patient may be precisely the detail sought at trial. In addition, there may be a long delay before a trial starts; therefore, without proper documentation, the provider may no longer be able to recall clearly the details of the interview and surrounding circumstances.

It is equally important to document all aspects of medical procedures performed on the child. For instance, if the child discloses sexual abuse and a rape/trauma kit is used, it is crucial to include not only the details of the interview and examination but also to note to whom the kit was given, so that the attorney(s) can trace the chain of custody at trial. Documentation of the proper handling of physical evidence helps to affirm that there has been no tampering with the evidence.

While medical providers are accustomed to speaking and writing in medical shorthand, the average layperson is not accustomed to such language. The testimony of a medical witness/expert can be difficult for the jury to understand. If the medical provider must use technical language, he or she should always define and explain the terms. If the testimony is complicated and/or confusing, ask the attorney to provide visual aids, which can facilitate the jury's understanding and focus their attention on the topic at hand.

BIBLIOGRAPHY

Hanes M, McAuliff T: Preparation for child abuse litigation: perspectives of the prosecutor and the pediatrician. *Pediatr Ann* 1997;26:288–295.

Palusci VJ, Hicks RA, Vandervort FE: "You are hereby commanded to appear": pediatrician subpoena and court appearance in child maltreatment. *Pediatrics* 2001;107:1427–1430.

ABANDONMENT
AND PHYSICAL NEGLECT

Abandonment of infants and small children is the most extreme form of parental neglect. Abandoned children may suffer physical and psychological harm unless there is immediate, appropriate intervention. Other significant forms of neglect include parents failing to meet a child's need for food, clothing, shelter, medical care, education, or supervision. The long-term effects of neglect may be more injurious than those of abuse, since the indolent nature of neglect causes it to be underreported and uncorrected.

Clinical Presentation and Diagnosis

Every abandoned child must undergo a thorough physical examination, with particular attention to a general assessment of the state of hydration, nutrition, body temperature, and hygiene. Undress and examine the child thoroughly for physical stigmata of abuse or neglect.

ED Management

The first priority is to try to locate the parent or another family member known to the child. Then perform the physical examination and obtain appropriate laboratory studies to document any harm resulting from abandonment and to find any treatable conditions.

The next step is to report this form of child neglect to the local CPS and/or police, depending on local child abuse reporting laws and protocols.

Disposition options in the management of an abandoned child include transfer to the custody of a relative who is judged suitable by the CPS worker or placement in a temporary shelter or in foster care. However, if medical care is necessary or if community-based resources do not exist, admit the child to the hospital. In most states, abandoned children who are referred to the local CPS may be legally placed, on a temporary basis, in another home without a court order. Proper court proceedings must follow to justify and continue an emergency placement.

In the ED, a parent who has abandoned a child may be extremely defensive and at times hostile to the ED staff. Do not induce further hostility by raising the levels of parental guilt or fear. Instead, focus on the mutual concern for the child.

For children with neglect short of abandonment, meticulously document the aspects and findings of neglect, consult a social worker, and refer the family to their primary care provider.

Indications for Admission

- Abandoned child who requires medical care
- Abandoned child when community placement resources do not exist

BIBLIOGRAPHY

Reece RM, Ludwig S: *Child Abuse: Medical Diagnosis and Management.* New York: Lippincott Williams & Wilkins, 2001.

DEATH IN
THE EMERGENCY DEPARTMENT

Clinical Presentation

The loss of a child has a devastating effect on a family, particularly when it is unexpected or without any readily identifiable cause. These families do not have the opportunity to experience "preparatory grief." Proper ED management is critical to the family's long-term adjustment.

Diagnosis

When the ED is notified of the transport of a child in extremis, assign a resuscitation team member to work with the parents. Take the parents to a quiet area not far from the resuscitation scene and have a team member shuttle between the two sites to keep the family informed. In some centers parents may be allowed in the resuscitation room, but a staff member who can interpret the events must accompany them.

At the time of the child's death, notify the parents privately, clearly, and directly. Specify the word "dead" to avoid any confusion. Avoid using euphemisms, such as "He has passed." Once the death has been announced, the management phase begins.

ED Management

Family members may display many emotional reactions, from hysterical screaming to anger to silence. All responses are normal. Once the immediate reaction has subsided, be available to answer any questions. There is no need for excuses, although parents may appreciate expressions of personal emotion and concern. Respond to parental expressions of guilt with a realistic appraisal of the circumstances. Gain history that may be helpful in establishing a diagnosis. If abuse is suspected, it will be confirmed at autopsy; there is no need to confront the grieving family.

Provide the family with assistance: phone, coffee, tissues. Do not assume that they want a particular relative or clergyman to be present unless they so request.

Encourage parents to see the child's body once it has been prepared for their viewing (removal of medical equipment, soiled linen, etc.). Allow parents to hold the child's body and say their farewells. A prayer said over the body is a good way to bring closure after a brief period of contact with the child.

Inform the family of any requirements concerning an autopsy. In most states an autopsy is not mandated if the child had a chronic condition in which death was expected. If there are no requirements, encourage autopsy in order to answer any questions pertaining to the cause of death. Instruct a trusted family member or friend about hospital policy on claiming the body and other necessary arrangements.

Give the parents your name and phone number for follow-up questions and concerns and document the chart and death certificate appropriately. Afterward, a brief staff meeting may pull staff members together and allow them to express their feelings.

BIBLIOGRAPHY

Krahn GL: Are there good ways to give bad news? *Pediatrics* 1993;91:578–582.
Leash RM: *Death Notification: A Practical Guide to the Process.* Hinesburg, VT: Upper Access, 1995.
Mandell F, McClain M, Reed RM: Suicide and unexpected death: the pediatrician's response. *Am J Dis Child* 1987;141:1748–1750.

PSYCHIATRIC EMERGENCIES

Although minor behavioral problems are common in pediatrics, true psychiatric emergencies are rare. However, with the relative lack of mental health services for children, the ED is often the portal of entry into the mental health system. The priorities in the ED are assessment of whether patients are dangerous to themselves or others and whether such patients' families can adequately care for their children at home.

Clinical Presentation

Depression   The depressed patient may present with recurrent somatic complaints (stomach aches, headaches, myalgias) for which no organic cause can be found. Sometimes depression can present with acting-out behavior (i.e., running away, stealing, fire-setting, or being accident-prone). Occasionally, the parent may be concerned about a loss of appetite, poor school performance, or a change in the patient's sleep pattern.

Psychosis   The psychotic patient, who cannot distinguish reality from fantasy, may present with a history of hallucinations, extreme variations in mood, and occasionally violent behavior. The adolescent with schizophrenia has delusions, auditory hallucinations, and inappropriate affect, although memory and orientation may remain intact.

Conduct Disorders   The child with a conduct disorder acts out or behaves in an antisocial way. There are many psychodynamic factors in conduct disorder, and often the child will be brought to the ED by police or by parents unable to provide supervision. Although use of drugs or alcohol may exacerbate conduct disorders, deviant or disruptive behavior usually occurs without intoxicants.

Diagnosis and ED Management

Depression   Somatic complaints with no identifiable organic basis or changes in the patient's normal behavior or mood suggest depression. Ask such patients how they are sleeping, whether they enjoy school, and what they do for fun. Ask about a family history of depression and suicide. Have patients name their best friends and tell you when they last were together.

Ask about future plans, hopes, and aspirations. When patients appear to be depressed (loss of interest in school, friends, usual hobbies, sports), ask whether they have ever thought of committing suicide. Far from putting thoughts in their minds, these types of questions may actually help patients to feel better, since they can now discuss something troubling. A patient who has considered suicide must be seen immediately by a psychiatrist or psychologist. If the suicidal ideation has reached the point of actual planning, hospitalization is indicated. Consider whether an organic disorder (*hypothyroidism, anemia*) may be making the patient depressed.

Psychosis   The first step is to rule out an organic origin for the psychosis. The most common organic cause is drug ingestion [lysergic acid diethylamide (*LSD*), phencyclidine (*PCP*), "Ecstasy," *amphetamines, cocaine, anticholinergics*]. Other causes are *hypoglycemia,* increased intracranial pressure (*tumor, brain abscess, arteriovenous malformation*), *temporal lobe seizures, encephalitis, porphyria, uremia,* and *Wilson's disease.*

Ask about possible drug ingestion, and have the family bring in all medications in the home and from the homes of friends or relatives the patient has visited recently. Inquire about a family history of schizophrenia, and try to determine when the symptoms were first noticed. With an organic psychosis, the onset is acute and the hallucinations are often visual, olfactory, tactile, or gustatory rather than auditory. With schizophrenia and other functional psychoses, the hallucinations are typically auditory and the onset is more insidious.

On physical examination, there may be fever (anticholinergic or amphetamine ingestion, brain abscess, encephalitis), tachycardia (sepsis or anticholinergic, hallucinogen, or amphetamine ingestion), and hypertension (anticholinergic, amphetamines, cocaine, LSD, or PCP ingestion). The vital signs may be normal in patients with psychosis of functional origin. Note the pupillary size and reactivity; there may be inequality (mass lesion, brain abscess), mydriasis (hypoglycemia or LSD, amphetamine, cocaine, or anticholinergic ingestion), or miosis (cholinergics, opiate, or PCP ingestion).

Immediately order a CT scan for a patient with any focal neurologic abnormalities, signs of increased intracranial pressure, or fever. A febrile patient requires a lumbar puncture after the CT (if it is normal). Also obtain a CBC, electrolytes, serum glucose, Dextrostix, liver function tests, and urinalysis.

Unless an organic cause for the psychosis can be definitely ruled out in the ED, admit the patient to a pediatric service to continue the evaluation after consultation with a psychiatrist. Do not initiate antipsychotic medications in the ED unless a psychiatrist, who can provide the necessary close follow-up, has examined the patient. If sedation is required for agitation or uncontrolled acting out, use an agent listed in Table 19-3.

Conduct Disorder   In managing a patient with a conduct disorder, the goals are to (1) ensure the safety of the child, family, and staff; (2) rule out medical conditions; and (3) gather information for appropriate disposition.

Table 19-3   Medications for Restraint of Uncontrolled Patients

DRUG	DOSE
Haloperidol (Haldol)	1–10 mg IM q 30 min*
Trifluoperazine (Stelazine)	10–15 mg IM q 30 min*
Thiothixene (Navane)	15–20 mg IM q 30 min*
Risperidone	0.25–0.50 mg PO

*Up to three doses may be given, as needed.

When the child is aggressive, the behavior must be controlled. If a medical condition or an intoxicant may be inducing the behavior, acute hospitalization is indicated. If the aforementioned conditions have been ruled out, psychiatric hospitalization is indicated to promote healthier ways of functioning.

Indications for Admission

- Suicide attempt or gesture
- Depression with concrete suicidal plan
- Depression with inability to function
- Psychotic episode thought to be organic
- Conduct that will harm self or others
- Complications of substance abuse

BIBLIOGRAPHY

Berenson CK: Frequently missed diagnoses in adolescent psychiatry. *Psychiatr Clin North Am* 1998;21:917–926.
Dorfman DH: The use of physical and chemical restraints in the pediatric emergency department. *Pediatr Emerg Care* 2000;16:1–6.
Halamandaris PV, Anderson TR: Children and adolescents in the psychiatric emergency setting. *Psychiatr Clin North Am* 1999;22:865–874.

SUDDEN INFANT DEATH SYNDROME

Sudden infant death syndrome (SIDS) is defined as the sudden death of an infant or young child, unexpected by history, in which a thorough postmortem examination and death scene investigation fails to demonstrate an adequate cause for death. SIDS is the leading cause of death during infancy after the first week of life.

Clinical Presentation

The peak incidence is at 2 to 4 months, although there have been autopsy-proven occurrences up to 12 months of age. The incidence is higher in males and in premature infants and if the mother is a smoker, drug addict, or of lower socioeconomic status. Most cases occur between midnight and 9 A.M. during the cold-weather months. Typically, a previously healthy baby either does not awaken for a morning feed or is found cold and lifeless in the crib.

On occasion, the infant is found pale or cyanotic, apneic, or limp, and resuscitation is initiated at home or en route to the ED. It is not clear whether these near-miss episodes are one end of the spectrum of SIDS.

There have been many theories that attempt to explain the cause of SIDS. Recently, prone positioning of infants during sleep has been strongly implicated. However, no single theory has been able to account for all cases of SIDS.

Diagnosis

The diagnosis of SIDS cannot be confirmed until an autopsy and other postmortem studies have ruled out other possible causes of sudden death in infancy, including *adrenal insufficiency, overwhelming pneumonitis, bacterial sepsis* (especially in sickle cell disease), *child abuse*, and *poisoning*. Near-miss episodes may also result from prolonged *sleep apnea, gastroesophageal reflux–induced apnea, cardiac dysrhythmias, metabolic disorders*, and *seizures*.

ED Management

The management of the SIDS victim requires a detailed history of the circumstances surrounding the infant's death. An autopsy must be performed by the medical examiner. The management of a bereaved family is discussed on pp 558–559.

If the resuscitation of a near-miss victim is successful, admit the infant to an intensive care unit (ICU) for continuous cardiopulmonary monitoring and further evaluation. Obtain an electrocardiogram (ECG) with rhythm strip, chest x-ray, and blood for a CBC with differential, electrolytes, glucose, and culture. Perform a lumbar puncture for cytology, chemistries, and culture and obtain a urinalysis and urine culture.

Indications for Admission

- Near-miss episode

BIBLIOGRAPHY

American Academy of Pediatrics Committee on Child Abuse and Neglect: Distinguishing sudden infant death syndrome from child abuse fatalities. *Pediatrics* 2001;107:437–441.

American Academy of Pediatrics Task Force on Sleep Position and Sudden Infant Death Syndrome: Changing concepts of sudden infant death syndrome: implications for infant sleep environment and sleep position. *Pediatrics* 2000;105: 650–656.

Leach CE, Blair PS, Fleming PJ, et al: Epidemiology and SIDS and explained sudden infant deaths. *Pediatrics* 1999;104:e43.

SUICIDE

Suicide is the third leading cause of death among teenagers, although it also occurs in younger children. Reported rates have steadily increased since the 1960s. Suicide gestures, which are seen more frequently in girls, are perhaps 100 times more common than successful suicides, which occur more often in boys. Girls are more likely to employ nonviolent methods (ingestion), whereas boys more often use violence (firearms, blades). Many suicides go undiagnosed, attributed to accidental trauma.

Clinical Presentation and Diagnosis

Suicide usually occurs in a depressed patient. The attempt is usually triggered by a "crisis" situation, such as the death or departure of a loved one, a fight with a boyfriend or girlfriend, or an argument with a parent. There are a number of danger signals that may signify that a patient is potentially suicidal (Table 19-4).

In the ED, these patients may present as trauma or overdose victims or in a coma of unknown origin. Every child above 6 years of age who takes a medication overdose or ingests a household product (caustics, hydrocarbons, insecticides) is making a suicidal gesture until proven otherwise.

ED Management

The patient's clinical condition and the method of attempted suicide determine the priorities of ED management. However, most patients are well enough to be interviewed when first seen. Assess the seriousness of the attempt; a suicidal patient requires continuous one-on-one nursing. Greater "lethality" of intent is suggested by a previous suicide attempt, a plan to commit suicide, no communication of intent to others, no request for help after the attempt (discovered accidentally), and taking action that is clearly lethal (jumping from a rooftop). Once the patient is medically stable, obtain psychiatric evaluation.

A child psychiatrist must screen every patient making a suicidal gesture or attempt. Hospitalize those with medical complications in a pediatric unit. Admit a patient who is medically stable to a psychiatric unit unless he or she has been cleared by a psychiatrist to be discharged home.

Table 19-4   Findings Suggesting a High Risk of Suicide

Recent previous suicide attempt
Multiple ED visits for trauma
Suicidal threat made
"Accidental" ingestion in a child over 6 years old
Signs of depression
Medical concerns accompanied by depression
Recent withdrawal behavior
Underlying psychiatric condition:
    Psychosis
    Conduct disorder
    Attention deficit disorder
    Substance abuse
    Mental retardation
    Family history of suicide
    Recent cluster of suicides in the community

Follow-up
- Primary care follow-up in 1 week

Indications for Admission
- Suicide attempt that requires medical care
- All other suicide attempts unless cleared for family-based care by a child psychiatrist

BIBLIOGRAPHY

Borowsky IW, Ireland M, Resnick MD: Adolescent suicide attempts: risks and pro-tectors. *Pediatrics* 2001;107:485–493.

Hirschfeld RMA, Russell JM: Current concepts—assessment and treatment of sui-cidal patients. *N Engl J Med* 1997;337:910–915.

Horowitz LM, Wang PS, Koocher GP, et al: Detecting suicide risk in a pediatric emergency department: development of a brief screening tool. *Pediatrics* 2001;107:1133–1137.

MUNCHAUSEN SYNDROME BY PROXY

Munchausen syndrome (MS) was first described in adults who subjected themselves to diagnostic tests and therapeutic procedures in order to gain the safety and security of being hospitalized. Munchausen syndrome by proxy (MSBP) is a subset of the child abuse syndrome in which signs or symptoms of medical illnesses are either feigned by the parent or pro-duced in the child so that the parent and child can be hospitalized. It is therefore an outgrowth of MS in adults. Similar psychopathology occurs in both; the difference is that in MSBP the child is used by the parent as the focus of medical attention.

Clinical Presentation

MSBP has many varied presenting signs and symptoms, including apnea, near-miss SIDS episodes, hematuria, hematochezia, hematemesis, fever, seizures, frequent infections, failure to thrive, hypoglycemia, and poison-ings. Virtually any complaint can be feigned or artificially produced in MSBP. In some series, MSBP has a 10% mortality rate.

Diagnosis

A high index of suspicion is required to diagnose MSBP. Suspect it in any clinical situation that has baffled physicians at other centers or has a "one of a kind" dimension. The identified parental characteristics include a parent (the mother in 90% of cases) who has some medical background, is often by the bedside, appears very devoted, and is invested in the illness. MSBP parents are usually very intelligent, ver-bal, and appealing to the medical staff. Generally, it is the parent who notes the episodic nature of the signs and symptoms. In addition, the parent is usually distant from her spouse, and she may have a history of being a patient herself.

ED Management

MSBP is rarely diagnosed in the ED, as careful observation over time is required. The ED staff should be alert to parents who seem to be frequent, inappropriate ED users or who seem to exaggerate their children's symptoms. If the diagnosis is suspected in the ED, admit the child and notify the child abuse team. Depending on the nature of the MSBP, there are many strategies for proving the diagnosis, including laboratory tests (blood type, insulin level, etc.), blood cultures, covert videotaping of the parent, monitoring devices, and limitation of parental visitation. If the ED staff can make the diagnosis of MSBP by direct observation, report the case to the CPS and place the child in a protected environment.

Indication for Admission

- Suspected victim of MSBP

BIBLIOGRAPHY

Levin AV, Sheridan MS: *Munchausen Syndrome by Proxy: Issues in Diagnosis and Treatment.* New York: Lexington Books, 1995.

Libow JA: Child and adolescent illness falsification. *Pediatrics* 2000;105:336–342.

Meadow R: False allegations of abuse and Munchausen syndrome by proxy. *Arch Dis Child* 1993;68:444–447.

INTERPERSONAL VIOLENCE

Interpersonal violence is an altercation between two or more noncaretaker individuals in which at least one of the participants intends to harm the other. These altercations frequently occur in the school, schoolyard, or street. However, it is not useful to apply the terms *victim* and *perpetrator*, as the "victim" who presents to the ED may have instigated the fight that he or she subsequently "lost." It has recently been reported that as many as 25% of all adolescents seen in a pediatric ED are treated for injuries resulting from interpersonal violence.

In contrast, in family violence, such as child abuse and domestic violence, one individual has significant power over another within the relationship. While most health care systems have protocols for the management of family violence, there is no mandated reporting system for interpersonal violence.

Clinical Presentation and Diagnosis

Violently injured patients present with a wide range of injuries and injury severity. Prior to the interview, assure the patient that all responses are confidential with the exception of suicidal or homicidal statements and the disclosure of child abuse. Let the patient tell the story in his or her own words, in private, and listen nonjudgmentally. After the interview, ask the youth's permission to involve the family in the discussion. Enlisting the help of the family can often facilitate follow-up and ongoing support for the patient.

The responses to a few suitable questions can determine the need for immediate referral to social work, mental health, or law enforcement

Table 19-5   Priorities in the Evaluation of the Violently Injured Patient

CIRCUMSTANCES	SAFETY ISSUES
What caused the event	Retaliation plans by patient, family, friends*
Relationship to the other participants	Suicidal ideation†
Use or appearance of weapons at the scene	Access to weapons
Police involvement	Depression: long-term plans,
Safety issues	presence of family and close friends
Retaliation plans by patient, family, or friend*	

*Require immediate referral to police.
†Requires immediate referral to psychiatry and social work.

(Table 19-5). Clearly document these responses in the medical record. However, the legality of access to the medical record by law enforcement agencies varies among communities. Contact the hospital's legal counsel regarding local statutes and recommendations pertaining to documentation.

A thorough evaluation of the violently injured patient includes a determination of what caused the violent event, the location and time of the event, the relationship of the patient to others involved in the incident, and the use or appearance of weapons at the scene. Explore issues related to the patient's safety. Ask specific questions regarding any intention to hurt self or others. Also inquire if a family member or friend plans to retaliate. Although open-ended questions such as, "Once you leave here, what are you going to do?" can clue a physician into potentially dangerous plans, ask directly about retaliation and suicidal thoughts. Similarly, ask the patient about drug selling and access to weapons. When present, these risk factors may predict the lethality of future actions. Inquire about the patient's friends and acquaintances when asking about substance use and abuse in order to ascertain exposure to this lifestyle. If the youth admits to using marijuana or other drugs, ask why. The patient's responses to these questions may indicate an adolescent who is self-medicating his or her stress, anger, or depression.

Assess the patient's present emotional state and reaction to the trauma. Since there is a strong correlation between depression and the risk of violent injury, ask about the patient's long-term plans for the future and the presence or absence of close friends or family members as confidants and allies.

ED Management

The primary goals of ED care of a violently injured youth are to stabilize the patient, ensure the immediate safety of the patient and other participants, and to assess the patient's risk for further injury. If the patient reveals suicidal or homicidal intent, contact a psychiatrist immediately.

Also, the medical staff is obligated to contact the police if there are legitimate concerns about retaliation.

It is also important to assess and address the psychosocial comorbidities, including depression, substance abuse, school failure, and family violence. Refer a depressed or hopeless patient to a psychiatrist urgently. However, provide psychosocial support to all violently injured patients, regardless of the situation that caused the injury. Consult a social worker, who can help provide access to available community resources. Give contact information for appropriate crisis hot lines, community support groups, and available local shelters. Information about these resources is often also available from municipal social service agencies.

If the patient is being admitted, communicate any safety concerns to the inpatient medical and nursing staff, security officers, and social workers. One-on-one observation is necessary for suicidal or homicidal patients.

Follow-up

- Primary care follow-up in 1 week

Indication for Admission

- Homicidal or suicidal ideation

BIBLIOGRAPHY

American Academy of Pediatrics Task Force on Adolescent Assault Victims Needs: Adolescent assault victims needs: a review of issues and a model protocol. *Pediatrics* 1996;98:991–1001.

Fein JA, Mollen CJ: Interpersonal violence. *Curr Opin Pediatr* 1999;11:588–593.

Ginsburg KR: Guiding adolescents away from violence. *Contemp Pediatr* 1997;14: 101–111.

CHAPTER 20

Pulmonary Emergencies

Carolyn Kercsmar
  • Sandra J. Cunningham (contributor—Pulse Oximetry)

ASTHMA

Asthma is defined as recurrent, reversible lower airway obstruction. More than 10% of children are affected, and despite recent therapeutic advances, morbidity continues to be substantial, especially among inner-city residents.

Inflammation contributes to airway edema, abnormal mucociliary clearance, and mucous plugging. The pathophysiology of the airway edema is multifactorial. Release of mediators (e.g., histamine, leukotrienes) from mast cells resident in the airways may initiate the process. Other cells, such as eosinophils, lymphocytes, and neutrophils, are recruited into the airways and also release proinflammatory mediators such as major basic protein, elastase, and cytokines. In addition, neuropeptides (e.g., substance P) may enhance the airway inflammation and bronchial smooth muscle hyperreactivity.

Common triggers include irritants (cigarette smoke, gases), viral infections, weather changes, allergens (dust, animals), exercise, cold air, and emotional stress. Children with a history of bronchopulmonary dysplasia (BPD) or other acute lung injury (smoke inhalation, hydrocarbon ingestion, near-drowning) are at increased risk for hyperreactive airways or asthma. The greatest risk of mortality is in children who have a history of respiratory failure or hypoxic seizures, are undertreated (at home or after a medical visit), or delay seeking medical attention.

Clinical Presentation

Acute asthma presents with dyspnea, cough, expiratory wheezing, and, to a lesser extent, inspiratory wheezing. Children with cough-variant asthma have recurrent episodes of dry or productive cough and little or no wheezing. Airway obstruction can lead to retractions and decreased air entry, with little or no audible wheezing. Tachycardia, tachypnea, and, in severe attacks, cyanosis may be present; altered mental status (agitation, lethargy) occurs with impending ventilatory failure. Findings of an upper respiratory infection (URI) are also often present.

Complications   Atelectasis is common. Other respiratory complications are pneumomediastinum, which requires no specific treatment, and, rarely, pneumothorax, which may be under tension and require immediate evacuation. Respiratory failure may occur suddenly from the collapse of large airways or from exhaustion.

Diagnosis

A trial of an inhaled beta$_2$ agonist may simultaneously confirm the diagnosis and provide clinical relief. Relief of airway obstruction occurs in less than 15 min (often <5 min), and peak flow improves by more than 20% from baseline (often >50%). Less improvement may occur with severe or prolonged episodes associated with more inflammation, leaving the diagnosis uncertain unless the patient has a history of previous wheezing episodes. Laboratory studies do not help in establishing the diagnosis of asthma, and chest x-rays are not necessary for most first episodes of wheezing. A chest x-ray may be indicated in the setting of localized posttreatment findings in association with significant tachypnea (rate >60/min in infants, >40/min in older children) or persistent tachycardia (rate >160/min) 20 to 30 min after the completion of a beta$_2$-agonist treatment in an afebrile child.

Inquire about a history of prematurity, mechanical ventilation, BPD, previous wheezing episodes, or heart disease. Check for a family history of asthma, recurrent bronchitis, eczema, allergic rhinitis, or other allergies.

Consider the possibility of complicating factors or a diagnosis other than asthma if a child or infant has protracted (>3 days), recurrent, or persistent localized wheezing in the face of adequate therapy for asthma. The differential diagnosis includes *upper airway obstruction* (pp 587–588) which presents with inspiratory stridor and drooling (*foreign body, retropharyngeal abscess*) or barking cough (*croup*), and *foreign body,* which is often associated with a history of aspiration and localized wheezing. A chest x-ray may reveal a radiopaque object, or inspiratory and expiratory films (bilateral decubitus films in children <3 years) may reveal differential hyperinflation. Air trapping on the obstructed side can be appreciated during expiration or when the affected side is dependent on decubitus views. Other conditions include infection due to *Mycoplasma pneumoniae* or *bronchiolitis* (pp 575–578), which cause wheezy illness in school-age children and infants, respectively. With mycoplasmal pneumonia, there may be patchy or diffuse interstitial infiltrates on chest radiograph, and cold agglutinins are positive in 50% of patients, although mycoplasmal titers are more specific. Adenovirus, influenza virus, and parainfluenza virus may also cause wheezy illnesses. Consider also tracheal or airway compression due to *congenital vascular rings* and *tracheo-* or *bronchomalacia.* These conditions may cause wheezing with variable degrees of reversibility. *Mediastinal masses* such as *lymphoma,* though rare, may also cause wheezing. *Bronchiectasis* is most commonly seen in *cystic fibrosis,* but other illnesses may induce chronic changes in small airways (*immune deficiency, chronic aspiration, tracheoesophageal fistula, gastroesophageal reflux, alpha$_1$-antitrypsin deficiency*). Children with cystic fibrosis generally have other findings, including malabsorption (85%), excessive salt loss, and failure to thrive. *Gastroesophageal reflux* typically presents in infancy and is associated with wheezing and night-time cough frequently unresponsive to bronchodilator therapy. Cardiac asthma may occur in children with *congestive heart failure* due to *left-to-right shunts, anomalous pulmonary venous return, or mitral stenosis* (cor triatriatum), but other features on the physical examination (tachycardia, murmur, hepatosplenomegaly) or chest x-ray (cardiomegaly, congestion) suggest the etiology.

ED Management

Acute Treatment

Rapidly assess the airway and breathing, measure the peak flow in all children over 5 to 6 years of age, and determine whether the patient has mild, moderate, or severe asthma (Table 20-1). Provide supplemental oxygen (40% by mask) to a patient with mild or moderate wheezing; use 100% oxygen if the attack is severe. The supplemental oxygen is important for treating hypoxemia; some patients may have an initial drop in Po_2 during beta$_2$-agonist therapy due to ventilation/perfusion mismatch, particularly if the aerosol is administered with room air rather than oxygen. Monitor a severely ill patient with pulse oximetry and consider obtaining an arterial blood gas (ABG) if the breath sounds are minimal and do not improve within 5 to 10 min following the initial therapy.

Inhaled βeta$_2$ Agonists   First-line treatment is an inhaled nebulized beta$_2$ agonist, such as albuterol 0.5%, 0.03 mL/kg (maximum 1.0 mL) in 3 mL of normal saline (NS). Administer the albuterol via either a snug-fitting face mask or mouthpiece, with oxygen (maximum flow rate 6 L/min), over 5 to 10 min. Levalbuterol, 0.63 mg/3 mL, may have less adverse effect. The efficacy of albuterol is comparable to that of epinephrine, but with fewer side effects and no painful injection. Onset of action is within 5 min, and duration is 4 to 6 h. In severe cases, repeat doses may be given continuously over 1 h, but frequent evaluations are essential. With mild or

Table 20-1   Classification of Severity of Asthma Attacks

	MILD	MODERATE	SEVERE
Symptoms	Cough, wheeze	Dyspnea, vomiting	+ Distress
Signs	None → wheeze Hyperinflation	+ Retractions ↓ Air entry	+ Pallor ↓ Sensorium
Chest X-ray	Mild hyperinflation ↑ Peribronchial markings	↑ Hyperinflation Variable atelectasis	↑↑Hyperinflation Variable pneumothorax/ mediastinum
Peak Flow	Normal to ↓	30–60% of predicted	<30% of predicted

moderate attacks, give the treatments every 20 to 30 min until no further improvement is noted in peak flow, oxygen saturation, or respiratory rate. Alternatively, give albuterol with a metered-dose inhaler (MDI) attached to a holding chamber or spacer device (e.g., InspirEase or Aerochamber) to a cooperative patient above 3 years of age. Administer 2 to 6 puffs every 20 min for 1 hour.

Subcutaneous Epinephrine and Terbutaline   Give a dose of subcutaneous epinephrine or terbutaline for severe attacks (peak flow <15% predicted or nearly absent breath sounds) when aerosolized medication may not reach the target small airways. For epinephrine, the dose is 0.01 mL/kg (0.3 mL maximum) of the 1:1000 preparation; for terbutaline, use 0.01 mL/kg (0.25 mL maximum). It is no longer recommended to give up to three repeated injections. Common side effects of epinephrine injection include nausea, palpitations, tachycardia, agitation, tremor, and, less frequently, hypertension and ventricular dysrhythmias. Terbutaline may cause less nausea and vomiting. Simultaneously begin treatment with a nebulized beta$_2$ agonist.

Corticosteroids   Promptly give an oral dose of a corticosteroid if the patient meets any of the following criteria: requires two or more treatments with a beta$_2$ agonist aerosol, has an oxygen saturation <93% on any assessment, chronically uses (daily or every other day) oral corticosteroids, has had an ED visit within the past 2 weeks, has had a past admission to an ICU, has been hospitalized within the past 2 weeks, or has had three or more hospitalizations during the past year. Use prednisone or prednisolone, 1 to 2 mg/kg (60 mg maximum) or dexamethasone 0.2 mg/kg (6 mg maximum). If the patient cannot tolerate oral medication, give IM dexamethasone (same dose as above).

For a patient with impending respiratory failure, give a bolus of IV methylprednisolone (2 mg/kg, 125 mg maximum), followed by 1 mg/kg q 6 h.

Ipratropium Bromide   Ipratropium bromide is a quaternary ammonium congener of atropine. Anticholinergic agents produce bronchodilation by antagonizing the activity of acetylcholine at the level of its receptors, particularly those found on airway smooth muscle. Compared to inhaled beta agonists, the effect on airway obstruction is modest and generally results in approximately a 10% improvement in FEV_1. Some asthmatics with severe airway obstruction may respond better to a combination of inhaled albuterol and ipratropium than to albuterol alone. Dilute albuterol (0.03 mL/kg) in a vial of ipratropium (250 μg <12 years of age; 500 μg >12 years of age). Give three consecutive ipratropium-albuterol inhalations to a patient whose asthma score or peak expiratory flow rate (PEFR) fails to improve after the initial albuterol treatment. The onset of action of ipratropium is relatively slow (20 min), and the peak effect occurs at about 60 min. Ipratropium, unlike atropine, is poorly absorbed across mucous membranes and has little toxicity at the recommended dose. In particular, it does not inhibit mucociliary clearance. However, there are infrequent reports of paradoxical bronchoconstriction with the administration of anticholinergic agents to some asthmatics. Monitor the patient carefully and stop the nebulization if there are any signs or symptoms of worsening asthma.

Magnesium Sulfate   The IV administration of magnesium sulfate may be useful for a patient whose condition worsens or fails to improve significantly (peak flow increases <50% from presentation and is <60% of predicted, intercostal retractions persist, or oxygen saturation is <93%) after administration of beta agonists and systemic corticosteroids. Mechanisms of action include inhibition of calcium channels in airway smooth muscle, blockade of calcium-mediated muscle contraction, reduction in acetylcholine release from neuromuscular end plates, parasympathetic-induced airway smooth muscle constriction, and inhibition of histamine-induced bronchospasm. The dose is 40 mg/kg (3 g maximum) in 50 mL of NS administered IV over 30 min. Side effects include hypotension, mild sedation, and cutaneous flushing. Do not use magnesium in a patient with significant hypotension or renal failure. Monitor the blood pressure every 10 min during the infusion and every 30 min thereafter for 4 h, but do not stop the infusion for mild reductions in blood pressure in the absence of hypotensive symptoms.

Hydration   Encourage oral fluids and provide IV hydration if the patient is seriously ill. However, limit IV hydration to maintenance plus replacement of ongoing losses. Assess the hydration status, obtain blood for electrolytes when placing the IV line, and monitor for the syndrome of inappropriate ADH excess (pp 169–170) in a patient with severe asthma (absent or minimal breath sounds, PEFR <15% of expected) who has been vomiting or drinking poorly.

Cromolyn Sodium   Cromolyn stabilizes mast cells and frequently helps prevent episodes of bronchospasm in patients with mild asthma, but it has no role in the treatment of an acute exacerbation. If the patient is already taking cromolyn, continue its use at home following treatment of an acute exacerbation; however, do not initiate it after ED treatment. The dose is 1 ampule via nebulizer q 6 h.

Intravenous Terbutaline   Although IV administration of beta agonists may not offer any significant advantage over continuously administered aerosols, consider IV terbutaline for a patient with impending respiratory failure as manifest by continued poor air exchange, central nervous system (CNS) depression, or rising Pco_2 (>50 mmHg with pH <7.3). A terbutaline infusion requires frequent ABGs as well as either continuous intraarterial or noninvasive blood pressure measurement. Start with 0.4 μg/kg/min, and increase by 0.1 to 0.2 μg/kg every 15 min until a clinical response is achieved (improved air entry or 10% reduction in Pco_2) or there is a serious complication (hypotension).

Mechanical Ventilation   If the above-described therapy fails to achieve adequate oxygenation, endotracheal intubation and mechanical ventilation are necessary. Use ketamine (1–2 mg/kg) to provide sedation and broncho-dilation. In general, use smaller tidal volumes than average (6–8 mL/kg instead of the standard 10 mL/kg) on a volume-preset ventilator, with respiratory rates normal to somewhat lower than normal for age, and long expiratory times. The required inspiratory pressures can exceed 50 to 60 cm. Assess breath sounds and obtain an ABG. Permissive hypercapnia may lessen the risk of barotrauma; limit the goal of mechanical ventilation to incomplete correction of the respiratory acidosis ($PCO_2 \geq 50–60$ mgHg). An intubated asthmatic patient will usually require a sedative (midazolam 0.1–0.3 mg/kg IV q 1–2 h, 5 mg maximum) and a neuromuscular relaxant (vecuronium 0.05–0.1 mg/kg IV q 1–2 h, 10 mg maximum) to minimize barotrauma.

Aminophylline   Aminophylline (85% theophylline) is a potent bron-chodilator, but it adds little to the effects of inhaled beta$_2$ agonists during an acute episode. Since frequent or continuous beta$_2$ agonist aerosol ther-apy is as effective, with fewer side effects, IV aminophylline is not indi-cated in the ED treatment of status asthmaticus. Aminophylline is now a second- or third-line drug because the clearance varies with age, the ther-apeutic window is narrow, and other, more effective and safer medications are available.

Discharge Management
A patient with acute asthma can be discharged home when the peak flow is >60 to 70% predicted for height, the oxygen saturation is >92% in room air, wheezing is minimal, and there are no signs of significant obstruction (retractions, tachypnea, decreased air entry). Ensure that the parent can give the medications confidently, monitor the child frequently, and return to the ED if necessary. Ongoing bronchodilator therapy is usually neces-sary for 2 weeks. Review all medications for home use with the parent and child and have the patient demonstrate proper use of the MDI (if one was prescribed). Be sure that the family has a written action plan for worsening symptoms and a follow-up appointment within a few days of the ED visit.

Beta$_2$ Agonist   Inhaled beta$_2$ agonists are preferred for all patients with documented asthma and are first-line therapy, sometimes as single-drug therapy, but more commonly in combination with steroids. An older child (>3 years) can use an MDI or an inhaler with a spacer (Aerochamber, InspirEase); an infant or younger child can use an MDI attached to a spacer with a face mask. For an inhaler (with or without spacer), use 2 puffs q 6 to 8 h of albuterol. For a nebulizer, use albuterol 0.5% (0.5–1.0 mL) or leval-buterol (0.63 mg) in 3 mL of NS given over 5 to 10 min. The oral prepara-tions have fair efficacy for young infants, but adverse effects (irritability) are common; therefore, oral beta$_2$ agonists are not recommended.

Corticosteroids   Give oral steroids if the patient required two or more acute albuterol treatments. In addition, prescribe steroids for a patient who has required acute therapy twice (or more) within 24 h or three times in the past week. Avoid steroids in a child who has been exposed to viruses in the herpes family (especially *varicella*). Give oral prednisone or methyl-prednisolone (2 mg/kg/day, 60 mg maximum qd or divided bid, half-life 12–36 h) for 5 days. Oral dexamethasone (0.6 mg/kg qd, 16 mg maximum, half-life 36–72 h) for 2 days is an alternative. Subtract the ED dose from the total to determine the number of days of home therapy required.

Follow-up

- Mild to moderate first wheezing episode >1 year of age, new or altered medications or steroids prescribed: primary care follow-up in 48 to 72 h

Indications for Admission

- Status asthmaticus: continued moderate or severe wheezing or other evidence of significant airway obstruction after therapy with nebulized beta$_2$ agonists or subcutaneous epinephrine, ipratropium, corticosteroids, or any wheezing after IV magnesium sulfate
- Repeated ED visits over several days when therapy is maximal or adherence uncertain
- Persistent tachypnea, inability to tolerate fluids or medications, altered mental status
- Hypercapnia: PCO_2>40 mmHg
- Hypoxemia: PO_2<60 mmHg or oxygen saturation <93% in room air despite aggressive therapy
- Pneumothorax, pneumomediastinum, or significant atelectasis

BIBLIOGRAPHY

Busse WW, Lemanske RF. Advances in immunology: Asthma. *N Engl J Med* 2001;344:350–362.

Chou KJ, Cunningham SJ, Crain EF: Metered-dose inhalers with spacers vs nebulizers for pediatric asthma. *Arch Pediatr Adolesc Med* 1995;149:201–205.

Ciarello L, Brousseau D, Reinert S: Higher-dose intravenous magnesium therapy for children with moderate to severe acute asthma. *Arch Pediatr Adolesc Med* 2000;154:979–983.

Quershi F, Zaritsky A, Poirer MP: Comparative efficacy of oral dexamethasone versus oral prednisone in acute pediatric asthma. *J Pediatr* 2001;139:20–26.

Smith SR, Strunk RC: Acute asthma in the pediatric emergency department. *Pediatr Clin North Am* 1999;46:1145–1165.

BRONCHIOLITIS

Bronchiolitis is the most common wheezing-associated respiratory illness in children below 2 years of age. Epidemics in the winter to early spring are most frequently caused by respiratory syncytial virus (RSV). Other etiologies are parainfluenza, influenza, and adenovirus, *Mycoplasma pneumoniae, Bordetella pertussis, Chlamydia pneumoniae*, and *Ureaplasma urealyticum*.

Clinical Presentation

Typically, there is a prodromal URI with rhinorrhea and coryza, followed by cough, audible wheezing, and varying degrees of respiratory distress.

An infant with severe disease has tachypnea (>50/min), subcostal and intercostal retractions, poor feeding, nasal flaring, and grunting. In all cases, symptoms are likely to be most prominent at night. An associated otitis media is present in more than 50% of cases, but fever is variable and usually of low grade. Although wheezing is the typical auscultatory finding, rhonchi and coarse rales may also be heard. In most patients, the condition worsens for 3 to 4 days and then rapidly resolves, although some patients may have a persistent cough for weeks afterward. Neonates and young infants may present with apnea and a sepsis-like picture.

Diagnosis

Acute wheezing, cough, and respiratory distress in a young infant are most often secondary to bronchiolitis.

Asthma   Asthma (reactive airway disease) can produce a clinical picture with wheezing that is indistinguishable from bronchiolitis. Some infants with a first RSV exposure may already manifest hyperreactive airways. Consider asthma if the patient has had previous episodes of wheezing that were responsive to bronchodilators, a history of bronchopulmonary dysplasia, eczema, or a family history of asthma or atopic disease.

Foreign-Body Aspiration   An infant (typically over 6 months of age) with an aspirated foreign body may present with wheezing after a coughing or choking episode. There is no URI prodrome. Unless there is acute infection distal to the foreign body, there is usually no fever. Auscultatory findings are often localized. An *esophageal foreign body* can impinge on the trachea and also cause respiratory distress.

Congenital Malformations   These conditions can cause airway obstruction and wheezing, which are exacerbated by a URI. Consider *congenital lobar emphysema* and *intrapulmonary cysts (bronchogenic* or *cystadenomatoid malformation)* when the wheezing is unilateral or localized. The chest x-ray is often diagnostic. With *tracheomalacia*, stridor from inspiratory collapse of a floppy trachea predominates over expiratory wheezing. Wheezing from a *vascular ring* is typically loudest over the trachea and midlung fields.

Cardiac Disease   Patients with *mitral stenosis* or obstruction (*cor triatriatum*) or myocardial dysfunction from other causes can occasionally present with pulmonary edema, which can mimic bronchiolitis. Usually there is significant tachycardia and a gallop, and cardiomegaly is seen on chest x-ray.

Gastroesophageal Reflux   The patient with gastroesophageal reflux (GER) presents with nighttime cough and wheeze typically unresponsive to bronchodilator therapy. There may be associated gagging with feeding or dysphagia, and, in some infants, intermittent or frequent episodes of apnea.

ED Management

Inquire about a history of wheezing, prematurity, or mechanical ventilation (BPD) and check for a family history of asthma or allergies. Perform the examination with the infant undressed from the waist up and sitting on the parent's lap. Obtain an accurate respiratory rate, note any signs of respiratory distress (flaring, grunting, retractions, cyanosis) or heart disease (murmur, hepatosplenomegaly), and assess the child's activity level and ability to drink.

Respiratory Rate >60/Min or Signs of Respiratory Distress   Check the oxygen saturation in room air by pulse oximetry and give supplemental oxygen. Suction the nares if necessary. Give a trial dose of nebulized epinephrine (1:1000, 0.5 mL/kg, 2.5 mL maximum, in 3 mL NS) or albuterol (0.5%, 0.25 mL in 3 mL NS) over 5 to 10 min. Occasional side effects in young infants include tachycardia and irritability. Assess the effectiveness of therapy by reevaluating the respiratory rate, signs of respiratory distress, and oxygen saturation. If there is no substantial improvement, admit the patient. If the respiratory rate slows to 40 to 60/min and the patient is not in distress, he or she may be discharged with a trial of a nebulized beta$_2$ agonist (see below) provided that oral intake is adequate and daily follow-up can be arranged. Oral corticosteroids are unlikely to be helpful except in patients with a past history of wheezing.

Respiratory Rate 40 to 60/Min   Supportive therapy (fluids, acetaminophen as necessary) is all that is needed if the infant is alert, is tolerating fluids well, and shows no signs of distress. Close follow-up is warranted. A trial of inhaled albuterol, via MDI and a spacer with a face mask (2 puffs q 4–6 h) may be useful if the child required mechanical ventilation as a newborn, has BPD or a family history of asthma or allergies, or improved following acute bronchodilator therapy in the ED. Oral theophylline has not been proven to be beneficial for patients with bronchiolitis.

Provide supplemental oxygen (usually 30–40% by oxygen hood or nasal prongs) to a hypoxic patient to maintain an oxygen saturation >95% or a PO$_2$ >85 mmHg. Start an IV and give maintenance fluids with D$_5$½ NS unless the patient is dehydrated (see pp 201–204). If the patient responded to nebulized albuterol, continue the nebulizations every 4 to 6 h, although albuterol can be administered as often as every hour if there is documented improvement and the patient is carefully monitored. If the patient did not respond to albuterol, give nebulized epinephrine, 0.5 mL/kg of 1:1000 (max 2.5 mL) in 3 mL NS every 4 to 6 h. Clinical deterioration, with persistent hypoxemia, elevation of PCO$_2$, or the development of acidosis may portend exhaustion and respiratory failure requiring mechanical ventilation.

Chest radiographs are not routinely indicated in patients with bronchiolitis. In general, obtain a chest x-ray if the infant has known underlying pulmonary or heart disease or does not respond to aggressive inpatient management.

Follow-up

- Persistent tachypnea (>60/min), difficulty feeding: return at once
- All infants in 24 h for reevaluation of feeding, respiratory effort, weight

Indications for Admission

- Respiratory rate >70/min after maximal ED therapy, regardless of clinical appearance
- Respiratory rate >50/min with lethargy or poor oral intake
- Infant below 3 months of age with a respiratory rate >60/min after maximal ED therapy
- Respiratory distress, oxygen saturation <93% or Po_2<65 mmHg in room air, or normal-to-elevated Pco_2 (>40 mmHg) in infant >6 months; O_2 sat <95% in infant <2 months
- Infant with congenital heart disease, chronic lung disease, or immunodeficiency (at risk for complications of RSV infection) in the progressive stage (first day or two) of the illness
- Parents uncomfortable with the severity of illness or with limited resources at home (especially if the infant is below 3 months of age)

BIBLIOGRAPHY

Bertrand P, Aranibar H, Castro E, Sanchez I: Efficacy of nebulized epinephrine versus salbutamol in hospitalized infants with bronchiolitis. *Pediatr Pulmonol* 2001;31:284–288.

Garrison MM, Chistakis DA, Harvey E, et al: Systemic corticosteroids in infant bronchiolitis: a meta-analysis. *Pediatrics* 2000;105:e44.

Klassen TP: Recent advances in the treatment of bronchiolitis and laryngitis. *Pediatr Clin North Am* 1997;44:249–261.

COUGH

Cough is a very common symptom that is most often caused by a minor URI. However, a cough may also signal a more serious problem, such as pneumonia, asthma, or congestive heart failure. A thorough clinical evaluation is necessary before assuming that the patient just has "a cold."

Clinical Presentation and Diagnosis

The clinical presentation varies, depending on the etiology (Table 20-2). Usually these cases can be differentiated with a careful history and physical examination, with only the occasional need for laboratory tests. Three features of a cough that help determine the cause are its *quality*, *timing*, and whether it is *productive of sputum*.

Quality   Quality refers to both the sound and pattern of the coughing episodes; it is best ascertained from hearing the cough rather than relying on the history. Coughs are often described as "wet" or "dry"; however, these descriptions may not be useful. A barking cough suggests *croup*, and a loud, honking cough is often associated with a *psychogenic cough*. Paroxysmal episodes (a series of coughs with no breathing between

Table 20–2 Differential Diagnosis of Cough

ANATOMIC SITE	EMERGENT/ POTENTIALLY EMERGENT	COMMON/ OTHER
Upper Airway	Croup (severe) Foreign-body aspiration Pertussis Aspiration Congenital anomalies (transesophageal fistula, etc.) Laryngeal edema	Upper respiratory infection Pharyngitis Sinusitis Noxious fumes Tracheal compression Gastroesophageal reflux
Lower Airway	Asthma Bronchiolitis Pneumonia Anaphylaxis Congestive heart failure	Foreign-body aspiration Cystic fibrosis Pulmonary hemosiderosis
Nonrespiratory	Impaired gag reflex	Aural foreign body Psychogenic cough Diaphragmatic irritation Phrenic or vagus nerve irritation

them), especially when followed by apnea, cyanosis, or a whoop, are consistent with a *pertussis syndrome*. A staccato cough (a series of coughs with short breaths between them) suggests an "afebrile pneumonia" (*Chlamydia, Mycoplasma*).

Timing   Cough that is related to feeds and includes either choking or emesis suggests *aspiration*. The possible causes include *GER* (cough may be the only symptom), mechanical abnormalities (*tracheoesophageal fistula*), and *neurologic abnormalities*. Night cough is consistent with *asthma, sinusitis, postnasal drip, GER*, and *croup*; an early-morning cough suggests a *suppurative process*. Seasonal cough, exercise-related cough, and cold air–related cough occur with *reactive airway disease*. Finally, "schoolday-only cough" suggests a *psychogenic* origin.

The patient's age suggests different causes. During infancy, consider *congenital anomalies, pertussis, bronchiolitis, chlamydial infection*, and *pulmonary edema* (usually cardiogenic). Cough during the first 2 months of life is more probably related to serious pathology than at any other age. Consider *foreign-body aspiration* in toddlers and older children. Among adolescents, consider *smoking* and *mediastinal masses*.

Sputum Production   Productivity is difficult to judge, as children tend to swallow sputum. Green sputum reflects leukocyte breakdown and not necessarily a bacterial process. Blood-streaked sputum suggests *pneumo-*

coccal pneumonia. Hemoptysis may reflect *foreign-body aspiration,* a chronic suppurative process (*cystic fibrosis*), *tuberculosis,* and, more rarely, *pulmonary hemosiderosis.*

Physical findings help localize the origin to a specific part of the respiratory tract. Pharyngitis, otitis media, rhinorrhea, swollen turbinates, sinus tenderness, snoring, and stridor are consistent with upper airway disease. Wheezing, rales, rhonchi, and decreased breath sounds occur with lower respiratory tract pathology. Also look for signs of *congestive heart failure* (gallop, hepatomegaly, jugular vein distention) and *diaphragmatic irritation* (right- or left-upper-quadrant tenderness).

ED Management

The priority is prompt recognition and treatment of respiratory distress and emergent conditions. Assess oxygenation and perfusion and initiate appropriate resuscitation, if necessary. Look for signs of upper airway obstruction, assess the patient's preferred position of breathing, and listen carefully for stridor (place the stethoscope on the side of the neck). If there are any signs of obstruction, maintain the patient in the position of maximal airway opening (see pp 4–5). If oxygenation and perfusion are not compromised, consider the potentially emergent and most common causes for each age group (Table 20-2). If the history and physical examination are not conclusive, obtain a chest x-ray and room-air pulse oximetry to screen for serious pathology.

Infants Below 2 Months of Age   Rule out serious pathology, as this age group is at relatively high risk for apnea. Serious etiologies include pneumonia, bronchiolitis, and pulmonary edema (cardiogenic and noncardiogenic). Potential emergencies include pertussis, chlamydial and other afebrile pneumonias (*Ureaplasma* and *Mycoplasma*), bronchiolitis, aspiration, and congenital mechanical obstruction. Measure the oxygen saturation, and obtain a chest x-ray and CBC looking for lymphocytosis (pertussis) or eosinophilia (chlamydial pneumonia).

URIs and GER are common nonemergent causes. Treat a URI with NS nose drops, but avoid neosynephrine nose drops, which may cause dysrhythmias (SVT) and rebound congestion. For reflux, consider obtaining an immediate upper GI series if there is associated apnea. Otherwise, further workup can be deferred to the outpatient setting.

Older Infants and Children   Emergent etiologies include pneumonia, reactive airway disease (bronchiolitis/asthma), and pulmonary edema. Upper airway obstruction in this age group is usually related to foreign-body aspiration or laryngeal edema (croup).

Common causes in this age group include asthma, sinusitis, postnasal drip, and GER. Asthma may have no corroborating physical findings, and the peak flow may be normal. If the history is suggestive (night cough, family history of atopy, other atopic symptoms, exercise-induced cough), a diagnostic/therapeutic trial of bronchodilators is warranted (pp 570–571). If the history and physical examination suggest sinusitis (rhinorrhea for more than 10 consecutive days, periorbital swelling, halitosis, swollen turbinates), treat with a 14-day course of antibiotics (pp 139–140). Finally, postnasal drip may cause a persistent cough. If sleep is disturbed, recommend a trial of an oral antihistamine such as chlorpheniramine (2–6 years: 1 mg per dose q 4–6 h, 4 mg/day maximum; 6–12 years: 2 mg per dose q 4–6 h, 12 mg/day maximum). Do not use sustained-release products in children under 6 years of age.

Since GER can cause persistent cough, despite the absence of GI symptoms, suspect it when systematic investigation for other common causes of cough are negative. Although a 24-h esophageal pH monitoring study can confirm the diagnosis, first assess the response to an empiric trial of antireflux medication (ranitidine, 4–5 mg/kg/day divided bid).

Older Children and Adolescents   ED management is similar to the approach outlined above. Emergency resuscitation and upper airway clearance are the priorities. Common causes are similar to those in younger children. If a patient presents with persistent symptoms, obtain a chest x-ray (mediastinal mass) and check for a history of exposure to tuberculosis.

Finally, treat the cause of the cough and not the cough itself. Consider cough suppression only when the cause is known and the cough severely impairs the patient's daily life (sleep deprivation, not permitted in school). In such cases, try a cough suppressant with 100% dextromethorphan or codeine (0.5 mg/kg q hs, 15–30 mg per dose; maximum 30 mg).

Follow-up

- Patient with chronic cough (>2 weeks): refer to primary care provider
- Bronchiolitis, croup, pneumonia <6 months old: 24h for reevaluation of feeding, respiratory effort, weight

Indications for Admission

- Respiratory distress or patient requires oxygen
- Pertussis (infant <6 months old)
- Bronchiolitis or chlamydial pneumonia in an infant <2 months (risk of apnea) if RR >60 or oxygen saturation <95%
- Interstitial pneumonia (infant <2 months)
- Lobar pneumonia (infant <6 months)
- Pulmonary edema
- Foreign-body aspiration
- Persistent upper airway obstruction from any cause
- Laryngeal edema
- Croup with significant upper airway obstruction and stridor at rest

BIBLIOGRAPHY

Chang AB, Asher MI: A review of cough in children. *J Asthma* 2001;38:299–309.
Irwin RS, Boulet LP, Cloutier MM, et al: Managing cough as a defense mechanism and as a symptom. A consensus panel report of the American College of Chest Physicians. *Chest* 1998;114(s):133–181.

Padman R: The child with persistent cough. *Del Med J* 2001;73:149–156.

CROUP

Laryngotracheobronchitis, or croup, is an acute subglottic inflammatory process, generally caused by parainfluenza virus types 1 and 3 during the late fall and early winter months. Other causes are influenza viruses A and B, measles, *M. pneumoniae*, and respiratory syncytial virus. Croup primarily occurs between 6 months and 3 years of age, but morbidity is greatest in the first year of life, when the subglottic airway is relatively narrow. Although exhaustion may lead to obstruction of the airway by mucus, death is infrequent.

Spasmodic croup is probably an allergic disease that occurs mainly in patients with a personal or family history of asthma and allergies.

Clinical Presentation

Croup causes varying degrees of acute upper airway obstruction. Clinically, this presents with inspiratory stridor, suprasternal retractions, tachypnea, and tachycardia. The illness usually begins with low-grade fever and rhinorrhea, followed by hoarseness and a barking, "seal-like" cough. The amount of stridor is highly variable, but with increasing obstruction there are suprasternal and intercostal retractions, decreased air entry, and increased work of breathing. The illness lasts 3 to 5 days, with the second or third day marking the peak of clinical symptoms. High fever, dysphagia, and drooling are usually absent. Exhaustion and respiratory failure ensue in a small number of cases (<2%). Patients with pre-existing upper airway problems (congenital or acquired subglottic stenosis, webs, tracheomalacia, choanal narrowing, micrognathia, macroglossia) are at particular risk.

Spasmodic croup presents in the middle of the night with the sudden onset of loud stridor and croupy cough, which resolve quickly and often improve with cool mist. There is little or no viral prodrome, and dysphagia, drooling, high fever, and toxicity are notably absent. The croup may recur on successive nights, and recurrent episodes are common. Some children have recurrent croup-like illnesses induced by infection or allergens that may have associated reversible lower airway obstruction suggestive of asthma.

Diagnosis

Croup is a clinical diagnosis based on history and physical findings. When epiglottitis cannot be ruled out clinically or when other entities are being considered, radiographs are helpful. A lateral neck film can exclude entities such as *epiglottitis* or a *retropharyngeal abscess*. With croup, on a posteroanterior (PA) view of the chest, the upper airway is narrowed to appear "like a steeple," and the infraglottic region is hazy.

Epiglottitis   The onset of epiglottitis (pp 584–586) is sudden, sometimes suggestive of spasmodic croup. However, a patient with epiglottitis is toxic, with high fever, dysphagia, and drooling. The barking cough is absent, and there is a tendency to adopt a characteristic "sniffing" position, sitting up with the neck extended. On lateral neck x-ray there is classic thumb-shaped epiglottis and swelling of the aryepiglottic folds, the normal cervical lordosis is lost, and the hypopharynx is distended with air.

Foreign Body   A foreign body in the upper airway can present with the sudden onset of stridor. The object may be seen only on radiograph or by direct visualization. However, hoarseness and the barking cough are not usually present.

Bacterial Tracheitis   Bacterial tracheitis is a form of acute subglottic obstruction usually caused by *S. aureus*. It generally occurs in patients who have had croup for several days and resembles epiglottitis, with the sudden onset of high fever, toxicity, and severe respiratory distress.

Laryngomalacia and Subglottic Stenosis   These are common causes of mild stridor in infants. The stridor is accentuated during respiratory infections and is not associated with hoarseness; the child's activity is usually normal.

Retropharyngeal Abscess   Fever is accompanied by drooling and dysphagia. Respiratory distress is variable but may be pronounced, and meningismus or torticollis may also be present. On examination, bulging of the posterior pharyngeal wall may be noted.

ED Management

Mild to Moderate Croup   Make a rapid assessment of color, perfusion, work of breathing, retractions, and air entry. If the patient is in mild to moderate distress, administer humidified oxygen, 4 L/min by face mask. Some infectious croup episodes and almost all spasmodic croup attacks will respond to mist with diminished stridor and lessened respiratory distress. Give a dose of dexamethasone (0.3–0.6 mg/kg PO or IM, 10 mg maximum) to a patient with stridor, a persistent barking cough, or cough with hoarseness or rhonchi.

Most often, the condition of a patient with spasmodic croup is markedly improved by the time of ED arrival; however, caution the parents that the illness may recur the following night.

Severe Croup   Administer humidified oxygen, 4 L/min by face mask; use 100% O_2 delivered by a nonrebreather mask for a patient in severe distress and continuously monitor with a pulse oximeter. Treat with either nebulized racemic epinephrine (Vaponephrine [0.01 mL/kg/dose (0.5 mL max) 1:1000] or L-epinephrine [1:1000, 0.5 mL/kg/dose (max ≤4 yrs 2.5 mL, >4 yrs 5 mL] in 3 mL NS over 5 to 10 min. Also treat a patient with stridor at rest with nebulized epinephrine. Epinephrine acts as a local vasoconstrictor that shrinks airway swelling; its effects last approximately 2 h unless steroids are given. Therefore, to prevent a rebound in the airway swelling, give dexamethasone to any patient who receives nebulized epinephrine treatment and observe for at least 2 h prior to discharge from the ED. Maintain the humidified oxygen after the treatment.

If the patient clearly has croup and there is no significant stridor at rest for at least 2 h after treatment with epinephrine and dexamethasone, discharge the patient. Arrange for follow-up in the next 24 h.

A patient whose severe respiratory distress persists despite racemic epinephrine or L-epinephrine and dexamethasone requires intubation. *Use a tube 0.5 mm smaller than usual* to prevent pressure necrosis of the airway lumen. Start an IV if the patient is not drinking adequately and administer a 20 mL/kg bolus of isotonic crystalloid if the patient appears dehydrated. Obtain an ABG after epinephrine treatment if the child is agitated or has increased work of breathing, as carbon dioxide retention can occur in a young infant with moderate to severe croup. In addition, obtain radiographs of the chest and lateral neck if the patient is in moderate to severe distress or the diagnosis is unclear.

Follow-up

- Immediately if stridor at rest develops at home, otherwise daily for the first 2 to 3 days

Indications for Admission

- Stridor at rest that fails to resolve with epinephrine and dexamethasone
- Rebound during a 2-h observation period following epinephrine and dexamethasone treatment for stridor at rest
- Inadequate fluid intake
- Impending respiratory failure ($Pco_2 > 40$ mmHg; O_2 saturation <93% in room air)

BIBLIOGRAPHY

Klassen TP: Croup: a current perspective. *Pediatr Clin North Am* 1999;46: 1167–1178.

Orlicek SL: Management of acute laryngotracheobronchitis. *Pediatr Infect Dis J* 1998;17:1164–1165.

Rittichier KK, Ledwith CA: Outpatient treatment of moderate croup with dexamethasone: intramuscular versus oral dosing. *Pediatrics* 2000;106:1344–1348.

EPIGLOTTITIS

Epiglottitis (supraglottitis) is a life-threatening bacterial infection of the upper airway almost always caused by *Haemophilus influenzae* type b (Hib). The incidence has declined dramatically as a result of the Hib vaccine. Other causes of supraglottic inflammation are *S. aureus,* herpesvirus, and *Candida albicans* infections as well as thermal injury from the aspiration of hot liquid. Immediate, aggressive management of the airway in a child with suspected epiglottitis is the first priority to ensure survival without morbidity from the complications of sudden upper airway obstruction.

Clinical Presentation

Most patients with epiglottitis are 3 to 8 years of age, although it occurs in young infants as well as adults. Typically there is a sudden onset of fever, lethargy, and respiratory distress with stridor. Drooling occurs in about 50% of patients, and the barking cough of croup is notably absent. Occasionally a patient (usually older child or teenager) presents in a more indolent fashion with mild stridor and a severe sore throat.

Most patients with epiglottitis will place themselves in the position of comfort, the sniffing position, sitting up with the neck extended. Physical findings include respiratory distress, tachypnea, stridor, and, often, retractions (suprasternal). Inspiratory breath sounds are prolonged but diminished throughout all lung fields. Adventitious breath sounds are uncommon in uncomplicated epiglottitis. If the obstruction is more severe, the child may have signs of respiratory failure, including obtundation, cyanosis, absent breath sounds, or apnea.

Diagnosis

The clinical picture is usually so characteristic that the diagnosis is suspected immediately. Epiglottitis is most safely and efficiently confirmed by direct visualization of the inflamed upper airway in an operating room. If a cooperative older child can open his or her mouth wide, direct visualization of the cherry-red epiglottis may be possible in the ED. However, do not use a tongue depressor; there is the potential danger of causing acute airway obstruction. When epiglottitis is *not* the primary suspected diagnosis, using a tongue depressor to visualize the oropharynx is generally safe. Be careful in evaluating a patient with an upper airway problem, especially when there may be secretions or a foreign body in the posterior pharynx.

If epiglottitis is *unlikely* (prolonged course, low-grade fever) but has not been ruled out clinically, order a lateral neck radiograph of the soft tissues. Obtain a portable film in the ED, with the emergency staff and airway equipment at the child's bedside. Allow the patient to remain in the sitting position for the x-ray, with the parent at the bedside. Radiographic findings include a distended hypopharynx, an obliterated vallecula, a large and indistinct epiglottis (thumbprint), thickened aryepiglottic folds, and loss of the normal cervical lordosis. The subglottic region appears normal.

Croup (pp 582–584) is most common in infants from 6 months to 3 years of age, although it does occur in older children. The onset is more indolent, with low-grade fever, hoarseness, a barking cough, and varying degrees of stridor. Often a normal supraglottic region can be seen during a careful examination of the oropharynx. If obtained, the lateral neck radiograph is normal in the supraglottic region, and there may be some subglottic haziness.

A *retropharyngeal or parapharyngeal abscess* most commonly occurs in a young child under 3 to 4 years of age. Fever is usually accompanied by excessive drooling and dysphagia. Respiratory distress is variable but may be pronounced, and meningismus or torticollis may also be present. Examination of the oropharynx reveals bulging of the posterior pharyngeal wall. The lateral neck radiograph shows a swollen prevertebral soft tissue space (much more than half the width of the vertebral bodies).

Foreign-body aspiration (pp 587–588) with upper airway obstruction is generally of very acute onset, with cough and varying degrees of stridor.

Aspiration is most common in children 6 months to 5 years of age. Fever is unusual, and the chest radiographs may be normal or a radiopaque density may be seen in the upper airway.

Bacterial tracheitis is an acute bacterial infection of the trachea associated with a membranous obstruction. It is usually caused by *S. aureus*, and it most often affects children 2 to 10 years of age. Most characteristic is the severe stridor. Diagnosis is usually made by direct visualization of the normal supraglottic region and intubation of the airway, with suctioning of thick inspissated secretions.

ED Management

The management varies according to the clinical presentation:

Epiglottitis Likely, Airway Stable   Place the patient in a position of comfort, with the parents, in a room with immediate access to airway equipment. Give supplemental oxygen if possible, but *do not agitate the child.* Pulse oximetry is advisable if it does not upset the patient. Immediately notify the operating room staff, and assemble the physician team best able to handle airway intubation (usually an attending anesthesiologist and otolaryngologist). Delay IV placement and laboratory studies until after the child is taken to the operating suite. The airway can best be secured under light general anesthesia without neuromuscular relaxation.

Epiglottitis Likely, Patient in Extremis with an Unstable Airway   Place the child supine and open the airway with a chin lift. Perform bag-valve-mask ventilation with a tight seal and 4 to 5 cm H_2O pressure to maximize air entry past the obstructing epiglottis. Occasionally this will not be sufficient and intubation will be necessary. Rarely, needle cricothyrotomy is required to provide a temporary airway until a team can assemble in the ED to manage the airway.

Mild Suspicion of Epiglottitis, Airway Stable   Obtain a lateral neck radiograph to differentiate among the other potential problems. If there is significant stridor or respiratory distress, perform the radiograph in the ED with the physician at the bedside. If epiglottitis is confirmed, proceed with operating room management.

Indications for Admission

- Suspected or confirmed epiglottitis
- Undiagnosed upper airway obstruction with stridor at rest

BIBLIOGRAPHY

Cressman WR, Myer CM III: Diagnosis and management of croup and epiglottitis. *Pediatr Clin North Am* 1994;41:265–276.

Lee SS, Schwartz RH, Bahadori RS: Retropharyngeal abscess: epiglottitis of the new millennium. *J Pediatr* 2001;138:435–437.

Mauro RD, Poole SR, Lockhart CH: Differentiation of epiglottitis from laryngotracheitis in the child with stridor. *Am J Dis Child* 1988;42:679–682.

FOREIGN BODY IN THE AIRWAY

Aspirated foreign bodies cause more deaths in the United States than croup and epiglottitis combined. Determining the presence of a foreign body requires an accurate history, a high degree of clinical suspicion, and often a direct look down the airway. The peak incidence coincides with the period of oral behavior, between 6 months and the early school years.

Clinical Presentation

Aspiration of a foreign body classically presents with an immediate episode of coughing, gagging, choking, or cyanosis. In infants and small children, a foreign body lodged in the esophagus can impinge on the trachea and cause respiratory embarrassment. Some foreign bodies will be promptly vomited or swallowed, eliminating the immediate risk of hypoxemia and the complication of a foreign body lodging in the pulmonary tree.

Extrathoracic (Laryngeal or Tracheal) The patient presents with stridor, a croupy cough, varying degrees of dyspnea, or acute hypoxemia and cyanosis. The symptoms may vary with the degree of obstruction of the airway. The sound elicited by air moving over the object varies with the size of the airway and degree of inflammation induced.

Intrathoracic (Lower Trachea and Bronchial) A patient with a foreign body in the lower airway presents with an initial choking episode and varying periods of quiescence, followed by persistent and often progressive symptoms. Commonly, there is cough, wheezing, and dyspnea. With inflammation or secondary atelectasis, fever and signs of pneumonia may predominate, leading to a misdiagnosis of asthma or recurrent pneumonia. A focal foreign body may produce unilateral hyperinflation with widening of intercostal spaces. On auscultation, localized or diffuse wheezing, rales, or decreased air entry may be appreciated.

Diagnosis

The only certain method for verifying the diagnosis is with bronchoscopy. However, if foreign-body aspiration is suspected and the patient is not in extreme respiratory distress, obtain radiographs, which can assist in the diagnosis.

Extrathoracic Radiographs of the lateral neck and chest are generally normal, as only a small number of aspirated foreign bodies are radioopaque. There may be signs of upper airway obstruction, such as ballooning of the hypopharynx, gastric distention, or diminished lung volumes. Esophageal foreign bodies can occasionally compress the trachea from behind; these tend to be larger objects that are more likely to be radiopaque. Orientation of a radiopaque foreign body in the sagital plane on the PA film of the chest (slit-like image) confirms its presence in the trachea or larynx.

The differential diagnosis of an extrathoracic foreign body includes *epiglottitis, croup, bacterial tracheitis, tracheomalacia, retropharyngeal abscess,* and *congenital anomalies of the airway.* While the abrupt onset suggests aspiration, bronchoscopy is required to confirm the diagnosis in cases with moderate symptoms.

Intrathoracic   Most intrathoracic foreign bodies are radiolucent, but there is a high incidence of abnormal chest radiographs (80%). Hyperinflation, atelectasis, and pneumonia are the most common abnormalities. In rare instances, a pneumothorax may be present. In the older child, inspiratory and expiratory chest films may reveal persistent hyperinflation of the ipsilateral side during expiration. Unilateral hyperinflation on the inspiratory film may be seen, but it is less common. For a toddler, when cooperation for an inspiratory film is unlikely, obtain bilateral decubitus films, which may reveal increased lucency on the affected side when that side is dependent. Fluoroscopy may sometimes be useful to distinguish small areas of air trapping or mediastinal shifting.

An intrathoracic foreign body is often confused with *asthma, pneumonia, congenital lobar emphysema,* or other syndromes associated with hyperinflation or atelectasis. History, clinical response to therapy (i.e., bronchodilators in asthma), and chronicity may help distinguish these entities.

ED Management

Assess the patency of the airway and breathing. Complete obstruction demands immediate BLS maneuvers: five back blows followed by five chest compressions in a patient <12 months of age and six to ten subdiaphragmatic abdominal thrusts (Heimlich maneuver, pp 13–14) for an older child. If there is an incomplete obstruction, place the child in the sniffing position (maximal airway opening), provide supplemental oxygen, and permit the child's own ventilation through a partly occluded airway to be maintained. Maneuvers that dislodge the foreign body may move the object to the central airways, causing complete obstruction. Continuously monitor the patient with pulse oximetry while awaiting an anesthesiologist and bronchoscopist (pediatric surgeon or otolaryngologist) to perform rigid bronchoscopy.

Foreign bodies in the lower airway generally present with less severe signs of obstruction. Chest physiotherapy, may cause occlusion of a major airway and hypoxemia, and is therefore contraindicated. Provide supplemental oxygen, and arrange for semielective removal by rigid bronchoscopy under general anesthesia.

Indications for Admission

- Clinical suspicion of an airway foreign body
- Respiratory symptoms after expulsion of an airway foreign body

BIBLIOGRAPHY

Burton EM, Brick WG, Hall JD, et al: Tracheobronchial foreign body aspiration in children. *South Med J* 1996;89:195–198.

Reilly JS, Cook SP, Stool D, et al: Prevention and management of aerodigestive foreign bodies in childhood. *Pediatr Clin North Am* 1996;43:1403–1411.

Skoulakis CE, Doxas PG, Papadakis CE, et al: Bronchoscopy for foreign body removal in children. A review and analysis of 210 cases. *Int J Pediatr Otorhinolaryngol* 2000;53:143–148.

HEMOPTYSIS

Hemoptysis is the expectoration of blood from the lower respiratory tract. It is uncommon in childhood; most suspected cases are actually the result of vomiting blood swallowed from the esophagus, nasopharynx, or oropharynx. The cause of true hemoptysis is usually a pulmonary infection or other pulmonary disease (Table 20-3).

Clinical Presentation

Hemoptysis usually presents with signs and symptoms of the underlying disease, an acute exacerbation of that process, or a pulmonary infection. For example, pneumonia presents with fever, cough, tachypnea, and rales or decreased breath sounds. A patient with cystic fibrosis may have chronic diarrhea and failure to thrive.

Bronchiectasis can occur with cystic fibrosis, tuberculosis, or fungal infections (e.g., coccidioidomycosis). Airway erosion leads to acute hemorrhage that is frightening but usually self-limited, although the bleeding may be life-threatening if a major vessel is affected. The usual presentation is fever, cough, and expectoration of blood.

A *foreign body* in the airway generally presents with cough, localized wheezing, and varying degrees of respiratory distress. A chronic foreign body may cause erosion of a bronchus or distal bronchiectasis.

Table 20-3   Etiologies of Hemoptysis

Infectious causes (bronchiectasis, airway erosion)
Bacterial infections
Measles
Tuberculosis
Coccidioidomycosis
Cystic fibrosis
Bronchopulmonary dysplasia

Noninfectious causes
Foreign-body aspiration
Rib fracture with pulmonary contusion
Airway compression: carcinoid, bronchogenic cyst,
cystadenomatoid malformation, mediastinal tumor
Pulmonary sequestration
Arteriovenous malformation
Bleeding diathesis
Pulmonary hemosiderosis
Wegener's granulomatosis
Pulmonary embolus

Trauma to the chest and airways is often associated with rib fractures and pulmonary contusion. In most instances there is point tenderness over the rib, pleuritic chest pain, and dyspnea in addition to the hemoptysis.

A patient with an intrinsic *pulmonary* or *endobronchial mass* may be relatively asymptomatic or may be coughing or wheezing. Weight loss or fatigue can also occur. A child with a *bleeding diathesis* will have other manifestations of bleeding (petechiae, ecchymoses, hematemesis, epistaxis, hematochezia).

Diagnosis

Initially, confirm that the blood is truly pulmonary in origin and exclude the *oral cavity, nasopharynx,* and *GI tract* as the site of the bleeding. If necessary, pass a nasogastric tube to exclude an upper GI bleed.

Inquire about a history of possible *aspiration of a foreign body, trauma, acute infection,* or exposure to a *fungus* or *TB.* Check for an underlying history of *bronchopulmonary dysplasia, cystic fibrosis,* or *bleeding dyscrasia.*

Perform a careful physical examination of the chest, including observation of any abnormality in chest excursion, palpation for external tenderness, and auscultation for air entry and adventitious sounds (rales or wheezes). The area of pulmonary hemorrhage may not alter the breath sounds heard over the chest wall.

Radiographs of the chest may be unchanged from previous films or may demonstrate an infiltrate, evidence of a foreign body (hyperinflation of the affected side, radiopaque foreign body, or infiltrate distal to the foreign body), or a mass or density. With *pulmonary hemosiderosis* there may be fluffy infiltrates that change location with each episode.

ED Management

Admit a patient with significant hemoptysis (>60 mL) and consult with a pulmonologist or thoracic surgeon. Obtain a chest radiograph, CBC, platelet count, PT, PTT, and type and cross-match. If the patient has tachypnea or respiratory distress, measure the oxygen saturation with either pulse oximetry or an ABG. Insert a large-bore IV and transfuse packed red blood cells (p 654) for volume depletion or evidence of significant ongoing blood loss. Place a 5TU PPD (0.1 mL) if the patient is not known to have a positive skin test.

Hemoptysis with blood-streaked mucus can be treated on an outpatient basis if the patient is not in respiratory distress. The ED management of pneumonia (pp 591–595), foreign-body aspiration (pp 587–588), and a bleeding diathesis (pp 304–305) is discussed elsewhere.

Follow-up

- Pulmonology or primary care follow-up within 1 week

Indications for Admission

- Hemoptysis >60 mL
- Hematocrit <30% or signs of acute, severe blood loss
- Underlying chronic disease requiring parenteral antibiotics or in-patient therapy

- Mediastinal mass or peripheral lung density
- Suspected foreign-body aspiration, pulmonary embolus, TB

BIBLIOGRAPHY

Batra PS, Holinger LD: Etiology and management of pediatric hemoptysis. *Arch Otolaryngol Head Neck Surg* 2001;127:377–382.

Painosi P, al-Sadoon H: Hemoptysis in children. *Pediatr Rev* 1996;17:34–48.

Thompson JW, Nguyen CD, Lazar RH, et al: Evaluation and management of hemoptysis in infants and children, a report of nine cases. *Ann Otol Rhinol Laryngol* 1996;105:516.

PNEUMONIA

Most pneumonias (90%) are viral in origin; the rest are bacterial but are responsible for a much higher rate of complications. This is especially true in young infants, in whom secretions can occlude the small airways, resulting in an increased work of breathing that can rapidly lead to exhaustion. Although pneumonias are believed to occur after microaspiration of oropharyngeal flora, organisms cultured from the oropharynx rarely represent the agents causing the acute pulmonary infection. Table 20-4 lists the most likely etiologies in each age group. *Streptococcus*

Table 20-4   Etiologies of Pneumonia

AGE	AGENT
<2 weeks	Group B *Streptococcus* Coliform bacteria Respiratory syncytial virus (RSV) *Staphylococcus aureus*
2 weeks–3 months	*Chlamydia trachomatis* RSV Parainfluenza virus *Streptococcus pneumoniae* *Haemophilus influenzae* type b (very rare if immunized) *S. aureus*
3 months–5 years	Viral (especially RSV, influenza) *S. pneumoniae* *H. influenzae* type b (inadequately immunized)
Over 5 years	Viral *Mycoplasma pneumoniae* *S. pneumoniae* *Chlamydia pneumoniae*
Other agents to consider	*Mycobacterium tuberculosis* Pertussis (<1 year old) *Pneumocystis carinii* (HIV+) *Legionella* sp.

pneumoniae is the most common bacterial pathogen, RSV is the most frequent viral cause, and *Pneumocystis carinii* is the most likely opportunistic infection in HIV-positive infants.

Clinical Presentation

Cough, tachypnea, and fever are the common symptoms of childhood pneumonia, while pallor, fatigue, and other constitutional symptoms are variable. Posttussive vomiting can be a common complaint in young children. A neonate or young infant may present with tachypnea, decreased activity, and poor feeding. With progression of the pneumonia, there may be signs of respiratory distress, including nasal flaring, intercostal or substernal retractions, dyspnea, cyanosis, or apnea. On auscultation, inspiratory rales may be heard or the breath sounds may be locally decreased or tubular, although adventitious sounds are harder to appreciate in a young child. Dullness and diminished breath sounds may indicate an effusion. Abdominal pain can occur with lower lobe pneumonia and meningismus with upper lobe infection.

Chlamydia trachomatis is the most common nonviral cause of pneumonia in infants between 2 weeks and 3 months of age. The classic presentation is a staccato cough in an afebrile, tachypneic infant with nasal congestion and fine rales. There may be a history of or concurrent conjunctivitis in approximately 50% of cases, as well as wheezing, bilateral patchy infiltrates on chest x-ray, and eosinophilia (>300/mm^3).

M. pneumoniae and *C. pneumoniae* present with the gradual onset of a nonproductive hacking cough in a school-age child. The patient does not appear very sick, wheezing is more common than rales, headache and myalgias may also occur, and other family members may have had a similar illness.

Infection with *B. pertussis* (pp 375–377) may also lead to a secondary lobar or diffuse pneumonia. Typically there is a URI with rhinorrhea (catarrhal stage), which progresses to a harsh, episodic cough (paroxysmal stage), followed by the resolution of the cough over weeks to months (convalescent stage). The primary illness is more common in children who have not received three primary immunizations or whose immunity has waned (patients over 10 years of age).

Diagnosis

Pneumonia can be diagnosed clinically when fever, cough, and rales are present; obtaining a radiograph does not usually alter the patient's management. Obtain a chest x-ray (PA and lateral) when the patient is in respiratory distress, the diagnosis is uncertain, there is concern about a pleural effusion, or an infant <2 months of age has respiratory signs (including cough). Also obtain a chest radiograph if a patient is not responding to appropriate therapy. Various patterns on the radiograph may help with the differential diagnosis (Table 20-5). Generally, pyogenic bacterial infections appear as bronchopneumonia or lobar infiltrates, sometimes with pleural effusion. Viral infections often present with diffuse airway involvement and hyperinflation.

Table 20-5   Chest X-Ray Pattern as a Guide to Etiology

Diffuse Pattern

Viral (90%) of cases

Chlamydia trachomatis (afebrile infant, eosinophilia common)

Mycoplasma pneumoniae and *Chlamydia pneumoniae*
    (school-age child)

Mycobacteria (uncommon)

Fungi (uncommon)

Rickettsia (uncommon)

Haemophilus influenzae type b (rare)

Pneumocystis carinii (usually central pattern, elevated LDH, hypoxia)

Lobar Pattern

Streptococcus pneumoniae (90%)

Staphylococcus aureus

H. influenzae type b (rare)

Other bacteria (uncommon)

Pneumonia with effusion

S. pneumoniae (commonest cause of effusion)

H. influenzae type b (empyema common)

Group A *Streptococcus*

Staphylococcus aureus (often cavitation and/or empyema)

Mycoplasma pneumoniae (effusion uncommon)

Mycobacteria (unilateral effusion can occur without pneumonia)

Adenovirus (small effusion)

The abdominal pain sometimes associated with pneumonia can suggest *gastroenteritis* or early *appendicitis*. However, a history of cough as an early symptom and a higher temperature suggest a primary respiratory disease.

Asthma   Asthma, which may be difficult to distinguish from pneumonia, can predispose to pneumonia, and accompanying atelectasis can lead to localized decreased breath sounds. Asthma is suggested by the presence of diffuse wheezing, coarse rales and rhonchi, and a response to bronchodilators.

Congestive Heart Failure   Congestive heart failure can present with tachycardia, tachypnea, rales, a gallop, and evidence of the primary cause (muffled heart sounds in myocardial disease, a murmur in volume overload shunts, poor perfusion or diminished pulses with left ventricular obstruction). Hepatosplenomegaly may be noted, and cardiomegaly and congestion can be seen on the chest radiograph.

Foreign-Body Aspiration   A foreign body can cause decreased breath sounds or predispose to pneumonia. The history and radiographs may be suggestive; bronchoscopy is often required for a definitive diagnosis.

Inhalation Injury   Inhalation injury or any pulmonary toxic agent may induce findings consistent with intrapulmonary inflammation, mimicking pneumonia.

Recurrent pneumonia is usually associated with *asthma* but may be caused by *immunologic dysfunction, cystic fibrosis, foreign body*, or *external airway compression* (tumor, node).

ED Management

Most children have infections with viral agents and require supportive care (fever control, fluids) only. Nonetheless, it is critical to immediately assess the adequacy of breathing. If the patient is dyspneic or in respiratory distress, assess the oxygen saturation with pulse oximetry. Obtain an ABG if the patient has poor breath sounds and is lethargic. Administer supplemental oxygen if the patient is in distress or has decreased oxygenation (oxygen saturation <95%; Po_2<80 mmHg). The goal is an oxygen saturation >95% or Po_2>80 mmHg. Obtain a chest radiograph if indicated (see above). Perform a lumbar puncture to exclude meningitis if there is fever and irritability, obtundation, lethargy, or meningismus. If the patient is febrile, give antipyretics to decrease the temperature and its effects on work of breathing (acetaminophen 15 mg/kg/dose; ibuprofen 10 mg/kg/dose). Place a PPD (0.1 mL, 5 TU) intradermally on the forearm unless the child is known to be positive for TB. If the patient is discharged from the ED, arrange follow-up to coincide with when the test needs to be read (48–72 h).

Below 6 Months Old   Admit all patients below 3 months of age with lobar pneumonia and all infants with interstitial pneumonia below 2 months of age. Obtain a CBC, blood culture, and chest radiograph; if the patient appears toxic or is under 2 months of age, perform a lumbar puncture and obtain serum electrolytes. Secure an IV if the patient appears toxic or is not taking oral fluids adequately. See pp 335–337 for the treatment of an infant under 8 weeks of age; treat a patient above 8 weeks of age with either cefuroxime (150 mg/kg/day divided q 8 h, IM or IV) or ceftriaxone (75 mg/kg/day divided q 12 h IV). If *C. trachomatis* pneumonitis seems likely, obtain a nasopharyngeal culture and treat with oral erythromycin (40 mg/kg/day divided q 6 h) for 14 days.

Above 6 Months Old   Obtain an oxygen saturation (pulse oximetry) if the patient is tachypneic (respiratory rate >60/min <2 years of age; 40–60/min >2 years of age) or has moderate retractions. For a patient with poor color and poor breath sounds, obtain an ABG. Indications for admission include a Po_2<80 mmHg, oxygen saturation <95%, or Pco_2>40–50 mmHg.

If the pneumonia is lobar, treat with amoxicillin (40 mg/kg/day divided tid for 10 days). Give an initial dose of parenteral ceftriaxone (50 mg/kg IM or IV, 500 mg maximum) before oral therapy if the patient is vomiting, although this does not hasten recovery. If the patient is being admitted to the hospital, treat with IV cefuroxime (150 mg/kg/day divided q 8 h) or ceftriaxone (50 mg/kg/day divided q 12 h). Penicillin G (150,000 U/kg/day divided q 6 h IV) is an alternative for a child above

5 years of age, depending on the prevalance of penicillin-resistant *Pneumococcus* in the community.

Treat a child >5 years of age with erythromycin (40 mg/kg/day divided qid, 1 g/day maximum), azithromycin (10 mg/kg, once on day 1, followed by 5 mg/kg/qd on days 2–5), or clarithromycin (15 mg/kg divided bid, 1 g maximum) for lobar or presumed mycoplasmal pneumonia.

If *P. carinii* pneumonia (PCP) is suspected (p 592), obtain a chest radiograph and LDH. Admit and treat with trimethoprim-sulfamethoxazole (TMP-SMX; 20 mg/kg/day TMP divided q 6 h) and prednisone (2 mg/kg/day divided q 6 h) if the LDH is elevated or the x-ray is consistent with PCP.

Significant pleural effusion is an indication for admission for diagnostic thoracentesis and parenteral antibiotics.

Follow-up

- Respiratory distress at home: at once
- Lobar pneumonia: 24 h
- Patient <2 years of age with suspected viral pneumonia: 24 to 48 h
- All patients: at the end of treatment or about 2 weeks after presentation to assess for improvement. However, chest x-ray abnormalities can persist for 8 to 12 weeks after the acute illness, and symptoms (especially cough) can persist for weeks. Therefore, wait at least 8 to 12 weeks after presentation to consider the need for a follow-up chest x-ray unless the patient is worsening

Indications for Admission

- Patient <2 months of age with pneumonia
- Patient <6 months of age with lobar pneumonia
- Patient with Po_2<65 mmHg, oxygen saturation <92%, Pco_2>40 mmHg
- Patient not taking fluids, exhausted, or with parents unable to comply with instructions
- Presence of significant pleural effusion
- Suspicion of PCP

BIBLIOGRAPHY

Hammerschlag MR: *Mycoplasma pneumoniae* infections. *Curr Opin Infect Dis* 2001;14:181-186.
Lerou PH: Lower respiratory infections in children. *Curr Opin Pediatr* 2001; 12:200–206.
Schidlow DV, Callahan CW: Pneumonia. *Pediatr Rev* 1996;17:300–309.

PULSE OXIMETRY

Pulse oximetry is a simple and noninvasive means of measuring the oxygen saturation of hemoglobin. It is based on the principle that deoxygenated blood absorbs more light in the red spectrum, while oxygenated blood absorbs more infrared light. The oximeter measures the two different light absorbencies and then calculates the oxygen saturation. When used appropriately, it provides a reliable assessment of a patient's

Table 20-6   Factors Affecting Accuracy of Pulse Oximetry

CONDITION	EFFECT ON OXYGEN SATURATION ESTIMATE
Anemia	False sense of adequate oxygenation
Carboxyhemoglobin	Overestimates
Methemoglobin	Over- and underestimates
Sickle cell anemia	May overestimate (not significantly)
Bilirubin	May underestimate
Dark nail polish	Underestimates
Profound hypoxia (O_2 saturation <80%)	Not reliable
Neonate	Accuracy varies with hemoglobin level

oxygen status. However, the light source and sensor of the oximetry probe must be placed opposite one another in an accessible area, such as a finger, toe, or earlobe. The pulse rate measured by the oximeter must reflect the patient's actual pulse rate to confirm the reliability of the reading. Verify the oximeter pulse rate reading by correlation with a manually obtained pulse rate. Several factors affect the accuracy of pulse oximetry and may limit its use (see Table 20-6).

BIBLIOGRAPHY

Blaisdell CJ, Goodman S, Clark K, et al: Pulse oximetry is a poor predictor of hypoxemia in stable children with sickle cell disease. *Arch Pediatr Adolesc Med* 2000;154:900–903.

Mower WR, Sachs C, Nicklin EL: Pulse oximetry as a fifth pediatric vital sign. *Pediatrics* 1997;99:681–686.

Villanueva R, Bell C, Kain ZN, et al: Effect of peripheral perfusion on accuracy of pulse oximetry in children. *J Clin Anesth* 1999;11:317–322.

RESPIRATORY DISTRESS AND FAILURE

Respiratory distress or respiratory failure may be the endpoint of a multitude of clinical disorders in children, both pulmonary and nonpulmonary in origin. Airway obstruction is the leading cause of life-threatening acute respiratory distress. Causes of upper airway obstruction include croup, epiglottitis, and foreign-body aspiration; asthma or bronchiolitis produce lower airway obstruction. Other disorders that can culminate in respiratory distress or failure are abnormalities of the neuromuscular control of breathing (seizures, central apnea, meningitis, encephalitis, head trauma), problems with the mechanics of breathing (congenital, acquired, or traumatic chest wall deformities), and alveolar disorders (pneumonia). Nonpulmonary disorders include cardiac disease and heart failure, sepsis, and disorders of oxygen delivery (CO poisoning, methemoglobinemia, severe anemia).

Clinical Presentation and Diagnosis

Respiratory distress is manifest by difficulty breathing, fatigue, diminished activity and/or feeding, varying degrees of exhaustion, and symptoms associated with the cause. Signs include pallor or cyanosis, tachypnea, retractions, diminished air entry, tachycardia (bradycardia with severe respiratory failure with hypoxemia), and/or signs of the specific etiology of the distress.

Upper airway obstruction usually presents with stridor. Radiographs may delineate supraglottic disorders such as epiglottitis or a foreign body, although direct visualization of the airway in a controlled setting is the diagnostic and therapeutic procedure of choice.

Lower airway obstruction presents with hyperinflation, expiratory prolongation, and wheezing. Localized signs are noted more with foreign-body aspiration.

Neurologic diseases lead to depressed level of consciousness, poor respiratory effort or apnea, depressed airway reflexes, and less effective cough.

Mechanical problems present with ineffective chest wall excursion or distorted lung inflation.

Alveolar causes present with general signs of respiratory distress, hypoxemia, and tachypnea. The findings on examination include rales or decreased breath sounds.

Congestive heart failure can present with tachycardia, a gallop, a murmur, diminished heart sounds, venous distention, and sometimes hepatomegaly. *Severe anemia* presents with pallor and a low hemoglobin.

Nonpulmonary disorders (CO poisoning, methemoglobinemia) require laboratory studies to confirm the diagnosis.

The criteria for respiratory failure areas follows:

- $P_{O_2} < 50$ mmHg (oxygen saturation <84%) on 60% FIO_2 (except in cyanotic congenital heart disease)
- $P_{CO_2} > 50$ mmHg and rising (with pH <7.30) or >40 mmHg with exhaustion
- In neuromuscular and central disorders, central apnea, or decreased vital capacity (<12–15 mL/kg) with exhaustion

ED Management

Provide 100% oxygen, rapidly assess airway patency, and check the stability of the airway (maintainable or unmaintainable). Count the respiratory rate, and evaluate color, breath sounds (air entry), heart rate, pulses, capillary refill, and blood pressure. Monitor the oxygen saturation. Ascertain the cause of respiratory failure and begin immediate therapy.

If the airway is not patent, use the jaw thrust for total airway obstruction and suction for partial obstruction. If respiratory failure is present, continue with 100% O_2 and institute bag-mask ventilation. Intubate a patient who is unable to maintain a stable airway for an extended period (pp 1–9). Establish IV access and give broad-spectrum antibiotics if infection is likely (cefuroxime 150 mg/kg/day divided q 8 h or ceftriaxone 100 mg/kg/day divided q 12 h).

Mechanical Ventilation
Under 10 kg   Use a pressure-limited ventilator. Adjust inspiratory pressure (IP) to obtain adequate chest movement and audible breath sounds. In disorders with minimal alteration of lung compliance, start with an IP of 20 cm and a rate of 20 to 25 breaths per minute. Higher pressures are required in more restrictive (less compliant) disorders.

10 kg and Over   Use a volume-preset ventilator set to deliver 8 to 10 mL/kg of tidal volume (lower in disorders with hyperinflation), a rate of 15 breaths per minute and an I:E ratio of 1:2.

With either ventilator, consider positive end-expiratory pressure (PEEP; 4–5 cmH$_2$O) to maintain end-expiratory lung volume and thereby minimize atelectasis and intrapulmonary shunting (except in a patient with hyperinflation). Assess the adequacy of ventilation by evaluating the chest excursions and breath sounds. Check an ABG after 15 min and obtain other laboratory studies as indicated to make the diagnosis [chest radiograph, lateral neck radiograph, serum electrolytes, respiratory cultures, electrocardiogram (ECG), lumbar puncture, electroencephalogram (EEG), CT scan]. Subsequent laboratory tests and changes in the ventilator settings are guided by the clinical status, pulse oximetry, and ABG results.

Indications for Admission

- Respiratory failure requiring mechanical ventilation or intensive monitoring
- Respiratory distress not reversible with definitive therapy
- New oxygen requirement
- Pulmonary infection requiring parenteral antibiotics

BIBLIOGRAPHY

Bateman ST, Arnold JH: Acute respiratory failure in children. *Curr Opin Pediatr* 2000;12:233–237.
Redding GJ: Current concepts in adult respiratory distress syndrome in children. *Curr Opin Pediatr* 2001;13:261–266.

CHAPTER 21

Renal Emergencies

Sandra J. Cunningham and Chester M. Edelmann, Jr.

ACUTE GLOMERULONEPHRITIS

Acute glomerulonephritis (AGN) is a clinical syndrome characterized by an acutely diminished glomerular filtration rate, oliguria or anuria, azotemia, proteinuria, hematuria with or without red blood cell (RBC) casts, pyuria, and evidence of volume overload (hypertension, peripheral edema, vascular congestion). Most cases of AGN result from deposition of preformed immune complexes in glomerular structures or *in situ* fixation of complement and specific antibody with antigen trapped within glomeruli. Etiologies include bacteria (group A *Streptococcus, Pneumococcus, Staphylococcus aureus*), viruses (Epstein-Barr virus, adenovirus), immune-related diseases [systemic lupus erythematosus (SLE), Henoch-Schönlein purpura (HSP), IgA nephropathy (Berger's disease), subacute bacterial endocarditis (SBE)], and disorders of undetermined origin (membranoproliferative glomerulonephritis).

Clinical Presentation

As the glomerular filtration rate (GFR) falls, oliguria/anuria ensues, leading to the clinical symptoms that are the hallmark of AGN: edema (particularly periorbital), weight gain, hypertension, decreased urine output, and gross hematuria (80% of patients). There may be constitutional symptoms, such as back or abdominal pain, and nausea and vomiting, in addition to the clinical features of the underlying disease. Central nervous system (CNS) symptoms such as lethargy, irritability, headache, mental status changes, and seizures may occur with minimal elevation in the blood pressure. Water and salt retention can lead to congestive heart failure, causing dyspnea and orthopnea in association with a systolic murmur, gallop, rales, and a pleural effusion.

Postinfectious Glomerulonephritis Postinfectious glomerulonephritis occurs primarily in children, with a peak between 2 and 6 years of age. Group A beta-hemolytic *Streptococcus* is the most common etiologic agent. Typically, manifestations of acute poststreptococcal glomerulonephritis follow a sore throat by 1 to 3 weeks or impetigo by 2 to 3 weeks. Onset of AGN synchronous with pharyngitis suggests an exacerbation of IgA nephropathy. For other infections there may be an upper respiratory infection (URI), a mononucleosis-like syndrome, or hepatitis with jaundice. The onset of the AGN is abrupt, with microscopic/macroscopic hematuria, periorbital edema, and mild to moderate hypertension.

Henoch-Schönlein Purpura   HSP occurs in preschool- and school-age children (peak incidence at 4–5 years of age) who present with one or more of the following: a purpuric rash on the extensor surfaces of the lower extremities and buttocks, abdominal pain, hematochezia, and arthralgias of the large joints, although not all of these features are present at the same time. There is often a history of a preceding URI. The majority of patients with HSP have nephritis, although it is usually mild (hematuria with or without low-grade proteinuria). Renal involvement may be the initial manifestation of HSP; alternatively, the nephritis can develop after other features of the disease have resolved.

Other   AGN or nephrotic syndrome can be the initial presentation of *SLE;* however, other manifestations of the disease are also usually present, including a butterfly rash, polyserositis, or arthritis. *Membranoproliferative glomerulonephritis* causes an illness that may be indistinguishable from postinfectious AGN at the onset of the disease. It is characterized, however, by persistent (>3–4 weeks) hypocomplementemia. *SBE* presents with persistent fever, splenomegaly, Roth's spots, Osler's nodes, splinter hemorrhages, and positive blood cultures. *Alport's syndrome*, characterized by sensorineural and ocular disorders, can cause an acute decline in renal function during an intercurrent URI.

Diagnosis

Obtain a careful history, including whether there is a family history of hematuria, hearing loss, or kidney failure. On physical examination, check the blood pressure, note the presence of edema, examine the fundi, skin, heart, lungs, and joints, and assess hearing, mental status, and neurologic function.

If AGN is suspected, order a urinalysis. In glomerular disease, dysmorphic RBCs and RBC casts are almost always present and are diagnostic of this disorder. In renal diseases associated with nonglomerular hematuria, such as *nephrolithiasis, trauma,* or a *bleeding diathesis,* the RBCs are eumorphic and RBC casts are not seen. If there is gross hematuria, examine an unspun urine specimen. White blood cells (WBCs) may predominate over RBCs early in the course of the disease (causing confusion with the diagnosis of urinary tract infection). Proteinuria is virtually always present. Obtain a complete blood count (CBC), platelet count, erythrocyte sedimentation rate (ESR), serum electrolytes, calcium, blood urea nitrogen (BUN), creatinine, total protein, albumin, cholesterol, triglycerides, and complement (C3, C4, C50). Hypocomplementemic forms of AGN include *postinfectious SLE, membranoproliferative glomerulonephritis,* and *embolic renal disease.*

If the clinical picture is compatible with *poststreptococcal AGN,* obtain an antistreptolysin O (ASLO) or streptozyme. If the illness is suggestive of *SLE,* obtain a fluorescent antinuclear antibody (FANA) and anti-dsDNA antibody titer. Obtain serial blood cultures to help rule out SBE in a patient with persistent fever and no obvious source.

If there are any signs of a *bleeding diathesis,* obtain a prothrombin time (PT), partial thromboplatin time (PTT), and bleeding time. Clotting studies and the platelet count are normal in HSP.

ED Management

Consult a nephrologist for all patients with AGN. Immediate priorities include management of hypertension and hyperkalemia. Because hypertensive encephalopathy can occur at a minimally increased blood pressure, especially in poststreptococcal AGN, treat hypertension promptly and aggressively. For an asymptomatic patient, use oral nifedipine (0.3 mg/kg, 10 mg maximum) or captopril (0.3–0.6 mg/kg, 6 mg/kg/day maximum). The onset of action of nifedipine can be accelerated by having the patient bite the capsule before swallowing the contents. Because captopril causes decreased aldosterone production, use it with caution in a hyperkalemic patient. For a patient with *acute* neurologic symptoms (headache, seizures, altered mental status), give IV labetalol or sodium nitroprusside (see Hypertension, pp 609–610). The goal of the initial antihypertensive therapy is a 20% reduction in the mean arterial pressure (MAP):

$$\text{MAP} = \text{diastolic BP} + \tfrac{1}{3} (\text{systolic BP} - \text{diastolic BP}).$$

The cornerstone of medical management is fluid and sodium restriction (see Acute Renal Failure, pp 602–605). Restrict fluids to insensible losses (400 mL/m2/day) plus urine output regardless of whether the patient is oliguric. Initiate IV therapy with NS but withhold potassium until the patient voids and eukalemia is documented. See p 605 for the treatment of hyperkalemia secondary to impaired renal excretion.

Conservative medical therapy is the rule, with hemo- or peritoneal dialysis reserved for severe volume overload with pulmonary edema, life-threatening hyperkalemia (≥ 7 mEq/L), intractable acidosis, intractable hypocalcemia with seizures, or symptomatic uremia [pleuritis, pericarditis, gastrointestinal (GI) bleeding, encephalopathy].

Follow-up
- AGN without hypertension, edema, or oliguria: next day for a BP check

Indication for Admission
- Acute glomerulonephritis with edema, hypertension, or oliguria

BIBLIOGRAPHY

Albright RC Jr: Acute renal failure: a practical update. *Mayo Clin Proc* 2001; 76:67–74.

Pan CG: Glomerulonephritis in childhood. *Curr Opin Pediatr* 1997;9:154–159.

Tizard EJ: Henoch-Schönlein purpura. *Arch Dis Child* 1999;80:380–383.

ACUTE RENAL FAILURE

Acute renal failure (ARF) is characterized by a decrease in the glomerular filtration rate (GFR), associated with increases in the serum urea nitrogen and creatinine concentrations. Oliguria (≤ 0.5 mL/kg/h) is a frequent but not invariable finding.

The causes of ARF can be divided into three pathophysiologic categories: prerenal, postrenal, and renal parenchymal disease. Prerenal azotemia reflects a functional decline in renal function in the absence of structural injury. It is a consequence of inadequate kidney perfusion secondary to hypovolemia (dehydration or blood loss), hypotension, or hypoxia. The GFR is rapidly restored to normal when renal blood flow is increased; however, severe renal hypoperfusion may lead to acute tubular necrosis (ATN). Postrenal azotemia is secondary to urinary tract obstruction. Renal parenchymal disease can result from glomerular diseases [AGN, hemolytic-uremic syndrome (HUS)], or ATN secondary to nephrotoxins, rhabdomyolysis, or tubular ischemia.

Clinical Presentation

The clinical presentation of acute renal failure is varied. There may be findings secondary to the renal insufficiency per se, such as edema, hypertension, nausea and vomiting, hypocalcemic tetany, and neurologic symptoms (coma, seizures). Alternatively, the presentation may reflect the primary pathologic process, such as hypotension and changes in orthostatic vital signs (hypovolemic shock), difficulty voiding, and an abnormal urinary stream (obstruction), lethargy and fever (sepsis), cutaneous burns, bleeding, jaundice (hemoglobinuria), myonecrosis due to trauma or heat illness (myoglobinuria), pallor and bloody diarrhea (HUS), abdominal pain and arthralgias (Henoch-Schönlein purpura), or an antecedent URI (postinfectious AGN).

Hemolytic-Uremic Syndrome   HUS is the most common cause of community-acquired ARF in children. Although the mortality from renal failure has decreased, renal sequelae occur in approximately 40% of patients. Late renal deterioration, with hypertension, proteinuria, and reduced renal function, after apparent resolution of the disease has been described. HUS is divided into two categories: epidemic or diarrhea-associated and nonepidemic or sporadic.

The epidemic form, which accounts for the majority of cases, is an abrupt illness that generally affects previously healthy children after the ingestion of foods contaminated with *Escherichia coli* O157:H7 (other bacteria have also been implicated). The peak incidence is from 6 months to 4 years of age, and there is a seasonal pattern, with most cases occurring between April and October. A generalized, toxin-mediated, thrombotic microangiopathy results, with diffuse colitis presenting as abdominal pain and hematochezia or bloody diarrhea. The diarrhea prodrome lasts for up to 12 days, followed by the onset of pallor and/or jaundice. Renal impairment is manifest by hematuria, proteinuria, and oliguria/anuria, but gross hematuria is rare. There may also be neurologic symptoms (coma, seizures, personality changes) and manifestations of fluid overload (edema, hypertension). The peripheral blood smear shows microangiopathic changes, including schistocytes and helmet cells, and thrombocytopenia (generally $<60,000/mm^3$) is a consistent feature. The Coombs test is negative, and the PT, PTT, and coagulation factors are normal.

Nonepidemic HUS accounts for fewer than 10% of cases and can occur at any age. There is no diarrheal prodrome, although an antecedent URI is often reported. Unlike epidemic HUS, the onset is slow and progressive.

Diagnosis

Make a rapid assessment of the patient's volume status, looking for clinical signs of dehydration (orthostatic changes in vital signs, poor capillary refill, weak peripheral pulses, hypotension) or volume overload (edema, rales, palpable liver, cardiac gallop). It is essential to identify the cause of oliguria as quickly as possible and to institute immediate treatment. Prerenal azotemia is a reversible condition early in its course; failure to recognize a prerenal etiology (hypovolemia) can lead to ATN.

If the patient is unable or unwilling to void spontaneously, insert a Foley catheter to obtain urine and monitor the urine output. To differentiate among the causes of oliguria, obtain urine for specific gravity, sodium and creatinine, and microscopy. Look for glomerular hematuria (*AGN*) or pyuria [>5 white blood cells (WBCs) per high-power field], which can be seen with *pyelonephritis* or *ATN secondary to drugs.*

Obtain blood for electrolytes, BUN, and creatinine, and calculate the fractional excretion of sodium (FENA) (Table 21-1):

$$FENA = (urine\ Na/plasma\ Na) / (urine\ Cr/plasma\ Cr)$$

If urine is unavailable or the urinary findings are pending and *there is no evidence of volume overload,* attempt to discriminate renal ARF from prerenal azotemia by rapidly infusing 20 mL/kg of an isotonic solution (normal saline, Ringer's lactate). If the oliguria persists and there are no signs of volume overload, repeat the bolus until it is clear that the patient is not volume-depleted (based on vital signs and capillary refill). If there is no diuresis, give one dose of IV furosemide (1–2 mg/kg). If oliguria continues, the diagnosis of *intrinsic renal disease* (frequently ATN) is probable. If urine output increases with these measures, the patient has *prerenal insufficiency* and the patient's condition will return to normal provided that adequate fluid therapy is given. A distended bladder suggests a *postrenal* problem. Confirmation of an obstructive cause requires a renal ultrasound.

ED Management

Renal ARF   Fluid restriction is required; limit fluids to insensible losses and urine output. Estimate insensible losses to be 400 mL/m²/day; losses are higher with fever and burns and lower with mechanical ventilation. The IV solution can be $D_5\frac{1}{2}NS$ or NS but remove potassium. A potassium >5 mEq/L requires an immediate ECG to look for peaked T waves (T wave height greater than or equal to one-half the R or S wave). The treatment of hyperkalemia entails enhancing potassium excretion or increasing

Table 21–1 Laboratory Findings in Acute Renal Failure

DIAGNOSIS	U_{SG}*	U_{Na}†(mEq/L)	BUN/Cr‡	FENA§(%)	U/A¶
Prerenal azotemia	>1.020	<20 μ	>20	<1%	Nonspecific
Acute glomerulonephitis (early)	>1.020	<20 μ	>20	<1%	RBC casts, dysmorphic RBCs
Acute tubular necrosis	1.008–1.012	>40 μ	<20	>1%	Tubular epithelial cells
Postrenal	1.008–1.012	>40 μ	<20	>1%	Nonspecific

*U_{SG} = urine specific gravity
†U_{Na} = urine sodium concentration
‡BUN/Cr = ratio of BUN to creatinine
§FENA = fractional excretion of sodium; $(U_{Na} \times P_{Cr})/(P_{Na} \times U_{Cr})$
¶U/A = typical urinalysis findings

the movement of potassium into cells and minimizing cardiac effects. In the absence of peaked T waves, treat with polystyrene sulfonate (Kayexalate), 1 g/kg dissolved in 4 mL of water, with sorbitol (PO or PR). This dose lowers the serum potassium by 0.5 to 1 mEq/L by enhancing GI excretion, but the onset is slow and duration is variable.

Hyperkalemia accompanied by ECG changes demands more aggressive IV therapy. Give 0.5 to 1.0 g/kg of glucose (2–4 mL/kg of a 25% dextrose solution) over 30 min *concurrently* with regular insulin (1 unit per 5 g of glucose given). The potassium-lowering effect occurs in 10 to 20 min, but carefully monitor the serum glucose for both hyperglycemia and hypoglycemia.

If there is a cardiac arrhythmia, give 10% calcium chloride (0.2–0.25 mL/kg) IV over 2 to 5 min, but do not administer calcium with a solution containing sodium bicarbonate, as calcium carbonate will be formed. The calcium-lowering effects are seen in 1 to 3 min. Complications include hypercalcemia and bradycardia; continuously monitor the ECG, and stop the calcium if the patient becomes bradycardic. Use the same regimen to treat hypocalcemia causing tetany, laryngospasm, arrhythmias, or seizures. When the symptoms have resolved, add maintenance calcium to the IV solution (100 mg of elemental calcium per kilogram per day). Administration of bicarbonate is not as effective as calcium in stabilizing the myocardium and does not reliably reduce the serum potassium.

Absolute indications for dialysis include life-threatening hyperkalemia (serum potassium ≥7 mEq/L), intractable acidosis, symptomatic volume overload [congestive heart failure (CHF), pulmonary edema], and symptomatic uremia (pleuritis, pericarditis, encephalopathy, GI bleeding).

Hypertension is frequent in ARF and may be mild and asymptomatic or life-threatening. Treat mild hypertension with salt restriction and oral antihypertensives; more severe hypertension requires IV therapy (p 610) and, in intractable cases, dialysis.

Postrenal ARF   If the patient has postrenal insufficiency, immediately consult with a urologist to determine the appropriate therapy.

Indications for Admission
- Acute renal failure
- HUS

BIBLIOGRAPHY

Bagga A: Management of acute renal failure. *Indian J Pediatr* 1999;66:225–239.
Brady HR, Brenner BM, Clarkson MR, et al: Acute renal failure, in Brenner BM (ed): *Brenner and Rector's the Kidney*, 6th ed. Philadelphia: Saunders, 1999, pp 1201–1246.
Flynn JT: Causes, management approaches, and outcome of acute renal failure in children. *Curr Opin Pediatr* 1998;10:184–189.

HEMATURIA

Hematuria is defined as 5 or more RBCs per high-power field of unspun urine or 1 to 2 RBCs per high-power field in a centrifuged specimen. Up to 5% of school-age children have microscopic hematuria on a single spe-cimen, and 1 to 2% have this finding subsequently confirmed. The inci-dence increases with age and is greater in girls.

Hematuria can be classified as either traumatic or nontraumatic in ori-gin. Nontraumatic hematuria can originate from the upper or lower geni-tourinary tract; upper tract bleeding may be further subdivided into glomerular and nonglomerular etiologies.

Clinical Presentation

Traumatic Bleeding
Because of their proportionately larger kidneys, less-developed abdominal musculature, and less perirenal fat, children are at increased risk for injury to the renal and genitourinary systems after blunt trauma. Up to 90% of children with significant renal or genitourinary trauma present with gross or microscopic hematuria. Findings may also include flank or lower abdominal pain, tenderness, abdominal rigidity, and, with bladder injuries, an inability to void. After blunt abdominal trauma, in the absence of obvious signs and symptoms of flank injury (abdominal tenderness, abrasions or contusions, fractured ribs or pelvis, penetrating wounds to the lower thorax/upper abdomen), microscopic hematuria with less than 50 RBCs per high-power field is not associated with significant renal injury.

Injury to the renal pedicle can be present without hematuria but is almost always associated with multisystem trauma and warrants further investigation.

Nontraumatic Bleeding
Lower Genitourinary Tract   Lower urinary tract bleeding is often accom-panied by suprapubic pain and dysuria. A *bacterial UTI* presents with urgency, frequency, pyuria, and bacteriuria, although these signs and symptoms may be absent in the infant or young child. *Viral cystitis* can occur in association with URI symptoms and is accompanied by fever and suprapubic tenderness. The urine culture will be negative, and the hema-turia resolves within 5 to 7 days without any specific treatment. A urethral *foreign body* presents with dysuria in an afebrile toddler. *Urolithiasis* can present with microscopic or gross hematuria and intense renal colic. Often the patient has a history of urinary tract abnormalities or infections. Some *drugs* (e.g., cyclophosphamide) are toxic to the bladder and can cause hemorrhagic cystitis.

Upper Genitourinary Tract: Glomerular   Hallmarks of glomerular bleeding include RBC casts, dysmorphic RBCs, and proteinuria in association with microscopic hematuria. In addition, edema, hyperten-sion, and oliguria can occur. There may be a history of a pharyngitis or impetigo in the previous 2 weeks (*poststreptococcal glomerulo-nephritis*) or URI in the previous 1 to 2 days (*IgA nephropathy, heredi-tary nephritis*). A family history of deafness and renal disease defines *Alport's syndrome* (hereditary nephritis). Palpable purpura of the lower extremities, abdominal pain, hematochezia, and arthralgias occur with

HSP. A history of a URI or diarrhea, followed by weakness, pallor, and CNS symptoms, is seen in *HUS*. Hematuria can be the presenting sign of *SLE,* or there can be associated findings (butterfly rash, polyserositis, arthritis, hematologic abnormalities).

Upper Tract: Nonglomerular   *Sickle cell trait* is associated with gross or microscopic hematuria without other obvious manifestations of renal disease. *Wilms' tumor* can cause brown or tea-colored urine in children under 6 years of age. However, hematuria is the presenting symptom in only 10% of cases of Wilms' tumor; most cases present with an abdominal mass. Congenital and anatomic abnormalities such as *polycystic kidney, renal hemangioma,* and *hydronephrosis* can also present with hematuria after minor blunt abdominal trauma. *Idiopathic hypercalciuria* in the absence of urolithiasis is a common cause of nonglomerular painless hematuria, usually gross. There is often a positive family history of renal stones.

Diagnosis

Hematuria must be confirmed by microscopic examination of the urine, since not all red urine contains blood. Foodstuffs such as *beets, red dyes,* and drugs such as *rifampin* and *phenazopyridine* can give the urine a red tint. A urine dipstick will detect RBCs in the urine, as well as *hemoglobin* and *myoglobin.* Also, hematuria may be incorrectly diagnosed when a *menstruating female* provides a voided urine specimen.

Gross hematuria can be bright red to brown. The urine sample from a patient with gross hematuria is always turbid, owing to the presence of RBCs. This is in contrast to pigmenturia, in which the urine is wine-colored but transparent. *Pigmenturia* due to myoglobin or hemoglobin can be differentiated by centrifugation of a sample of serum; a pink tinge is found with hemoglobin, whereas the serum is clear with myoglobin.

A careful urinalysis is critical for locating the source of the bleeding. With *nonglomerular hematuria*, the RBCs appear eumorphic. Gross nonglomerular hematuria is usually red and may be associated with clots. With *glomerular hematuria* there are usually RBC casts, and the RBCs are dysmorphic (distorted or fractured). In gross hematuria of glomerular origin, the urine is cloudy and dark brown (cola- or tea-colored) and never associated with clots.

Idiopathic hypercalciuria is suggested by a spot urine Ca:Cr ratio >0.21. However, confirmation requires a 24-h urine collection with a calcium excretion >4 mg/kg/day.

Microscopic hematuria that occurs only with fever or exercise is usually transient and does not indicate any underlying pathology.

ED Management

Obtain a thorough history, including current symptoms (fever, dysuria, suprapubic pain, URI, pharyngitis, gastroenteritis, joint pain), recent genitourinary trauma, medication use, previous episodes of hematuria or sickle cell trait or disease, and family history of renal disease or deafness [hereditary nephritis (Alport's syndrome) accounts for nearly 40% of patients with microscopic hematuria of glomerular origin]. Priorities on physical examination include measuring the blood pressure and evaluating the patient for rash or purpura, abdominal mass, signs of a bleeding disorder, edema, and arthritis.

Traumatic Hematuria   After blunt abdominal trauma, an intravenous pyelogram (IVP) or abdominal CT is indicated for gross hematuria or microscopic hematuria with more than 50 RBCs per high-power field. In the absence of hematuria, however, clinical evidence of renal injury (flank or lower abdominal tenderness or mass, difficulty voiding, low rib or pelvic fracture) demands an imaging study. Conservative management and careful follow-up are recommended for asymptomatic patients with isolated microscopic hematuria (less than 50 RBCs per high-power field). Hematuria caused by penetrating abdominal trauma is an indication for immediate imaging studies or laparotomy, depending on the clinical situation (see Genitourinary Trauma, pp 258–262).

Nontraumatic Hematuria   In the absence of edema, hypertension, an abdominal mass, proteinuria, or oliguria, the workup of nontraumatic hematuria can be performed on an outpatient basis. If the bleeding is non-glomerular, obtain a urine culture, sickle prep, and measurement of urinary calcium excretion. Order an ultrasound if there is gross hematuria. When there is isolated hematuria of glomerular origin, minimal testing is warranted. Obtain a BUN, creatinine, and C3 and C4 levels if there is a history of hematuria for more than 6 months.

Admit any patient with signs of acute glomerulonephritis (edema, hypertension, oliguria, proteinuria in association with microscopic hematuria). In addition to the initial workup outlined above, further evaluation includes total protein and albumin, serology (ANA, ASLO, VDRL), and consultation with a nephrologist.

Follow-up

- Asymptomatic patient with traumatic hematuria: next day
- Nontraumatic hematuria (<50 RBCs per high-power field) with a normal PE and without signs of glomerulonephritis or renal failure: primary care or nephrology follow-up in 2 to 4 weeks

Indications for Admission

- Posttraumatic hematuria with abnormal IVP (renal contusion, laceration, collecting system injury, major-vessel injury)
- Renal failure or acute glomerulonephritis with edema, hypertension, or oliguria
- Hematuria associated with an abdominal mass

BIBLIOGRAPHY

Ahn JH, Morey AF, McAninch JW: Workup and management of traumatic hematuria. *Emerg Med Clin North Am* 1998;16:145–164.

Diven SC, Travis LB: A practical primary care approach to hematuria in children. *Pediatr Nephrol* 2000;14:65–72.

Feld LG, Waz WR, Pérez LM: Hematuria. *Pediatr Clin North Am* 1997;44: 1191–1210.

HYPERTENSION

Hypertension is defined as a blood pressure that is equal to or greater than the 95th percentile for age and gender on three measurements. Hypertension is estimated to occur in 1 to 3% of children under the age of 13 years. In the ED, hypertension can be divided into two categories: nonemergent and emergent. In nonemergent hypertension (>95th percentile but <99th percentile), the blood pressure elevation is mild and is detected as an incidental finding. Further diagnostic evaluation can usually be deferred until a later, scheduled visit.

Emergent hypertension in children is unusual; the most common causes are renal parenchymal disorders, renal vascular lesions, pheochromocytoma, and drugs. The patient has symptoms (headache, disorientation, seizures) that can be ascribed to the increase in blood pressure, the blood pressure exceeds the 99th percentile in both upper extremities on at least three successive readings by two examiners over 10 min, or the primary disease demands emergency treatment (increased intracranial pressure, renal failure). In these cases, urgent therapy is required. The detailed diagnostic evaluation can be deferred to the inpatient setting.

Clinical Presentation and Diagnosis

It is imperative that the blood pressure cuff is the correct size. A cuff that is too narrow gives a falsely high reading. The appropriate width of the inflation bladder is at least two-thirds the distance from the acromion to the olecranon, and the bladder should be long enough to encircle the arm completely. Use age-specific blood pressure tables adjusted for height (e.g., the *Harriet Lane Handbook*) to confirm the normal ranges of blood pressure in children.

In general, defer the diagnostic evaluation of asymptomatic hypertension to a primary care setting, where further testing can be delayed until sustained hypertension is confirmed by repeated measurements. However, elicit a hypertension-oriented history: neonatal history (prematurity, umbilical line catheterization), *congenital anomalies*, medication or herbal remedy use (*sympathomimetics, ephedra, oral contraceptives*), illicit drug use (*cocaine*), *cardiac or renal disease* (especially hematuria), the nature of any previous hypertensive episodes (particularly if episodic), and a *family history of hypertension*. Useful physical examination findings include height and weight, differential blood pressure and pulses between upper and lower extremities, heart murmur, abdominal mass and bruits, virilization, skin lesions (purpura in HSP), and signs of increased intracranial pressure.

In general, the younger the child and the higher the blood pressure, the more likely that the hypertension is secondary to some other cause. Sixty to 80% of secondary hypertension in children is renal in origin.

ED Management

Urgent parenteral therapy is required for life-threatening hypertension, especially if there are neurologic symptoms (visual changes, headache, seizures). Give IV labetalol (0.2–1.0 mg/kg, 20 mg per dose maximum, 100–150 mg/day maximum). Repeat the dose every 10 min as needed or, after the initial bolus, start a continuous infusion of 0.4 to 1.0 mg/kg/h. The onset of action is in 2 to 5 min. Labetalol is contraindicated if the patient has asthma, since it is a combined alpha/beta blocker. IV nifedipine (0.25–0.5 mg/kg/dose, maximum 10 mg/dose) may also be used, and limited data support the IV use of nicardipine (0.5–5 μg/kg/min). As an alternative, give sublingual nifedipine (0.25–0.5 mg/kg, 10 mg maximum). Puncture the capsule first and drop the liquid into the child's mouth; the onset of action is in 5 to 10 min. The goal of acute antihypertensive therapy is a 20% reduction in the mean blood pressure [diastolic + ⅓ (systolic − diastolic)]. If the blood pressure responds, admit the patient to an intensive care unit (ICU), consult a nephrologist, and start maintenance therapy with an angiotensin converting enzyme (ACE) inhibitor such as captopril (0.3–0.6 mg/kg q 6–8 h over 6 months; 0.05–0.1 mg/kg for an infant under 6 months of age).

If the blood pressure does not respond within 30 min and the patient has life-threatening hypertension, begin a sodium nitroprusside continuous infusion with an initial dose of 0.3 to 0.5 μg/kg/min and titrate to an effective dose (maximum 10 μg/kg/min). Advantages include immediate onset of action, ease of titration, and immediate cessation of antihypertensive activity when the drip is discontinued. Cover the IV tubing with foil to avoid exposure to light. Side effects include thiocyanate poisoning, which presents with a progressive metabolic acidosis; this generally occurs with rapid infusion or long-term use (several days).

Before admission, obtain a urinalysis, serum electrolytes, BUN and creatinine, chest x-ray, and ECG, and schedule a renal ultrasound. If an adrenal cause is suspected (virilization, cushingoid appearance), obtain a serum cortisol and 17-hydroxyprogesterone. If there are symptoms suggestive of a pheochromocytoma (headache, sweating, nausea, vomiting), obtain a 24-h urine collection for catecholamine excretion.

Follow-up

- Asymptomatic or mild to moderate hypertension: primary care follow-up in 1 to 2 weeks

Indications for Admission

- Symptomatic or severe hypertension (sustained systolic and/or diastolic >99th percentile for age)
- Hypertension of any degree associated with acute glomerulonephritis or any other urgent underlying condition

BIBLIOGRAPHY

Bartosh SM, Aronson AJ: Childhood hypertension. An update on etiology, diagnosis, and treatment. *Pediatr Clin North Am* 1999;46:235–252.

Harriet Lane Handbook, 16th ed. Philadelphia: Mosby, 2002, pp 128–131.

National Heart, Lung, and Blood Institute: Update on the 1987 Task Force on High Blood Pressure in Children and Adolescents: A working group from the National High Blood Pressure Education Program. *Pediatrics* 1996;98:649–658.

Norwood VF: Hypertension. *Pediatr Rev* 2002;23:197–208.

Sinaiko A: Hypertension in children. *N Engl J Med* 1996;335:1968–1973.

PROTEINURIA

Normal urine contains no protein (as detected by the usual clinical tests), while proteinuria is present in many renal diseases. However, with vigorous exercise, stress, or fever, or when the urine is highly concentrated (specific gravity >1.025) or alkaline (pH >8.0), small amounts of protein may be present as an incidental finding in an otherwise healthy child. Because the urine dipstick is very sensitive (particularly to albumin, but not to low-molecular-weight proteins) and detects protein concentrations as low as 10 to 15 mg/dL, qualitative proteinuria is prevalent in 5 to 15% of normal individuals. Significant proteinuria (>2+ on dipstick) is defined as follows:

$$\text{Urinary protein (mg/dL)} / \text{urinary creatinine (mg/dL)} > 0.2$$

Fewer than 2% of patients with dipstick proteinuria will have significant proteinuria. When proteinuria is ≥1+ by dipstick on several occasions, further investigation is warranted. False-negative results on urine dipstick can occur with very dilute urine.

Nephrotic Syndrome   The nephrotic syndrome is defined as edema, hypoalbuminemia, hyperlipidemia, and heavy proteinuria with a urinary protein/creatinine ratio >2. A glomerular protein leak is the primary disturbance in this syndrome. In contrast to AGN, the GFR is usually normal. Although there are numerous causes of nephrotic syndrome, minimal change nephrotic syndrome (MCNS) is the most common type in children (75%), with a peak incidence between 2 and 5 years of age. Other primary etiologies are focal segmental glomerulosclerosis, membranoproliferative glomerulonephritis, and membranous nephropathy. Secondary causes include systemic disorders such as HSP, SLE and sickle cell disease, chronic infections (syphilis, HIV, hepatitis B), and medications (captopril, penicillamine, nonsteroidal anti-inflammatory medications). Children with nephrotic syndrome are at risk for electrolyte disturbances, infections (cellulitis, spontaneous bacterial peritonitis), and thromboembolism.

Clinical Presentation

Most often, proteinuria is an unexpected finding in a child being examined for fever, vomiting, or diarrhea. Edema, hypoalbuminemia (<3 g/dL), hypercholesterolemia, apparent hypocalcemia (secondary to the decreased albumin), and peritonitis (rare) are findings in the nephrotic syndrome. In patients with *isolated proteinuria* or the nephrotic syndrome, the blood pressure and renal function are generally normal, although urine output may be decreased. With renal disease such as *glomerulonephritis*, there may be edema, hypertension, oliguria, or associated microscopic hematuria. *Orthostatic proteinuria* occurs only in samples voided in the upright position. This is a variant of normal and is usually found in adolescents.

Diagnosis

Very few patients with dipstick proteinuria truly have renal disease. In the absence of edema, hypertension, oliguria, or associated hematuria, merely repeat the urinalysis in 2 to 4 weeks. Examine urine obtained with the patient upright and also with the patient recumbent. If the proteinuria persists, test an early-morning specimen. If this sample is negative, the patient is either normal or has *orthostatic proteinuria.* Consider causes other than MCNS if the child is below 1 year of age or above 10 years of age or if there are associated clinical findings, such as fever, rash, or arthralgias. A patient with associated microscopic hematuria is more likely to have *glomerular disease.*

Although edema is a cardinal feature of the nephrotic syndrome, extrarenal causes of edema include *cirrhosis, congestive heart failure,* and *protein-losing enteropathy.* Significant proteinuria is absent in these conditions.

The most expeditious method of measuring urinary protein excretion is a determination of the protein:creatinine ratio in an early-morning (first void) specimen. This determination correlates well with the 24-h urinary protein excretion in patients with renal disease. Moreover, it simplifies the diagnosis of orthostatic proteinuria and eliminates the need for a cumbersome 24-h collection. Normally, this ratio is below 0.2; with nephrotic-range proteinuria, it is above 2.

ED Management

Children with edema, hypertension, oliguria, or associated hematuria require an immediate and more complete evaluation, including serum electrolytes, BUN, calcium, creatinine and creatinine clearance, cholesterol, total protein and albumin, complement (C3, C4), ANA, ASLO, VDRL, serology for hepatitis B and C, and HIV testing (if indicated). However, follow a patient with isolated subnephrotic proteinuria (urinary protein:creatinine ratio of 0.2–2.0) for at least 6 to 12 months before arranging a renal biopsy.

Nephrotic Syndrome   Admit a patient with nephrotic syndrome who has moderate to severe edema or complications associated with nephrotic syndrome (e.g., peritonitis) and consult with a pediatric nephrologist to decide whether corticosteroid therapy and a renal biopsy are necessary.

Follow-up

- Nonnephrotic proteinuria: primary care follow-up in 2 to 4 weeks

Indications for Admission

- Proteinuria in association with signs or symptoms of renal disease (moderate to severe edema, hypertension, oliguria, electrolyte disturbances, infection, thromboembolism)
- Infant with nephrotic syndrome
- Nephrotic syndrome with fever or abdominal complaints

BIBLIOGRAPHY

Hogg RJ, Portman RJ, Milliner D, et al: Evaluation and management of proteinuria and nephrotic syndrome in children: recommendations from a pediatric nephrology panel established at the National Kidney Foundation Conference on Proteinuria, Albuminuria, Risk, Assessment, Detection, Elimination (PARADE). *Pediatrics* 2000;105:1242–1249.

Leung AK, Robson WL: Evaluating the child with proteinuria. *J R Soc Health* 2000;120:16–22.

Loghman-Adham M: Evaluating proteinuria in children. *Am Fam Physician* 1998; 58:1145–1159.

URINARY TRACT INFECTIONS

Urinary tract infections (UTIs) occur in approximately 4 to 7% of febrile infants and 3 to 5% of febrile school-age children (predominantly girls). Extensive epidemiologic evidence suggests that uncircumcised boys under 1 year of age have a 10-fold relative risk of having a UTI compared to circumcised boys. The two most common types of infection are cystitis (infection confined to the bladder) and pyelonephritis (infection in the renal parenchyma). The most frequent etiology is *E. coli;* other causative organisms include *Klebsiella, Pseudomonas, Enterococcus, Staphylococcus saprophyticus,* and *Staphylococcus epidermidis,* which is not a contaminant if cultured repeatedly, particularly in adolescent girls. *Proteus* is an important pathogen in uncircumcised boys, but it is less common in girls and may be a contaminant.

Clinical Presentation

The presentation in infancy is nonspecific and includes poor feeding, vomiting, diarrhea, irritability, jaundice, and seizures. From 1 month to 2 years, fever is more common, and some urologic symptoms (change in voiding pattern, foul-smelling urine) occur. Preschool- and school-age children usually have specific urologic complaints, such as frequency, urgency, dysuria, suprapubic pain, and enuresis. However, less specific symptoms, such as abdominal pain and vomiting, may also be seen in this age group. Fever ($>38.5°C$, $101.3°F$), flank (CVA) tenderness, and systemic toxicity are consistent with pyelonephritis.

Diagnosis

Traditionally, the amount of bacterial growth required for the diagnosis of UTI is $\geq 10^5$ colony-forming units (CFU) per milliliter in a midstream clean-catch urine, and $>10^4$ in a catheterized specimen. Any growth in a urine culture obtained by suprapubic bladder tap is considered significant. However, the concept of "significant bacteriuria" is a statistical one, indicating an 80% chance of true infection; two consecutive positive cultures increase the likelihood of infection to 95%. In fact, a culture with a pure growth of $>10^2$ CFU/mL from a catheterized or voided specimen, in the context of symptoms associated with UTI may be indicative of infection. Prompt plating of the specimen is as important as compulsive cleaning of the perineum and urethral meatus for reducing the frequency of false-positive urine cultures. If the urine specimen cannot be plated immediately, refrigerate at 4°C (39.2°F) to prevent overgrowth of contaminating bacteria. A bagged urine specimen is unreliable unless the culture demonstrates no growth.

Urinalysis findings are not sufficient for a definitive diagnosis. However, the urinalysis is a useful screening test in the ED. If a complete urinalysis is normal (including dipstick testing for leukocyte esterase and nitrite and microscopic examination for bacteriuria), the likelihood that the patient *does not* have a UTI exceeds 95%. With a UTI, the urinalysis usually has more than 10 WBCs per high-power field of centrifuged urine, although pyuria may be absent in some culture-proven UTIs. Alternatively, only 50% of patients with WBCs in the urine have a culture-proven UTI, as pyuria can occur with infections near but outside the urinary tract. With a UTI, proteinuria and hematuria are often present, and the leukocyte esterase is generally positive on dipstick testing. The dipstick nitrite test has a low sensitivity in infants and young children who void frequently; urine must remain in the bladder for at least 4 h for bacteria to produce the nitrite. The presence of any organisms on Gram's stain of an uncentrifuged urine correlates with a colony count $>10^5$/mL and is presumptive evidence of a UTI, with higher sensitivity, specificity, and positive predictive value than urinalysis and dipstick. However, the urine culture remains the definitive diagnostic test.

WBC casts (not clumps) are usually diagnostic of *pyelonephritis.* Other laboratory findings with pyelonephritis are leukocytosis (WBCs $>15,000$/mm^3) and an elevated sedimentation rate (>30 mm/h). There are no reliable laboratory tests to discriminate cystitis and pyelonephritis, although a DMSA scan may prove to be the best method of verifying renal parenchymal infection. Pyelonephritis causes patchy uptake of the radionuclide during the acute infection.

Symptoms of a UTI are not sufficient for a definitive diagnosis. Dysuria, frequency, and urgency among patients with suprapubic tenderness and gross hematuria without pyuria or bacteriuria suggest *viral cystitis* or *idiopathic hypercalciuria.* The same findings in a patient with pyuria but no hematuria are compatible with the *dysuria-pyuria (acute urethral) syndrome.* The symptoms of *vaginitis* and *balanitis* can mimic a UTI. Negative urine cultures are necessary to confirm these diagnoses.

ED Management

Inspect the external genitalia for signs of inflammation or infection, and measure the blood pressure. Obtain a catheterized or suprapubic urine culture specimen from a patient who lacks bladder control, has evidence of vaginitis, or is unable to provide an adequate midstream specimen. A bagged specimen can be used for a screening urinalysis when the clinical condition of the child does not warrant immediate antimicrobial therapy. If the urinalysis suggests an infection, obtain a suprapubic or catheterized urine specimen for culture. In an older child or adolescent, when a midstream specimen is used, collect samples from two separate voids to increase the likelihood of a noncontaminated culture. A large number of epithelial cells in these specimens suggests contamination.

After urine cultures are obtained, treat a nontoxic patient with signs or symptoms and microscopy results consistent with a lower tract infection on an outpatient basis with a 10-day course of trimethoprim-sulfamethoxazole (TMP-SMX; 8 mg/kg/day of TMP divided bid, 160 mg/dose TMP maximum). Use cefixime 8 mg/kg/day divided bid (400 mg/day maximum) or loracarbef 15 to 30 mg/kg/day divided bid (400 mg/day maximum) when there is a known high level of resistance to TMP-SMX in the community. Treat an afebrile, nonpregnant adolescent girl with an uncomplicated lower tract infection (symptoms for <3 days and no history of urinary tract abnormality), with ciprofloxacin 250 mg twice a day for 3 days or TMP-SMX DS (160 mg/tab TMP) twice a day for 3 days. This therapy may be especially useful when compliance with a 10-day oral regimen is not assured. However, 3-day treatment is inadequate for infants and children.

Indications for admission and IV antibiotics include toxic appearance, inability to tolerate oral intake (including antibiotics), dehydration, or immunocompromise as well as in cases where adequate adherence to treatment and/or follow-up seems unlikely. Also admit an infant less than 3 months old regardless of clinical appearance. Treat as follows:

Below 4 weeks of age: Since a young infant with a UTI is at risk for sepsis, treat with ampicillin (<1 week of age: 100 mg/kg/day, divided q 12 h; >1 week of age: 200 mg/kg/day, divided q 6 h) *and* cefotaxime (<1 week: 100 mg/kg/day, divided q 12 h; 1–4 weeks: 150 mg/kg/day, divided q 8 h).

Between 4 and 8 weeks of age: ceftriaxone 100 mg/kg/day divided q 12 h

Above 8 weeks of age: ceftriaxone 75 mg/kg/day divided q 12 h

Continue parenteral therapy until the patient is afebrile and the urine culture is sterile (usually 2–3 days). Obtain a follow-up urine culture after 48 h if the patient does not have the expected clinical response to the appropriate antibiotic, the organism has intermediate sensitivity or resistance to the selected antibiotic, or the sensitivities of the organism are not available.

It is important to determine whether there is anatomic or functional uropathology, particularly vesicoureteral reflux (VUR). Radiographic evaluation is indicated following a UTI in a girl under 3 years of age, after two or more episodes in a girl over 3 years of age, in boys at any age, and in any patient after an episode of pyelonephritis or an atypical UTI with hypertension or a flank mass.

For a child under 3 years of age, obtain an ultrasound to evaluate urinary tract anatomy and a voiding cystourethrogram (VCUG) under fluoroscopy to detect VUR. Although an ultrasound may be performed at any time after a UTI is diagnosed, a sterile urine culture must be obtained before the VCUG is performed. If VUR of grade 2 or worse is found, a DMSA scan is necessary. In a child with VUR or suspected pyelonephritis, a DMSA scan is indicated 2 to 4 months after resolution of the UTI. The delay is necessary to distinguish acute, reversible changes related to the episode of pyelonephritis from permanent renal parenchymal scarring. With the widespread use of radionuclide scans an IVP is rarely needed to visualize the kidneys after a UTI.

For a child over 3 years of age, ultrasonography is sufficient. Also obtain a VCUG if there are findings suggestive of reflux. Siblings of patients with VUR require urinary tract imaging, as this is a heritable abnormality.

Recurrences are common in children with abnormal urinary tracts; 80% occur in the first year after a UTI. Patients must have follow-up cultures monthly for 3 months, then every 3 months for a year, and then every 6 months for 2 years. Routine surveillance cultures are unnecessary in children with normal urinary tracts.

Follow-up

- Persistent symptoms on appropriate antibiotic therapy: within 2 days to repeat a urine culture
- Imaging studies required for evaluation of the urinary tract: at the completion of antibiotic therapy for the infection to institute antibiotic prophylaxis

Indications for Admission

- Upper tract infections (pyelonephritis) in a patient under 3 months of age
- Any age: toxic-appearing, dehydrated, inability to tolerate oral intake, immunocompromised, at risk for nonadherence to treatment or follow-up plan
- UTI with fever in a patient at risk for decreased renal function (decreased GFR, single kidney)

BIBLIOGRAPHY

American Academy of Pediatrics. Committee on Quality Improvement. Subcommittee on Urinary Tract Infection: Practice parameter: the diagnosis, treatment, and evaluation of the initial urinary tract infection in febrile infants and young children. *Pediatrics* 1999;103:843–852.

Lindert KA, Shortliffe LM: Evaluation and management of pediatric urinary tract infections. *Urol Clin North Am* 1999;26:719–728.

MacNeily AE: Pediatric urinary tract infections: current controversies. *Can J Urol* 2001;8:18–23.

Tran D, Muchant DG, Aronoff SC: Short-course versus conventional length therapy for uncomplicated lower urinary tract infections in children: a meta-analysis of 1279 patients. *J Pediatr* 2001;139:93–99.

CHAPTER 22

Sedation and Analgesia

Alison Brent

In the emergency department, sedation and analgesia are required for a wide variety of procedures. The ideal drug or drug combination has a rapid and predictable onset of action, short duration, and minimal side effects. It is readily reversible and has a reasonable margin of safety. Currently, there is no perfect drug or drug combination for all situations; it is necessary to tailor the choice of drug to the procedure, child, and institution. *The use of these drugs requires that personnel skilled in pediatric resuscitation be immediately available.* Always provide sedation or analgesia in accordance with the 1992 American Academy of Pediatrics *Guidelines for Monitoring and Management of Pediatric Patients During and After Sedation for Diagnostic and Therapeutic Procedures.*

To maximize patient safety, each ED should generate protocols and flow sheets for all patients treated with sedative and analgesic drugs. Obtain written consent before the procedure, in accordance with institutional requirements. Document the health history, including dietary and fasting information, physical examination, vital signs, and weight in kilograms. Only patients who can be assigned to American Society of Anesthesiologists (ASA) Physical Status Classification ASA I to III should receive sedation and analgesia in the ED (Table 22-1). All others require consultation with anesthesia.

Fasting Guidelines

The use of sedative and analgesic agents always poses a risk of loss of protective airway reflexes, resulting in regurgitation of gastric contents and aspiration into the airway. This risk is increased in the ED because of underlying medical conditions (e.g., head trauma) and frequent uncertainty of fasting history (e.g., multiple trauma victim; nonverbal, unconscious, or frightened child; transported without parents or guardians). In a nonurgent situation, strict adherence to fasting guidelines should be maintained. However, an emergent procedure may take precedence over the risk for aspiration. Current recommendations for preprocedure restrictions

Table 22-1   American Society of Anesthesiologists (ASA) Physical Status Classification System

ASA CLASS	PATIENT DESCRIPTION
I	Healthy, no underlying organic disease
II	Mild or moderate systemic disease that does not interfere with daily routines (e.g., well-controlled asthma, essential hypertension)
III	Organic disease with definite functional impairment (e.g., severe steroid dependent asthma, insulin-dependent diabetes, uncorrected congenital heart disease)
IV	Severe disease that is life-threatening (e.g., head trauma with increased intracranial pressure)
V	Moribund patient, not expected to survive
E (suffix)	Physical status classification appended with an "E" connotes a procedure undertaken as an emergency (e.g., an otherwise healthy patient presenting for fracture reduction is classified as ASA physical status 1 E)

are as follows: clear fluids 2 h, breast milk 4 h, formula 6 h, and solids 8 h. In urgent or emergent situations, the need to proceed must be weighed against the benefit of delaying the procedure to allow for gastric emptying. If a window of opportunity to prescribe drugs is available, give metoclopramide, 0.15 mg/kg IV, which increases gastric emptying and improves lower esophageal sphincter tone, and ranitidine, 1.0 mg/kg IV, to decrease gastric acidity, plus a nonparticulate antacid, such as sodium citrate (2 to 3 mEq/kg/day divided tid or qid) Give these drugs expeditiously. However, pharmacologic emptying of the stomach does not guarantee an empty stomach or eliminate the risk of aspiration.

SEDATION

Chloral Hydrate

Indications for Use   Chloral hydrate is a sedative hypnotic agent used for sedation and anxiolysis for electroencephalograms (EEGs), CT or MRI scans, and other painless studies.

Equipment   Pulse oximeter.

Technique of Administration   Chloral hydrate is well absorbed after PO or PR administration. It may be given rectally in suppository form or dissolved in cottonseed oil or olive oil as a retention enema.

Monitoring   Use continuous pulse oximetry and recheck the vital signs hourly. Neonates require close observation for paradoxical excitation.

Dose   Chloral hydrate sedative dose: 50 to 75 mg/kg (maximum 500 mg); hypnotic dose: 75 to 100 mg/kg (maximum 1 g).

Advantages   Chloral hydrate is easy to administer PO or PR and, at therapeutic doses, has minimal effect on the patient's cardiovascular or respiratory status.

Disadvantages   Chloral hydrate has an unpredictable onset and duration of action, is irreversible once it takes effect, and has a 30 to 40% failure rate (patient either does not fall asleep or becomes more agitated). In the presence of pain, it may produce excitement or delirium. This drug does not produce conscious sedation but rather renders patients unconscious. Contrary to popular belief, it is not a "safe" drug. Airway compromise can occur secondary to positioning, such as neck hyperflexion, while the patient is in a car seat or carrier, while en route to an outpatient procedure. Chloral hydrate has an unpleasant taste and may cause gastrointestinal irritation. Therapeutic doses may cause epigastric distress, nausea, vomiting, and flatulence, while overdosage may result in gastric necrosis. In rare instances, arrhythmias [sinus arrhythmias, wandering atrial pacemaker, multifocal premature ventricular contractions (PVCs)] occur with therapeutic doses. Recovery can be prolonged, with "hangover" and light-headedness.

Conclusion   Despite the risk of mechanical airway obstruction, chloral hydrate remains one of the most popular sedative agents used for procedures. Do not allow the family to give chloral hydrate at home. It must be administered under a physician's supervision. Afterwards, patients must be monitored until the presedation level of consciousness is reached (which may take hours).

Chloral hydrate is easy to administer and, if used with a careful delivery and monitoring protocol, has some utility in the ED setting for nonpainful procedures, including CT and EEG. Typically, it is not useful for MRI. The unpleasant taste, GI irritation, long and unpredictable onset and duration of action, high failure rate, significant degree of "hangover," and mechanical airway obstruction that chloral hydrate may cause decrease its utility in the ED setting.

BENZODIAZEPINES

Benzodiazepines cause sedation, antegrade amnesia, and skeletal muscle relaxation; they also reduce anxiety. Doses used for sedation have a minimal effect on respiratory and cardiovascular function.

Midazolam (Versed)

Indications for Use   Midazolam is a short-acting benzodiazepine indicated for conscious sedation, anxiolysis, skeletal muscle relaxation, and amnesia for painful procedures.

Equipment   IV or IM equipment, pulse oximeter, flumazenil, oxygen, and resuscitation equipment and medications.

Technique of Administration   Midazolam may be administered IV, IM, IN/SL, PO, or PR.

Monitoring   Use continuous pulse oximetry and recheck the vital signs every 15 min. With the onset of medication effect, there is a normal slowing of the rate and depth of respirations.

Dose   Until recently, only the IV preparation was available for all routes of administration, which was unsatisfactory for oral administration because of the bitter aftertaste. A cherry flavored oral preparation is now available (2 mg/mL). Doses for the various routes of administration are as follows:

IV	0.1 to 0.3 mg/kg (5 mg maximum)
IM	0.2 to 0.4 mg/kg (5 mg maximum)
IN/SL	0.2 to 0.5 mg/kg (6 mg maximum)
PR	0.3 to 0.6 mg/kg (7 mg maximum)
PO	0.4 to 0.9 mg/kg (8 mg maximum)

Advantages   Midazolam has a rapid and predictable onset of action and a short recovery time. It provides amnesia for the event and is reversible. The new oral formulation has made PO administration attractive in the ED.

Disadvantages   The primary concerns with midazolam are respiratory suppression and laryngospasm. Other disadvantages are hallucinations, difficulty with spatial relations, and mild hypotension. Flumazenil reverses the effects and side effects of midazolam; however, use flumazenil as an adjunct to appropriate airway management; not as a substitute for it. Owing to the short half-life of flumazenil as compared with midazolam, there is a risk of resedation.

Conclusion   Midazolam is an effective drug for sedation when used with a monitoring protocol. It has a rapid and predictable onset of action, and patients recover rapidly with little residual "hangover." The added benefits of reversibility and amnesia surrounding the unpleasant event and muscle relaxation make it attractive for use in the ED.

Alternative Benzodiazepines
These are diazepam (Valium) and lorazepam (Ativan) (see Table 22-2).

Benzodiazepine Reversal
See Table 22-2.

Table 22-2 Sedative Agents

DRUG	ROUTE OF ADMINISTRATION	DOSE	MAXIMAL DOSE	TIME TO ONSET (MIN)	DURATION OF ACTION
Chloral hydrate	PO/PR	Sedative: 50–75 mg/kg	500 mg	30–100	4–8 h
		Hypnotic: 75–100 mg/kg	1 g	30–100	4–8 h
Benzodiazepines					
Midazolam	PO	0.4–0.9 mg/kg	8 mg	3–15	1.5–3.0 h
(Versed)	IV	0.1–0.3 mg/kg	5 mg	15	1.5–3.0 h
	IM	0.2–0.4 mg/kg	5 mg	10–15	1.5–3.0 h
	IN/SL	0.2–0.5 mg/kg	6 mg	3–15	1.5–3.0 h
	PR	0.3–0.6 mg/kg	7 mg	3–15	1.5–3.0 h
Diazepam	PO	0.05–0.2 mg/kg	5 mg	15–45	7–8 h
(Valium)	IV	0.05–0.2 mg/kg slowly over 3 min	5 mg	1–5	15–60 min
Lorazepam (Ativan)	IM	0.05 mg/kg	20 mg	15–30	2–8 h
	IV	0.03 mg/kg	5 mg	1–5	2–8 h
Benzodiazepine reversal					
Flumazenil (Mazicon)	IV	0.01 mg/kg initial dose then 0.005 mg/kg/min	1.0 mg (0.2 mg/min)	1–2	10–20 min
Barbiturates					
Pentobarbital	PO	2–6 mg/kg	200 mg	15–60	2–4 h
(Nembutal)	PR	2–6 mg/kg	200 mg	15–60	2–4 h
	IM (deep)	2–6 mg/kg	150 mg	5–15	2–4 h
	IV	0.5–1.0 mg/kg initial dose titrate to 6.0 mg/kg	150 mg	1–10	1–4 h
Methohexital (Brevital)	PR	20–30 mg/kg	1 gram	7–10	30–90 min

PO = by mouth; PR = per rectum; IV = intravenous; IM = intramuscular; SL = sublingual; IN = intranasal;

621

BARBITURATES

Pentobarbital

Indications for Use   Pentobarbital (Nembutal) is an intermediate-acting sedative-hypnotic that can be used to sedate children undergoing nonpainful studies in which motion is an issue (e.g., diagnostic imaging studies).

Equipment   Material for IV, IM, PO, and PR administration.

Technique of Administration   Pentobarbital may be given by the PO, PR, deep IM injection, or IV routes. The PO, PR, and IM routes have a fairly prolonged onset of action, whereas the IV route is rapid and can be titrated to effect.

Monitoring   Use continuous pulse oximetry and recheck vital signs every 15 min.

Dose   Doses for the various routes of administration are as follows:

IV   Initial dose: 0.5 to 1.0 mg/kg. Titrate to a maximum of 6 mg/kg or 150 mg.

IM   Initial dose: 2 to 6 mg/kg (150 mg maximum)

PO   Initial dose: 2 to 6 mg/kg (200 mg maximum)

PR   Initial dose: 2 to 6 mg/kg (200 mg maximum)

Advantages   The advantages of pentobarbital are its effective and predictable production of sedation and immobility.

Disadvantages   The disadvantages are a relatively slow onset of action and prolonged duration of sedation. Irritation at the injection site may occur after deep IM administration. When pentobarbital is given intravenously, the risks of apnea, respiratory depression, and laryngospasm are increased. Pentobarbital is not effective in patients who are taking barbiturates regularly.

Conclusion   Pentobarbital is an effective sedative that is a popular choice for patients undergoing CT scanning and MRI. It is relatively safe via the PO, PR, and IM routes. Although its onset of action is relatively slower than that of other sedatives, it is superior to chloral hydrate with regard to versatility in administration, which makes it an alternative in many settings. All barbiturates are associated with significant and potentially life-threatening side effects, including respiratory depression, apnea, airway obstruction, coma, paradoxical excitement, and residual sedation or "hangover," which may impair behavior, mood, and judgment for 24 h or longer.

Methohexital

Indications for Use   Methohexital (Brevital) is a short-acting general anesthetic. When used IV, it induces general anesthesia; but when given rectally, it causes deep sedation. It can be used for sedation of children who must remain still during nonpainful studies (e.g., diagnostic imaging).

Equipment   Materials for rectal administration.

Technique of Administration   Methohexital is given by the PR route only. It is reconstructed from powder and administered as a 10% solution (100 mg/mL).

Monitoring   Use continuous pulse oximetry and recheck vital signs every 15 min.

Dose   This ranges from 20 to 30 mg/kg PR (1 g maximum).

Advantages   The advantages of methohexital include its production of rapid, effective, and predictable sedation and immobility.

Disadvantages   Patients who take anticonvulsants may require higher doses.

Conclusions   Although methohexital has excellent efficacy for preprocedure sedation and immobility for nonpainful procedures, all barbiturates are associated with significant and potentially life-threatening side effects, including respiratory depression, apneas, and airway obstructions as well as coma, paradoxical excitement, and residual sedation or "hangover," which may impair behavior, mood, and judgment for 24 h or longer.

ANALGESIA

See Table 22-3.

OPIATES

The opiate agonists provide relief of moderate to severe pain.

Codeine

See Table 22-3.

Meperidine (Demerol)

The usefulness of meperidine is limited by its side effects [myocardial depression, accumulation of the toxic metabolite normeperidine, interactions with other drugs (MAO inhibitors)]. Except in the case of sickle cell vasoocclusive crisis, use alternative medications.

Morphine

See Table 22-3.

Table 22-3   Agents Used for Analgesia

DRUG	ROUTE OF ADMINISTRATION	DOSE	MAXIMAL DOSE	TIME TO ONSET	DURATION OF ACTION
Opiates					
Codeine	PO, SC, IM	0.5–1.0 mg/kg	30 mg	15–30 min	4–6 h
Meperidine	IM/SC	0.8–1.0 mg/kg	100 mg	10–15 min	2–4 h
	IV	0.8–1.3 mg/kg	100 mg	10 min	2–4 h
Morphine	SC	0.1–0.15 mg/kg	30 mg	10 min	4–5 h
	IM	0.1–0.15 mg/kg	30 mg	10 min	4–5 h
	IV	0.1–0.15 mg/kg	30 mg	2–5 min	4–5 h
Fentanyl	IV	1–4 µg/kg*	400 µg	90 s	30–60 min
	Oralette	10–15 µg/kg	an Oralette	10–15 min	60–90 min
Opiate reversal					
Naloxone	SC	Initial (all routes):	2 mg	2–5 min	30–45 min
	IM	0.01–0.02 mg/kg	2 mg	1–5 min	30–45 min
	IV	If no response: 0.1 mg/kg	2 mg	1–2 min	30–45 min

*Give in 0.5 µg/kg aliquots over 1 min (25 µg/min maximum). Rate of delivery more important than maximum dose.

SC = subcutaneous; IM = intramuscular; PO = by mouth; IV = intravenous.

Fentanyl (Sublimaze)

Indications for Use Fentanyl is a potent synthetic opiate agonist, estimated to be 25 to 100 times more potent than morphine. It is highly lipid-soluble and readily enters the CNS, leading to a rapid onset of action. In the outpatient setting, fentanyl provides relief of moderate to severe pain.

Equipment

Intravenous: IV materials, T-connector, pulse oximeter, naloxone, resuscitation equipment, and medications.

Oral: Omit the IV materials only.

Technique of Administration

Intravenous Give fentanyl slowly IV to allow careful titration of effect. Because the rate of infusion appears to be a major factor in respiratory depression, the drug must always be instilled close to the hub of the angiocatheter. Naloxone reverses the side effects and analgesia of fentanyl.

Oral The Oralette comes on a plastic mold that the child or parent holds.

Monitoring Use continuous pulse oximetry, and recheck the vital signs every 15 min. When fentanyl is given PO, a dedicated observer is required while the patient utilizes the Oralette.

Dose

Intravenous: Dose ranges from 1 to 4 μg/kg. Give IV in 0.5 μg/kg/min aliquots (25 μg/min maximum), titrating against mental status and the degree of relaxation. Use slow, small boluses until the desired effect is achieved while watching for respiratory depression.

Oralette: Dose ranges from 10 to 15 μg/kg.

Advantages The major advantages of fentanyl are rapid onset of action, short duration of action, potent analgesia, and complete, permanent reversibility of side effects with a single dose of naloxone. Unlike other opiates, the half-life of fentanyl is shorter than that of naloxone. The advantages of the Oralette are painless administration without the need for IV access.

Disadvantages The major disadvantages are respiratory depression and apnea, which may begin before alteration in consciousness. Patients with severe pain may tolerate two to four times the usual dose; as soon as the painful stimulus subsides, however, side effects may evolve. Fentanyl can cause thoracic and abdominal muscular rigidity ("wooden chest syndrome"), impairing ventilation. This can occur with low doses if the drug is given too rapidly; there is not complete consensus that it is reversible with naloxone. A relatively common side effect is facial pruritus, of unknown origin, which is a useful indicator of drug activity.

Conclusion Fentanyl is an extremely potent narcotic analgesic, with a rapid onset and relatively short duration of action; it is reversible with naloxone. Because of the potential for respiratory depression, fentanyl must be used in a controlled clinical setting by personnel experienced in its use.

Opiate Reversal

Naloxone (Narcan)   See Table 22-3.

TOPICAL ANALGESIA

Several topical anesthetics are now available that effectively relieve the pain of a needle stick.

EMLA Cream

Indications for Use   EMLA cream is a eutectic mixture of lidocaine and prilocaine. It is effective up to a depth of 5 mm and is indicated for topical anesthesia before venipuncture, arterial puncture, IV, LP, laser treatment for port-wine stains, injections, immunizations, accessing subcutaneous drug reservoirs, release of penile adhesions, myringotomy, and postherpetic neuralgia.

Equipment   None.

Technique of Administration   Apply EMLA cream directly to the smallest possible area requiring anesthesia. Use a thick coat, and cover with an occlusive dressing for a minimum of 30 to 60 min. In a young child, apply a secondary gauze wrap over the occlusive dressing to decrease the risk of accidental oral or ocular contact with the drug.

Monitoring   No specific monitoring is indicated.

Dose   The dose of EMLA cream is based on the child's weight and the amount of skin surface covered:

WEIGHT (KG)	MAXIMUM AREA COVERED (CM^2)
0–10	100
10–20	600
>20	2000

Advantages   EMLA cream provides local anesthesia without painful application that lasts after removal of the cream. It can make procedures pain-free, and this is a unique benefit for the child who may need repeated procedures.

Disadvantages   For maximum topical anesthesia, EMLA cream must remain in place for a minimum of 30 to 60 min. This long delay makes its use less attractive in an acute care setting. EMLA cream may potentially induce methemoglobinemia if a large amount of drug is applied and left in place for a prolonged period. There have also been case reports of methemoglobinemia in infants less than 6 months of age; therefore it is not recommended in this age group.

Avoid ocular contact, which may cause severe eye irritation or a corneal abrasion secondary to loss of protective reflexes. If ingested, the lidocaine or prilocaine can cause CNS excitation or depression.

Conclusion   EMLA cream is a safe topical anesthetic when used in children over 6 months of age. The major drawback is the prolonged time to onset of action.

ELA-Max

Indications for Use   ELA-Max cream is a 4% lidocaine cream in a liposomal vehicle. The liposomal encapsulation uses lipid bilayers to deliver the anesthetic into the epidermal and dermal layers of the skin, where the lidocaine accumulates in areas of nerve endings and pain receptors. ELA-Max has the same indications as EMLA (see above); in addition, it can be used for the pain associated with minor cuts, abrasions, burns, and sunburns. EMLA and ELA-Max have similar efficacy.

Equipment   None.

Technique of Administration   Apply a thick layer of ELA-Max cream for 30 min directly to the smallest possible area requiring anesthesia. No occlusive dressing is required, although young children need either observation or a secondary gauze dressing to decrease the risk of accidental oral or ocular contact with the drug.

Monitoring   No specific monitoring is indicated.

Dose   The dose of ELA-Max is the same as for EMLA (see above) and is based on the child's weight and the amount of skin surface to be covered.

Advantages   ELA-Max cream provides all the advantages of a topical analgesic (see EMLA), with the added benefit of a shorter application time of 30 min.

Disadvantages   While the likelihood of adverse reactions to lidocaine is low because of the small dose absorbed, systemic adverse reactions to lidocaine include CNS excitation and/or depression, including euphoria, light-headedness, confusion, dizziness, drowsiness, tinnitus, blurred or double vision, vomiting, twitching, tremors, seizures, unconsciousness, and respiratory depression or arrest. Potential cardiovascular complications include bradycardia, hypotension, and cardiovascular collapse (see Lidocaine, pp 631–632).

Conclusion   ELA-Max is a safe topical anesthetic, which is equal in efficacy to EMLA cream but has the added benefit of a shorter onset of action, making it a more attractive alternative in the ED.

TAC (Tetracaine/Adrenaline/Cocaine)

Indications for Use   Tetracaine/adrenaline/cocaine (TAC) is a topical local anesthetic that acts by preventing both the generation and conduction of nerve impulses at a cellular level. It is used for the repair of lacerations located in well-vascularized areas. Never use TAC on mucous membranes or in areas in close proximity to mucous membranes, where passive drainage is possible. TAC is also contraindicated for lacerations of end-artery areas, such as the fingers, toes, penis, nose, or ears.

Equipment   Sterile cotton balls or swabs, disposable glove, and pulse oximeter.

Technique of Administration   Apply a few drops of TAC directly on the wound and place the rest on sterile cotton balls or a sterile swab. Do not use gauze, or it will absorb the TAC. Give the TAC applier (parent, child, or medical personnel) a disposable glove to wear, with instructions to hold the TAC-soaked cotton balls or swabs directly over the wound with firm pressure for 10 min. After that time, observe the wound for blanching, which correlates with analgesia. The wound can then be irrigated, draped, and prepared for repair. Assess for analgesia by pinprick using a 25-gauge needle gently applied to the area. If the patient notes a sharp sensation or if an infant responds with a grimace, withdrawal, or crying, infiltrate with 1% buffered lidocaine intradermally. (1 mL sodium bicarbonate + 9 mL 1% lidocaine).

Monitoring   Record the vital signs initially and every 30 min thereafter until the procedure is over. Observe for euphoria, irritability, fussiness, hyperactivity, or seizures. Observe the patient for 1 h, including wound repair time, after application of TAC.

Dose   The dilute solution of TAC is prepared as follows:

Tetracaine 1%

Epinephrine 1:4000

Cocaine 4% + saline = 3 mL

The dose of the dilute solution of TAC is 1.5 mL/kg (consistent with 1.5 mg/kg of tetracaine and 6.0 mg/kg of cocaine). Never repeat TAC; if analgesia is inadequate, use supplemental lidocaine.

Advantages   TAC is a topical anesthetic with painless application and excellent pain control. It decreases the time for surgical repair and the need for restraints and the presence of additional ED personnel. There is no increased risk of wound infection with TAC as compared with lidocaine. In addition, lack of distortion of wound margins facilitates an improved cosmetic outcome.

Disadvantages   TAC cannot be used on mucous membranes because of the risk of systemic absorption, There have been several case reports of death after the use of TAC, but in each case appropriate guidelines were not followed. TAC is effective only on nonintact skin and is not effective for abscess drainage or the cleansing and debridement of "road tattoos." Cocaine requires the use of schedule II drug-control measures and is a costly ingredient.

Conclusion   For wound repair, TAC is superior to lidocaine in terms of patient compliance, and there is no increased risk of wound infection. TAC may be the optimal anesthetic for the repair of pediatric lacerations located in well-vascularized, non-end-artery areas that are not on or near mucous membranes.

Lidocaine-Epinephrine-Tetracaine (LET)

Indications for Use   This combination topical dermal anesthetic is an alternative to TAC in situations where a non-cocaine-containing compound is desirable. LET is contraindicated in end-artery areas, such as the pinna, penis, tips of the fingers, nose, and toes and in patients allergic to any of its ingredients. LET can be prepared in a gel or liquid formulation.

Equipment   Sterile cotton balls or swab

Technique of Administration   Use 1 to 3 mL of the gel or liquid formulation. Put part of the dose directly on the wound and the remainder on sterile cotton balls or swabs. Do not use gauze, which absorbs LET. Hold the cotton balls or swabs in place with firm pressure (gloved hand or occlusive dressing) for 20 to 30 min. The blanching that occurs after 20 to 30 min correlates with analgesia. Assess the wound for analgesia by pinprick, using a 25-gauge needle gently applied to the area. If pain persists, use supplemental 1% buffered lidocaine intradermally, but do not exceed a total dose of 3 to 5 mg/kg.

Monitoring   Check vital signs every 30 min.

Dose   LET *gel* (400 mL) contains 80 mL of 20% lidocaine, 40 mL of racemic 2.25% epinephrine, 100 ML of 2% tetracaine, 252 mg of sodium metabisulfite, 10 g of methylcellulose, and 180 mL of sterile water. LET *liquid* contains 10 mL of 20% lidocaine, 5 mL of 2.25% racemic epinephrine, 12.5 mL of 2% tetracaine, 31.5 mg of sodium metabisulfite, and 22.5 mL of sterile water. The gel expires 6 months from the date of preparation, and the liquid is stable for 3 weeks at room temperature and 5 months if refrigerated.

Advantages   The benefits of LET include improved patient compliance, no need for physical restraint, and lack of physical wound distortion that occurs with injected anesthetics.

Disadvantages   Potential lidocaine toxicity, including confusion, seizures, coma, respiratory, depression, vasomotor collapse, and cardiac arrest.

Conclusion   LET is as effective as TAC and without the problems associated with the cocaine component of TAC.

LOCAL ANALGESIA

Iontocaine

Indications for Use   Iontocaine (2% lidocaine hydrochloride and epinephrine 1:100,000 topical solution), or "Numby Stuff," is a local anesthetic delivered to the tissues by iontophoresis, an active form of transdermal drug delivery. A low-level electric current is used to rapidly transport drug molecules to the tissues. Iontocaine can be used on intact skin for procedures including phlebotomy, vascular access (peripheral), lumbar puncture, accessing SC ports, and injections; it is an alternative to EMLA and ELA-Max creams.

Equipment   An IOMED Phoresor (Iomed, Salt Lake City, UT) iontophoretic drug-delivery unit, Numby Stuff electrodes (drug delivery and dispersive electrode), alcohol preparatory pad, and 1 mL Iontocaine topical solution. Confirm that the patient is not allergic to lidocaine or any other local anesthetics of the amide type, epinephrine, sulfites, or plastic tape.

Technique of Administration/Dose   The 1 mL of Iontocaine is usually administered by the nurse, following the directions in the kit. The patient may feel a tingling, prickly, or warm sensation, which usually disappears within a few minutes. After the total dose of Iontocaine has been delivered, the phoresor will ramp the current down and stop. There may be erythema or blanching of the electrode sites, which generally resolve within hours or days.

Advantages   For the emergency medicine setting, Numby Stuff provides rapid (5–15 min) dermal analgesia with little systemic absorption, and no monitoring is required.

Disadvantages   The primary disadvantage is that many children do not like the tingling, itching, or burning sensation from the electric current. It cannot be used over denuded, damaged, or nonintact skin, new scar tissue, or in patients with electrically sensitive support systems (e.g., pacemakers). Do not use Numby Stuff over the temporal or orbital regions.

Conclusion Numby Stuff is a good alternative to EMLA cream. Although it is not a totally painless application and the tingling sensation is frightening to younger children, it is well tolerated by older children and adolescents. The rapid time to onset, 10 min, is a major advantage in the ED setting. For older children, Numby Stuff may be the preferred topical anesthetic when time to onset of action is critical.

Lidocaine

Lidocaine is available in several forms:

Viscous: 2%

Aerosol: 10% spray

Solutions: 0.5% solution (0.5 mg/mL lidocaine)

          1% solution (10 mg/mL lidocaine)

          2% solution (20 mg/mL lidocaine)

The higher concentration prolongs the effect. The 0.5% solution is useful for large wounds requiring greater amounts of lidocaine. Mixing lidocaine with epinephrine provides vasoconstriction, delays absorption, decreases lidocaine toxicity, and increases duration of effect. Mixing the solution with sodium bicarbonate (44 mEq/50mL), in a ratio of 10 parts lidocaine to 1 part sodium bicarbonate, raises the pH and decreases the burning sensation during infiltration.

Indications for Use
Topical Lidocaine jelly diminishes the pain of urethral catheterization and scrubbing of a "road tattoo," and it provides analgesia for gingivostomatitis. Absorption of topical lidocaine in extensive gingivostomatitis (e.g., herpetic) can produce systemic toxicity. The spray can provide anesthesia to the vocal cords and larynx before intubation.

Local Local lidocaine infiltration is indicated for wound repair, lumbar puncture, arterial puncture, IVs, and incision and drainage of an abscess.

Regional Regional nerve blocks are indicated for complex wound repairs and may be less painful and more practical when extensive local infiltration is necessary.

Equipment and Technique of Administration
Topical Apply the jelly with a cotton-tipped swab to the gums or urethra. Use it on a gauze pad before scrubbing a wound with embedded dirt or road tattoo.

Jet Injector This provides almost painless infiltration of 0.05 to 0.2 mL of lidocaine to a depth of about 1.4 cm. It can be used for laceration repair, lumbar puncture, and incision and drainage of abscesses. Clean the target surface, and put the injector lightly but firmly at the skin site and squeeze the trigger. Repeat if a wider area of analgesia is needed.

Local   A 20-gauge needle is recommended to draw up the solution. For infiltration, use a smaller gauge (25, 27, or 30) and preferably longer [4–5 cm (1½–2 in)] needle to produce "fanning," which causes less pain and fewer needle punctures. For deeper penetration, a larger needle (22 gauge) is preferred. First, drip a few drops of lidocaine on the wound. Next, pull the skin taut, insert the needle, aspirate for blood, and then slowly infiltrate the lidocaine through the wound margins at a rate of 2 mL/min. Wait 5 to 10 min for maximal effect.

Regional   A nerve block is a useful technique when the nerve supply to the wound is superficial. Anesthetize the site of infiltration with the jet injector and then infiltrate around the nerve, aspirating frequently to be sure a vessel has not been punctured.

Monitoring
Topical   No special monitoring.

Local   VS q 30 min.

Regional   VS q 15 min.

Dose   The dose of lidocaine used depends on the route of administration and whether epinephrine is used (Table 22-4).

Advantages
Topical   Local analgesia without special monitoring requirements.

Local   Lidocaine takes effect rapidly (5–10 min) and lasts long enough for most procedures (90–200 min). It can be mixed with epinephrine for vasoconstriction and sodium bicarbonate to diminish pain.

Regional   Avoids tissue disruption at the site of repair.

Disadvantages
The jelly is not recommended for infants who are teething or in young children who cannot expectorate. The jet injector can cause a hematoma or bleeding at the site of injection, but no significant tissue damage results. Side effects are unusual when lidocaine is used as recommended for wound repair. Toxicity from overdose includes confusion, seizures, coma, respiratory depression, vasomotor collapse, and cardiac arrest.

Conclusion   Lidocaine is highly effective for many situations and procedures in the ED when used with appropriate guidelines and monitoring.

Table 22-4 Topical and Local Analgesia

DRUG	ROUTE OF ADMINISTRATION	DOSE	MAXIMAL DOSE	TIME TO ONSET (MIN)	DURATION OF ACTION
TAC	Topical	1.5 mL/kg	Cocaine 6.0 mg/kg Tetracaine 1.5 mg/kg	10–15	1 h
LET	Topical	1–3 mL	3 mL	30 min	30–60 min
EMLA Cream	Transdermal	Maximal area to be covered: $0-10$ kg $= 100$ cm^2 $10-20$ kg $= 600$ cm^2 >20 kg $= 2000$ cm^2		60 min	3–4 h
ELA-Max Cream	Transdermal	Maximal area to be covered: $0-10$ kg $= 100$ cm^2 $10-20$ kg $= 600$ cm^2 >20 kg $= 2000$ cm^2		30 min	3–4 h
Numby Stuff (Iontocaine)	Phoresor unit and electrode kit	Iontocaine: 1 mL Current $= 2-4$ mA		5–15 min	1 h
Lidocaine Topical	Jelly Aerosol	2% gel 10% spray		2–5 min 2–5 min	30–60 min 30–60 min
Local	Jet injector	1% w/epinephrine 1% w/out epinephrine	300 mg	5–10 min	30–60 min
Local	Needle, syringe	Rate: 1 mL/30 s 1% w/epinephrine: 7 mg/kg 1% w/out epinephrine: 4–5 mg/kg	300 mg	4–10 min	90–200 min
Regional	Needle, syringe	1% w/out epinephrine	300 mg	5–10 min	90–200 min

NONSTEROIDAL
ANTI-INFLAMMATORY DRUGS
Ketorolac (Toradol)

Indications for Use   Ketorolac is a relatively new nonsteroidal anti-inflammatory drug that has greater analgesic properties than acetaminophen and as such provides an effective alternative to opioids for the treatment of moderate to severe pain.

Equipment   IV or IM materials.

Technique of Administration   Initially formulated for PO and IM use, it is now also approved for IV use.

Dose   The dose of ketorolac is the same for all routes of administration: 1.0 mg/kg loading dose, followed by a maintenance dose of 0.5 mg/kg every 6 h. Ketorolac can be combined with acetaminophen or low-dose opioids to produce greater analgesia.

Advantages   Ketorolac is an effective alternative to opioid analgesia. There is no respiratory depression or vomiting.

Disadvantages   Uncommon side effects of ketorolac include bleeding diathesis, hyperkalemia, and depression of renal function.

Conclusion   Ketorolac provides an alternative to opioids for moderate to severe pain without the side effects of respiratory depression and vomiting. It is very effective for postoperative musculoskeletal pain as well as headaches.

Aspirin
See Table 22-5.

Ibuprofen
See Table 22-5.

Acetaminophen
See Table 22-5.

SEDATION AND ANALGESIA
Midazolam + Morphine
Midazolam + Fentanyl

Indications for Use   Midazolam combined with opiates is useful for sedation and analgesia for moderate to severe pain.

Table 22-5   Miscellaneous Analgesic Agents

DRUG	ROUTE OF ADMINISTRATION	DOSE	MAXIMAL DOSE	TIME TO ONSET (MIN)	DURATION OF ACTION
Ketorolac (Toradol)	IV	All routes:	60 mg	5	4–6 h
	IM	Load: 1 mg/kg	30 mg q 6 h	30	4–6 h
	PO	Maintenance: 0.5 mg/kg q 6 h	40 mg/day	30–60	4–6 h
Acetaminophen	PO/PR	15 mg/kg q 4 h	60 mg/kg/day	10–60 min	3–4 h
Ibuprofen	PO	10 mg/kg q 6–8 h	2.4 g/day (adult)	20–60 min	3–4 h
Aspirin	PO	10 mg/kg q 4 h	65 mg/kg/day	10–20 min	3–4 h

Equipment and Technique of Administration   IV or IM materials, appropriate dose of narcotic (fentanyl, morphine), naloxone, flumazenil, pulse oximeter, resuscitation equipment and medications.

Monitoring   Use continuous pulse oximetry and recheck the vital signs every 10 min. With the onset of medication effect, there is a normal slowing of rate and depth of respirations.

Dose

IV midazolam/morphine:	0.05 to 0.3 mg/kg midazolam (5 mg maximum) plus
	0.1 to 0.2 mg/kg morphine (10 mg maximum)
IV midazolam/fentanyl:	0.05 to 0.3 mg/kg midazolam (5 mg maximum) plus
	1 to 4 μg/kg (0.001–0.004 mg/kg) fentanyl (100 μg maximum)

Give midazolam 5 to 10 min before starting the fentanyl infusion.

Advantages   Midazolam, an effective sedative, also provides analgesia when combined with a narcotic. The effects and side effects of both the midazolam and the narcotic can be reversed with flumazenil and naloxone, respectively. This combination has a rapid and predictable onset of action and short recovery time and provides amnesia for the event.

Disadvantages   The primary disadvantages are synergistic respiratory depression, apnea, laryngospasm, and wooden chest syndrome. Although flumazenil reverses the effects and side effects of midazolam, use it as an adjunct to, and not a substitute for, appropriate airway management. Because of the short half-life of flumazenil as compared to midazolam, there is a risk of resedation.

Conclusions

Midazolam in combination with a narcotic is effective for sedation and analgesia. It has a rapid and predictable onset of action and children recover rapidly, with little residual "hangover." The added benefits of amnesia surrounding the unpleasant event and muscle relaxation make it ideal for many procedures in the ED. Since there is a potential for respiratory depression, this combination must be used only by experienced personnel.

Ketamine + Midazolam + Atropine

Indications for Use   The combination of ketamine, midazolam, and atropine is excellent for sedation, anxiolysis, analgesia, and amnesia for painful procedures. Since ketamine is a sialogogue, atropine must be added to control secretions. While ketamine can produce emergent reactions, this effect is rare in children under 6 years of age and may be diminished by the use of midazolam.

Equipment   IV or IM equipment, pulse oximeter, oxygen, flumazenil, and resuscitation equipment and medications.

Technique of Administration   The combination may be administered PO, IV, or IM, although optimal results are seen with IM administration because of a depot effect and steady absorption.

Monitoring   Continuously monitor with pulse oximetry, and check vital signs every 15 min.

Dose   The dose varies based on the route of administration:

PO: ketamine 3 to 4 mg/kg + midazolam 0.5 mg/kg + atropine 0.02 mg/kg
IM: ketamine 2 to 3 mg/kg + midazolam 0.1 mg/kg + atropine 0.01 mg/kg
IV: ketamine 0.5 mg/kg + midazolam 0.05 mg/kg + atropine 0.01 mg/kg

Advantages   Ketamine produces little respiratory depression. When used IM, this combination provides excellent sedation and analgesia for relatively long (45–60 min), painful procedures.

Disadvantages   The main disadvantage of ketamine is that it is not reversible. While there is always a risk of emergent reactions and hallucinations, this risk is minimized with the addition of midazolam. Do not use ketamine in a child with an upper respiratory infection or requiring intraoral laceration repair because of the risk of increased secretions. It is also contraindicated in a child with a history of psychosis or with any condition associated with increased intracranial pressure. Atropine is required to decrease secretions and prevent hypersalivation.

Conclusion   This combination provides a safe and effective method of sedation and analgesia for long, painful procedures.

INHALED AGENTS

Nitrous Oxide

Nitrous oxide is a colorless gas that is heavier than air and has a sweet odor. It diffuses rapidly across membranes, resulting in a rapid onset and short duration of action. It has both sedative and analgesic properties and is a relatively weak anesthetic agent. Most children experience a sense of euphoria with inhalation of the gas as well as a detached attitude toward their surroundings.

Indications for Use   Nitrous oxide can be used for any short-term painful procedure in children age 4 and older. Do not use nitrous oxide in cases of impaired mental status, respiratory distress, abdominal distention or suspicion of abdominal obstruction, significant nausea or vomiting, hypotension, or pregnancy.

Equipment and Technique of Administration   The delivery device is a Nitronox machine. The gas is delivered by a demand valve mask, which the patient holds and breathes through normally. This requires a child who is old enough to cooperate and is physically able to generate a negative pressure of 1 to 5 cmH_2O for the gas to flow. The mask is weighted, so as the patient becomes too lethargic to hold the mask, it falls away from the face, automatically discontinuing the administration of nitrous oxide. The system comes with a scavenger device that attaches to wall suction, minimizing environmental exposure.

Additional recommended equipment includes a pulse oximeter, oxygen, and resuscitation equipment and medications.

Monitoring   Use continuous pulse oximetry and check vital signs every 15 min. In addition, closely monitor the patient's color and response to verbal commands. Indications to terminate gas delivery include a lack of verbal response to a command, difficulty arousing the patient, nausea, vomiting, gagging, and a significant change in vital signs.

Dose   The Nitronox delivers a 50% nitrous oxide/50% oxygen mixture. After the procedure, give the patient 100% oxygen for at least 5 min.

Advantages   The advantages of nitrous oxide include a completely painless system that is self-administered and has a rapid onset of action. It allows the patient to remain alert and responsive throughout the procedure. In addition to providing some analgesia, it also produces an amnestic and a dissociative effect, making the patient's recall of the event more pleasant than the actual occurrence. The duration of action is short, with complete elimination within 10 min after the procedure. Nitrous oxide has a wide margin of safety, and the Nitronox machine has many built-in safety features. First, true anesthesia cannot be achieved because the maximum amount of nitrous oxide delivered is limited to 50%; the patient remains alert and responsive throughout the procedure. Second, if the oxygen tank becomes empty, the machine shuts off automatically. Third, because the patient holds the demand valve mask, one is assured of having a responsive patient with adequate respiratory effort. Fourth, the scavenging device reduces environmental exposure to negligible amounts.

Disadvantages   In approximately 10% of the general population, nitrous oxide is an inadequate analgesic. Because of the need for cooperation, nitrous oxide can usually be used only in children older than 4 years of age. Although nitrous oxide has few side effects, it may, with prolonged exposure (>48 h), suppress bone marrow activity. This is reversible when the gas is discontinued. At a concentration of 50%, the main physiologic effect is an elevation of the respiratory minute volume.

Conclusion   Nitrous oxide is safe, painless, effective, fast-acting, and rapidly eliminated. It is unique compared with other methods of sedation or analgesia in that it is an inhaled agent and its administration is titrated by the patient for the duration of the procedure.

BIBLIOGRAPHY

Brent AS: The Management of pain in the emergency department. *Pediatr Clin North Am* 1994;41:31–58.

Ferrari LR, Rooney FM, Rockoff MA: Preoperative tasting practices in pediatrics. *Anesthesiology* 1999;90:978–980.

Kennedy RM, Luhman JD: The "ouchless emergency department." *Pediatr Clin North Am* 1999;46:1215–1247.

Zempsky, WT, Anand KJS, Sullivan RM, et al: Lidocaine iontophoresis for topical anesthesia before intravenous line placement in children. *J Pediatr* 1998;132:1061–1063.

CHAPTER 23

Trauma

Anthony J. Ciorciari

CERVICAL SPINE INJURIES

Cervical spine injuries are uncommon in children, occurring in only 1 to 2% of cases of pediatric blunt trauma. However, approximately 1000 children per year suffer paralysis from injuries to the spinal cord. Cervical spine injuries may accompany serious head trauma, such as severe deceleration injuries caused by high-speed motor vehicle accidents or falls from extreme heights. Sports injuries are also a common mechanism for cervical spine injury. Less often, they may result from injuries to the top of the head or the back of the neck.

Clinical Presentation

Cervical spine injuries are most common in patients with severe head injuries. Therefore cervical spine injury is always a possibility in a child who is unconscious or has an altered mental status after head trauma. This is especially true in younger children, whose horizontally aligned facet joints and more elastic intervertebral ligaments can predispose to subluxation without bony injury. This occurs when the angular momentum resulting from forceful impact levers the proportionately larger head on the fulcrum of the upper cervical spine. The result is a condition known as spinal cord injury without radiographic abnormality (SCIWORA), which predisposes the victim to paraplegia and neurogenic shock or respiratory arrest. Approximately 20% of all pediatric spinal injuries are of the SCIWORA type.

In the alert patient, the most common symptoms are midline cervical tenderness, paraspinous muscular tenderness, and cervical muscle spasm. Less often, there is weakness, pain, or paresthesia along the affected nerve roots. In the unconscious patient with high-grade partial or complete transections, common findings include spinal shock (flaccidity and areflexia instead of spasticity, hyperreflexia, and Babinski's sign) and neurogenic ("warm") shock (hypotension that is poorly responsive to volume resuscitation but is paradoxically associated with bradycardia, "normal" urine output, and warm extremities).

Diagnosis

Assume that a cervical spine injury may have occurred in a patient who is unconscious or has an altered mental status after head trauma. Spinal cord injury is sometimes overlooked during the initial evaluation of a comatose patient with severe traumatic brain injury.

See pp 649–658 for the general approach to the patient with multiple trauma and pp 461–467 for the general approach to the patient with head trauma.

Often an awake, alert patient arrives in the emergency department (ED) immobilized on a backboard in a semirigid extrication collar. Ask about the presence of pain at the top of the head (C2–3) or back of the neck and about paresthesias of the hands, arms, or legs. If none of these are present, without moving the patient, carefully remove the cervical restraint while maintaining in-line stabilization of the neck. Palpate the spinous processes for local tenderness, associated interspinous muscle spasm, or obvious deformity. The first spinous process that can be palpated is C2; C6 and C7 are the largest. Ask the patient to move the fingers and hands, the feet and toes, and to raise the arms and legs. If there is no tenderness, hyperesthesia, or paresthesia in the extremities or evidence of trauma and the patient moves all extremities easily, ask him or her to move the neck gently from side to side, then up and down. *Do not attempt to move the patient's neck yourself; insist that the patient stop immediately if any movement causes pain.*

Suspect a cervical spine injury in a patient with any of the following: unresponsiveness after head trauma, paresthesias or weakness, hyperesthesia, limitation of neck motion, inability to cooperate with the examination, pain on top of the head, neck trauma, or injury above the clavicles. Consider a patient who has a distracting injury that interferes with response to pain or is intoxicated to have a cervical spine injury until proven otherwise.

ED Management

Begin by performing an assessment of the airway, breathing, and circulation (the ABCs), the initial component of the primary survey (see Resuscitation, pp 9–13). Immediately stabilize the head and neck of every patient suspected of having a cervical spine injury if temporary immobilization was not accomplished earlier in the field. The preferred method is with an appropriate-size semirigid extrication collar and head immobilizer. Place a thin layer of padding beneath the torso from shoulders to hips in a young child; the prominent occiput predisposes the neck to slight flexion unless this precaution is taken. A soft collar, sandbags, or large IV bags placed on both sides of the patient's head (even if well secured with tape across the forehead) do not provide adequate immobilization of the head and neck. Finally, because ventilation may be impaired by the very techniques required to achieve adequate immobilization, monitor the patient carefully for signs of respiratory compromise.

If intubation is necessary, apply bimanual in-line stabilization to the sides of the head and remove the extrication collar. Have an assistant apply slight downward pressure over the larynx (the Sellick maneuver), if necessary, to bring the vocal cords into view. Avoid hyperextending or flexing the neck during the procedure. *Never delay intubation because a cross-table lateral cervical spine x-ray has not been obtained or interpreted.*

Once the airway has been secured and the head and neck have been properly immobilized, order a cross-table lateral x-ray of the cervical spine. The base of the skull, all seven cervical vertebrae, and the top of the first thoracic vertebra must be visualized. Continuity of the normal lordotic curves of the cervical spine and important anatomic measurements (Table 23-1) must be confirmed by a physician experienced in interpretation of pediatric cervical spine radiographs. Be aware of certain anatomic features of young children that mimic vertebral injuries, including unfused epiphyses (particularly at the base of the dens), widening of the prevertebral soft tissue spaces on forced expiration (crying), and hypermobility of the upper cervical spine (resulting in the slight forward shifting of C2 on C3 and C3 on C4, known as *pseudosubluxation*).

However, a lateral cervical spine radiograph alone can miss certain vertebral fractures. Thus, once this film is obtained and interpreted as normal and if the child's vital signs are stable, transport the patient to the x-ray suite, for AP and open-mouth views. An open-mouth view permits visualization of the odontoid process (dens) of the axis (C2) and the ring of the atlas (C1). A CT scan of the cervical spine to look for additional fractures is indicated when it is impossible to obtain a full radiographic series, there is a suggestion of fracture on radiograph without the actual fracture being seen (e.g., increased prevertebral soft tissue), or a fracture has been identified by x-ray.

There is no immediate need to ascertain the integrity of the cervical spine in the comatose patient. Normal x-rays cannot definitely exclude spinal cord injury because of SCIWORA, while the patient's inability to relate symptoms compromises the reliability of the physical examination. Thus, it is safest to presume that spinal cord injury may be present, maintain full spinal immobilization, and defer comprehensive evaluation of the cervical spine to a later time.

When a cervical spine injury is diagnosed clinically or radiographically, immediately call the appropriate surgical specialist (neurosurgeon, orthopedist) to assist in further management (e.g., application of Gardner-Wells tongs). Admit any patient in whom cervical spine injury cannot be definitively ruled out in the ED.

Table 23-1 Normal Cervical Spine Measurements

MEASUREMENT	<8 YEARS	≥8 YEARS
Predental space	4–5 mm	3 mm
C2-3 override (flexion)	4–5 mm	3 mm
Prevertebral space	⅔ thickness of C2	5–7 mm
Spinal cord area	Varies with age	10–13 mm
Most commonly injured	C1-3	C5-7

Indications for Admission

- Cervical spine fracture
- Focal neurologic deficit
- Inability to exclude cervical spine injury

BIBLIOGRAPHY

Baker C, Kadish H, Schunk JE: Evaluation of pediatric cervical spine injuries. *Am J Emerg Med* 1999;17:230–234.

Eleraky MA, Theodore N, Adams M, et al: Pediatric cervical spine injuries: report of 102 cases and review of the literature. *J Neurosurg* 2000;92:12–17.

Medina FA: Neck and spinal cord trauma, in Barkin RM (ed): *Pediatric Emergency Medicine,* 2nd ed. St. Louis, Mosby-Year Book, 1997, pp 287–317.

HAND INJURIES

The injured hand requires a thorough evaluation, as improper management may lead to permanent disability. A systematic approach is essential to avoid overlooking subtle injuries.

Clinical Presentation

Lacerations   Hand lacerations may affect the skin only or may be deep and involve underlying structures. Active extension of a digit may be possible despite partial laceration of the extensor tendon. However, a dorsal hand laceration associated with pain on extension of the digit against resistance suggests a partial tendon injury.

Bites   Bites (pp 664–666) are actually lacerations combined with crush injuries. Suspect that an irregular laceration over the metacarpophalangeal (MCP) joint is a human bite sustained by punching another person in the mouth. This is a serious injury, as oral flora can be inoculated into the MCP joint.

Fractures and Dislocations
Phalangeal Fractures   These fractures are common but not serious unless they are malrotated or the joint, volar plate, or collateral ligament is affected.

Wrist Fractures   Wrist fractures are less common in children than in adults. The most commonly fractured carpal bone is the scaphoid. Key findings include tenderness on deep palpation in the anatomic snuffbox area distal to the radial styloid and radial pain on pronation followed by ulnar deviation of the affected wrist.

Metacarpophalangeal Joint Dislocations   MCP dislocations are rare. They cause fixed digit hyperextension and a swollen, painful joint. There can be an associated volar laceration through which the metacarpal head can be seen.

Proximal and Distal Interphalangeal (PIP and DIP) Joint Dislocations
PIP and DIP joint dislocations present with obvious deformity unless already reduced at the scene by the patient or an onlooker.

Tendon Injuries
Gamekeeper's (Skier's) Thumb   Gamekeeper's thumb is caused by acute radial deviation of the thumb at the MCP joint, tearing the ulnar collateral ligament. Typically the injury occurs when a patient falls with the thumb abducted. Findings include tenderness along the ulnar aspect of the thumb MCP joint, associated with laxity of the joint on passive radial abduction (performed under local anesthesia).

Mallet (Baseball) Finger   A mallet finger results from a direct blow to the tip of an extended digit, rupturing the DIP extensor tendon or avulsing it from the base of the distal phalanx. The finger is flexed at the DIP joint. X-rays, which must contain a view of the PIP joint, may reveal an avulsed bone chip remaining attached to the extensor tendon.

Boutonniere (Buttonhole) Deformity   A boutonniere deformity follows violent flexion of the PIP joint. It presents with PIP flexion and DIP hyperextension. The lateral bands of the intrinsic muscles are pulled volar to the PIP axis, such that the lateral bands become PIP flexors while hyperextending the DIP. As a result, the PIP "buttonholes" through the torn extensor hood.

Nail Bed Injuries   Blunt trauma to the nail can cause a subungual hematoma, or bleeding between the nail and the nail bed. A very tender nail with blue-black subungual discoloration is seen.

Infections
Paronychia   A paronychia is an infection of the soft tissues around the fingernail. It usually begins as a hangnail and is more common in patients with a history of finger sucking or nail biting. There is exquisite tenderness to palpation of the nail as well as erythematous swelling along the nail margin. There may also be a purulent collection or discharge and/or an associated felon (see below).

Felon   A felon is a serious infection of the distal pulp space. Tense, tender, erythematous swelling of the volar surface of the distal phalanx is seen.

Purulent Tenosynovitis   This infection of the flexor tendon sheath is a true surgical emergency. There is usually a history of penetrating trauma. Kanavel's four cardinal signs of tenosynovitis are (1) symmetric swelling, (2) slight flexion of the finger, (3) tenderness over the tendon sheath, and (4) exquisite pain on passive finger extension. Tenosynovitis may progress to a palmar space infection.

Palmar Space Infection   This infection presents with tense, tender, erythematous swelling of the palmar surface with pain and decreased mobility of the third and fourth fingers (midpalmar space) or thumb (thenar space). In certain circumstances, the dorsum of the hand may be more swollen than the palmar surface. These infections can spread to the flexor tendon sheaths. Associated signs may include fever, lymphangitis, and lymphadenitis.

Ganglion   A ganglion is a benign, well-defined, smooth cystic lesion of synovial origin. It is fixed to the deep tissues, typically tendon sheaths, or less commonly, herniated joint lining. Usually less than 3 cm in diameter, it is most often found on the volar or dorsal surface of the wrist or on the volar surface at the base of a digit.

Traumatic Amputations   Most traumatic amputations involve the distal fingertip only. Loss of the entire nail bed results in a more significant injury. However, children have remarkable regenerative ability, so consider reattachment of virtually any amputated part.

Diagnosis

The evaluation begins with a careful history, including hand dominance, tetanus immunization status, and description of any previous hand injuries. Inquire about the mechanism of injury, including the hand position at the time of injury, the time elapsed since injury, and whether the trauma occurred in a clean or dirty environment.

Expose and inspect the entire upper extremity. Note any discrepancy between active and passive mobility of upper extremity joints. Inspect the hand and evaluate the vascular status. Look for an alteration in the usual resting cascade of the digits, suggestive of a tendon or nerve injury. Check the color and temperature of the injured digit, and assess capillary refill (compress the distal fingertip pulp).

Before anesthetizing the hand in preparation for a surgical procedure, assess sensory function by evaluating two-point discrimination with two points of a paper clip. Apply both points to the radial side of each digit. Then move the points closer together until the patient can no longer distinguish between them. The normal range is 3 mm static or 6 mm moving, but use an uninjured digit as a control. Repeat the examination on the ulnar side. Then evaluate the median (volar index fingertip), radial (dorsal web space between the thumb and index finger), and ulnar (volar fifth fingertip) sensory nerves. The "immersion test" can substitute when an adequate two-point discrimination test cannot be obtained. Failure of the skin to wrinkle after immersion for 5 to10 min in water suggests sensory nerve injury.

Motor (nerve, muscle, and tendon) function must be evaluated in a systematic manner. First, test the extrinsic flexors: the IP joint of the thumb (flexor pollicis longus), the DIP joints of the fingers while the PIP joints are held in extension (flexor digitorum profundus), and then the PIP joints of each finger while the other fingers are held completely extended (flexor digitorum superficialis). Next, have the patient flex the wrist against resistance, and palpate the three tendons (flexor carpi ulnaris, palmaris longus, and flexor carpi radialis, from medial to lateral) at the base of the wrist. The palmaris longus is best seen by flexing the wrist against resistance with the thumb and fifth finger opposed; however, it is absent in approximately 15 to 20% of children.

Evaluate the thenar muscles and median motor function by opposing the pulp of the thumb with that of the other four fingers. Test thumb adduction (adductor pollicis) and ulnar nerve function by having the patient grasp a piece of paper between the thumb and radial surface of the proximal index finger. Weakness is indicated by Froment's paper sign, contraction of the flexor pollicis longus with flexion of the IP thumb joint when a sheet of paper is held between the thumb and index finger. To check the hypothenar muscles, ask the patient to abduct the small finger. Evaluate the interosseus muscles (ulnar nerve) by having the patient spread the fingers apart. Test the lumbricals (median and ulnar nerves) by asking the patient to flex the digits at the MCP joints while keeping the PIP and DIP joints extended. Assess motor function of the radial nerve by having the patient extend the wrist against resistance.

ED Management

Manage profuse bleeding with elevation and pressure. *Never use clamps for hemostasis,* as the nerves traveling with the blood vessels can be damaged.

Palpate for localized bony tenderness or soft tissue swelling, and examine for obvious deformities, ecchymoses, and functional deficits. Obtain x-rays if any of these findings are present over the wrist or hand. Radiographs of the fingers are indicated for gross deformities, lacerations in association with crush injuries, or loss of IP joint mobility.

Instill local anesthesia for surgical procedures only after a satisfactory sensory examination has been completed. If a digital block is required, allow the skin to dry after preparing it with povidone-iodine. Use a 25- or 27-gauge needle to inject 2 to 4 mL of 2% lidocaine *without* epinephrine into both medial and lateral sides of the digit at the level of the metacarpal head. The maximum allowable dose of lidocaine is 4 to 5 mg/kg (without epinephrine). Before administration, be sure to inquire about personal or family history of previous reactions to local anesthetics.

Lacerations and Bites   Carefully debride and irrigate these wounds after administration of local anesthesia (see pp 626–633). Close with 5-0 or 6-0 nylon, using simple sutures that are left in place for 7 days. Do not use deep sutures because of the risk of infection. A drain may be needed if the laceration is large. Carefully evaluate human bite wounds adjacent to MCP joints for evidence of joint capsule violation. Open irrigation in the operating room is necessary if the wound has penetrated the capsule.

All deep lacerations and bite injuries require prophylactic antibiotics for 7 days. Treat human and animal bite wounds with an IV dose of ampicillin/sulbactam (45 mg/kg). Follow this with amoxicillin/clavulanate alone (875/125 formulation, 45 mg/kg/day of amoxicillin divided bid). Alternatively, give penicillin VK (50 mg/kg/day divided qid) *plus* 40 mg/kg/day of either cephalexin (divided qid) *or* cefadroxil (divided bid) for 5 days. For other deep or potentially contaminated lacerations, discharge the patient with cephalexin or cefadroxil, as above. Provide tetanus prophylaxis if indicated (pp 682–683).

Fractures and Dislocations   Refer patients with *fractures* (except distal tuft), *MCP dislocations,* or *nonradiographic suspicion of a scaphoid fracture* to an appropriate surgical specialist (orthopedic, plastic, or hand surgeon). Treat *distal tuft phalangeal fractures* with a hairpin splint or bulky dressing.

A *PIP dislocation* can be reduced with traction and splinted after x-rays rule out an associated avulsion fracture. To reduce a dorsal (most common) PIP joint dislocation, first anesthetize the finger with a digital block. Hold the finger proximal to the injury, then use a distracting force to hyperextend at the PIP joint to bring it back to its normal anatomic position. If successful, repeat the examination of active and passive range of motion and immobilize the joint for 3 weeks. If reduction was unsuccessful, consult with a hand specialist. Reduce a *dorsal DIP joint dislocation* using distracting force at the involved joint.

Tendon Injuries   Refer a patient with a *gamekeeper's thumb* or *boutonniere deformity* to an appropriate surgical specialist. Treat a *mallet finger* with a short dorsal splint, ensuring mild DIP joint hyperextension with free PIP joint mobility, for 6 to 8 weeks. A paper clip or tongue blade wrapped in tape can serve as a temporary splint for a mallet finger.

Nail Bed Injuries   To drain a *subungual hematoma,* first soak the digit in warm water for 20 min. Then, "screw" through the nail with an 18-gauge needle. After several holes have been made, soak the digit in warm water to permit blood to escape. Remove the nail only if there is disruption of the nail or nail margin. Repair lacerations of the nail bed with 6.0 absorbable sutures to prevent abnormal growth of the new nail. If the nail is present, suture it in place to act as a dressing and splint. With crush injuries, however, it may be necessary to remove the nail in order to identify and repair occult lacerations to the nail bed. If the nail cannot be used as a splint, insert petrolatum gauze into the eponychial fold until the wound heals and the nail begins to grow.

Infections   Treat a *paronychia* without fluctuance with warm soaks every 2 to 3 h, elevation, and 40 mg/kg/day of cephalexin (divided qid) or cefadroxil (divided bid) for 3 to 5 days. If fluctuance is present, soak the digit, then lift the edge of the eponychial fold with a no. 15 scalpel blade in order to remove pus from the eponychium. If it is not clear whether all of the pus was removed, place a wick under the eponychium. Warm soaks and elevation are also necessary. If pus extends under the nail, partial nail removal is indicated.

Refer a patient with a *felon* to an appropriate surgical specialist (orthopedic, plastic, or hand surgeon) for immediate drainage. Admit patients with *purulent tenosynovitis* (culture for gonococcus) and *palmar space infections* for IV ampicillin/sulbactam (200 mg/kg divided qid) or, if allergic to beta-lactams, IV clindamycin (40 mg/kg/day divided q 6 h). Immediately consult with an appropriate surgical specialist.

Ganglion   Elective surgical removal is indicated if the lesion is painful or very disfiguring.

Traumatic Amputations   Rinse the amputated part gently in saline, wrap it in saline-soaked (but not dripping) gauze, and place it in a sealed plastic bag immersed in ice (do not allow direct contact with the ice). *Distal fingertip amputations* may require wrapping in petrolatum gauze. For more serious injuries, obtain a complete blood count (CBC), type, and cross-match; start an IV line with maintenance fluids; treat pain with morphine sulfate (0.1–0.15 mg/kg IV or IM); and give IV ampicillin/sulbactam (200 mg/kg divided qid). Gently cleanse the wound and cover it with petrolatum gauze or saline-soaked gauze until the patient can be taken to the operating room. Obtain an x-ray if there is suspicion of a crush injury to the distal phalanx.

Follow-up

- Bite wound or laceration being treated with prophylactic antibiotics: 2 to 3 days
- Drained subungual hematoma: 2 days
- Paronychia with wick in eponychial fold: 1 to 2 days; without wick: 3 to 5 days

Indications for Admission

- Felon, purulent tenosynovitis, or palmar space infection
- Any fracture requiring open reduction in the operating room
- Intraarticular fracture (>25% articular surface) or MCP dislocation
- Amputations other than distal fingertip
- Extensor tendon laceration that requires operative repair
- Flexor tendon laceration

BIBLIOGRAPHY

Henretig FM, King C (eds): *Pediatric Emergency Procedures,* Baltimore: Williams & Wilkins, 1997, pp 1205–1215.
Innis PC: Office evaluation and treatment of finger and hand injuries in children. *Curr Opin Pediatr* 1995;7:83–87.
Jebson PJ: Infections of the fingertips. Paronychias and felons. *Hand Clin* 1998; 14:547–555.

MULTIPLE TRAUMA

Trauma is the leading cause of death in children 1 to 14 years of age, exceeding all other causes combined. Blunt injuries are most common at all ages, although the incidence of penetrating trauma increases in adolescence. The main factors contributing to early morbidity and mortality are upper airway compromise and respiratory failure or arrest due to central neuraxis injury (brain and cervical spinal cord). Intracranial and intraabdominal hemorrhages are less common. Late deaths are caused chiefly by traumatic brain injury. Posttraumatic pulmonary insufficiency, respiratory distress syndrome, or "shock lung," and multiple organ system failure are not common.

Children are subject to unique mechanisms of injury that interact with their immature anatomic features and physiologic responses to produce distinct patterns of trauma. They are struck by cars or fall from heights while playing, are propelled into the windshields or ejected through the windows of moving vehicles in which they ride as unrestrained passengers, and fall while bicycle riding, in-line skating, scooter riding, or skateboarding. Because the head is proportionately larger and heavier in the child than in the adult, it bears the brunt of the forces of injury, even if other body regions are involved. Thus, serious head injury is more common in multiple blunt trauma in childhood, while internal organ injury is less common. It is estimated that at least 80% of multiple injury cases involve the head. Therefore, pediatric trauma is more often a disorder of airway and breathing than of bleeding and shock. The mortality associated with neuroventilatory derangements (concomitant abnormalities in mental status and respiratory function) approaches 25%. Hypotensive (decompensated) shock is present in fewer than 10% of all cases of major pediatric trauma, but mortality in those cases exceeds 50%.

Initial management of the injured child must be expeditious, in accordance with consensus protocols with which all participants in the resuscitative effort must be thoroughly familiar. This is best accomplished through the use of an aggressive team approach, with one member serving as the team leader, who takes responsibility for directing and coordinating the resuscitative effort. Although trauma resuscitation may be initiated in the ED, major trauma is a surgical illness that requires the immediate participation of experienced surgeons. The most common cause of preventable trauma death in children is inadequate initial resuscitation. Other preventable deaths are due to missed internal injuries, both intracranial and intraabdominal. Surgical interventions are ultimately required in more than 50% of victims of major pediatric trauma, despite the greater reliance on nonoperative management in children as opposed to adults.

Clinical Presentation

The presentation usually depends on the extent of central neuraxis injury, respiratory compromise, and blood loss. Head injuries are the most common anatomic findings, followed by injuries involving the axial skeleton; injuries to internal organs are least common. Abnormalities in level of consciousness and respiratory status are the most common physiologic findings. While hypotensive shock is uncommon in the pediatric trauma victim, particularly after blunt injury, a child may be in early shock with little or no external evidence (see Shock, pp 18–22), leading to what may be called the "deceptive" presentation of shock.

Diagnosis and ED Management

Primary Survey

The first priority is the primary survey, a rapid initial assessment that combines rapid cardiopulmonary assessment (the foundation of pediatric advanced life support) with rapid cranial-truncal examination, to *identify life-threatening problems that require immediate intervention* (Table 23-2). Note the patient's general condition, and take the following actions (*A, B, C, D, E*):

1. Assess the *Airway* for patency and maintainability. Confirm spontaneous air movement and listen for gurgling or stridor while protecting the cervical spine from flexion and extension.

Table 23-2   Management Options for Life-Threatening Conditions

FINDING	PROBLEM	MANAGEMENT
Noisy breathing, stridor	Upper-airway obstruction	Jaw thrust/C-spine control, intubation
Difficulty breathing	Respiratory failure	Bag-valve-mask ventilation, intubation
Unconsciousness	Severe traumatic brain injury	Intubation, mild hyperventilation
External bleeding	External wound	Direct pressure
Neck pain, spasm, tenderness; head injury	Possible C-spine fracture	Immobilize neck (semirigid extrication collar, tape, and head immobilizer)
Asymmetric breath sounds and hyper-resonant percussion note	Possible tension pneumothorax	Insert over-the-needle plastic catheter (2nd ICS in MCL) or chest tube
Asymmetric breath sounds and dull percussion note	Possible massive hemothorax	Chest x-ray; insert chest tube through separate incision in midaxillary line at level of nipple
Penetrating chest wound with difficulty breathing	Possible sucking chest wound	Apply occlusive dressing; insert chest tube through separate incision in midaxillary line at level of nipple
Penetrating chest wound with muffled heart sounds or distended neck veins	Possible pericardial tamponade	Pericardiocentesis (subxiphoid or 4th ICS 1cm lateral to left sternal border)
Paradoxical chest wall movement	Flail chest	Positive-pressure ventilation for respiratory failure
Orthostasis (pale, cool skin)	Compensated shock	Establish 2 large-bore IVs and give 20 mL/kg crystalloid boluses (may repeat once)
Hypotension	Decompensated shock Transient response to volume resuscitation	Tranfusion emergency: type O (Rh-neg for ♀) urgent: type-specific
Upper abdominal distention, hyper-resonant percussion note	Gastric dilatation	Insert nasogastric tube (orogastric tube if major orofacial trauma or an infant)

2. Check the adequacy of *Breathing* by simultaneously watching chest excursions, listening for breath sounds, and evaluating respiratory effort and rate. Palpate the trachea and ribs, and search for other signs of immediate life-threatening chest injuries.

3. Evaluate the *Circulation* for signs of shock by obtaining the pulse (tachycardia is the earliest measurable response to hypovolemia). In addition, examine the skin for pallor, cyanosis, mottling, and moisture. Check for the presence of active bleeding and delayed capillary refill (>2 s). Obtain a core temperature to assess for hypothermia.

4. Estimate the degree of *Disability* by noting the response to verbal and painful stimuli using the "AVPU" score (A = alert, V = responsive to verbal stimuli, P = responsive only to painful stimuli, U = unresponsive). Record pupillary size and reaction to light.

5. Fully *Expose* the patient, taking quick note of all external signs of injury (especially in penetrating trauma) before covering him or her to prevent heat loss.

6. Resuscitation. Trauma resuscitation is conducted concurrently with the primary survey. If life-threatening problems are identified, the team leader must immediately begin treatment, summon surgical assistance, and organize a sequence of therapy corresponding to the alphabetical order listed below.

A: Airway/Cervical Spine   As described in the section on cardiopulmonary resuscitation (pp 9–18), establish and maintain a patent airway. Noisy or stridulous breathing suggests airway obstruction, most often due to the tongue falling against the posterior pharyngeal wall. Perform a modified jaw thrust while maintaining bimanual in-line stabilization of the cervical spine in a neutral position (place a thin layer of padding beneath the torso of the young child). If the child is *A* (alert) or *V* (responsive to verbal stimuli) and is breathing spontaneously, administer humidified 100% oxygen. Use a nonrebreathing mask with a flow rate high enough to keep the nonrebreathing bag inflated throughout the respiratory cycle. If the child is *P* (responsive only to painful stimuli) or *U* (unresponsive), insert an oropharyngeal airway and ventilate with humidified 100% oxygen via a bag-valve-mask device. If these measures are unsuccessful in effectively maintaining or immediately restoring spontaneous ventilation and oxygenation or if the child is comatose as determined by a score of ≤8 on the Glasgow Coma Scale (GCS), perform orotracheal intubation while continuing to apply bimanual in-line stabilization to the head and neck.

If severe orofacial injuries prevent orotracheal intubation and bag-valve-mask ventilation is unsuccessful, perform needle cricothyroidotomy by inserting a large-bore (16- to 18-gauge) over-the-needle catheter through the cricoid membrane (located between the thyroid cartilage and the cricoid ring). Then attach oxygen tubing containing a side hole or a Y-connector to the hub of the catheter, and insufflate oxygen by intermittently occluding (1 s) and releasing (4 s) the open end of the side hole or Y-connector, thereby avoiding chest overexpansion. Alternatively attach the Luer-Lok tip of a 3.0-mL syringe from which the plunger has been removed to the hub of the catheter. Administer oxygen by ventilating with a bag-valve device through a no. 7.5 endotracheal tube adaptor inserted into the open end of the barrel of the syringe.

Severe multiple trauma, significant head or neck trauma, neck pain and tenderness, cervical muscle spasm, or a history of a sudden deceleration suggests the possibility of cervical spine and spinal cord injury. Immobilize the neck once the airway has been secured with a semirigid cervical extrication collar and a head immobilizer (soft collar or sandbags or large IV bags and tape are inadequate) until anteroposterior (AP), lateral, and open-mouth radiographic views of the cervical spine and a careful neurologic examination rule out an injury (see Cervical Spine Injuries, pp 641–644). Note that a lateral x-ray of the cervical spine, by itself, is insufficient to rule out cervical spine injury because of possible SCIWORA. Therefore it is neither necessary nor indicated as part of the initial management of the multiply injured child. Despite the importance of early control of the cervical spine, however, do not sacrifice the airway by efforts to maintain neck immobilization; never delay intubation because a radiologist or neurosurgeon has not reviewed the radiographs and confirmed that the films show no fracture.

B: Breathing/Chest Injuries   Administer humidified 100% oxygen to all victims of major trauma without waiting for arterial blood gas (ABG) results. Immediately intubate a patient who is unconscious, has decreased breath sounds, or has persistent evidence of respiratory failure after the airway is opened.

Examine for signs of a tension pneumothorax (see Pneumothorax, pp 660–662), including contralateral tracheal deviation, a hyperresonant percussion note, subcutaneous emphysema, distended neck veins, and continued respiratory distress after intubation. If any of these are found, immediately decompress by inserting a large-bore (16- to 18-gauge) over-the-needle catheter into the second intercostal space, above the third rib, in the midclavicular line on the affected side, without waiting for x-ray confirmation.

Asymmetric breath sounds associated with a hyperresonant percussion note and subcutaneous emphysema but without tracheal deviation or distended neck veins suggest a simple pneumothorax. Asymmetric breath sounds associated with a dull percussion note suggest a simple hemothorax. Tube thoracostomy is indicated for both after the ABCs have been adequately addressed.

Hypotension after a penetrating chest wound suggests the possibility of pericardial tamponade. Tachycardia is the most common finding. Muffled heart sounds, distended neck veins, and pulsus paradoxus are variable. Emergency thoracotomy is required, but pericardiocentesis (see Pericardial Tamponade, pp 659–660) is indicated if emergency thoracotomy is not initiated in the ED.

Also examine the patient for rib fractures, subcutaneous emphysema, and signs of penetrating chest trauma. A flail chest can cause paradoxical chest wall movement after blunt chest trauma. Positive-pressure ventilation is required if large flail segments are impairing ventilation. Small flail segments are associated with enough muscle spasm that they rarely impair ventilation. They require supportive treatment only, primarily for the underlying pulmonary contusion that is invariably present. Once the patient is stable, give analgesics as necessary.

Penetrating chest trauma can cause an open pneumothorax (sucking chest wound). Cover penetrating chest wounds completely with petrolatum gauze and perform tube thoracostomy to prevent the subsequent development of tension pneumothorax.

After securing the airway, obtain a chest radiograph if any of the above abnormalities are found on examination of the chest (except tension pneumothorax, which must be treated immediately). Review the film carefully for intrapleural air (simple or tension pneumothorax), intrapleural fluid (hemothorax), rib fractures, lung densities (pulmonary contusion), mediastinal emphysema, and widened mediastinum and loss of aortic contour (traumatic dissection of the aorta). Do not rely on normal chest radiographs when there is a suspicion of traumatic dissection of the aorta; obtain a CT of the chest.

C: Circulation/Bleeding and Shock   Cardiopulmonary arrest in a pediatric trauma victim may be an indication for emergency thoracotomy with pericardiotomy in the ED for relief of pericardial tamponade, cross-clamping of the descending aorta, or both if personnel experienced in these techniques are available. ED thoracotomy is not indicated for victims of blunt trauma but is occasionally successful in victims of penetrating trauma, particularly those who have pericardial tamponade or develop profound hypotension during the course of the resuscitative effort. ED thoracotomy is also indicated for victims of penetrating trauma who have lost pulses en route to the hospital. A patient with penetrating parasternal chest wounds or pericardial tamponade who is not in hypotensive shock should immediately be transported to the operating room for urgent thoracotomy. Summon the surgical team immediately upon the arrival of any such patient, and notify the operating room that the need for surgery may be imminent.

Control external bleeding with direct digital or manual pressure, pressure dressings, or pneumatic splints, but do not use tourniquets or clamps. Secure two large-bore (16- to 18-gauge) peripheral IV lines using over-the-needle catheters. Substitute a tibial intraosseous line if initial attempts at IV access fail, provided that the extremity is uninjured. The distal femur (3 cm above the external condyle) can be used if the tibia is fractured. Give 20 mL/kg of warmed isotonic crystalloid (normal saline or Ringer's lactate) as a rapid IV bolus after obtaining blood for type and cross-match, spun hematocrit, and CBC. Monitor the blood pressure carefully, and repeat the bolus every 5 to 10 min as needed. If 40 mL/kg does not raise the blood pressure, give a transfusion of 10 mL/kg of packed red blood cells. In an emergency, when there is evidence of hypotensive shock, use type O blood, which is available immediately: O positive or negative for males, O negative for females; transfusion reactions are extremely rare. Type-specific blood that is not cross-matched can be available in 10 min; it can be used in urgent but not emergency circumstances.

Base ongoing volume resuscitation on the response to the initial fluid challenge. Remember that fewer than 10% of children present in hypotensive shock after major trauma. Also, for most seriously injured children, excessive fluid administration is as detrimental as inadequate fluid administration because of the potential for further increases in the elevated intracranial pressures associated with traumatic brain injury, the most common internal organ injury sustained from pediatric blunt trauma.

However, cerebral hypoxia due to inadequate cerebral perfusion is the most common cause of secondary brain injury, and it dramatically worsens cerebral swelling. Thus, never restrict fluid until hemodynamic stability has been completely restored.

Attempt to identify sources of potential or ongoing blood loss. Following a careful physical examination, obtain a chest x-ray to rule out hemothorax and obtain a pelvic x-ray, since a pelvic fracture is a common cause of retroperitoneal hemorrhage. Obtain urine for urinalysis. Hematuria (>50 cells per high-power field) may indicate urinary tract injury (see Genitourinary Trauma, pp 258–262) or injury to other intraabdominal organs, as 80% of blunt renal injuries are associated with damage to adjacent organs. Although isolated hematuria is rarely a life-threatening problem, expeditious radiographic evaluation of the urinary tract is indicated.

If the patient remains in shock or has a falling hematocrit, reassess for occult blood loss in the pleural cavities, abdomen, retroperitoneum, and pelvis; repeat diagnostic tests if indicated; and transport the patient to the operating room.

Diagnostic peritoneal lavage is not routinely employed for injured children with suspected intraabdominal bleeding to determine the need for urgent laparotomy. Conservative, nonoperative management of solid-organ (liver, spleen, kidney) injury is standard, so a positive result (RBCs >100/mm^3) does not constitute an automatic indication for surgery. Abdominal CT with IV contrast enhancement is the diagnostic procedure of choice for identifying injuries and bleeding sites in a hemodynamically stable patient. For an unstable patient, use the focused abdominal sonography for trauma (FAST). It is noninvasive and does not interfere with resuscitation. It is accurate for the identification of free abdominal fluid as well as pericardial fluid. Reserve abdominal paracentesis for a patient with unstable vital signs in whom the source of the bleeding is unknown or the abdominal sonogram is suboptimal and/or the child with stable vital signs who is going immediately to the operating room for treatment of intracranial or musculoskeletal injuries. If necessary, the paracentesis can be performed in the operating room.

D: Disability (Neurologic)   Once vital signs have been stabilized, direct the resuscitative efforts toward the diagnosis and treatment of injuries to the central neuraxis (see Head Trauma, pp 461–467, and Cervical Spine Injuries, pp 641–644). Priorities in the neurologic evaluation are accurate determination of the level of consciousness, pupillary size and reactivity, eye movements and oculovestibular responses, and motor, sensory, and reflex responses. Asymmetry in pupillary size and reactivity or in motor, sensory, or reflex responses suggests the possibility of an intracranial hematoma, while areflexia, even in deep coma, suggests the possibility of spinal cord injury.

Request neurosurgical assistance and arrange for an immediate CT scan of the head for any patient with a history of prolonged unconsciousness (>5 min) or a seizure occurring more than 3 s after impact, GCS score ≤14, focal neurologic signs, or symptoms of increased intracranial pressure, such as nausea, vomiting, or persistent headache or dizziness. Monitor the patient fully (ECG, Doppler sphygmomanometry, pulse oximetry) throughout the study, and ensure that someone (emergency physician, trauma surgeon, anesthesiologist, nurse-anesthetist) capable of emergency management of the pediatric airway is present. The leading cause of the increased intracranial pressure commonly observed after pediatric closed head injury is not intracranial hematoma, as in adults, but cerebral swelling due to the secondary brain injury caused by cerebral hypoxia. For this reason, and because the outcome of traumatic brain injury in children is far better than it is in adults, children with traumatic brain injury who present in coma require aggressive resuscitative efforts.

A number of factors contribute to the development of cerebral hypoxia in the child with severe closed head injury. Unconsciousness produces hypotonia in the muscles supporting the soft tissues of the larynx and oropharynx, resulting in passive closure of the upper airway. Both primary brain injury (direct trauma) and secondary brain injury (cerebral hypoxia) can cause temporary paralysis of cerebrovascular autoregulation, resulting in cerebral vasodilation and hyperemia, leading to progressive increases in intracranial pressure. These, in turn, decrease cerebral perfusion pressure and disrupt medullary control of breathing, thereby worsening cerebral hypoxia and leading to further increases in intracranial pressure.

Immediate intubation and mild hyperventilation, if instituted promptly, may interrupt this vicious cycle, which otherwise leads to uncal herniation and brain death. Intubation reopens the airway, permitting oxygen to reach the circulation and facilitating hyperventilation. Hyperventilation induces alkalosis, normalizing cerebral blood flow and allowing blood to perfuse the brain. Immediately intubate any child who presents with a GCS score ≤8, extensor posturing, asymmetric or unreactive pupils, or progressive neurologic deterioration (decrease in GCS of more than 2 points from patient's best). Initiate mild hyperventilation with a tidal volume of 8–10 mL/kg, at a rate that lowers the Pco_2 to between 35 and 40 mmHg. Mild hyperventilation is preferred owing to the risk of cerebral ischemia associated with aggressive hyperventilation.

Rapid-sequence intubation is indicated for the head-injured child who presents in coma; it must be performed only by personnel experienced in emergency intubation of the pediatric patient and familiar with the use of neuromuscular blockers. It is technically more difficult in the trauma patient whose neck must remain in a neutral position throughout the procedure because of the possibility of spinal cord injury. A number of therapeutic regimens are in common use (see Airway Management, pp 1–9).

Treat ongoing seizures with lorazepam (0.05–0.1 mg/kg) or diazepam (0.1–0.3 mg/kg) slowly over 2 min, followed by fosphenytoin [20 phenytoin equivalents (PE)/kg IV over 10–15 min) or phenytoin (20 mg/kg IV over 20–30 min). If cervical or thoracic spinal cord injuries are suspected treat any associated focal neurologic deficits within 8 h with IV methylprednisolone (30 mg/kg/15 min loading dose, followed 45 min later by a constant infusion of 5.4 mg/kg/h for 23 h). Corticosteroids have no established role in the acute management of head injuries or penetrating spinal trauma. Avoid the use of diuretic agents such as IV mannitol (0.5–1 g/kg) or furosemide (1 mg/kg) unless there is evidence of uncal herniation (unilateral dilated pupil or other lateralizing signs). Carefully document key neurologic findings before rapid-sequence intubation or other treatments that alter neurologic status, but never delay treatment of life-threatening neurotrauma while awaiting arrival of neurologic or neurosurgical consultants.

E: Expose (Examine)   Expose the patient completely, and perform a rapid but thorough physical examination (including the back, buttocks, and all skin creases), looking for associated injuries. Palpate all bones, including the pelvic and facial bones, and palpate and percuss the teeth. Check the extraocular movements and corneal clarity, and recheck pupillary reactivity and symmetry. Look for signs of depressed (scalp hematoma or laceration with underlying deformity or crepitance) and basilar (hemotympanum, clear rhino- or otorrhea, infraorbital and retroauricular ecchymoses) skull fractures. Once the examination is completed, cover the patient with a blanket to prevent hypothermia. The diagnosis and management of other traumas is detailed elsewhere: ocular (pp 489–495), dental (pp 67–71), orthopedic (pp 509–522), genitourinary (pp 258–262), and soft tissue (pp 677–684).

F: Foley Catheter   Insert a catheter into the bladder to monitor the urine output closely in all multiple trauma patients. The sole exception is a patient with suspected urethral disruption, suggested by blood at the urethral meatus, and males with scrotal hematoma or a "high-riding" or "boggy" prostate. These injuries are usually associated with a pelvic fracture, straddle injury, or penetrating wound. Call a urologist immediately to perform a retrograde urethrogram; urine output can be monitored with a suprapubic catheter if needed. The desired urine output is at least 2 mL/kg/h in an infant, 1 mL/kg/h in a child, and 0.5 mL/kg/h in an adolescent. Gross or significant microscopic hematuria (>50 RBCs per high-power field) requires radiologic evaluation to rule out renal injury.

G: Gastric Decompression   Insert a nasogastric tube and attach to intermittent (Levin tube) or continuous (sump tube) suction to prevent aspiration and improve ventilation by reducing gastric dilatation. Use an orogastric tube instead if there is evidence of significant orofacial trauma.

Secondary Survey
Once the primary survey has been completed and the resuscitation phase is under way, proceed with the secondary survey: a careful, complete head-to-toe examination of the trauma patient to determine the full extent of tissue injury. Be sure to perform a rectal examination to exclude GI bleeding and evaluate anal sphincter tone. If life-threatening problems are not identified during the primary survey but the mechanism of injury indicates that the patient is potentially at risk for life-threatening problems, secure a large-bore IV, check vital signs frequently, arrange for initial blood and x-ray studies, order a urinalysis as a screen for occult intra-abdominal injury, and admit the patient for observation.

Obtain a CBC, ABG, and type and cross-match for any patient admitted for observation to a critical care unit. In addition, obtain serum lipase (pancreatic injury) and hepatic transaminases for a patient admitted for evaluation of abdominal trauma. CPK and urine myoglobin are indicated for the child with suspected crush injury, as well as electrolytes, blood urea nitrogen (BUN), and creatinine. The last three, as well as serum glucose, are useful as baseline studies in a child with severe traumatic brain injury.

Victims of multiple trauma require x-rays of the chest and pelvis if an adequate physical examination cannot be performed. A lateral x-ray of the cervical spine may be obtained (see pp 642–643), although, as discussed previously, it cannot reliably rule out spinal cord injury. Therefore maintain full spinal immobilization of any patient in whom spinal cord injury has not been or cannot be properly ruled out. If the vital signs are stable but intraabdominal injury is suspected (based on physical signs of internal hemorrhage, such as abdominal tenderness, distention, bruising, or gross hematuria), prepare the patient for a CT scan of the abdomen with IV and oral contrast (to follow CT scan of the head when obtained). For oral contrast, the dose of Gastrografin for a child over 10 years of age is 15 mL in 485 mL of water. Give 8 to 10 mL in 350 mL water to a patient 8 to 10 years of age and 5 mL in 245 mL water to a child 1 to 5 years of age. Oral contrast is not helpful in children unless the full dose can be given (usually requiring a nasogastric tube). If this is not possible, obtain the CT scan with IV contrast only. Plain x-rays may then be ordered as necessary. Victims of minor trauma with stable vital signs who are awake, alert, and able to ambulate normally require x-rays only if indicated by historical and physical findings.

Indications for Admission

- Spine injury
- Respiratory distress or compromise
- Hypotension or orthostatic changes in vital signs
- Suspected intrathoracic or intraabdominal injury
- Serious fracture or soft tissue injury
- GCS < 14, increased intracranial pressure, compound/depressed skull fracture
- Stab wound unless surgical evaluation determines it to be superficial

BIBLIOGRAPHY

American Academy of Pediatrics and American College of Emergency Physicians Joint Task Force on Advanced Pediatric Life Support: Traumatic emergencies, in *APLS: The Pediatric Emergency Medicine Course,* 2d ed. Elk Grove Village, IL and Dallas: American Academy of Pediatrics and American College of Emergency Physicians, 1993, pp 59–115.

Kevill K, Wong AM, Goldman HS, Gershel JC: A complete trauma series indicated for all pediatric trauma victims. *Pediatr Emerg* Care 2002;18:75–78.

Rothrock SG, Green SM, Morgan R: Abdominal trauma in infants and children: prompt identification and early management of serious and life-threatening injuries. Part I: injury patterns and initial assessment. *Pediatr Emerg Care* 2000; 16:106–115.

Rothrock SG, Green SM, Morgan R: Abdominal trauma in infants and children: prompt identification and early management of serious and life-threatening injuries. Part II: specific injuries and ED management. *Pediatr Emerg Care* 2000;16:189–195.

Sanchez JI, Paides CN: Trauma care in the new millennium. *Surg Clinics North Am* 1999;79:1503–1535.

PERICARDIAL TAMPONADE

Pericardial tamponade is a life-threatening emergency requiring immediate intervention. The most common cause is penetrating thoracic trauma, when blood accumulates in the pericardial sac and interferes with cardiac filling. Tamponade is rare after blunt thoracic trauma.

Clinical Presentation

Suspect pericardial tamponade if there are failing vital signs or pulseless electrical activity is noted after penetrating chest trauma, especially following a poor response to tube thoracostomy. Shock associated with tachypnea, clear lungs with equal breath sounds bilaterally, neck vein distention (if the patient is not hypovolemic), and distant or muffled heart sounds suggest the diagnosis. The pulse pressure is usually narrowed, and pulsus paradoxus (a drop of more than 10 mmHg in the systolic blood pressure on inspiration) may be present but is not necessary to establish the diagnosis.

Diagnosis

See pp 649–658 for the approach to the multiple trauma patient. The clinical presentation of pericardial tamponade may resemble that of other life-threatening chest injuries; often, they occur simultaneously. Distended neck veins and pulsus paradoxus can both be seen in a patient with nontraumatic disorders such as *congestive heart failure*. Pulsus paradoxus may also be noted in a patient with severe *asthma* (wheezing, poor air movement). Tachypnea and tachycardia with normal heart sounds are frequent in patients with *pneumothorax* or *hemothorax*.

In acute pericardial tamponade, the chest x-ray frequently reveals a normal heart or a water-bag cardiac shadow. Emergency transthoracic ultrasound can demonstrate fluid in the pericardium and poor left ventricular wall motion.

Insert a right atrial catheter or central venous pressure (CVP) line if the diagnosis is uncertain. The CVP is usually elevated (>15 cmH$_2$O) unless the patient is hypovolemic from other injuries. The ECG in pericardial tamponade may reveal low voltage and nonspecific ST-T wave changes. Electrical alternans (alternating variations in the height of the QRS complex due to shifts in the QRS axis from beat to beat as the heart swings to and fro in the pericardial sac) is diagnostic of a pericardial effusion.

ED Management

Once the diagnosis is made, immediately consult a surgeon to perform a thoracotomy or pericardiotomy in the operating room. If an experienced surgeon is not available, pericardiocentesis is indicated. Monitor the patient's vital signs and ECG before, during, and after the procedure. Use a large-bore (16- to 18-gauge) over-the-needle catheter, attached by three-way stopcock to a 30-mL syringe and by an alligator clip (placed just beyond the hub of the needle) to the chest lead (V) of an ECG machine. Puncture the skin inferior to the xiphoid process, directing the needle toward the tip of the left scapula, at a 45-degree angle to the skin. Free flow of nonclotted, nonpulsatile blood suggests that the pericardium has been entered. If the needle touches the epicardial surface, a "current-of-injury pattern" (ST segment elevation) will be seen on the ECG; in that case, withdraw the needle slightly. An improvement in vital signs may follow removal of as little as 10 to 20 mL of blood. After aspiration is complete, withdraw the needle but leave the catheter in with the stopcock closed in case fluid reaccumulates. A negative tap does not rule out tamponade, since blood in the pericardial sac clots rapidly.

Indications for Admission

- Pericardial tamponade
- Pericardial effusion

BIBLIOGRAPHY

Cooper A, Foltin GL: Thoracic trauma, in Barkin RM (ed): *Pediatric Emergency Medicine: Concepts and Clinical Practice,* 2nd ed. St Louis: Mosby-Year Book, 1997, pp 318–331.

Kosta K, Krinzon I: Electrical alternans in cardiac tamponade. *Echocardiography* 2000;17:575–576.

Scarpinato L: Pericardial effusion and cardiac tamponade diagnostic methods. Where are we headed? *Chest* 1996;110:308–310.

PNEUMOTHORAX

Pneumothorax can result from blunt or penetrating thoracic trauma. It can also occur in asthmatics, in newborns, in association with smoking "crack" cocaine or marijuana, and occasionally in otherwise healthy adolescents without trauma.

Clinical Presentation

Pneumothorax presents with signs of respiratory distress, including tachypnea, nasal flaring, accessory muscle use, and anxiety or altered mental status. Breath sounds may be decreased or absent on the affected (ipsilateral) side. The percussion note can be tympanitic. Pulsus paradoxus (>10 mmHg drop in the systolic blood pressure on inspiration) may be noted.

Signs of a tension pneumothorax may include all of the above, along with deviation of the trachea away from the affected side and, if severe, may include cyanosis, jugular vein distention (if the patient is not hypovolemic), and deterioration of the vital signs, leading to pulseless electrical activity and death. Pneumomediastinum can occur with or without pneumothorax. Although a pneumomediastinum requires no immediate treatment, its presence suggests the possibility of barotrauma and an associated pneumothorax.

Diagnosis

See pp 649–658 for the general approach to the patient with multiple trauma. Always be suspicious of the possibility of pneumothorax in a trauma victim. Air can leak from the lung, the tracheobronchial tree, or

Table 23-3   Diagnosis of Immediate Life-Threatening Chest Injuries

	TENSION PNEUMOTHORAX	MASSIVE HEMOTHORAX	CARDIAC TAMPONADE
Breath Sounds	Ipsilateral decrease	Ipsilateral decrease	Normal
Percussion note	Hyperresonant	Dull	Normal
Tracheal location	Contralateral shift	Midline	Midline
Neck veins	Distended	Flat	Distended
Heart tones	Normal	Normal	Muffled

the esophagus or through a sucking wound in the chest wall. Trauma can produce pneumothorax directly in penetrating injury or indirectly in blunt injury (by fracturing ribs). However, a pneumothorax can occur in the absence of either.

Tension pneumothorax may be confused with other immediate life-threatening chest injuries (Table 23-3). In *massive hemothorax,* breath sounds are decreased on the affected side, as in tension pneumothorax, but the percussion note is dull and the neck veins are flat. In *pericardial tamponade,* the neck veins may be distended (if the patient is not hypovolemic), but breath sounds are adequate, heart sounds are diminished or muffled, and ECG monitoring may reveal low voltage. In *hypovolemic shock,* vital signs will have deteriorated, but breath and heart sounds are usually normal and the neck veins flat.

The diagnosis of tension pneumothorax is made on clinical grounds alone. *Treat immediately if it is suspected,* without waiting for a confirmatory chest x-ray. A chest x-ray is indicated to confirm the diagnosis of simple pneumothorax. A *pleural effusion* in the asthmatic patient with pneumonia can mimic hemopneumothorax.

ED Management

Immediately give humidified 100% oxygen with a flow rate high enough to keep the nonrebreathing bag inflated throughout the respiratory cycle and, unless the patient has severe respiratory distress, secure a large-bore (16- to 18-gauge) IV line.

Tension Pneumothorax   Decompress immediately, without waiting for x-ray confirmation. Insert a large-bore over-the-needle plastic catheter into the chest above the top of the third rib, in the midclavicular line of the affected side. A rush of air and improvement in the patient's ventilatory status confirm both the diagnosis and the adequacy of the therapy. Remove the needle and leave the catheter in place. Then insert a chest tube in the fifth intercostal space above the sixth rib in the anterior to midaxillary line, attach it to an underwater seal device once the tube has been properly secured, and remove the over-the-needle catheter used for decompression.

Simple Pneumothorax   Treat after x-ray confirmation. Insert a chest tube in the fifth intercostal space above the sixth rib in the anterior to midaxillary line and attach it to an underwater seal device once the tube has been properly secured.

Indication for Admission

- Any pneumothorax or hemothorax

BIBLIOGRAPHY

Cooper A: Critical management of chest, abdomen, and extremity trauma: management of systems for chest drainage and suction, in Holbrook PR (ed): *Textbook of Pediatric Critical Care.* Philadelphia: Saunders, 1993, pp 1060–1081.

Cooper A, Foltin GL: Thoracic trauma, in Barkin RM (ed): *Pediatric Emergency Medicine: Concepts and Clinical Practice,* 2nd ed. St Louis: Mosby-Year Book, 1997, pp 318–331.

Sarihan H, Abes M, Akyazici R, et al: Blunt thoracic trauma in children. *J Cardiovasc Surg (Torino)* 1996;37:525–528.

CHAPTER 24

Wound Care
and Minor Trauma

Anthony Ciorciari and Michael Touger

ABSCESSES

A cutaneous abscess is a localized collection of pus, usually secondary to disruption of skin integrity. The organisms most often involved are *Staphylococcus aureus* and group A *Streptococcus*.

Clinical Presentation and Diagnosis

An *abscess* presents as a discrete, well-circumscribed swelling with central fluctuance. It is tender and is usually associated with erythema and warmth of the overlying skin. Lymphangitis and lymphadenitis are complications that can herald hematogenous dissemination and sepsis. *Cellulitis* presents with localized swelling, tenderness, erythema, and warmth, but there is no fluctuance.

ED Management

The definitive treatment of an abscess is incision and drainage, which can usually be performed in the ED. When the abscess is in immediate proximity to neurovascular structures, however, first perform needle aspiration to confirm purulence and avoid incising a vascular aneurysm. This precaution specifically applies to abscesses in the neck, supraclavicular fossa, antecubital fossa, popliteal fossa, and inguinal and axillary areas.

Maintain strict aseptic technique to prevent the spread of the infection; prepare the skin with a povidone-iodine solution. Although total anesthesia may be difficult to achieve, use a combination of a regional field block (a ring of 1% lidocaine outside the perimeter of the abscess and erythema) and a linear injection of 1% lidocaine into the roof of the abscess along the planned incision. If this technique is unsuccessful, provide sedation and analgesia (pp 617–639).

Make the incision along the natural skin tension lines to prevent excessive scarring. After incision, obtain culture specimens if the patient appears ill, is an IV drug user, or is immunocompromised. Routine cultures are not necessary for immunocompetent patients. Explore the abscess cavity with a blunt instrument or sterile gloved finger to break up any loculated pockets of purulence. Copiously irrigate the cavity with normal saline (NS) under moderate pressure; and pack it loosely with iodoform gauze to promote drainage and ensure hemostasis; and apply a sterile dressing. Instruct the family to irrigate the cavity under running warm water three times a day or to apply warm wet soaks three times a day. Prescribe daily dressing changes, for 3 to 5 days. Oral antibiotics are of no additional benefit after incision and drainage of uncomplicated abscesses in otherwise healthy children; antibiotics are indicated if there is an area of cellulitis surrounding the abscess. Use cephalexin (40 mg/kg/day divided qid), cefadroxil (40 mg/kg/day divided bid), amoxicillin-clavulanate (875/125 formulation; 45 mg/kg/day of amoxicillin divided bid), or if the patient is allergic to penicillin, clindamycin (20 mg/kg/day divided tid). Have the patient return in 24 h to evaluate for complications, remove the packing, and repeat the irrigation. Loosely repack the cavity only if pus is again found. Usually, by 48 h, the incision remains open without packing while the cavity heals from below.

Refer breast, perirectal, fingertip (pulp), hand, and deep abscesses of the neck to an experienced surgeon.

Follow-up

- After abscess drainage: daily for 2 to 3 days

Indications for Admission

- Abscess associated with lymphangitis, fever >38.9°C (102°F), or signs of toxicity
- Abscess in an immunocompromised patient

BIBLIOGRAPHY

Simon RR, Brenner BE: *Emergency Procedures and Techniques,* 4th ed. Baltimore: Lippincott Williams & Wilkins, 2001.

Wind CG, Rich NM: *Principles of Surgical Technique,* 2d ed. Baltimore: Urban & Schwarzenberg, 1989.

BITE WOUNDS

About 1% of all ED visits are for bites, about 80% of which are caused by dogs. More than one-half of bite victims are children, most of them toddlers. While a patient may seek medical attention because of cosmetic concerns, bleeding, or fear of rabies, the most common complication is infection. An increased risk of infection occurs with puncture wounds, hand wounds, or when there has been a delay (>24 h) in seeking medical attention.

Clinical Presentation and Diagnosis

Usually, the history of an animal bite is readily obtained, so the diagnosis is evident. The three major types of bite wounds are puncture wounds, lacerations, and closed-first injuries (CFIs). Puncture wounds are of particular concern, as the small break in the skin belies the significant risk of infection. Suspect that a laceration over the metacarpophalangeal joint of an adolescent represents a CFI, sustained when the patient punched another person in the mouth.

ED Management

General Measures Thoroughly clean every bite wound with soap and water. Moderate-pressure irrigation in the ED is indicated for lacerations and CFIs, but it is probably ineffective for punctures. Use an 18- or 20-gauge IV catheter attached to a 1-L bag of NS, around which a blood transfusion cuff is inflated to 300 mmHg. If the irrigation is not tolerated, anesthetize the intact skin margins of the wound with 1% lidocaine and then irrigate. Debride devitalized tissue, which is an excellent culture medium. This is particularly important with dog bites, which are in part crush injuries.

Suturing The suturing of bite wounds remains controversial. When the wound can be thoroughly cleaned, primary closure is acceptable. This is particularly important with facial lacerations, for which cosmesis is a priority. Close these lacerations whenever possible. Puncture wounds and CFIs cannot be adequately cleaned, so suturing is contraindicated.

Antibiotics Prophylactic antibiotics are indicated for puncture wounds, CFIs, hand wounds, all cat bite wounds, and any bite-wound laceration that is sutured. *Staphylococcus aureus* and group A *Streptococcus* are implicated in infected human, cat, and dog bite wounds. Species of gram-negative bacteria—such as *Pasteurella, Moraxella,* and *Enterococcus* from dog and cat bites and *Eikenella corrodens* and *Corynebacterium* from human bites—can also cause infections. Use amoxicillin-clavulanate (875/125 formulation; 45 mg/kg/day of amoxicillin divided bid). Give a penicillin-allergic patient clindamycin (20 mg/kg/day divided tid) and trimethoprim-sulfamethoxazole (TMP-SMX; 10 mg/kg/day of TMP divided bid).

Tetanus *Clostridium* can be present in the mouths of coprophagic animals. Give tetanus toxoid (0.5 mL) unless a booster was received in the previous 5 years.

Rabies Decisions regarding rabies treatment depend on the prevalence of the disease in the species in the area where the animal lives. See pp 670–672 for the indications for prophylaxis.

Follow-up

- Bite wound: daily for 2 to 3 days. Give antibiotics if the patient develops fever, increasing pain or erythema, or a purulent discharge.

Indications for Admission

- Bite wounds unresponsive to oral antibiotics
- Infected bite wounds in patients who initially seek attention >24 h after the bite
- Bite wounds in immunocompromised patients

BIBLIOGRAPHY

Kelleher AT, Gordon SM: Management of bite wounds and infection in primary care. *Cleve Clin J Med* 1997;64:137–141.

Presutti RJ: Prevention and treatment of dog bites. *Am Fam Physician* 2001; 63:1567–1572.

Talan DA, Citron DM, Abrahamian FM, et al: Bacteriologic analysis of infected dog and cat bites. *N Engl J Med* 1999;340:85–92.

FOREIGN-BODY REMOVAL

Small fragments of wood or pieces of glass are the most common foreign bodies embedded in the skin. A fresh wound is usually tender, and the foreign body is often seen or palpated just below the skin surface. Delayed presentations are associated with induration and tenderness, often with purulent or serosanguinous drainage.

Fishhooks embedded in the skin merit special consideration, as there may be more than one barb. The barb may completely penetrate a finger or earlobe, emerging from the other side and leaving the hook shaft still embedded.

Diagnosis

Radiographs can be helpful in identifying and locating foreign bodies. A radiopaque marker, such as a bent paperclip taped to the overlying skin, can be used as a reference point for estimating the exact location of the object. A radiograph is also indicated when the presence of a foreign body cannot be ruled out, as when an old wound does not heal, continues to drain serosanguineous or purulent material, or remains tender. Virtually all glass is radiopaque, and wooden splinters can occasionally be seen if they are covered with dirt particles. Obtain an ultrasound to locate a non-radiopaque foreign body such as a thorn or piece of plastic.

ED Management

Attempt to remove a foreign body in the ED only if it is close enough to the surface to be seen or palpated. Cleanse the skin with povidone-iodine and anesthetize the area by local infiltration, field block, or regional nerve block. Using the paperclip marker and x-rays for reference, make a stab incision with a no. 11 blade directed at the foreign body. Carefully explore the wound with a small hemostat to find and remove the object. Then gently palpate over the wound with a gloved finger to identify any remaining fragments. Obtain a repeat x-ray if there is a question of a retained fragment.

When removal attempts are prolonged or unsuccessful, consult with a surgeon to plan for a definitive operative procedure under fluoroscopic or sonographic guidance. Foreign bodies in the plantar surface of the foot are especially difficult to remove in the ED. Refer patients with foreign bodies in the face or hand to a surgeon, and consult with a surgeon before attempting to remove a foreign body from the neck unless it is clearly superficial.

When the foreign body is small or cannot be palpated, it is usually fruitless to probe the wound. If the wound is tender and crusted over, however, unroof it with the point of an 18-gauge needle to facilitate the drainage of any pus; the object may emerge over the next several days. Continue with warm soaks at home, and reevaluate the wound in 48 h.

To remove a fishhook, advance the barbed end until the skin is tented and anesthetize that area with 1% lidocaine. Then advance the point until the barb leaves the skin, sever the barbed point with wire cutters, and pull the shaft of the hook back out through the original entrance wound. If the fishhook has several barbs, separate them with wire cutters and remove each one individually. If the barb is already through the skin, cut it off and pull the shaft out without using any anesthetic.

Give tetanus toxoid (0.5 mL) to any patient who has completed a primary series but has not received a booster in the previous 5 years. Use DT for children under 6 years of age and dT for older patients.

Follow-up
- Small or nonpalpable foreign body: 48 h

Indication for Admission
- Foreign body in plantar surface of foot causing inability to bear weight, requiring surgical removal

BIBLIOGRAPHY

Gammons MG, Jackson E: Fishhook removal. *Am Fam Physician* 2001;63: 2231–2236.
Horton LK, Jacobson JA, Powell A, et al: Sonography and radiography of soft-tissue foreign bodies. *AJR* 2001;176:1155–1159.
Trott A: *Wounds and Lacerations: Emergency Care and Closure,* 2nd ed. St. Louis: Mosby, 1997.

INSECT BITES AND STINGS

Insect bites and stings usually cause a local reaction. However, systemic anaphylactoid reactions can occur after Hymenoptera stings (honeybees, wasps, hornets, yellow jackets, harvester and fire ants) in susceptible patients.

Clinical Presentation

Reactions can be classified as immediate (within 2 h) or delayed (after 2 h). Immediate reactions may be local or systemic.

Immediate Local Reactions   These include local pain, erythema, swelling, tingling, warmth, and pruritus at the sting site. Local reactions usually last 24 to 48 h; they can be extensive, although all affected skin is contiguous with the sting site.

Delayed Reactions   These can occur after a 1- to 2-week interval. They present as large local reactions, serum sickness (fever, arthralgia, urticaria, lymphadenopathy), and, rarely, peripheral neuritis, vasculitis, nephritis, or encephalitis.

Immediate Systemic Reactions   The hallmark of a systemic reaction is swelling that occurs at locations not contiguous with the sting site. The reaction may be mild, with itching and urticaria. More severe anaphylactoid reactions can occur with hypotension, wheezing, laryngeal edema, and shock. Some 85% of sensitive patients manifest symptoms within 5 min; all have symptoms within 1 to 2 h.

Diagnosis

The diagnosis is suggested by the history of a sting or by the typical appearance of a local reaction in the warm-weather months. Stings, as opposed to *insect bites,* are always painful. *Cellulitis* may look similar, but a bacterial infection usually does not develop abruptly. Also, a cellulitis may be associated with fever, lymphangitic streaking, and local lymphadenopathy.

Consider other causes of systemic allergic reactions, such as *drugs* (penicillins, sulfonamides, contrast dyes) and *foods* (shellfish, eggs). Try to ascertain whether the insect was a member of the Hymenoptera order, and inquire about a history of allergies and any previous systemic reactions to insect stings.

ED Management

Local Reactions   Among the Hymenoptera, only honeybees lose their stingers, which may remain at the sting site. Remove the stinger (if it is still in place) by grasping it as close to the puncture site as possible with a small forceps. Cleanse the site, apply ice or cool compresses to the area, and give oral diphenhydramine (5 mg/kg/day divided qid, 50 mg/dose maximum) or hydroxyzine (2 mg/kg/day divided tid, 50 mg/dose maximum). If the erythema continues to spread during the 24 h after the bite or sting, consider the wound to be infected (see Cellulitis, pp 86–87). Treat with 40 mg/ kg/day of either cephalexin (divided qid) or cefadroxil (divided bid), warm compresses every 2 h, and elevation.

Systemic Reactions   Treat mild reactions (itching, urticaria) with oral diphenhydramine or hydroxyzine. The management of severe systemic reactions is the same as for anaphylaxis (see pp 23–26). Prescribe an EpiPen and refer the patient to an allergist for evaluation and possible immunotherapy.

Follow-up

- Local reaction: 24 h if the erythema is spreading
- Systemic reaction (not anaphylaxis): 2 to 3 days

Indications for Admission

- Systemic anaphylactoid reaction
- Severe local reaction associated with inability to drink

BIBLIOGRAPHY

Bahna SL: Insect sting allergy: a matter of life and death. *Pediatr Ann* 2000;29: 753–758.

Graft DF: Stinging insect hypersensitivity in children. *Curr Opin Pediatr* 1996;8: 597–600.

Schexnayder SM, Schexnayder RE: Bites, stings, and other painful things. *Pediatr Ann* 2000;29:354–358.

MARINE STINGS AND ENVENOMATIONS

Marine stings and envenomations can be caused by both invertebrates and vertebrates. Invertebrates such as the jellyfish, Portuguese man-of-war, sea anemone, and coral can contain thousands of stinging cells (nematocysts); others contain a toxin that can be transmitted by contact (certain sponges, sea urchins).

Envenomation from vertebrates results from contact with toxin on the dorsal spines of the Scorpaenidae family (scorpionfish, stonefish, lionfish) or the spines on the tail of a stingray.

Clinical Presentation and Diagnosis

Invertebrates   Symptoms correlate with the number of nematocysts coming into contact with the skin. The clinical presentation ranges from mild dermatitis with pain, burning, swelling, and erythema at the site of the sting to anaphylactoid reactions. The *Portuguese man-of-war* can cause generalized muscular cramps, vomiting, and cardiovascular collapse.

Sponges deposit silica spicules, causing pruritic or irritant dermatitis that can lead to epidermal desquamation. The barbs of *sea urchins* can become deeply embedded. The toxin causes severe pain, swelling, erythema, and occasionally muscular paralysis.

Vertebrates   Contact with the dorsal spines of scorpionfish, stonefish, and lionfish causes excruciating pain, associated with erythema, swelling, and paresthesias of the affected extremity. The tail of a *stingray* can cause a severe laceration, without venom release. If venom is released from the tail spines, local pain and burning ensue, followed by muscular cramping and weakness and, on occasion, cardiac arrhythmias and seizures.

ED Management

As a rule, the venoms are heat-labile. Soaking the affected area in hot water (43.4–46.1°C, 110–115°F) may greatly reduce the pain. Additional therapy consists of local wound care, analgesia, tetanus prophylaxis (if indicated), antihistamines (hydroxyzine 2 mg/ kg/day divided tid, 50 mg/dose maximum, or diphenhydramine 5 mg/kg/day divided qid, 50 mg/dose maximum) for itching, and antibiotics (40 mg/kg/day of cephalexin divided qid or cefadroxil divided bid) for lacerations.

Invertebrates   Before immersion in hot water, remove any unruptured nematocysts by rinsing with sea (salt) water for 30 to 90 min. Do not use fresh water, which will cause them to activate. Then remove any remaining tentacles with a forceps or gloved hand. If any tentacles persist, first fix them by pouring vinegar over the area, then dust with talcum powder and remove by shaving or scraping with a sterile blade.

Treat the dermatitis from *sponges* by removing the stingers and soaking the contact area in dilute acetic acid, vinegar, or isopropyl alcohol. *Sea urchin* spines may require surgical removal.

Vertebrates   Immerse the area in hot water for at least 1 h. Other therapy consists of local wound care and systemic support as necessary. Stonefish antivenin is available via the regional poison control center for your area.

Follow-up

- 1 to 2 days to assess for infection and evaluate healing

Indication for Admission

- All marine animal envenomations associated with signs or symptoms of systemic toxicity

BIBLIOGRAPHY

Fenner PJ: Dangers in the ocean: the traveler and marine envenomation. I. Jellyfish. *J Travel Med* 1998;5:135–141.
Fenner PJ: Dangers in the ocean: the traveler and marine envenomation. II. Marine vertebrates. *J Travel Med* 1998;5:213–216.
Hawdon GM, Winkel KD: Venomous marine creatures. *Aust Fam Physician* 1997; 26:1369–1374.

RABIES

Most rabies viruses are transmitted by the bites of infected mammals. Rabies is virtually universally fatal once the virus becomes established in the central nervous system (CNS). The issue of rabies postexposure prophylaxis is considered most often after domestic animal (dog and cat) bites. However, wildlife (skunks, raccoons, bats, foxes, ferrets, opossums, weasels, wolves, woodchucks) now constitutes the major reservoir of rabies in the United States. Rodents (squirrels, hamsters, rats, mice) and rabbits can be infected, but they do not secrete the virus in their saliva, so they rarely transmit the disease. The local health department is the best resource for current information about epizootic outbreaks.

Clinical Presentation

The most common scenario in which rabies is considered is when a patient comes to the ED after an unprovoked bite (as while attempting to feed an animal). On occasion, abnormal behavior on the part of the animal is noted. Exposure can be by bite (any penetration of the skin by the animal's teeth) or by scratch, abrasion, or saliva. Petting alone or contact with blood, urine, or feces does not constitute exposure.

The incubation period of rabies ranges from 4 days to 1 year, with an average of 20 to 90 days. Clinical rabies presents with a nonspecific 2- to 10-day prodrome of fatigue, anxiety, fever, headache, anorexia, nausea and vomiting, and abdominal pain. Pain, paresthesias, and fasciculations may occur at the site of the injury. This is followed by increasing agitation, incoordination, hyperactivity, hallucinations, seizures, pharyngeal spasm, and hydrophobia.

Diagnosis

The definitive diagnosis is made from examination of the animal's brain. Unfortunately, the specimen is not always available, so management decisions must be based on the likelihood of rabies in that species in the particular locale. The best information will come from the local health authorities. However, postexposure prophylaxis for any bat contact is recommended, even if there is no evidence of soft tissue injury.

Clinical rabies can be confused with a variety of neurologic conditions, including *poliomyelitis, Guillain-Barré syndrome, herpes simplex virus infection, brain abscess, vaccine reaction, sepsis,* and *psychosis.*

ED Management

Recommend confinement and observation of healthy domestic animals for 10 days. If any signs of rabies develop, the animal must be sacrificed and the head sent to an appropriate laboratory. Contact the local veterinary public health service to arrange for transportation of stray domestic animals to the American Society for the Prevention of Cruelty to Animals (ASPCA).

Regardless of the nature of the attack, clean all wounds thoroughly. Infiltrate high-risk wounds with 1% lidocaine, then irrigate thoroughly to the depth of the wound. Give prophylactic antibiotics if indicated (see Bite Wounds, pp 664–666).

The indications for postexposure prophylaxis are summarized in Table 24-1. Use human rabies immune globulin (HRIG) and human diploid cell

Table 24-1 Guide to Rabies Postexposure Prophylaxis

ANIMAL SPECIES	CONDITION AT TIME OF ATTACK	TREATMENT
Dog, cat, ferret	Healthy (observed for 10 days)	None*
	Rabid or suspected rabid	HRIG and HDCV
	Unknown (escaped)	Consult local public health officials†
Bats, skunks, raccoons, foxes, and most other carnivores; woodchucks	Regard as rabid unless area is free of rabies or laboratory tests prove otherwise	HRIG and HDCV
Livestock, rodents, lagomorphs (rabbits and hares)	Consider individually	Consult local public health officials

Bites of squirrels, hamsters, guinea pigs, gerbils, chipmunks, rats, mice and other rodents, rabbits, and hares almost never require antirabies prophylaxis.

HRIG = human rabies immune globulin; HDCV = human diploid cell vaccine.
*During the holding period, immediately begin prophylaxis if the dog or cat develops any signs of rabies. Sacrifice the animal and test its brain.
†The incidence of rabies in the community determines the need for prophylaxis.
Adapted from: Committee on Infectious Diseases: Rabies, in *Red Book 2000: Report of the Committee on Infectious Diseases,* 25th ed Elk Grove village, IL: American Academy of Pediatrics, 2000, p 477.

vaccine (HDCV) at the initial time of presentation. Give a single dose of 20 IU/kg of HRIG; infiltrate one-half (or as much as is anatomically possible) of the dose locally around the wound, and inject the remaining one-half IM in the gluteal area. Give 1 mL IM of HDCV, with subsequent doses 3, 7, 14, and 28 days after the first. Use the deltoid area for adolescents and older children; the outer thigh may be used in younger children. Do not give the vaccine in the gluteal region or at the same site as HRIG (may cause prophylaxis failure).

Follow-up
- Rabies prophylaxis initiated: 3 days

Indication for Admission
- Clinical rabies

BIBLIOGRAPHY

Committee on Infectious Diseases, American Academy of Pediatrics: Rabies, in *Red Book 2000: Report of the Committee on Infectious Diseases,* 25th ed. Elk Grove Village, IL: American Academy of Pediatrics, 2000, pp 475–482.
Jackson AC: Rabies. *Can J Neurol Sci* 2000;27:278–282.
Wilkerson JA: Rabies update. *Wilderness Environ Med* 2000;11:31–39.

SCORPION STINGS

There are 650 species of scorpions worldwide. Most are found in tropical and warm temperate zones; they hibernate in winter. Scorpions are nocturnal and will frequently enter houses to feed on cockroaches. Although all species are venomous, most do not cause fatal reactions. In North America, the *Centruroides* genus may cause significant envenomation; all others typically cause only local pain and erythema.

Clinical Presentation

The *Centruroides* bite is acutely painful, with surrounding hyperesthesia. There may be cholinergic signs, including diaphoresis, nausea, hypersalivation, and blurred vision. Movement disorders including restlessness and seizure-like activity may occur. Rarely, life-threatening sympathetic signs—including hypertension, tachyarrhythmias, and respiratory failure—have been reported.

Diagnosis

In most cases, there is a definite history of a scorpion sting. When the history is lacking, consider a scorpion bite when local pain and numbness are accompanied by sympathetic symptoms such as tachycardia, hypertension, diaphoresis, and cholinergic findings.

ED Management

As soon as the patient arrives in the ED, apply an ice bag to the area of the sting. Treat anxiety with diazepam (0.05–0.2 mg/kg IV), hypertension with phentolamine (5–20 mg slow IV push at 1 mg/min) or diaz-oxide (1 mg/kg mini bolus IV push), and the parasympathetic effects with atropine (0.01 mg/kg IV). Opiates and barbiturates are contrain-dicated, as they can potentiate the toxin. Monitor IV fluids carefully; these patients are at risk for pulmonary edema and hypertension. Although commercially prepared antivenin is produced in other parts of the world for endemic scorpions, there is no commercially prepared scorpion antivenin available in the United States. One experimental *Centruroides* antivenin is distributed as part of a research protocol only in the state of Arizona.

Follow-up
- *Centruroides* bite: 24 hours

Indication for Admission
- *Centruroides* bite if the patient is symptomatic after 4 h of ED obser-vation

BIBLIOGRAPHY

Amitai Y: Clinical manifestations and management of scorpion envenomation. *Public Health Rev* 1998;26:257–263.

Bond GR: Snake, spider, and scorpion envenomation in North America. *Pediatr Rev* 1999;20:147–150.

Kemp ED: Bites and stings of the arthropod kind. Treating reactions that can range from annoying to menacing. *Postgrad Med* 1998;103:88–102.

SNAKEBITES

Most snakes in the United States are not venomous. However, snakebites cause approximately 5 to 15 deaths annually. Poisonous snakes indige-nous to the United States include the *Crotalidae* (rattlesnakes, water moc-casins, copperheads) and the *Elapidae* (coral snake). *Crotalidae* account for 99% of venomous snakebites occurring in the wild and *Elapidae* for the remaining 1%. Victims will occasionally be bitten by exotic snakes that are kept as pets.

Clinical Presentation

Snake venom reactions can be divided into three presentations: cytotoxic, hemotoxic, and neurotoxic. In North America, most venomous snakebites in the wild are from crotalids and cytotoxicity predominates, with variable hemotoxicity. The coral snake and the Mojave rattlesnake are exceptions; local signs are minimal but are followed several hours later by severe neurologic toxicity.

Cytotoxicity presents with local pain, swelling, and ecchymoses; a com-partment syndrome may develop in severe cases. Hematologic toxicity can include ecchymoses, coagulopathy, and thrombocytopenia. Neuro-logic toxicity can include taste abnormalities, local paresthesias, and, in severe cases, bulbar and respiratory muscle weakness.

Diagnosis

It is helpful to determine the type of snake. Any snake with a large triangular head and vertically oriented elliptical pupils is likely a venomous *viper. Copperheads* and *rattlesnakes* have diamond-shaped patterns of varying colors. *Coral snakes* are brightly banded with red, yellow, and black rings and are found in Florida and Arizona. Inside the continental United States, it is useful to remember the adage "Red on yellow, kill a fellow; red on black, venom lack."(There are Central American coral snakes that don't follow the color pattern.)

ED Management

Nonvenomous   Clean the wound, give tetanus prophylaxis, if necessary (pp 682–683), and appropriate pain medication. Give oral antibiotic therapy for 5 days, using either amoxicillin/clavulanic acid (875/125 formulation; 45 mg/kg/day of amoxicillin divided tid) or the combination of penicillin VK (50 mg/kg/day divided qid) and cephalexin (40 mg/kg/day divided qid). If there is any uncertainty about the identity of the snake, contact poison control, and observe for venomous symptoms for at least 3 to 4 h.

Venomous   In the field, the priority is expedient transfer to a medical facility. Splint the affected extremity and remove jewelry that could cause a tourniquet effect. Do not apply cold packs or tourniquets. Remember that up to 20% of bites from venomous snakes are "dry" bites and are therefore asymptomatic.

Once the patient arrives in the medical facility, the decision to use antivenin is based on the type of snake and the duration and progression of symptoms. Contact the local poison control center to consult with someone experienced in managing snakebites. For all patients, start an IV in the contralateral extremity, elevate the affected body part, and begin warm soaks. Antibiotics and pain medication should be administered as for nonvenomous snakebites. Obtain blood for CBC, electrolytes, BUN, creatinine, PT, PTT, fibrinogen level, and a blood type. Also obtain a urinalysis to look for hematuria and proteinuria.

Most commercially available snake antivenin is produced from horse serum, so be prepared for possible allergic reactions. Skin testing prior to treatment is contraindicated and may sensitize the patient. Pretreat with diphenhydramine (1–2 mg/kg, 50 mg maximum) before starting a continuous infusion of the antivenin diluted in saline. Pulse therapy or starting and stopping the infusion can sensitize the patient and lead to an allergic reaction. The volume of antivenin is based on the presumed degree of envenomation (see Table 24-2). During the infusion, reassess the progression or regression of symptoms to determine the need for continued antivenin administration.

A new crotalid antivenin produced from sheep serum (CroFab) has been approved for treatment of mild to moderate crotalid envenomations. It is clearly indicated for patients known to be allergic to horse serum.

Debridement is often necessary after the first 48 h, but fasciotomy is rarely required for treatment of compartment syndrome. Warn the patient that serum sickness may occur 10–14 days after treatment. This presents

Table 24-2 Antivenin Therapy

SEVERITY	CLINICAL FEATURES	VIALS
None	Fang punctures, only	0
Mild	Local swelling (<10 cm), not progressive	0
	No systemic symptoms or evidence of coagulopathy	
Moderate	Swelling progressive beyond bite site (10–30 cm)	5–10
	Systemic reaction (coagulopathy, fever, vomiting, weakness)	
Severe	Marked progressive swelling	15–20
	Severe coagulopathy	
	Proteinuria, hematuria, azotemia, hypertension	

with a pruritic urticarial rash, which can be associated with fever, nausea, headache, arthralgias, and adenopathy. Admit all symptomatic patients for at least 24 h, regardless of whether antivenin was given.

Follow-up

- Nonvenomous: 2 days to assess wound healing
- Venomous: 1 day to assess wound healing and for bleeding diathesis

Indication for Admission

- Snakebite with signs of envenomation or requiring antivenin treatment

BIBLIOGRAPHY

Bond GR: Snake, spider, and scorpion envenomation in North America. *Pediatr Rev* 1999;20:147–150.

Dart RC, McNally J: Efficacy, safety, and use of snake antivenoms in the United States. *Ann Emerg Med* 2001;37:181–188.

Holve S: Treatment of snake, insect, scorpion, and spider bites in the pediatric emergency department. *Curr Opin Pediatr* 1996;8:256–260.

SPIDER BITES

There are 50 species of North American spiders with fangs capable of penetrating human skin. However, only two species (black widow and brown recluse) can cause fatalities.

The black widow (*Latrodectus*) is distinguished by a red hourglass marking on the abdomen. The spiders are found in temperate climates. The female is twice as large as the male and therefore more dangerous. Black widow envenomation has a 5% mortality.

The brown recluse (*Loxosceles*) is the most common cause of serious spider bites in the United States. It is distinguished by a dark-orange violin-shaped marking on the cephalothorax. It generally lives in dark, dry environments such as abandoned houses or vacation homes.

Clinical Presentation

Black Widow The bite causes a pinprick sensation with slight local erythema and swelling. Within 10 to 60 min there are systemic symptoms, including muscle cramps, especially in the abdomen, after bites of the lower extremities. There may be spasms with intense pain, paresthesias (particularly intense in the soles of the feet), headache, dysphagia, dizziness, nausea and vomiting, facial edema, and hypertension. A venom dose that may cause only pain in an adult may lead to respiratory and cardiac arrest in a child.

Brown Recluse The bite of this spider is generally trivial. Within 6 to 8 h there is sharp, stinging pain at the bite site, followed by an aching pain and pruritus. The lesion becomes an irregular violaceous blister surrounded by an erythematous halo. Over 2 to 3 days the blister becomes an eschar that later sloughs, leaving an ulcer that is very slow to heal. The larger South American *Loxosceles* genus produces a more pronounced cutaneous picture, with intense pain and accompanying facial edema. Systemic involvement is rare but can occur in any *Loxosceles* envenomation. The manifestations include fever, chills, nausea, vomiting, malaise, and a confluent scarlatiniform rash with an associated hemolytic anemia presenting as hemoglobinuria. The systemic response is usually not seen until 24 h after the bite, making the diagnosis difficult.

ED Management

Assess the ABCs and treat as necessary (see Shock, pp 18–22). Start an IV with D5½ NS (use NS if the patient has signs of shock), and obtain a CBC, electrolytes, CPK, calcium, PT, and PTT. Apply ice to the bite site to reduce toxin absorption and decrease the pain.

Black Widow Treat muscle cramps and spasms with 10% calcium gluconate (0.1 mL/kg by slow IV infusion). If necessary, also give diazepam (0.05–0.2 mg/kg IV) or methocarbamol [1 g (10 mL) IV at 50–100 mg/min, followed by an infusion of 200 mg/h or 500 mg PO q 6 h]. Use a slow IV drip of equine antivenin for severe envenomations (1 vial diluted in 50 mL NS).

Brown Recluse Apply repeated ice compresses for 2 to 3 days; these will reduce pain and the local cutaneous inflammation. There is no demonstrable benefit for any specific treatment of brown recluse bites other than routine wound care. Persistent ulceration may require skin grafting.

Follow-up

- Black widow: daily until the patient is asymptomatic
- Brown recluse: daily, until the wound is healing well

Indication for Admission

- Systemic symptoms

BIBLIOGRAPHY

Forks TP: Brown recluse spider bites. *J Am Board Fam Pract* 2000;13:415–423.
Kemp ED: Bites and stings of the arthropod kind. Treating reactions that can range from annoying to menacing. *Postgrad Med* 1998;103:88–102.
Koh WL: When to worry about spider bites. Inaccurate diagnosis can have serious, even fatal, consequences. *Postgrad Med* 1998;103:235–250.

WOUND MANAGEMENT

Most lacerations can be treated in the ED using basic principles of aseptic technique and wound closure. Plastic surgical consultation may occasionally be required for complex wounds, cosmetic concerns, functional deficits, or loss of subcutaneous tissue.

Clinical Presentation and Diagnosis

History   Determine the elapsed time since the injury. Most wounds less than 8 h old may be closed primarily without an increased risk of infection; scalp and face wounds can be sutured up to 12 to 24 h after injury.

Knowing the mechanism of injury is helpful in predicting the likelihood of infectious complications: wounds resulting from compressive forces (blunt scalp trauma) often cause stellate lacerations, which are more susceptible to infection than linear lacerations due to shearing forces (razor). Assess the general health of the patient, and ask about any possible immunocompromise that may increase the risk of an infection, such as underlying chronic illnesses (diabetes, vasculitis), steroid use, or chemotherapy.

Examination   Determine the extent of the injury, and evaluate sensation, general strength, vascular supply, motor function, and range of motion with and without resistance (looking for tendon injuries). This is difficult in an uncooperative young child, but if an extremity is involved, observe the patient moving it normally through a full range of motion before closing the wound. During the assessment, keep the wound edges moist by applying gauze pads moistened with NS.

Radiology   Radiographs are indicated when the mechanism of injury or physical examination suggests a bony injury or a retained foreign body. Metal fragments and glass can be seen, and wood fragments are visible if coated with radiopaque particles of dirt. Obtain radiographs of a crush injury to rule out a compound fracture.

Shaving   Infection rates in surgical patients are increased with razor prepping. Therefore, clip the hair around a wound with scissors only if it interferes with wound closure. Never shave eyebrows, since there is no guarantee that they will grow back.

Anesthesia   To prepare the wound for anesthesia, apply povidone-iodine solution twice to the skin surrounding the wound, allowing it to dry for 4 min between applications. Lidocaine is the usual anesthetic agent. To minimize the possibility of a toxic reaction, use the 1% strength in children, although 2% can be used when only a limited volume of anesthetic is to be injected (small child's finger). Use lidocaine with epinephrine for vascular areas (scalp, face). Do not exceed a total dose of 5 mg/kg of lidocaine (7 mg/kg when used with epinephrine). Procaine is the alternative in the patient allergic to lidocaine (extremely rare). In unquestionably clean wounds, inject the lidocaine through the open wound (less painful); but in wounds likely to be dirty, administer it through the surrounding skin to avoid injecting debris into the deeper tissues. Local anesthesia may be required to perform adequate irrigation and debridement. Apply a solution of either TAC or LET (see Topical Analgesia, pp 626–630) prior to administering the local anesthetic. Topical anesthesia is especially useful for lacerations of the face and scalp.

Debridement and Irrigation   After anesthesia has been achieved, debride any devitalized tissue, including fat. Irrigate the wound with a large (35 mL) syringe attached to an 18-gauge IV catheter tip. Avoid high-pressure irrigation, as this may increase tissue injury. The least toxic solution for irrigation is NS; use copious amounts (often more than 1 L, depending on the wound size). An alternative irrigating solution is povidone-iodine, diluted to 1% in NS. This dilute solution retains its bactericidal properties without being toxic to tissues. Use bacitracin irrigating solution (50,000 U anhydrous bacitracin in 100–1000 mL normal saline) for wounds likely to be very dirty (animal bites, wounds filled with particles of dirt and debris). It can also be used to irrigate abscess cavities just before insertion of the packing.

Exploration   Examine every wound for foreign substances and any associated trauma to blood vessels, ligaments, tendons, and bone. Remove

Table 24-3   Suggested Suture Size

SITE	SUTURE SIZE
Scalp (consider wounds at the hairline to be facial)	3–0, 4–0
Face, orbit	5–0, 6–0
Neck	
Ventral	5–0, 6–0
Dorsal	4–0, 5–0
Arms, legs, trunk	4–0, 5–0
Hands and fingers	5–0, 6–0
Feet	
Dorsum	4–0, 5–0
Plantar	3–0, 4–0
Toes	5–0, 6–0
Deep (absorbable)	
Hemostasis	4–0, 5–0
Deep closure	3–0, 4–0, 5–0*

*The more superficial the subcutaneous suture, the smaller the size.

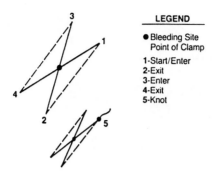

LEGEND

- Bleeding Site
  Point of Clamp

1-Start/Enter
2-Exit
3-Enter
4-Exit
5-Knot

Figure 24-1 Figure-eight suture.

fragments of hair, pieces of clothing, other debris, and blood clots, which may camouflage other injuries and be a source of infection. For scalp wounds, examine with a sterile gloved finger to determine any disruption of the galea and the outer table of the skull.

Suturing For skin closure, nonabsorbable suture material is indicated, the least reactive of which is monofilament nylon. For typical outpatient wounds, deep sutures must be absorbable. Synthetics (Dexon) are less reactive than naturally occurring substances (gut). The appropriate suture size for different areas is given in Table 24-3. For areas where there is an increase in tension, as over joints, choose the next heavier size.

Hemostasis may be accomplished with a simple ligature, a loop of absorbable suture either around the bleeder or tied in a small figure eight (Fig. 24-1). Never use a hemostat to clamp blindly, as a tendon, tendon sheath, or nerve may be clamped and destroyed.

Close deep wounds in two layers to obliterate dead space (Fig. 24-2). When using deep sutures, bury the knot (Fig 24-3) except where it will cause friction (fascia, tendon sheaths), and cut the ends fairly short.

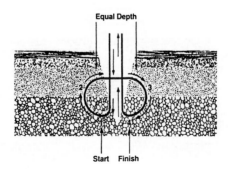

Figure 24-2 Suture for a deep wound.

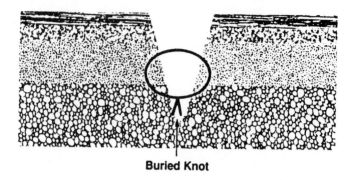

Buried Knot

Figure 24-3   Suture for a deep wound—burying the ends.

Most wounds can be closed with simple interrupted sutures (Fig. 24-4). The skin edges must be everted and touching. Inverted edges result in poor healing but can be avoided by ensuring that the suture is at equal depth on both sides of the wound, that the depth is greater than the width (B>C), and that the width at the bottom of the suture (C) is greater than at the top (A). Evenly space the sutures so that the tension is distributed equally.

A vertical mattress (Fig. 24-5) is a good method of closing a wound when there are problems with wound edge eversion or tension on the wound edge or when a wound is deep but does not require a two-layer closure. The area inside the suture has all the tension, leaving the edges with none. The suture must be of equal depth on the two sides of the wound, to prevent a stepping scar.

Employ a horizontal mattress (Fig. 24-6) when there are problems with wound edge eversion; do not use it where there will be any tension or to

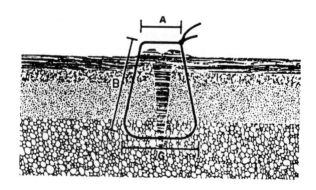

Figure 24-4   Interrupted suture.

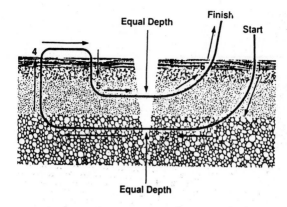

Figure 24-5   Vertical mattress suture.

eliminate a two-layer closure. Note that each horizontal mattress takes the space of two sutures, so this is a fast way to close a wound.

The half-buried horizontal mattress is the best way to handle any sharp corner (Fig. 24-7A and B) and can be used for a "v," "y," "t," "z," or stellate type of wound (Fig. 24-7C to F).

In wounds of the lip, the first suture must bring together the edges of the vermilion border; otherwise, a noticeable scar results.

Wound Adhesives   Cyanoacrylates, such as Dermabond, can be used for minor facial lacerations that are small (<5 cm), clean, under minimal

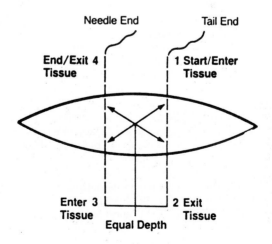

Figure 24-6   Horizontal mattress suture.

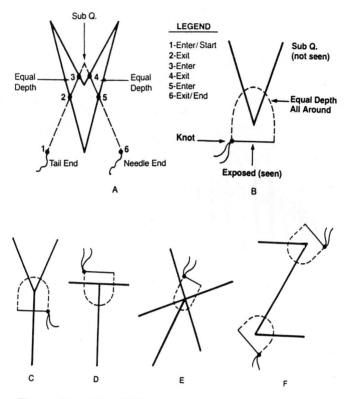

Figure 24-7 A–F   Half-buried horizontal mattress sutures.

tension, with sharp edges. Anesthesia may not be necessary and wound closure time can be decreased by as much as 50%. The adhesive polymerizes in about one second; hold the wound margins together with forceps or the wooden ends of swabs placed about 3 to 5 mm from the edges.

Referral   Refer complex wounds, in which underlying structural injury is a possibility, to a surgeon. Among these are deep lacerations of the wrist or hand, chest, abdomen, perineum, or anterior neck. Also refer ear and eyelid wounds.

Tetanus   Clean minor wounds require tetanus prophylaxis only if the patient has not had at least three documented previous doses of tetanus toxoid or if a previously immunized patient has not had a tetanus dose in at least 10 years. Serious wounds at greater risk for tetanus include contaminated (dirt, feces, saliva) and puncture wounds and wounds with devitalized tissue. With these wounds, give tetanus toxoid to patients who have had three previous doses if more than 5 years has elapsed since the last dose. For patients with fewer than three previous doses, use toxoid and tetanus immune globulin (250 to 500 U IM). When tetanus toxoid is indicated for patients under 7 years of age, use 0.5 mL of diphtheria-pertussis-tetanus vaccine (DPT) or DaPT unless pertussis vaccination is contraindicated [use diphtheria and tetanus toxoids (DT)]. For patients over 7 years of age, use 0.5 mL of dT.

Other Measures   Splint wounds in areas of great mobility (across joints, on the hand) using a thick wrapping of gauze for 2 days, until healing is under way. Advise the patient to avoid getting the wound wet for the first 24 h; after that, it can be cleaned gently and allowed to air-dry. Give the parents dry bandages to apply in case the original dressing becomes wet.

No antibiotics are necessary for small, uncomplicated wounds that are not a result of an animal or human bite. Give antibiotics for facial wounds less than 24 h old; other wounds more than 12 h old; contaminated wounds; and wounds in immunosuppressed patients. Use amoxicillin-clavulanate (875/125 formulation; 45 mg/kg/day of amoxicillin divided bid). For penicillin-allergic patients, give clindamycin (20 mg/kg/day divided tid) or erythromycin (40 mg/kg/day divided qid).

Suture Removal   Remove sutures according to Table 24-4. When sutures are removed, cut them just below the knot with suture scissors or a curved blade and pull them out. This prevents pulling contaminated material through the tissue. After sutures are removed, apply Steri-Strips to provide additional strength for a few days without the risk of infection or a foreign-body reaction.

Table 24-4   Approximate Timetable for Removing Sutures*

LOCATION	DAYS TO SUTURE REMOVAL
Scalp	8 ± 2
Face	4 ± 1
Orbit	4 ± 1
Neck	
Dorsal	6 ± 1
Ventral	5 ± 1
Chest, arms, legs	7 ± 1
Back	11 ± 1
Hands	7 ± 1
Fingertips	9 ± 1
Feet	
Dorsal, toes	9 ± 1
Plantar	10 ± 2
Skin over joints	10 − 14

*Remove any packing in 24 h and reevaluate the wound.

Follow-up

- Immediately for signs of infection (fever, erythema, proximal streaking, induration, purulence). Otherwise, return for suture removal.

Indications for Admission

- Location or extent of wound requires continual nursing care
- Evidence of associated systemic injury.

BIBLIOGRAPHY

Jackimczyk K, Pollack ES: Management of pediatric wounds. *Pediatr Ann* 1996; 25:440–447.

Singer AJ, Hollander JE, Quinn JV: Evaluation and management of traumatic lacerations. *N Engl J Med* 1997 337;1142–1148.

Trott A: *Wounds and Lacerations: Emergency Care and Closure,* 2nd ed. St. Louis: Mosby, 1997.

CHAPTER 25

Special Considerations in Pediatric Emergency Care

- Frank Maffei (contributor—The Crying Infant)
- Linda Volpe (contributor—Emergency Care of the Child with a Chronic Disorder)
- Frank Maffei (contributor—The Approach to the Critically Ill Infant)
- Kirsten Roberts (contributor—Failure to Thrive)
- Kirsten Roberts (contributor—The Cross-Cultural Encounter)
- Loren Yellin (contributor—Telephone Triage)
- Alfred DeSimone and Jeremy Halberstadt (contributors— Special Instructions on Drug Administration)
- Dan Barlev, Diane Rhee, and Melissa Sheinker (contributors— Radiology)
- Fred Henretig (contributor—Biological and Chemical Terrorism)

THE CRYING INFANT

For infants, crying is an essential means of communication. The infant may cry in response to an unmet primary need, because of discomfort, or as a sign of distress. The reason for the crying can usually be readily identified and the infant can subsequently be consoled. Occasionally, the infant's cry may be excessive or uncharacteristic, prompting the caretaker to seek medical attention.

Clinical Presentation and Diagnosis

Crying frequency increases from birth and peaks at about 6 to 8 weeks of age. Crying episodes can last for up to 2 h at a time and may cluster during the early afternoon and late evening. For infants with excessive, unexplained crying or with an acute change in the character or pattern of their crying, a careful history, meticulous physical examination, and a period of observation are paramount in the evaluation.

Obtain a description of the infant's baseline feeding, sleeping, and crying patterns. Ask about any infectious symptoms (fever, tachypnea, rhinorrhea, or ill contacts), feeding intolerance (*gastroesophageal reflux with esophagitis*), vomiting, diarrhea, or *constipation*. Make specific inquiries regarding trauma, recent immunizations (*vaccine reaction*), and the possibility of *drug reactions*, including maternal drugs taken during pregnancy (*neonatal withdrawal syndrome*) and drugs that may be transferred via breast milk. An inconsistent history, a pattern of numerous emergency department (ED) visits, and/or a high-risk social situation raises the concern of *abuse*. Perform a thorough head-to-toe physical examination (Table 25-1) with the infant completely undressed.

Table 25-1   Physical Examination Findings and Related Diagnoses in a Crying Infant

ORGAN SYSTEM	EXAMINATION FINDINGS	POSSIBLE DIAGNOSES
HEENT	Bulging fontanelle	Meningitis, shaken baby syndrome
	Blepharospasm, tearing	Corneal abrasion
	Retinal hemorrhage	Shaken baby syndrome
	Oropharyngeal infections	Thrush, herpangina, gingivostomatitis, otitis media
Cardiovascular	Poor perfusion	Sepsis, meningitis, CHF Anomalous coronary artery Myocarditis
	Tachycardia	Supraventricular tachycardia
Respiratory	Tachypnea	Pneumonia, CHF
	Grunting	Respiratory disease, response to pain
Abdomen	Mass, empty RLQ	Intussusception
Genitourinary	Scrotal swelling	Incarcerated hernia, testicular torsion
	Penile/clitoral swelling	Hair tourniquet
Rectal	Anal fissure	Constipation or diarrhea
	Hemoccult positive stool	Intussusception, volvulus, NEC
Musculoskeletal	Point tenderness or decreased movement	Fracture, osteomyelitis, syphilis toe/finger hair tourniquet
Neurologic	Irritability or lethargy	Meningitis, shaken baby syndrome

Specific Diagnostic Considerations
Colic   Often, after a normal examination and period of ED observation, the infant will be consoled and return to baseline. If the history is suggestive of paroxysmal crying episodes, consider a diagnosis of colic (pp 234–235), particularly if the "rule of threes" is satisfied: colic typically begins at 3 weeks of age, the crying episodes can last 2 to 3 h at a time, in severe cases the infant can experience two to three occurrences per day, the episodes can occur three or more days per week, and usually resolve by 3 to 4 months. Crying episodes are concentrated in the late afternoon or early evening and are sometimes associated with drawing up of the infant's knees against a sometimes tense, distended abdomen. Fever, vomiting, constipation, and diarrhea are notably absent.

Hair Tourniquet   Strangulation of a digit, penis, or clitoris by a hair or piece of synthetic fiber is a rare but serious cause of acute crying in infancy. The hair or fiber initially entwines around the appendage, usually during a bath. Subsequently, as the hair dries, it shortens, producing a tourniquet effect.

Corneal abrasion   If results of the examination are normal but the infant remains irritable and crying, proceed with further evaluation. Evert the eyelids and carefully examine the cornea. Perform fluorescein staining regardless of the presence of ocular signs and symptoms. *Corneal abrasions* may be present despite the absence of eye findings.

GI Disease   Test the infant's stools for occult blood to evaluate for gastrointestinal (*GI*) *disease*. Esophagitis may be associated with reflux.

Other   Obtain a urinalysis and culture to look for occult *urinary tract infection*. Obtain further studies based on the degree of clinical suspicion for specific diagnoses. These tests may include blood work [complete blood count (CBC), culture, electrolytes, calcium, lactate, ammonia], lumbar puncture, toxicologic testing, and imaging studies [skeletal survey, computed tomography (CT) scan of the head, air enema).

ED Management

Management may be as simple as counseling and reassurance, or it may require the prompt institution of ED therapy and subsequent admission: [supraventricular tachycardia (SVT; pp 32–38), urinary tract infection (UTI; pp 613–616), meningitis (pp 366–369), osteomyelitis (pp 527–529), intussusception (pp 239–240), incarcerated hernia (pp 266–269), testicular torsion (pp 265–269), and inflicted injuries (pp 543–547)]. Other diagnoses may be treated in the outpatient setting if clinical and social situations allow: otitis media (pp 121–126), oral infections (pp 65–67), constipation (pp 236–238), gastroesophageal reflux (pp 214–215), anal fissures (pp 243–247), and corneal abrasion (pp 490–494).

Colic   The treatment is discussed on pp 234–235. In summary, reassure the family that the baby is normal and that they are not bad parents. Discuss methods for soothing the infant, including increased holding, gentle rocking, using an infant swing or pacifier, car rides, and avoidance of noxious stimuli (secondhand smoke, loud noises, bright lights). Educate the parents about the devastating effects of shaking an infant vigorously, suggest asking other family members, such as grandparents, to assist with the infant's care if possible, and arrange for primary-care follow-up.

Hair Tourniquet   Carefully examine the affected digit and locate the constricting material. Remove it with a fine-tipped forceps, skin hook, and scissors. Occasionally a loupe is needed to isolate the strand. If there is any question of a remaining band, make a perpendicular incision over the area of constriction. Though lateral incisions have been described, making the incision over the extensor surface of the digit may best avoid underlying neurovascular structures. Consult a surgeon if the external genitalia are involved and the hair cannot be removed easily and completely.

Follow-up

- Primary care follow-up in 1 to 2 days

Indications for Admission

- Surgical emergencies (incarcerated hernia, testicular torsion, intussusception)
- Infectious disease emergencies (sepsis, meningitis, UTI, osteomyelitis)
- Cardiac emergencies (SVT, anomalous coronary artery)

- Suspected child abuse
- Parents no longer able to cope with crying infant

BIBLIOGRAPHY

Barr RG: Colic and crying syndromes in infants. *Pediatrics* 1998;102:1282–1286.
Oberklaid F: Persistent crying in infancy: a persistent clinical conundrum. *J Paediatr Child Health* 2000;36:297–298.
Poole SR: The infant with acute, unexplained, excessive crying. *Pediatrics* 1991; 88:450–455.

CHILDREN WITH CHRONIC OR COMPLEX MEDICAL CONDITIONS

Children with chronic illnesses, especially those with complex or unusual conditions, pose special challenges for the emergency physician. Technology dependence or the presence of multisystem disorders such as spina bifida often compound the difficulty in evaluation. In some cases, the child's baseline medical status obscures the acute problem.

Clinical Presentation and ED Management

The initial assessment and treatment follows the ABC's of emergency care. If the child has stable ventilatory function and vital signs, the history, and answers to the following questions, can help guide management:

What is the child's underlying medical status?   In general, the caregiver is the best resource for the accurate assessment of how the child's appearance and behavior differ from baseline. If the caregiver is unavailable, check to see if the child is wearing a medic alert bracelet, which may provide the child's underlying diagnosis. Ask the caregiver for any medical documentation which they may carry with them such as an emergency information form or outpatient DNR form. Because allergy status and medications change frequently, reconfirm information on these topics with the caregiver.

What is the history of recent illness, and what were the outcomes? Knowledge of the child's recent or frequent illnesses may be a clue to a pertinent sign or symptom that would otherwise go unnoticed or be minimized.

What doses of medications has the child been taking, and what allergies does the child have?   Remember that latex and other environmental allergies, and herbal and home remedies, are important and often forgotten by the caregiver.

Is the support system at home adequate to deal with the child's present condition?   Any medical discharge plan needs to be carried out in the home environment. Inadequate home support, inaccessible resources, or caregiver fatigue can be serious barriers to competent outpatient health care.

Special Concerns for Technology Dependent Children   More children with chronic disorders and congenital malformations survive the neonatal period and serious illness. Many return to the home environment and require significant technological support. The physician must be able to evaluate and occasionally replace certain types of life-sustaining equipment:

Gastrostomy tubes/Buttons: These are surgically placed tubes used for total or partial nutritional supplementation that bypass the esophagus. The clinician must be able to determine the type and size. In general, the size is written on the button or tube. Buttons or tubes anchored with an inflatable balloon (i.e., Mic-Key button™) can be removed and replaced with relative ease; other types of tubes (i.e., Bard type™) require a specific introducer or must be replaced endoscopically. Common problems involving gastrostomy tubes/buttons include the following:

The tube is blocked so fluid will not pass.   If an appropriate size replacement tube or button is not available, attempt to unblock the tube by instilling 10 to 30 mL of warm water or any carbonated beverage (seltzer or soda). Allow the fluid to remain in the tube for 30 to 40 minutes, and then flush the tube with approximately 30 mL of any nutritionally tolerated fluid. Use a large (20–30 mL volume) syringe for the flush, as moderate force may be required to dislodge the clog. If the tube remains blocked, repeat the procedure a second time. If unsuccessful, replace the tube with a same sized tube or button. If the same size is unavailable, use the largest passable size. The stoma can close very quickly; if the tube is not replaced within a mater of hours, the child may require a dilatation procedure.

Formula is leaking around the tube.   Small, intermittent leaks around the tube are usually secondary to post-prandial bloating or intestinal gas; no intervention is needed. If a large amount of leakage is noted, the balloon or anchor may be broken. The balloon volume is noted on the valve. Attach the appropriate syringe (generally 5 mL) to the valve and aspirate any fluid or air in balloon. This should allow easy removal of the tube or button. Then refill the balloon with fluid and inspect for leaks. If no leaks are noted, replace the same tube or button. Note that although the tube is often discolored, and even blackened from gastric acid, discoloration is not a contraindication to replacement in the stoma site. If the tube, balloon, or anchor is broken, replace the tube. If a replacement button or tube is not available, use a Foley catheter of the same diameter (or French size). An x-ray may be needed to evaluate a tube or button with hard anchors. If replacement is necessary, the appropriate introducer is required for removal; consult with a surgeon or pediatric gastroenterologist.

There is erythema around the stoma.   The tube or tape around the stoma can irritate the skin. Prescribe a barrier cream such as zinc oxide. While many caregivers apply a dressing to the gastrostomy site, encourage them to defer this until the area is healed. Treat any minor cutaneous irritation with an antibacterial cream such as bacitracin or mupirocin. True cellulites is rare.

Tracheostomy tubes: The caregiver should know the size of the patient's tracheostomy tube and may even have a spare one with them. The size is usually written on the wings of the tracheostomy tube itself. Many children with a tracheostomy are not chronically oxygen dependent. Do not mistake the use of humidified air to keep secretions fluid with chronic oxygen use. An acute requirement for supplemental oxygen may indicate the need for hospital admission. Common problems involving a tracheostomy include the following:

Signs and symptoms of respiratory distress.   Set the wall suction to ≤ 100 mm Hg, inject 1–3 mL of saline into the tube to dilute secretions, insert a 6 to 10 Fr catheter into the tracheostomy tube, and suction. A mucous plug may be easily cleared. If suctioning does not adequately resolve the symptoms, change the tube. Prior to the procedure, secure one same-sized tracheostomy tube and a second one that is one size smaller. Irritation from local trauma or infection can cause edema that may make tube replacement with the same size difficult or impossible. If the ED does not have the necessary sizes, check if the caregiver has a replacement. If the existing tube has a cuff, deflate it. Place ties in the flanges of the replacement tube, and then cut the ties that hold the old tube in place and remove the obstructed tube. Insert the new tube into the stoma with the curve pointing downward. If the tracheostomy tube cannot be inserted, use a smaller tube or an endotracheal tube. If the ET tube has a cuff, inflate it once the tube is in place. Confirm the position of the tube by clinical examination and capnography.

Fever associated with increased respiratory rate and sputum production. A patient with a tracheostomy tube is at increased risk for respiratory infections due to the lack of upper airway protection. Aspirate sputum through the tracheostomy for culture and Gram's stain, but initiate antibiotic therapy prior to obtaining the culture report. If the results of a previous tracheostomy culture are available, use that to guide your antibiotic choice. Otherwise give a first line antibiotic, such as amoxicillin (40 mg/kg/day divided tid, 500 mg tid maximum), until the culture results and antibiotic sensitivities are known.

Home ventilators: Since home ventilators now come in a variety of rapidly changing models, it is unlikely that ED staff will be familiar with them. Ask the caregiver to demonstrate how to work the ventilator. Be aware that home and hospital ventilators do not directly correlate so that many settings will need to be adjusted if the patient needs to be changed to a bedside hospital ventilator. If a ventilator-dependent child is in respiratory distress, remove the ventilator and provide assisted manual ventilations until the cause can be determined and corrected.

Follow-Up

- Erythema around a gastrostomy stoma: 24–48 hours
- Mild pneumonia (oxygen saturation ≥ 95% on room air or the patient's baseline supplemental oxygen, minimal or no retractions, baseline respiratory rate) with antibiotic and pulmonary therapy: 24 h for reevaluation of respiratory effort, hydration, feeding.

Indications for Admission

- Inability to replace a feeding tube for nutrition and hydration
- Patient with a tracheostomy: Acute increase in oxygen requirement, persistent respiratory distress after suctioning, or the need for frequent and/or increased tracheal suctioning
- Patient using a home ventilator: Persistent respiratory distress or need for a major ventilatory setting change (increased rate, pressure, oxygen requirement)
- Inability to return for care, caregiver fatigue or inability to provide required care

BIBLIOGRAPHY

Nakamura CT, Ferdman RM, Keens TG, et al. Latex allergy in children on home mechanical ventilation. *Chest* 2000; 118:1000–1003.

Day AS, Beasley SW, Meads A, Abbott GD. Morbidity associated with gastrostomy placement in children demands an ongoing integrated approach to care. *New Zealand Med J* 2001;114:164–167.

Hazinski MF (ed). *PALS Provider Manual,* Ch. 11: Children with Special Healthcare Needs, pp. 287–304, Dallas: American Heart Association, 2002.

THE APPROACH TO
THE CRITICALLY ILL INFANT

The ongoing maturation of the young infant creates a unique state of physiologic transition. The infant may develop signs of severe illness due to a congenital disorder that was not initially apparent (i.e., congenital heart disease, inborn errors of metabolism) or become ill due to environmental forces or infectious agents that produce severe disease because of the infant's physiologic immaturity. Establishing the correct diagnosis is challenging owing to the variety of disorders that can produce toxicity in a young infant. Additionally, the initial stabilization can be difficult and requires expertise in airway, respiratory, circulatory, and neurologic support. The approach to the critically ill-appearing infant demands simultaneous initiation of diagnostic and therapeutic measures.

Clinical Presentation

The clinical presentation of the critically ill infant is dependent upon the patient's previous health, the primary organ system affected, and when in the course of the illness the infant is brought to medical attention. Often, with severe disease, the infant may present with derangements in respiratory, cardiovascular, and/or neurologic function. A meticulous and ordered examination can quickly narrow the diagnostic possibilities and allow for the timely initiation of specific therapies. While stabilization is the priority, begin gathering data simultaneously with the initial therapeutic measures. Physical examination findings are summarized in Table 25-2.

Diagnosis and ED Management

A basic tenet when dealing with any critically ill infant is to assume sepsis (pp 335–339) and administer antibiotics quickly. Obtain blood and urine cultures, preferably before antibiotics are given, but defer a lumbar puncture, if necessary, until the patient is stabilized (do not wait to initiate the antibiotics). For any critically ill infant, obtain a CBC, electrolytes, liver function tests, coagulation profile, and a urinalysis. Also send for cultures, rapid antigen testing, and polymerase chain reaction (if available) for viral pathogens if a serious viral infection is suspected clinically (*respiratory syncytial virus, herpes simplex virus, enterovirus*). Other laboratory tests to consider include an arterial blood gas (to assess acid-base and ventilatory status); *methemoglobin* level (unexplained cyanosis); blood for lactate, pyruvate, ammonia, and amino acids; as well as urine for amino and organic acids (*inborn error of metabolism*); cortisol and 17-hydroxyprogesterone (*adrenal insufficiency*); blood and urine for toxicologic testing (*accidental or intentional ingestion*); and imaging studies

Table 25-2   Physical Examination Findings
in the Critically Ill-Appearing Infant

ORGAN SYSTEM	EXAMINATION FINDING	POSSIBLE DIAGNOSES
General appearance	Cyanosis	Congenital heart disease, respiratory failure, sepsis, methemoglobinemia
	Hypotonia	Sepsis, botulism
	Dehydration/emesis	Gastroenteritis, insufficient intake, pyloric stenosis, volvulus, congenital adrenal hyperplasia
HEENT	Bulging fontanelle	Meningitis, shaken baby syndrome, inborn error of metabolism, increased ICP
	Retinal hemorrhages	Shaken baby syndrome
	Ptosis/mydriasis	Botulism
	Miosis	Toxic ingestion
Cardiovascular	Tachycardia	Hypovolemia, sepsis, tachyarrhythmia, myocarditis, toxic ingestion
	Bradycardia	Increased ICP (meningitis, shaken baby syndrome), sepsis, toxic ingestion
	Poor perfusion	Hypovolemia, sepsis, congenital heart disease, tachyarrhythmia, myocarditis
Respiratory	Apnea	Bronchiolitis, sepsis, increased ICP
	Wheeze/rales	Bronchiolitis, congenital heart disease, myocarditis
Gastrointestinal	Distention/tenderness	Hirschsprung's enterocolitis, volvulus, necrotizing enterocolitis
	Mass	Pyloric stenosis, intussusception
	Hepatomegaly	Congenital heart disease, myocarditis, inborn error of metabolism
Skin	Vesicles	Herpes simplex
	Purpura	Sepsis, inflicted trauma
Neurologic	Irritability/lethargy	Meningitis, shaken baby syndrome, inborn error of metabolism
	Bulbar findings	Increased ICP, botulism

as indicated by the clinical presentation (chest and/or abdominal radiographs, head CT, skeletal survey, echocardiogram).

Proceed with stabilization in a systematic manner. Adherence to an expanded "ABCDs" (airway, breathing, circulation, and disability) format can aid in stabilization and early initiation of lifesaving therapies.

Airway The small infant has a proportionately larger tongue and a smaller, more compliant subglottic airway than an older child or adult. As a result, an infant is at greater risk for upper airway obstruction. Note the presence or absence of airway protective reflexes and anatomic features that may predispose to a difficult intubation (i.e., micrognathia). If the airway needs to be secured, choose an appropriate-sized endotracheal tube (see Airway Management, pp 1–9).

Breathing Note the rate, depth, and work of breathing. Assess the oxygen saturation quickly, but obtain an ABG if there is any question of inadequate ventilation. If there is evidence of respiratory failure or insufficiency, begin bag-mask ventilation with 100% oxygen and prepare for endotracheal intubation (see Respiratory Failure, pp 596–598). If there is coexisting hemodynamic compromise, provide volume expansion while preparing for intubation in case positive-pressure ventilation impairs venous return.

Circulation Assess pulse rate, rhythm, and the quality of distal perfusion. Note the mental status and urine output. If necessary, begin volume resuscitation with boluses of normal saline, 20 mL/kg (see Shock, pp 18–22). To help differentiate a primary pulmonary process versus congenital heart disease (CHD) with restriction of pulmonary blood flow, obtain an ABG after hyperoxygenation with 100% oxygen for 10 min (see Cyanosis, pp 50–52). With a pulmonary process, the Po_2 is above 150 mmHg, while in CHD it remains below 50 mmHg). Consider a left-sided heart lesion with duct-dependent systemic blood flow (i.e., *coarctation of the aorta, critical aortic stenosis, hypoplastic left heart syndrome*) in an infant with poor to absent distal pulses, a gallop rhythm, enlarged liver, abnormal chest radiograph, and acidosis. This is in contrast to right-sided lesions with duct-dependent pulmonary blood flow (*pulmonary stenosis/atresia, tricuspid atresia*), which often present shortly after birth with cyanosis as the primary abnormality. Give prostaglandin E_1 (0.05–0.1 μg/kg/min) early and consult with a pediatric cardiologist. Continuous cardiopulmonary monitoring is essential during prostaglandin infusion, as apnea is a known side effect.

A rapid (>220 bpm), regular, narrow-complex tachycardia is suggestive of *supraventricular tachycardia.* The P waves may be normal, inverted, or absent. In a hemodynamically stable infant, attempt vagal maneuvers (see Supraventricular Tachycardia, pp 32–38).

The 3 D's

Disability An infant with *meningitis,* intracranial injury (*shaken-baby syndrome*), or certain metabolic disorders (*Reye's syndrome, inborn error producing hyperammonemia*) may have progressively increased intracranial pressure (ICP). Perform a rapid neurologic assessment looking for signs of increased ICP (i.e., altered mental status, hypertension, hyperpnea, bradycardia, bulging fontanel). See pp 468–470 for the treatment.

Dextrose Promptly obtain a rapid glucose determination; treat hypoglycemia (pp 165–168) with 0.5 to 1 g/kg of dextrose (2–4 mL/kg of D_{25} or 1–2 mL/kg of D_{50}). Inadequate intake, limited glycogen stores, and an increase in glucose utilization during stress (*gastroenteritis, pneumonia, sepsis*) can lead to clinically significant hypoglycemia. A primary endocrine or metabolic abnormality (*congenital adrenal hyperplasia, fatty acid oxidation disorders*) may also lead to hypoglycemia.

Drugs   Inquire about medications given to the infant and those taken by a breast-feeding mother. Also consider specific medications needed for further stabilization (i.e., antibiotics, intubation medications, prostaglandin, inotropes and/or pressors).

Euthermia/Equipment   Because of its relatively large surface area, reduced subcutaneous fat stores, and immature thermoregulatory mechanisms, a young infant is at risk for significant heat loss. Hypothermia leads to increased oxygen consumption and pulmonary and systemic vasoconstriction, and it impedes effective resuscitation. Use a radiant warmer to maintain the patient's temperature, but avoid hyperthermia, especially if neurologic injury exists.

Check equipment for proper functioning. An acute decompensation during stabilization may be secondary to equipment failure rather than a true physiologic change.

Foley   A bladder catheter is necessary to assess urinary output during volume resuscitation. Use a 5-Fr feeding tube in an infant from birth to approximately 2 months of age, and an 8-Fr feeding tube in infants from 2 months to 1 year of age. If the tube must remain in place, use an 8-Fr Foley catheter.

Gastric Tube   If the airway is secured, insert a gastric tube and decompress the stomach. This is especially important if prolonged bag-mask ventilation was employed prior to intubation.

Hemoglobin/Hydrocortisone   Consider the need for packed red blood cell infusion in infants with ongoing blood loss or the need for surgery (see Transfusion Therapy, pp 306–307). Consider the need for corticosteroid replacement in an infant with suspected adrenal insufficiency (i.e. *congenital adrenal hyperplasia, hypopituitarism, adrenal hemorrhage from overwhelming infection*). Give fresh frozen plasma, 10 mL/kg, to ill-appearing infants with suspected sepsis.

Indication for Admission

- Critically ill infant: generally to a pediatric intensive care unit unless the primary process was easily identified and stabilized in the ED

BIBLIOGRAPHY

Burton BK: Inborn errors of metabolism in infancy: a guide to diagnosis. *Pediatrics* 1998;102:e69.
Conway EE: Nonaccidental head injury in infants: "The shaken baby syndrome revisited." *Pediatr Ann* 1998;27:677–690.
Pickert CB, Moss MM, Fiser DH: Differentiation of systemic infection and congenital obstructive left heart disease in the very young infant. *Pediatr Emerg Care* 1998;14:263–267.

FAILURE TO THRIVE

Failure to thrive (FTT) represents an inability to maintain appropriate growth for age. It is essentially a sign of undernutrition and not a diagnosis per se. By definition, a patient under 2 years of age is found to have a weight that is below the third percentile for age (or <80% of the ideal weight for age) or has a history of crossing two major percentiles (90th, 75th, 50th, 25th, 10th, and 5th) downward on a standardized growth chart. While weight is the usual concern, in severe cases height and head circumference can also be affected. The possible etiologies of FTT can be divided into three major categories (Table 25-3), although a patient may have more than one problem contributing to growth failure.

Clinical Presentation

Inadequate Caloric Intake
Lack of Appetite   This usually occurs in the toddler age group. The parents report a refusal of food and frustration with their inability to get their child to eat. Psychosocial stressors, including lack of food/resources, domestic violence, and parental mental illness can play an important role. Anemia, lead poisoning, and chronic infections (recurrent otitis media) may also contribute to poor appetite.

Difficulty Ingesting   Infants with congenital anomalies, such as cleft palate or choanal atresia, as well as toddlers with poor dentition or severe tonsillar hypertrophy may have difficulty ingesting adequate calories. Dyspnea due to congestive heart failure or bronchopulmonary dysplasia can interfere with oral intake. The parents may report that the patient seems to be exhausted during feeds and needs to rest frequently. Neurodevelopmental problems such as cerebral palsy and oral motor dysfunction

Table 25-3   Etiologies of Failure to Thrive

INADEQUATE CALORIC INTAKE	
Lack of appetite	*Difficulty ingesting food*
Anemia	Craniofacial anomaly
Psychosocial	CP/CNS disorder
Chronic infection	Dyspnea
Gastrointestinal disorder	Tracheoesophageal fistula
	Oral-motor dysfunction
Unavailability of food	*Vomiting*
Insufficient food	CNS pathology
Inappropriate feeding	Gastrointestinal obstruction
Withholding of food	Gastroesophageal reflux

INADEQUATE CALORIC ABSORPTION	
Malabsorption	Diarrhea

INCREASED CALORIC REQUIREMENTS	
Increased metabolism	*Inefficient use of calorics*
Chronic infection	Metabolic disorders
Chronic cardiopulmonary disease	Diabetes mellitus
Malignancy	Renal tubular acidosis
Endocrine disease (hyperthyroidism)	
Toxins (lead)	

are among the most common causes of FTT. In such a case, growth may be adequate the first 6 to 8 months, then FTT develops after solid foods are introduced. The child often has difficulty with textures and finds solid foods aversive, thereby making eating an unpleasant experience. The parents report prolonged mealtimes and a preference for liquids. The patient commonly also presents with speech and language delays. An infant who was critically ill and therefore not given oral feeds during the first months of life may have difficulty acquiring oral feeding skills.

Recurrent Vomiting   Gastroesophageal reflux with subsequent esophagitis can lead to refusal to eat because of pain upon swallowing. The parents may report irritability and grimacing with feeds, but there may not be a history of frank vomiting. Increased ICP of any etiology can cause recurrent vomiting, leading to inadequate intake. Gastrointestinal obstruction in an infant (pyloric stenosis, malrotation) can present as poor weight gain and recurrent vomiting. The infant typically appears very hungry, since appetite is unaffected.

Lack of Available Calories   Inadequate availability of calories is a common cause of FTT and may be due to economic problems, stresses within the family, mental health problems (maternal depression, leading to neglect), and intentional abuse. Improper breast-feeding technique or mixing of formula and feeding primarily foods that are nutritionally empty ('junk food') can result in inadequate caloric intake.

Inadequate Calorie Absorption

Once ingested, foods may be inadequately digested, malabsorbed, or eliminated too rapidly. Malabsorption generally presents with a history of failure to grow, accompanied by chronic diarrhea. Enzyme deficiencies, severe food allergies, and celiac disease are possible etiologies. The parents may be able to correlate onset of symptoms with the introduction of specific foods. Cystic fibrosis can cause malabsorption, usually in association with other manifestations of the disease, but FTT may be the initial presentation. Inflammatory bowel disease can also lead to chronic malnutrition through malabsorption. Diarrhea due to bacterial or parasitic infection can interfere with nutritional uptake by shortening transit time as well as leading to the consumption of nutrients by the parasites. Hepatic dysfunction secondary to biliary atresia, cirrhosis, or hepatitis can also result in malabsorption of nutrients.

Increased Caloric Requirements

Conditions that lead to an increased metabolic rate or inefficient use of calories resulting in FTT typically are secondary to a disorder that is not difficult to diagnose. Chronic infection with tuberculosis or HIV, malignancy, hyperthyroidism, chronic cardiac or pulmonary disease, metabolic diseases, renal tubular acidosis, and diabetes mellitus can all cause defective or inefficient use of calories and subsequent FTT.

Diagnosis

Obtain a complete, detailed history, including a feeding history: adequacy of breast feeding, formula preparation, amounts consumed, feeding techniques, child's feeding behaviors, what types of food the child can and cannot tolerate, timing of solid foods introduction, and any parentally imposed dietary restrictions such as sugar-free, fat-free, or vegan diet. Ask about the perinatal and developmental history (prematurity, delayed oral feeds, intrauterine growth restriction, congenital infections, developmental milestones, child's temperament), psychosocial history (ability to buy food, household stresses such as illness or domestic violence, history of abuse or neglect, environmental exposure to lead or other toxins, and travel to areas with high rates of intestinal parasites, TB, or hepatitis). Ask about the details of the FTT, including the age of onset and rate of growth deceleration, and history of diarrhea, vomiting, food intolerance, and recurrent infections.

On physical examination, observe a feeding to assess the quality of child–caregiver interaction, the quality of suck/swallow, abnormal use of tongue and lips, aversion to oral stimulation, and any evidence of pain during or after feeding. Plot the weight, height, and head circumference on an appropriate, gender-specific growth chart. Whenever possible, include previous measurements to assess changes in growth velocity. Examine an infant for dysmorphic features and congenital facial anomalies. Check the oral cavity of a toddler, looking for dental caries and tonsillar hypertrophy. Other priorities on physical examination are the cardiopulmonary (tachypnea, cyanosis, murmur, rales, hepatosplenomegaly), gastrointestinal (hepatomegaly, jaundice), and neurologic (micro- or macrocephaly, asymmetric tone, hyperreflexia, developmental milestones, mental status) examinations as well as signs of abuse or neglect (unexplained bruises or burns, poor hygiene, inappropriate behavior).

Except for renal disease, laboratory testing is very unlikely to establish a diagnosis in the absence of specific abnormalities noted on history or physical examination. If no likely diagnosis is suggested, obtain a limited battery of routine laboratory tests (CBC, urinalysis and pH, urine culture, serum electrolytes and pH, and a TB skin test) to reassure the family that there is no immediate life-threatening pathology. Further tests—such as a sweat test, chest radiograph, or stool analysis—are indicated only if the history or physical suggests a particular diagnosis.

The majority of cases of FTT in infants and toddlers represent "failure to feed" secondary to the provision of inadequate food (quantity or quality) or improper feeding technique. In such a case, the best diagnostic test is hospital admission, with feeding supervised or performed by the nursing staff. Appropriate weight gain while under close supervision confirms the diagnosis; however, this may require up to 7 to 10 days.

ED Management

The goal of ED management is to rule out the presence of an immediately life-threatening condition, assess the severity of the malnutrition, and ensure that adequate outpatient services (medical subspecialist, speech or occupational therapist, nutritionist, family support services) and follow-up with a primary provider are arranged. As noted above, the results of a thorough history and physical usually indicate the diagnostic and therapeutic course to follow.

Follow-up

- Primary care or subspecialty follow-up in 3 to 5 days

Indications for Admission

- Infant below 4 months of age with FTT
- Severe malnutrition or ill appearance
- Underlying disease that requires hospitalization
- Suspicion of abuse or neglect in a child with moderate or severe malnutrition
- Poor response to outpatient management

BIBLIOGRAPHY

Careage MG, Kerner JA Jr: A gastroenterologist's approach to failure to thrive. *Pediatr Ann* 2000;29:558–567.

O'Connor ME, Szekely LJ: Frequent breastfeeding and food refusal associated with failure to thrive. A manifestation of the vulnerable child syndrome. *Clin Pediatr (Phila)* 2001;40:27–33.

Zenel JA Jr: Failure to thrive: a general pediatrician's perspective. *Pediatr Rev* 1997;18:371–378.

THE CROSS-CULTURAL ENCOUNTER

Providing health care that is consistent with the perceived and real needs of patients is particularly challenging when the provider and the patient's family come from different cultural backgrounds. Sociocultural differences can lead to misunderstandings, which, in turn, can lead to distrust, lack of cooperation, refusal of care, and poor compliance. Sociocultural differences include style of communication (e.g., amount of eye contact), roles of various family members in decision making, expectations of the provider's role, customs relating to physical contact, and gender issues. Past experiences with medical care can also have a great impact on the cross-cultural encounter.

While effective provider-patient communication is the foundation of the therapeutic relationship, the chances for miscommunication, poor medical outcomes, and patient dissatisfaction multiply as the "cultural distance" between individuals increase. Since one in every five children in the United States is an immigrant or the child of immigrant parents, it is necessary to have a set of effective, efficient tools to minimize cross-cultural issues and foster the therapeutic alliance.

Language   Being able to communicate with a family on the basic level of language is an essential first step to a successful cross-cultural interaction. If there is language discordance between provider and family, interpreter services must be used. Patients with limited English have a legal right, through Title VI legislation, to free interpreter services if the institution receives federal money of any type. There are several acceptable options for interpreter services, including trained interpreters, bilingual staff members, and remote interpreter services (i.e., telephone-based language banks). Trained, physically present interpreters are best. It may be difficult, however, to have an interpreter available for every potential language, especially in emergency situations. Telephone language banks can be somewhat awkward to use but are readily available, and can generally handle any language.

Interpreters that are considered inadequate include unrelated, untrained people from the waiting room as well as juvenile family members. Without proper training, these ad hoc interpreters often cannot fully understand the nuances of the medical interview and may summarize or misinterpret questions and answers. Use of an ad hoc interpreter also breaches patient confidentiality.

In using interpreter services, it is important to speak to and maintain eye contact with the patient/parent, not the interpreter. Note any nonverbal cues and use visual aids whenever possible. Ask important questions in more than one way and request that the family repeat key instructions to ensure understanding. Avoid using medical terminology and idiomatic expressions. Inquire about the family's ability to read written instructions and medication labels. It is necessary to continue the interpreter services throughout the ED encounter, including during treatment and discharge.

Health Beliefs   Providers need to develop skills to assess the role and impact of each patient's culture and background. Given the vast diversity of individuals and cultures, it is impossible to become familiar with the health beliefs of every group. This type of categorical approach can also lead to stereotyping and misguided assumptions about a patient of any cultural background. Regard each patient and family as unique in their perception of any given chief complaint and their expectations for treatment. The most accurate and relevant sources of information about health beliefs are patients and their families themselves. A health belief history (see Table 25-4) can give insight into the patient's and family's understanding of the importance and ramifications of the chief complaint. The answers to these straightforward questions can be enlightening when asked in an open, nonjudgmental manner.

Negotiation   The final step in a successful cross-cultural encounter is negotiation of an acceptable treatment plan. Acknowledge and show respect for the family's views and practices whenever medically possible. Build common ground by describing your perception of the problem and treatment options in terms consistent with the family's explanatory model. Develop the priorities of management from both the medical and family viewpoints. Confirm the family's understanding of the problem and acceptance of the course of treatment. The cross-cultural negotiation, if successful, can optimize compliance and outcomes.

Table 25-4   Health Belief Questions

What do you think is wrong with your child?
Why do you think your child has gotten this illness?
What do you think caused the problem?
Why and when do you think the illness began?
What do you think is going on inside your child's body?
What symptoms make you think that your child has this particular problem?
What are you most worried about?
How long do you think the illness might last?
How have you tried to treat the problem?
What home remedies have you tried?
What will happen if the illness is not treated?
What do you expect the treatments to do?
How will you know when your child is better?

Cross-cultural encounters require optimizing communication (through interpreters if necessary), obtaining a health belief history, and negotiation of an acceptable treatment plan, while at the same time avoiding the pitfalls inherent in sociocultural differences. This template can be helpful in any clinical encounter but especially in the ED, where there is generally no previous therapeutic alliance between provider and patient/family. It is important to remember that essentially every provider-patient encounter is cross-cultural; some are just more obviously so.

BIBLIOGRAPHY

Carillo JE, Green AR, Betancourt JR: Cross-cultural primary care: a patient-based approach. *Ann Intern Med* 1999:130:829–834.

Pachter LM (ed): *Child Health in the Multicultural Environment,* Report on the Thirty-First Ross Roundtable on Critical Approaches to Common Pediatric Problems. Columbus, Ohio, Ross Products Division, Abbott Laboratories, 2000, pp 36–43.

Pachter LM: Parent's participation and perspectives regarding clinical judgment and clinical guideline development. *Curr Opin Pediatr* 1998;10:476–479.

TELEPHONE TRIAGE

Telephone triage is the process of conducting a verbal interview without being able to assess the patient in person. Parents and caregivers may call the ED to obtain information and advice regarding an acute or chronic illness, clarify prior explanations or instructions, review medication-related issues, and ask questions about primary care.

The goal of the telephone triager is to be an interviewer and communicator who, by collecting focused data, quickly and competently triages ill patients into an appropriate disposition category. Recognition of serious, sometimes subtle symptoms is critical, but it is also important to manage high frequency, nonurgent symptoms such as nasal discharge.

Priorities   In order for a telephone triage system to function efficiently, calls must be prioritized, with possibly life-threatening situations handled immediately by activation of the 911 system. In particular, keep an acutely suicidal or intoxicated caller on the line while help is summoned. Handle urgent calls (e.g., fever in a young infant) next, followed by nonurgent calls, to be returned in the order received.

Protocols   As telephone triage duties are often delegated by the physician to other medical staff, many EDs use established protocols to accurately assess, evaluate, and advise. Many pediatric protocol systems exist and can be reviewed and modified to fit individual settings. It is particularly helpful for training purposes to use protocols that list the reasoning behind each question or decision. These protocols enable the triager to give consistent, targeted advice, while minimizing variability among personnel.

Selecting the appropriate protocol is a critical step in the telephone triage process. Employing an incorrect protocol can lead to serious errors in evaluation and disposition. Telephone protocols are symptom-driven. Therefore, to use the protocols properly, the primary concern of the caller must be identified expeditiously. When there are multiple complaints, it is useful to focus on the one with the highest likelihood of requiring an office or ED visit. Ask the caller which symptom or complaint is of most concern, then use the most specific protocol available. Inquire about each symptom, from the most serious or significant to the least urgent, as well as any associated complaints (for example, is diarrhea associated with decreased urine output?). A positive response to one of the protocol questions may place the patient into a specific triage category and expedite the patient's care.

Demographic and Basic Information   In conducting a telephone interview, obtain demographic information: patient's name, caller's name and relationship to the patient (is this the mother of the child or the babysitter, who may be unaware of past medical history), patient's age and approximate weight (for medication advice), and callback number. Past medical history or birth history (for a newborn) is vital, as it may change the advice and triage disposition.

Interview Technique   In conducting a telephone interview, it is helpful to do so in a quiet area, so that the triager can concentrate and the caller is not asked to repeat information. Callers are often stressed, and differences in educational level and cultural idiosyncrasies affect the ability of the triager to give, and the caller to understand, telephone advice. Telephone triage is a subtle balance of listening and inquiring, with the triager guiding the caller to serve as the "eyes and ears" in order to focus the interview and reach a timely conclusion. Ask the caller to measure a lesion or compare it to a known object (such as a coin) or to gently touch a painful or injured area to elicit the child's response. If there is cough, noisy breathing, or respiratory distress, have the caller hold the phone in front of the patient for 30 to 60 s. However, do not accept the caller's suggested diagnosis (i.e., croup, streptococcal pharyngitis) unless it clearly meets the diagnostic criteria.

In addition to the fact that the usual visual clues used to assess severity of illness are not available, there may be a language or cultural barrier or an evasive or uninformed caller. Therefore, special attention must be paid to aural cues, such as tone of voice, rapidity of speech, and the manner in which questions are answered. With experience, the triager can become adept at sensing that "something doesn't sound right." In such a case, request that the caller bring the patient to the ED.

Disposition   By interviewing the caller, using protocols as guidelines to ask focused, selected questions, and evaluating the information obtained, the triager can establish a working diagnosis. The triager can then place the patient into a disposition category, thus directing the child to the level of care best suited to the current need. Depending on the practice setting and the acuity and severity of the complaints, these categories include immediate activation of the 911 emergency response system, seeing the patient immediately, referring the patient to the primary care setting later that day, giving an appointment for a future time, or giving home care advice. However, both the triager and the caller can elect to move a patient to a more urgent disposition, advising or requesting that a child be seen despite negative responses to "be seen" indicators. Possible examples include symptoms in a very young infant, a patient with multiple or vague complaints, significant past medical history, multiple previous telephone calls for the same illness, or if no protocol can be found that pertains to the patient. "Up-triaging" is medically harmless. "Down-triaging" a patient to a less urgent disposition, for example, agreeing with a caller that an ill child can remain home despite the triager's medical judgment that the symptoms warrant a visit, should be done only with great caution and with clear follow-up in place.

Home Care   Home care can be arranged for patients not needing a visit or who will be seen at a later time. Ask about any treatments or remedies the caller may have already tried and how they are working; if appropriate, encourage the caller to continue. Change or add to the home treatments if they are incomplete or inadequate based on the recommendations in the protocol. When the treatment or remedy being used is potentially harmful, be nonjudgmental but firm in recommending to change it. A phrase such as "I suggest you do not do that; try this instead," is useful.

It is helpful to have the caller write down the information, especially if medication dosages will be given. Give three or four instructions or recommendations consisting of two or three sentences each. Be clear when moving from one instruction to another. The triager may need to recap the conversation, particularly medication advice, as communication errors with numbers are common. After giving advice, ask whether the caller has any questions, then have him or her repeat the instructions. If there is any question as to the caller's ability to understand the instructions, recommend that the patient be seen. End each telephone triage encounter with callback instructions: advise the caregiver to call back if the symptoms worsen or do not improve within a finite time, as dictated by the symptom complex. Assess the caller's comfort level with the plan; if the caller is not comfortable, arrange for a callback or for the patient to be seen. Give reassurance that the problem can be handled at home. This is helpful in calming stressed or nervous callers.

Documentation   A documentation system for all telephone triage calls is useful for both ongoing quality improvement review and record keeping for medicolegal purposes. A preprinted documentation sheet is extremely useful in allowing the triager to document as the conversation is taking place, as delayed documentation leads to errors and omissions. At a minimum, the sheet should include space for demographic information, chief complaint, protocol used for assessment, disposition category, and medication dosages. Check boxes are useful for indicating the caller's understanding of the recommendations, callback instructions, and the caller's agreement with the plan discussed, with space to elaborate reasons for deviation from the protocol if applicable. Sign, date, and time the form. It is also helpful to have space for documentation of a follow-up phone call if needed.

BIBLIOGRAPHY

Barber JW, King WD, Monroe KE, et al: Evaluation of emergency department referrals by telephone triage. *Pediatrics.* 2000;105:819–821.

Ottolini, MC, Greenberg L: Development and evaluation of a CD-ROM computer program to teach residents telephone management. *Pediatrics* 1998;101:e2.

Philipp BL, Wilson C, Kastner B, et al: A comparison of suburban and urban daytime telephone triage calls. *Pediatrics* 2000;106:231–233.

SPECIAL INSTRUCTIONS
ON DRUG ADMINISTRATION

Parents frequently ask questions about the administration of medications (whether to give on an empty stomach, side effects, etc.). While pharmacists are very useful resources, they are not always available. Table 25-5 provides general information about the use of the most common oral pediatric medications. Most important, carefully instruct caregivers about the common symptoms of allergic reactions, including rash, changes in breathing, vomiting/diarrhea, or joint pain. In the event of a suspected reaction, advise the parent to discontinue the medication and seek medical attention for their child.

Table 25-5   Common Pediatric Oral Medications

GENERIC DRUG NAME	COMMENTS
Acetaminophen	No effect of food Overdose can be very serious The infant drop preparation is more potent and should only be dosed with the dropper
Albuterol	Oral: Take with food MDI: Shake before using and rinse mouth with water following each dose
Amoxicillin	No effect of food
Amoxicillin/clavulanate	Take with food May be associated with GI upset or diarrhea
Azithromycin	Take on empty stomach Do not take with antacids
Cefadroxil	No effect of food, but take with food if GI upset occurs Use with caution in a penicillin-allergic patient
Cefixime	No effect of food, but take with food if GI upset occurs Use with caution in a penicillin-allergic patient
Cefuroxime	Take with food Use with caution in a penicillin-allergic patient
Cephalexin	No effect of food, but take with food if GI upset occurs Use with caution in a penicillin-allergic patient
Cefpodoxime	Tablet: take with food Suspension: no effect of food Avoid concurrent use of an antacid or H_2 blocker Use with caution in a penicillin-allergic patient
Cefprozil	No effect of food, but take with food if GI upset occurs Use with caution in a penicillin-allergic patient
Clarithromycin	No effect of food Do not refrigerate Potential for "metallic" aftertaste
Clindamycin	No effect of food Take with a full glass of water Do not refrigerate

Table 25-5   Common Pediatric Oral Medications *(continued)*

GENERIC DRUG NAME	COMMENTS
Dexamethasone	Take with food Avoid alcohol and limit caffeine
Diphenhydramine	Take with food Avoid alcohol May cause drowsiness
Doxycycline	No effect of food, but take with food if GI upset occurs Do not take with dairy products or antacids Avoid prolonged sunlight exposure
Erythromycin	Take with food May be associated with GI upset Do not crush enteric-coated tablets Do not swallow chewable tablets whole
Erythromycin-acetylsulfisoxazole	No effect of food Maintain adequate fluid intake
Griseofulvin	Take with fatty foods (peanut butter, ice cream, etc.) Avoid prolonged sunlight exposure Follow-up required to monitor blood work
Hydroxyzine	No effect of food Avoid alcohol May cause drowsiness
Ibuprofen	Take with food or milk
Metronidazole	Strictly avoid alcohol Take on empty stomach If GI upset occurs, take with food
Nystatin	No effect of food Shake well before using Older children: Swish and retain suspension before swallowing Neonates/infants: swab into recesses of the mouth
Penicillin VK	Take on empty stomach If GI upset occurs, take with food
Prednisolone	Take with food Avoid alcohol and limit caffeine
Prednisone	Take with food Avoid alcohol and limit caffeine
Trimethoprim-sulfamethoxazole	Take with food Maintain adequate fluid intake

RADIOLOGY

Ordering Radiologic Examinations

To maximize the value of ED radiographic imaging, adhere to the following guidelines:

- Order a study if the results will alter the care and management of the patient. For example, the clinical diagnosis of sinusitis is evident in a child who has fever, several days of cough, purulent nasal discharge, and tenderness over the maxilla, so that sinus films will not affect the ED management. However, radiographs might confirm (or help eliminate) the diagnosis of acute sinusitis in a patient with frontal headache and infraorbital swelling but without purulent rhinorrhea or facial tenderness.

- Consult with a member of the radiology department prior to ordering a test, particularly when the patient's presentation is not straight-forward. Discuss the child's signs and symptoms to determine, with the radiologist, the best test or sequence of tests to perform. This may vary by institution or time of day, based on the availability of equipment and expertise of the personnel.
- Inform the radiologist, either in person or when ordering the test, of the location of the patient's findings as well as the tentative diagnosis. Never simply write, for example, "rule out pneumonia" when ordering a chest radiograph. Instead, specify the pertinent history and the nature of the physical findings.

Table 25-6 contains suggested radiologic examinations when a patient presents with a particular finding or when a specific diagnosis is being considered.

BIOLOGICAL AND CHEMICAL TERRORISM

Most authorities anticipate that a terrorist attack with biological or chemi-cal agents would utilize an aerosol route of exposure. A chemical attack would combine elements of a mass-casualty disaster with a hazardous materials incident. Most of the victims would be managed initially by emergency medical services personnel. A biological event would likely present similarly to a natural infectious disease epidemic, with numerous patients becoming ill at points distant in time and place from the expo-sure. However, an intentional epidemic would likely be more compressed in time, and the patients would exhibit a particularly high degree of mor-bidity and mortality. Pediatricians and ED physicians would likely be "first responders" in this context. A heightened anticipation of such an epidemic and efforts at its early recognition would be advantageous in mitigating the number of casualties and provide some protection for treat-ing physicians.

A concise overview and summary of current knowledge follows. How-ever, consult recent publications and the websites referenced below for more details, as new information is being reported almost weekly.

Major Biological Agents

The primary agents of concern are anthrax, smallpox, plague, and botu-linum toxin (see Table 25-7). Other agents, such as the viral hemorrhagic fevers (VHFs), are described in some of the references. All these illnesses have a characteristic incubation period from time of exposure, ranging from 1 to 5 days for anthrax, plague, and botulism; 7 to 17 days for small-pox; and 4 to 21 days for the VHFs. All of these infections begin with a

(text continued on page 712)

Table 25-6 Suggested Radiologic Procedures by Presentation or Suspected Diagnosis

	PROCEDURE	FINDINGS	NOTES
Neurology			
Head trauma	Noncontrast CT of brain	Epidural bleed: convex (lens-shaped) density	Do not give IV contrast
	Skull films	Subdural bleed: crescentic density which could cross suture lines	Acute blood is dense (white) on CT
		Subarachnoid bleed: blood within sulci	Calvarial fractures easier to see on plain films
		Brain contusion: focal bleed or edema (hypodense)	Basilar fractures easier to see on CT
VP shunt evaluation	Shunt series	Plain films: identify breaks or kinks in shunt	IV contrast not needed for CT
	Noncontrast CT of brain	CT: evaluate ventricular size	Compare CT to prior studies to assess change in ventricular size
	Abdominal ultrasound (AUS)	AUS: identify CSF pseudocyst	
Acute ataxia	CT of brain	CT: quickly assesses for hydrocephalus, cerebral lesions or acute blood	CT and MRI can be done pre/post IV contrast
Acute hemiparesis	MRI of brain	MRI: more sensitive for posterior fossa (cerebellar) lesions	
Nonfebrile seizure			
Headache			No imaging for febrile seizure
ENT			
Orbital cellulitis	CT of orbits	CT: distinguish preseptal from postseptal disease	Noncontrast CT usually sufficient
		CT: orbital abscess easily seen	May give IV contrast, however, on case-by-case basis if necessary
Mastoiditis	CT of temporal bones and mastoids	Opacification of mastoid air cells may be seen	IV contrast not usually necessary, but may be administered if epidural abscess suspected
		Coalescence of air cells represents bony septal destruction	
Sinusitis	Sinus films	Plain films: opacification of sinus or air fluid level	Limited CT is sufficient (coronal images only, one slice through each sinus)
	Sinus CT	CT: more sensitive in select cases	IV contrast not needed

Table 25-6 Suggested Radiologic Procedures by Presentation or Suspected Diagnosis (*continued*)

	PROCEDURE	FINDINGS	NOTES
Retropharyngeal abscess	Soft tissue neck film	Abnormal retropharyngeal soft tissue swelling with/without gas bubbles	IV contrast may not be needed for diagnosis
	CT of neck	CT: low density center may be seen (IV contrast: ring enhancement)	Obtain CT only if there is no clinical improvement on IV antibiotics
Epiglottitis	Clinical diagnosis	Edematous epiglottis and aryepiglottic folds	Do not leave patient unattended
	Soft tissue neck film only if diagnosis *unlikely*	Pharyngeal distention	Emergent intubation/tracheostomy may be needed
Croup	Airway films (usually not necessary)	Steeple sign on frontal view	
		Infraglottic edema on lateral view	
Peritonsillar abscess	Imaging not indicated		
Cervical adenitis	Imaging usually not indicated		Consider ultrasound if node is enlarging or resistant to antibiotic therapy
Pulmonary			
Foreign-body aspiration	Chest x-rays in inspiration and expiration	Airway obstruction could cause atelectasis, hyperinflation, or hyperlucency	Forced exhalation using careful abdominal pressure with a lead-gloved hand is more useful than decubitus films in a young child
Pneumonia	Chest x-rays	Bacterial (pneumococcal) pneumonia presents as a unifocal pleural-based opacity (usually)	Decubitus views useful in evaluating for pleural effusion
Asthma Bronchiolitis	Imaging usually not indicated		
Tuberculosis	Chest x-rays	Lung opacities	
		Hilar and mediastinal adenopathy	

Table 25-6 Suggested Radiologic Procedures by Presentation or Suspected Diagnosis (*continued*)

	PROCEDURE	FINDINGS	NOTES
Cardiology			
Congestive failure	Chest x-rays	Large heart and increased central pulmonary blood volume with indistinct vessels	
Endocarditis	Chest x-ray	May be normal	
Pericarditis	Chest x-ray	May be normal	
Abdomen			
Appendicitis	Abdomen film Abdominal ultrasound (AUS) CT of abdomen	Plain film may be normal Presence of appendicolith associated with perforation AUS: blind-ending noncompressible structure >6 mm CT: nonfilling of appendix (with oral or rectal contrast), >6 mm in diameter, with thickened wall	No imaging necessary if clinically positive CT done with either: • rectal contrast (with/without IV contrast) • PO and IV contrast
Intussusception	Abdominal films Abdominal ultrasound (AUS) Contrast/air enema for therapy	Plain films: crescent or target sign and lack of gas in transverse colon AUS: target or pseudokidney sign Enema for reduction	Hydrate patient prior to reduction attempt Hydrostatic reduction contraindicated if peritoneal signs are present
Malrotation/ volvulus	Abdominal films Abdominal ultrasound (AUS) Upper GI series (UGI)	Plain films may be normal AUS: May show reversal of SMA and SMV or whirlpool sign UGI: may show corkscrew sign with dilatation of duodenum	Plain films may be normal UGI always done through a nasogastric tube
Pyloric stenosis	Abdominal ultrasound (AUS)	Pyloric muscle thickness >4 mm Pyloric channel length >16 mm	Not an emergency study, can wait until the next morning if presentation is in the middle of the night

Table 25-6 Suggested Radiologic Procedures by Presentation or Suspected Diagnosis (*continued*)

	PROCEDURE	FINDINGS	NOTES
Meckel's diverticulum	Meckel's scan	Gastric mucosa takes up radiotracer	Findings can be easily obscured by previous nuclear studies
Cholecystitis	Abdominal ultrasound (AUS) HIDA scan	AUS: stones or thickened GB wall or common bile duct HIDA scan: cystic duct obstruction	
Gynecology			
Ectopic pregnancy	Transvaginal ultrasound	Extrauterine gestation Fluid in cul-de-sac	Study can confirm an intrauterine pregnancy Twin ectopic pregnancy is very unlikely
Ovarian torsion	Pelvic ultrasound	Enlarged ovary with peripheral follicles	Blood flow may be seen, since ovaries have a dual blood supply
Genitourinary			
Testicular torsion	Scrotal ultrasound (US) Testicular (nuclear) scan	US: enlarged testicle with absent flow using color Doppler Nuclear scan: absent uptake, but a missed torsion may appear as a doughnut sign	If diagnosis is clear, do not delay surgery to obtain imaging studies
Epididymitis	Scrotal ultrasound (US)	US: enlarged epididymis with increased color Doppler flow	
Orthopedics			
Osteomyelitis	Plain films Bone scan	Plain film: periosteal elevation, bone destruction Bone scan: hot focus	Plain film not positive for ≥10 days Nuclear scan positive in 24–48 hours
SCFE	AP and frog-leg lateral hip x-rays	Widening of the proximal femoral growth plate with irregularity of the metaphysis may be the earliest sign of the entity (pre-slip slip)	Always image the contralateral side for comparison since SCFE can be bilateral

Table 25-6 Suggested Radiologic Procedures by Presentation or Suspected Diagnosis (*continued*)

	PROCEDURE	FINDINGS	NOTES
Trauma			
Cervical spine	Lateral neck x-rays	Interruption of anterior vertebral, posterior vertebral, or spinal-laminal lines Prevertebral soft tissue swelling Widening of space between dens and anterior arch of C1	Lateral neck: must see C1-C7 and top of T1 Once lateral neck is normal, obtain AP, open-mouth views Pseudosubluxation seen at C2-3 and C3-4 Normal films do not exclude major injury
	CT		Do not obtain a CT if the patient is unstable
Abdomen	Abdominal film	May see free air or loss of normal fat stripes on plain film	
	CT	CT with IV contrast (no PO contrast) is very sensitive for visceral organ injury	
Pericardial tamponade	Chest x-rays Echocardiogram	Enlarged heart may be seen on plain film Echocardiogram can better evaluate size of fluid collection	
Chest	Chest x-ray	Pneumothorax, pulmonary contusion, rib fractures, pleural effusion, pneumomediastinum	
	CT	CT can better delineate injury seen on plain films	CT is contraindicated if patient is unstable
Renal	CT with contrast	Renal laceration, fracture or pedicle avulsion	Consider delayed scans or delayed abdominal film (after IV contrast injection) to assess bladder (Foley must be clamped beforehand)
Soft-tissue foreign body	Plain films Ultrasound		Most glass is radiopaque and will be seen on x-ray

Table 25-7 Biological Agents of Terrorism

AGENT	CLINICAL FINDINGS	INCUBATION PERIOD	DIAGNOSTIC SAMPLES	DIAGNOSTIC ASSAY	ISOLATION PRECAUTIONS	TREATMENT*	PROPHYLAXIS
Anthrax	Inhalational: flu-like prodrome with rapid progression to mediastinitis (widened mediastinum/scant pneumonia), sepsis, shock, and/or meningitis Cutaneous: papule progressing to vesicle, then ulcer, then depressed black eschar with marked edema	1–5 days (up to 60 days)	Blood	Culture Ag-ELISA Gram's stain	Standard	Ciprofloxacin: 10–15 mg/kg (max 500 mg) IV q 12 h Doxycycline: 2.5 mg/kg (max 100 mg) IV q 12 h	Ciprofloxacin: 10–15 mg/kg (max 500 mg) PO bid × 60 d Doxycycline: 2.5 mg/kg PO bid (max 100 mg) × 60 d
Plague	Flu-like prodrome with rapid progression to fulminant pneumonia with bloody sputum, sepsis, DIC	2–3 days	Blood Sputum Lymph node aspirate	ELISA, IFA Gram's or Wright-Giemsa stain Ag-ELISA Culture	Pneumonic: droplet until patient treated for 3 days	Gentamicin: 2.5 mg/kg IV q 8 h × 10–14 days Doxycycline: 2.2 mg/kg IV (max 100 mg) q 12 h Chloramphenical: 25 mg/kg (max 1 g) q 6 h × 10–14 days	Tetracycline: 10 mg/kg (max 500 mg) PO qid × 7 days Doxycycline: 2.2 mg/kg (max 100 mg) PO bid × 7 days Ciprofloxacin: 20 mg/kg (max 500 mg) PO bid × 10 days
Smallpox	Flu-like prodrome Synchronous vesicopustular eruption, predominantly on face and extremities	7–17 days	Pharyngeal swab Scab material	ELISA, PCR Virus isolation	Airborne	Cidofovir (experimental; effective *in vitro*)	Vaccination within 3 d of exposure
Botulism	Afebrile Descending flaccid paralysis Cranial nerve palsies Sensation and mentation intact	1–5 days	Nasal swab?	Ag-ELISA	Standard	CDC trivalent antitoxin (serotypes A, B, E) 1 vial IV Dept. of Defense heptavalent antitoxin (serotypes A–G) 1 vial (10 mL) IV	None

Adapted from Henretig FM, Cieslak TJ, et al: Bioterrorism and pediatric emergency medicine. *Clin Pediatr Emerg Med* 2000; 211–222.

*See text: For systemic infections (e.g. anthrax), the CDC may recommend additional antibiotics when resources allow.

flu-like prodrome of fever, fatigue, malaise, and headache that can last 1 to 3 days before more characteristic signs and symptoms evolve. The diagnosis of the first presenting patients would thus be very difficult. However, early recognition of those presenting later, once the unique clinical syndromes have evolved, might allow earlier treatment of those who follow at a more treatable stage, particularly for anthrax and plague.

Anthrax   Anthrax is caused by *Bacillus anthracis,* a gram-positive rod. Naturally occurring anthrax is a rare bacterial disease in the United States and is usually contracted by contact with infected animals or animal products, such as unprocessed wool or animal hides, or by eating contaminated meat. Cutaneous anthrax begins as a papular lesion, evolving rapidly through stages of vesicle, then ulcer, to deep, black eschar, with marked surrounding edema. Inhalational anthrax causes a hemorrhagic, necrotizing mediastinitis, which may progress to sepsis and meningitis. Inhalational anthrax is not contagious to health care providers, though contact precautions are recommended for a patient with cutaneous disease.

Plague   Plague is caused by *Yersinia pestis,* a gram-negative bacterium. It occurs infrequently in the southwestern United States, where it can present in bubonic, septic, or pneumonic forms. Pneumonic plague is a severe, hemorrhagic bacterial pneumonia, also with the potential to progress to sepsis, meningitis, or disseminated intravascular coagulation. A patient with plague pneumonia typically has hemoptysis and progresses rapidly to respiratory failure. The patient is highly contagious, so droplet precautions are required.

Botulism   Botulism is caused by intoxication with the very potent botulinum toxin (see pp 329–330). It may occur naturally after ingestion of toxin in contaminated food (food-borne form) or spores (infant form) and rarely when *Clostridium botulinum* infects a wound. The patient is afebrile and presents with a symmetric, descending, flaccid paralysis. There typically are marked bulbar findings, but sensation and mental status are unaffected. Botulism is not contagious, so special precautions are unnecessary. Patients poisoned by inhaling weaponized botulinum toxin would present very similarly to those with natural disease.

Smallpox   Smallpox is a viral infection that was thought to be eradicated in the late 1970s. However, bioterrorism experts fear that during the collapse of the former Soviet Union, weaponized forms of this agent might have survived. Smallpox presents with a characteristic vesiculopustular exanthem, similar to varicella, except that the lesions are all in the same stage and are concentrated centripetally on the face and extremities.

Smallpox is accompanied by high fever and prostration. This disease is highly contagious, and airborne precautions are necessary.

Viral Hemorrhagic Fevers   The VHFs (Ebola, Marburg, etc.) begin with a febrile prodrome that may also include facial flushing and conjunctival injection. The clinical picture rapidly evolves into shock, with widespread mucous membrane hemorrhage. The VHFs are also highly contagious, and contact precautions are necessary as well as airborne precautions for patients with massive hemoptysis and/or hematemesis.

Chemical Agents

The primary chemical agents of concern (Table 25-8) are nerve agents, cyanide, the vesicants (mustard, Lewisite), and pulmonary agents such as chlorine and phosgene. Most of these cause a rapid onset of clinical effects, ranging from seconds or minutes (potent nerve agents) to several hours (e.g., pulmonary edema after phosgene exposure).

Nerve Agents   These organophosphate compounds cause a clinical syndrome very similar to that seen after a pesticide poisoning (pp 416–417). However, there typically is greater immediate CNS toxicity in addition to the expected cholinergic effects, and fatalities are more common. Exposure to a high concentration of vapor causes the rapid onset of rhinorrhea, miosis, and dyspnea, followed shortly—if immediate antidotal therapy is not given—by coma, seizures, paralysis, and apnea. A patient exposed to nerve agent vapor may pose a modest hazard to health care providers, since slight off-gassing can occur from contaminated hair or clothing.

Cyanide   Cyanide inhibits mitochondrial oxidative metabolism and therefore most severely affects highly metabolically active tissues, especially the brain and heart. After a high vapor exposure, a patient rapidly loses consciousness, then develops seizures and becomes apneic, although without the muscarinic signs of the comparably poisoned nerve agent victim.

Diagnosis and Management

ABCDEs   If a biological or chemical exposure is suspected, first attend to the basic ABCs. Then, *D* represents critical *drug* interventions (e.g., glucose, anticonvulsants, antiarrhythmics, antidotes, etc.) *E* stands for *epidemiology,* including three "little *e*" questions: Are there *epidemic* numbers of patients, identifiable *exposure* sources, or *exotic* disease presentations? A large number of sick patients, out of proportion to time of year and expected clinical syndromes; a history of geographic proximity among patients; or an observation of an unusual source of exposure (e.g., an explosion or cloud of vapor in an enclosed area) raises the possibility of a deliberate attack. In this setting, an exotic disease means that the syndromes caused by these agents are relatively unusual and characteristic. Identification of an exotic illness may assist in the early recognition of a new or reemerging natural infectious disease epidemic and expedite reporting to local and regional public health authorities before a specific diagnosis can be confirmed.

Document any possible exposure history or febrile prodrome and ascertain the acuity of illness onset. On physical examination, note the vital signs and look for respiratory, neurologic, or dermatologic signs. While specific laboratory tests exist for many of the relevant biological and chemical agents, few are readily available on a stat basis. Instead, obtain a focused laboratory assessment, including a CBC, chest x-ray, and, in a patient with a purpuric rash, coagulation studies. These agents all cause clinical illnesses that can be primarily characterized as acute or subacute respiratory, neurologic, or dermatologic syndromes (Table 25-9).

Table 25-8 Principal Chemical Agents

AGENT	TOXICITY	CLINICAL FINDINGS	ONSET	DECONTAMINATION	MANAGEMENT
Tabun Sarin Soman VX	Nerve agents (anticholinesterase)	Vapor: miosis, rhinorrhea, dyspnea Liquid: diaphoresis, vomiting Both: apnea, coma, paralysis, seizures	Vapor: seconds Liquid: minutes to hours	Vapor: fresh air, remove clothes Liquid: remove clothes Skin: soap and water	ABCs Atropine: 0.02–0.05 mg/kg (min 0.1 mg, max 2–5 mg) IV, IM Pralidoxime: 25–50 mg/kg (max 1–2 g) IV, IM Seizure control (lorazepam)
Mustard	Vesicant Alkylation	Skin: erythema, vesicles Eye: inflammation Resp: inflammation	Resp: hours	Skin: soap and water Eyes: water (within 2 min)	Symptomatic
Chlorine Phosgene	Pulmonary agents (liberate HCL, alkylation)	ENT: irritation (esp chlorine) Resp: bronchospasm, pulmonary edema (esp phosgene)	Pulmonary edema: hours	Fresh air Skin: water	Symptomatic
Cyanide	Cellular anoxia	Tachypnea, coma, seizures, apnea	Seconds	Fresh air Skin: soap and water	ABCs, 100% O_2 Na bicarbonate, 1–2 mEq/kg IV bolus for severe acidosis Na nitrite (3%): 0.33 mL/kg (10 mL max) for Hgb>12 g/dL Na thiosulfate (25%): 1.65 mL/kg (max 50 mL)
CS CN Capsaicin	Lacrimators Alkylation	Eye: tearing, pain, blepharospasm Nose and throat irritation Pulmonary failure (rare)	Irritation: seconds	Fresh air Eyes: lavage	Symptomatic Eyes: topical ophthalmics

Adapted from Henretig FM, Cieslak TJ, et al: Bioterrorism and pediatric emergency medicine. *Clin Pediatr Emerg Med* 2000; 211–222.

Table 25-9   Clinical Syndromes Secondary to Aerosol and/or
Cutaneous Exposure to Biological or Chemical Agents

Respiratory predominance
Acute onset, afrebrile: chemical agents
   Nerve agents (organophosphates): dyspnea, rhinorrhea, wheezing, rales,
      coma, seizures
   Chlorine: eye, nose, throat irritation; progressing to wheezing
   Phosgene: wheezing, pulmonary edema (onset over several hours)
Subacute onset, febrile: biological agents
   Anthrax, inhalational: flu-like prodrome (1–3 days), chest pain, widened
      mediastinum with/without infiltrates on chest x-ray, cyanosis, shock,
      meningitis
   Plague, pneumonic: flu-like prodome (1 day), then fulminant pneumonia
      (typically with bloody sputum), bilateral infiltrates on chest x-ray, sepsis,
      DIC
Neurologic predominance
Acute onset, afebrile: chemical agents
   Nerve agents (organophosphates): cholinergic syndrome (miosis, rhinorrhea,
      lacrimation, dyspnea, wheezing and rales) progressing to coma, seizures,
      paralysis, apnea
   Cyanide: tachypnea, apnea, coma, seizures
Subacute onset, ± fever: biological agents
   Botulism: afebrile; bulbar dysfunction, progressive descending flaccid
      paralysis, intact sensation and mental status, CSF negative
Dermatologic predominance
Acute onset, afebrile: chemical agents
   Vesicants (mustard, arsenicals): erythema, vesicles, ocular inflammation,
      respiratory tract inflammation in severe cases after a few hours
Subacute onset, ± febrile: biological agents
   Anthrax, cutaneous: papule progressing to vesicle then ulcer then black
      depressed eschar, often with marked surrounding edema, typically
      relatively painless
Subacute onset, febrile: biological agents
   Smallbox: flu-like prodrome (2–3 days), centrifugal synchronous vesiculo-
      pustular exanthem
   Plague, septicemic: febrile prodrome, often with prominent gastrointestinal
      symptoms, then shock, petechiae, purpura, gangrene
   Viral hemorrhagic fevers: flu-like prodrome, with rapid progression to
      shock, purpura, bleeding diathesis

General Measures   If a terrorist attack is suspected, immediately initiate the hospital's disaster plan and notify the hospital's infection control
officers (biological attack) or toxicology service/Poison Control Center
(chemical attack). In addition, alert the local and regional public health
resources, and consider contacting the U.S. Centers for Disease Control
and Prevention (CDC) at (770) 488-7100.

Biological Agents   The treatment of the major biological agent threats is
summarized in Table 25-7; the mainstays of therapy for most of the treat-

able infections are ciprofloxacin and doxycycline. In contained casualty circumstances, when adequate capacity is available, treat severe anthrax and plague infections with multiple parenteral antibiotics (see updated CDC guidelines available at the CDC bioterrorism website). In the setting of either mass casualties or mass prophylaxis, when maximal therapy would be impossible, a single oral drug might have to suffice.

Chemical Agents   Disrobe the patient and decontaminate with a brief shower. If the patient was exposed to a liquid agent, a more scrupulous decontamination is indicated, with thorough scrubbing with soap and water, possibly preceded by a 0.5% sodium hypochlorite wipe-down. Contaminated skin and clothing are highly toxic to unprotected caregivers.

The treatment of the major chamical agents is summarized in Table 25-8. Treat a nerve agent exposure emergently with atropine, pralidoxime, and anticonvulsants (if needed) as well as intensive supportive care. Cyanide antidotal therapy includes the potential use of sodium nitrite, sodium thiosulfate, sodium bicarbonate, and supportive care. Treatment of the vesiculating and pulmonary agents is primarily supportive.

Indication for Admission

- Significant symptoms: fever, respiratory distress, arrhythmias, seizures, altered level of consciousness

Useful Websites

AAP: www.aap.org
CDC: www.cdc.gov; special site for bioterrorism in particular:
  www.bt.cdc.gov
NACHRI: www.childrenshospital.net
U.S. Army Medical Research Institute of Chemical Defense:
  http://ccc.apgea.army.mil
U.S. Army Medical Research Institute of Infectious Diseases:
  www.amriid.army.mil
Association of Professional Infection Control: www.apic.org
Johns Hopkins University Civilian Biodefense Center:
  www.hopkins-biodefense.org

BIBLIOGRAPHY

American Academy of Pediatrics: Chemical and biological terrorism and its impact on children: a subject review. *Pediatrics* 2000;105:662–670.

Henretig FM, Cieslak TJ: Bioterrorism and pediatric emergency medicine. *Clin Pediatr Emerg Med* 2001;2:211–222.

Henretig FM, Cieslak TJ, Madsen JM, et al: The emergency department response to incidents of biological and chemical terrorism, in Fleisher GR, Ludwig S (eds): *Textbook of Pediatric Emergency Medicine,* 4th ed. Philadelphia: Lippincott Williams & Wilkins, 2000, pp 1763–1784.

Index

Note: Page numbers followed by f indicate figures; those followed by t indicate tables.

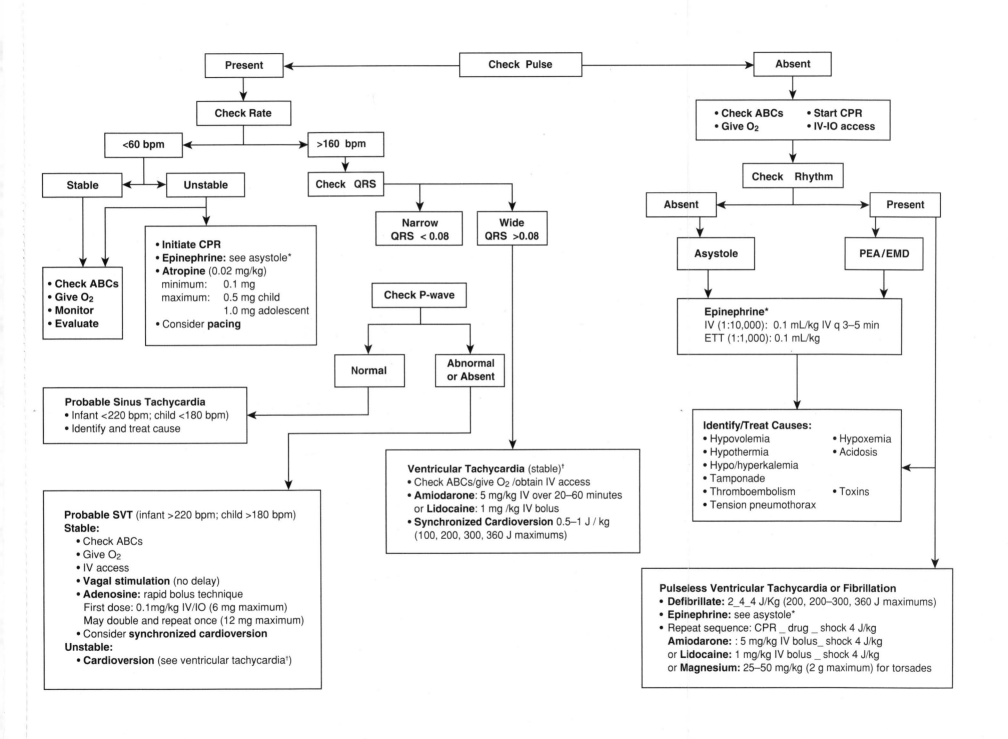

Check Pulse

Present ← Check Pulse → **Absent**

Present:

Check Rate

<60 bpm ← Check Rate → **>160 bpm**

<60 bpm:

Stable ↔ **Unstable**

Stable:
- **Check ABCs**
- **Give O₂**
- **Monitor**
- **Evaluate**

Unstable:
- **Initiate CPR**
- **Epinephrine:** see asystole*
- **Atropine** (0.02 mg/kg)
  minimum: 0.1 mg
  maximum: 0.5 mg child
            1.0 mg adolescent
- Consider **pacing**

>160 bpm:

Check QRS

Narrow QRS < 0.08 ← Check QRS → **Wide QRS >0.08**

Narrow QRS:

Check P-wave

Normal ← Check P-wave → **Abnormal or Absent**

Probable Sinus Tachycardia
- Infant <220 bpm; child <180 bpm)
- Identify and treat cause

Probable SVT (infant >220 bpm; child >180 bpm)
Stable:
- Check ABCs
- Give O₂
- IV access
- **Vagal stimulation** (no delay)
- **Adenosine:** rapid bolus technique
  First dose: 0.1mg/kg IV/IO (6 mg maximum)
  May double and repeat once (12 mg maximum)
- Consider **synchronized cardioversion**
Unstable:
- **Cardioversion** (see ventricular tachycardia†)

Wide QRS:

Ventricular Tachycardia (stable)†
- Check ABCs/give O₂/obtain IV access
- **Amiodarone:** 5 mg/kg IV over 20–60 minutes
  or **Lidocaine:** 1 mg /kg IV bolus
- **Synchronized Cardioversion** 0.5–1 J / kg
  (100, 200, 300, 360 J maximums)

Absent:

- **Check ABCs**   • **Start CPR**
- **Give O₂**   • **IV-IO access**

Check Rhythm

Absent ← Check Rhythm → **Present**

Absent:

Asystole

Present:

PEA/EMD

Epinephrine*
IV (1:10,000): 0.1 mL/kg IV q 3–5 min
ETT (1:1,000): 0.1 mL/kg

Identify/Treat Causes:
- Hypovolemia   • Hypoxemia
- Hypothermia   • Acidosis
- Hypo/hyperkalemia
- Tamponade
- Thromboembolism   • Toxins
- Tension pneumothorax

Pulseless Ventricular Tachycardia or Fibrillation
- **Defibrillate:** 2_4_4 J/Kg (200, 200–300, 360 J maximums)
- **Epinephrine:** see asystole*
- Repeat sequence: CPR _ drug _ shock 4 J/kg
  Amiodarone: : 5 mg/kg IV bolus_ shock 4 J/kg
  or **Lidocaine:** 1 mg/kg IV bolus _ shock 4 J/kg
  or **Magnesium:** 25–50 mg/kg (2 g maximum) for torsades

PEDIATRIC EMERGENCY MEDICATIONS

		AGE	Newborn	3-6 mo	1 Yr	2-3 Yrs	4-6 Yrs	7-9 Yrs	10-12 Yrs	13-15 Yrs	>15 yrs
ETT size = 4 + 1/4 Age	Depth = 3 X ETTsize										
Preemie < 30 wk = 2.5	30-35 wk = 3.0	Weight	3 kg	5 kg	10 kg	15 kg	20 kg	25 kg	30 kg	40 kg	>50 kg
> 35 wk = 3.5	40 wk = 3.5-4.0	ETT	3-3.5	3.5-4.0	4-4.5	4.5-5.0	5.0-5.5	5.5-6.0 cuff	6.0-6.5 cuff	7.0-7.5 cuff	7.5-8.0 cuff
Syst BP min = 70 + 2xAge	BP max = 110 + 2xAge	L. Blade	Miller 0-1	Miller 0-1	Miller 0-1	Miller 1-2	Miller 2	Mil / Mac 2	Mil / Mac 2-3	Mil / Mac 3	Mil / Mac 3
$PO_2 = 7 \times FiO_2 - 1.2 \times PCO_2$	$AG = Na - (Cl + HCO_3)$	Suction	6-8 F	8-10 Fr	10 Fr	10 Fr	10 Fr	10 Fr	10 Fr	12 Fr	12-14 Fr
Osm = 2xNa+Glu/18+	BUN / 2.8	NG Tube	5-8 Fr	5-8 Fr	8-10 Fr	10-12 Fr	12-14 Fr	12-14 Fr	14-16 Fr	14-16 Fr	16-18 Fr
Burn = 4mL/kg/%BSA burn+	Maint or $5L/m^2 + 2L/m^2$	Foley	6-8 Fr	6-8 Fr	8-10 Fr	10-12 Fr	10-12 Fr	12 Fr	12 Fr	12-14 Fr	12-14 Fr
PRBC / Platelet / Albumin /	FFP = 10 mL / kg	Chest Tube	10-12 Fr	12-16 Fr	16-20 Fr	20-24 Fr	24-32 Fr	28-32 Fr	28-32 Fr	32-40 Fr	32-40 Fr
		LMA (cuff)	1 (4 mL)	1.5 (7 mL)	2 (10 mL)	2 (10 mL)	2-2.5 (14 mL)	2.5 (17 mL)	3 (20 mL)	3 (20 mL)	4-6 (30-50mL)

DRUG	DOSE	ROUTE									
Atropine	0.02 mg/kg	IV/ETT	0.1 mg	0.1 mg	0.2 mg	0.3 mg	0.4 mg	0.5 mg	0.6 mg	0.8 mg	max 1 mg
Amiodarone	5 mg/kg X 3 max	IV	15 mg	25 mg	50 mg	75 mg	100 mg	125 mg	150 mg	200 mg	250-300 mg
Calcium Chloride 10%	20 mg/kg = 0.2 mL/kg	IV-SLOW	60 mg	100 mg	200 mg	300 mg	400 mg	500 mg	500 mg	500 mg	max 500 mg
Epinephrine 1 : 10,000	0.01mg/kg = 0.1mL/kg	IV/ETT	0.3 mL	0.5 mL	1 mL	1.5 mL	2 mL	2.5 mL	3 mL	4 mL	max 10 mL
Epinephrine 1 : 1,000	0.1mg/kg = 0.1mL/kg	IV/ETT	X	0.5 mL	1 mL	1.5 mL	2 mL	2.5 mL	3 mL	4 mL	max 10 mL
Glucose (D25W)	0.5 g/kg = 2mL/kg	IV	X	10 mL	20 mL	30 mL	40 mL	50 mL	60 mL	80 mL	100 mL
Glucose (D10W)	0.5 g/kg = 5mL/kg	IV	15 mL	25 mL							
Lidocaine	1 mg/kg	IV/ETT	3 mg	5 mg	10 mg	15 mg	20 mg	25 mg	30 mg	40 mg	max 100 mg
Sodium bicarb 4.2%	1 mEq/kg = 2mL/kg	IV	6 mL	10 mL							
Sodium bicarb 8.4%	1 mEq /kg = 1mL/kg	IV	X	X	10 mL	15 mL	20 mL	25 mL	30 mL	40 mL	50 mL
SEDATION											
Etomidate	0.3 mg/kg	IV	0.9 mg	1.5 mg	3 mg	4.5 mg	6 mg	7.5 mg	9 mg	12 mg	15-20 mg
Fentanyl	1-4 ug/kg	IV-SLOW	3-12 ug	5-20 ug	10-40 ug	15-60 ug	20-80 ug	25-100 ug	30-120 ug	40-150 ug	50-200ug (max 400)
Ketamine	1-2 mg/kg	IV	3-6 mg	5-10 mg	10-20 mg	15-30 mg	20-40 mg	25-50 mg	30-60 mg	40-80 mg	100-150 mg
Midazolam	0.1-0.3 mg/kg	IV	0.03-0.6 mg	0.5-1.5 mg	1-3 mg	1.5-4.5 mg	2-5 mg	2.5-5 mg	3-5 mg	4-5 mg max	max 5 mg
Thiopental	4-6 mg/kg	IV	12-18 mg	20-30 mg	40-60 mg	60-90 mg	80-120 mg	100-150 mg	120-180 mg	160-240 mg	200-300 mg
PARALYZING											
Rocuronium	0.6-1.0 mg/kg	IV	1.8-3.0 mg	3-5 mg	6-10 mg	9-15 mg	12-20 mg	15-25 mg	18-30 mg	24-40 mg	30-50 mg
Succinylcholine	2 mg/kg	IV	6 mg	10 mg	20 mg	30 mg	40 mg	50 mg	60 mg	80 mg	100mg (max 150mg)
Vecuronium	0.1mg/kg	IV	0.3 mg	0.5 mg	1 mg	1.5 mg	2 mg	2.5 mg	3 mg	4 mg	5 mg (max 10 mg)
REVERSAL AGENTS											
Flumazenil	0.01 mg/kg	IV	0.03 mg	0.05 mg	0.1 mg	0.15 mg	0.2 mg	0.25 mg	0.3 mg	0.4 mg	0.5 mg (1 mg max)
Naloxone	0.1 mg/kg	IV / ETT	0.3-6 mg	0.5 mg	1.0 mg	1.5 mg	2.0 mg	2.0 mg	2.0 mg	2.0 mg	2.0 mg
NEUROLOGY											
Lorazepam	0.05-0.1 mg/kg	IV SLOW	0.15-0.3 mg	0.25-0.5 mg	0.5-1 mg	0.75-1.5 mg	1-2 mg	1.25-2.5 mg	1.5-3.0 mg	2-4 mg	max 4 mg
Diazepam Rectal	0.2-0.5 mg/kg	Rectal	2.5 mg	5 mg	5 mg	5-10 mg	10 mg	12.5 mg	15 mg	15 mg	20 mg
Fosphenytoin	PE = 20 mg/kg	IV 30 min	X	100 mg	200 mg	300 mg	400 mg	500 mg	600 mg	800 mg	1 g
Phenobarbital	PE = 20 mg/kg	IV infusn	60 mg	100 mg	200 mg	300 mg	400 mg	500 mg	600 mg	800 mg	1 g
Mannitol 20%	0.5-1 g/kg	IV SLOW	1.5-3 g	2.5-5 g	5-10 g	7.5-15 g	10-20 g	12.5-25 g	15-30 g	20-40 g	max 50 g
CARDIAC											
Adenosine	0.1-0.3 mg/kg	IV rapid	0.3-0.9 mg	0.5-1.5 mg	1-3 mg	1.5-3 mg	2-6 mg	2.5-7.5 mg	3-9 mg	4-12 mg	max 6-12 mg
Furosemide	1 mg/kg	IV	3 mg	5 mg	10 mg	15 mg	20 mg	25 mg	30 mg	40 mg	50 mg
Labetalol	0.2-1.0 mg/kg	IV	X	1-5 mg	2-10 mg	3-15 mg	4-20 mg	5-20 mg	6-20 mg	8-20 mg	10-20 mg max
Nifedipine	0.25-0.5 mg/kg	PO	X	1.25-2.5 mg	2.5-5 mg	3.75-7.5 mg	5-10 mg	6.25-10 mg	7.5-10 mg	8-10 mg	max 10 mg

INFUSIONS	DOSE in ug/kg/min	PREPARATION
Dopamine/Dobutamine	Dopamine: 2-20/Dobutamine 5-20	[6 X (wgt in kg)] = mg to add to 100 mL D5W/IV rate of 1 mL/hr = 1 μg/kg/min
Epinephrine/Norepinephrine	Epinephrine: 0.1-1/Norepi: 0.1-2	[0.6 X (wgt in kg)] = mg added to 100 mL D5W/IV rate of 1 mL/hr = 0.1 μg/kg/min
Inamrinone	5-10 (load 0.75-1.0 mg/kg)	[6 X (wgt in kg)] = mg to add to 100 mL D5W/IV rate of 1 mL/hr = 1 μg/kg/min
Lidocaine	20-50	[120 X (wgt in kg)] = mg to add to 100 mL D5W/IV rate of 1 mL/hr = 20 μg/kg/min
Milrinone	0.5-0.75 (load 50-75 μg/kg)	[0.6 X (wgt in kg)] = mg added to 100 mL D5W/IV rate of 1 mL/hr = 0.1 μg/kg/min
Nitroprusside/Nicardipine	Nitro: 1.0-8.0/Nicardipine: 0.5-3	[6 X (wgt in kg)] = mg added to 100 mL D5W/IV rate of 1 mL/hr = 1 μg/kg/min
Terbutaline	0.4	[0.6 X (wgt in kg)]= mg added to 100 mL D5W/IV rate of 1 mL/hr = 0.1 μg/kg/min